# Nurse as Educator

# Principles of Teaching and Learning for Nursing Practice

## Second Edition

### Susan B. Bastable, Ed.D., R.N.

*Le Moyne College, Syracuse, NY*

**JONES AND BARTLETT PUBLISHERS**

*Sudbury, Massachusetts*

BOSTON    TORONTO    LONDON    SINGAPORE

*World Headquarters*
Jones and Bartlett Publishers
40 Tall Pine Drive
Sudbury, MA 01776
978-443-5000
info@jbpub.com
www.jbpub.com

Jones and Bartlett Publishers
Canada
2406 Nikanna Road
Mississauga, ON L5C 2W6
CANADA

Jones and Bartlett Publishers
International
Barb House, Barb Mews
London W6 7PA
UK

**Library of Congress Cataloging-in-Publication Data**

Nurse as educator : principles of teaching and learning for nursing
practice / [edited by] Susan B. Bastable.— 2nd ed.
    p. ; cm.
Includes bibliographical references and index.
 ISBN 0-7637-1441-0
 1. Health education. 2. Teaching. 3. Learning.
 [DNLM: 1. Education, Nursing—methods. 2. Learning—Nurses'
Instruction. 3. Patient Education—methods. 4. Teaching—Nurses'
Instruction.  WY 18 N9715 2002] I. Bastable, Susan Bacorn.
RT90 .N86 2002
613—dc21

                              2002016194

Acquisitions Editor: Penny M. Glynn
Production Manager: Amy Rose
Associate Production Editor: Tara McCormick
Editorial Assistant: Karen Zuck
Production Assistant: Karen Ferreira
Marketing Associate: Joy Stark-Vancs
Manufacturing Buyer: Amy Bacus
Composition: Northeast Compositors
Text Design: Anne Flanagan Graphic Design
Cover Design: Night & Day Design
Printing and Binding: Transcontinental Printing
Cover printing: Transcontinental Printing

This book was typeset in Quark 4.1 on a Macintosh G4. The font families used were Palatino and Stone Sans.

Printed in Canada
06 05        10 9 8 7 6

# Dedication

*To the past, present, and future nursing students in my nursing education courses,*

*and*

*In memory of Dr. Stephen Bastable, who never failed to express his obvious pride in my professional endeavors.*

# Contents

# About the Author

Susan B. Bastable earned her M.Ed. in community health nursing and her Ed.D. in nursing with a concentration in curriculum and instruction at Teachers College, Columbia University, in 1976 and 1979, respectively. She received her diploma from Hahnemann Hospital School of Nursing in Philadelphia in 1969 and her BSN from Syracuse University in 1972. Dr. Bastable began her academic career in 1979 as an assistant professor at Hunter College, Bellevue School of Nursing, where she remained on the faculty for two years. From 1987 to 1989, she was an assistant professor in the College of Nursing at the University of Rhode Island. In 1990, she joined the faculty of the College of Nursing at the State University of New York (SUNY) Health Science Center at Syracuse, now known as Upstate Medical University, and has been Chair of the Undergraduate Program for the past 12 years. As an Associate Professor, she teaches undergraduate-level courses in nursing research and in the role of the nurse as educator, and courses in the nurse educator role and in educational evaluation at the master's and post-master's programs. For the past six years, she has co-tutored an ethics course to first- and second-year medical students in her campus' College of Medicine. Dr. Bastable is currently serving a second elected term as a SUNY Senator in the statewide faculty governance unit of the University Faculty Senate. For the past 21 years, she has been a consultant and external faculty member for Excelsior College (formerly known as Regents College of the University of the State of New York). Her clinical practice includes experience in community health, oncology, rehabilitation and neurology, occupational health, and medical/surgical nursing. Dr. Bastable is the recipient of her campus' 1996 President's Award for Excellence in Teaching, the SUNY 1999 Chancellor's Award for Excellence in Teaching, and the 2001 Nursing Education Alumni Association Award from Teachers College, Columbia University.

# Foreword

American nursing's pivotal role in the health education of the community is rooted in the history of nursing practice and the social and temporal context of which it was a part. Long before the preparation of nurses took place in institutions of higher education, nursing evolved into a practice that included teaching and demonstrating healthcare actions to patients, their families, other healthcare workers, and the community at large. This historical precedent is most vividly demonstrated by the history of public health and of visiting nurses and through the vast wealth of data that exists about the health needs of diverse cultural groups who emigrated to this country at the end of the nineteenth century up to the present day. It is reflected in the experience of nurses at home and abroad during two world wars and their aftermath, other military conflicts, dramatic social movements, and scientific breakthroughs. These events resulted in a heightened need for consumer education and the participation of people in their own health decision making and care. Nurses responded to this need by becoming educators of the community.

Today, education of the community about health promotion, wellness, and illness is recognized as an essential component of nursing practice. There has been continuous development and emphasis on the leadership role of nurses in this arena over the last century, as evidenced by the focus on patient teaching and the increasing sophistication of health consumers as full participants in decision making. Another dimension relates to the public's increasing conversance with healthcare policy and the effect of changes in health delivery and financing that affect all members of society as citizens and consumers.

*Nurse as Educator: Principles of Teaching and Learning,* first published in 1997, represented a response to the need to prepare nurses for their educative roles commensurate with the changing healthcare scene and the emergence of a technological age that supports greater access to health information. The quality of substantive information included a balanced treatment of theory and application, which enhanced nurses' ability to meet the challenges confronting the profession and addressed strategies for promoting the health of the community. The response to this award-winning book has already contributed significantly to the professional healthcare literature and the text is acknowledged as an exemplary work of scholarship.

This second edition of *Nurse as Educator* increases the value of the original work in several important ways. A significant change is the refocus of the teaching-learning process to place primary emphasis on the learner as an active participant and the nurse as the enabler, resource person, and mentor. Another enhancement is the inclusion of important content about technology and the ways that it supports the education of the public about health care. The role of the nurse in the design of learning experiences for consumers that can be supported by state-of-the-art technology is a well-developed theme. A third major emphasis and enhancement in this new edition is increased attention to outcomes as the basis for evaluation of the teaching-learning experience and improvement in patient care.

*Nurse as Educator* reflects the knowledge, expertise, and experience of its contributors as well as their insights into contemporary and future challenges that nurses face as primary healthcare educators in the community. The book meets a compelling need to continue to prepare nurses for leadership in making health concerns a public priority.

M. Louise Fitzpatrick, Ed.D., R.N., F.A.A.N.
*Dean and Professor, College of Nursing*
*Villanova University*

# Preface

Educating others, whether the learners are patients and their families, fellow staff nurses, or nursing students, has been a professional responsibility of registered nurses at all levels of education for many years. It is the aim of nurses to assist patients, well or ill, to become independent in managing their own health and to help our fellow colleagues and future nurses to deliver the highest possible quality of health care to those whom we serve.

Although nurses recognize their legal, ethical, and moral responsibility to teach clients, colleagues, and prospective nurses, most of us acknowledge that we have not had the formal preparation to successfully and securely assume this role. It is imperative that nurses be prepared to carry out their role as educators competently and confidently, based on a solid understanding of the principles of teaching and learning. In today's healthcare arena, the unique holistic perspective of nursing practice mandates that nurses possess the knowledge and skills necessary to educate various audiences in a variety of settings with efficiency and effectiveness.

This text is intended to be a primary resource for graduate students, upper-level undergraduates, and professional nurses for whom the role of educator is an essential component of practice. It is designed to help them become proficient in educating others, taking into consideration the basic foundations of the education process, the needs and characteristics of the learner, and the appropriate instructional techniques and strategies for teaching and learning.

This second edition provides many new features that reflect a balance between current theoretical perspectives in the field and the application of these theories to practice. There is an increased emphasis on the nurse functioning as a "guide by the side" and as a "facilitator" of learning, rather than serving in the traditional role as primarily the "giver of information." With respect to patients as a population of learners, there is a noticeable shift in focus in this text from teaching those who are ill to teaching clients to maintain optimal health and prevent disease. Some of the significant revisions and additions to this second edition, based on the expertise of each contributor and suggestions of external reviewers, follow.

New to this edition is a chapter on Technology in Education (Chapter 13), written by an expert in computers and distance education, that describes the impact of technology on the teacher and the learner, the latest technological strategies available to the nurse educator, and the issues related to the use of technology in patient and professional education. It is a very readable chapter, even for those who are novices in the application of computers for teaching and learning.

Chapter 1 emphasizes the new educational paradigm of partnership in the teaching and learning process. Chapter 2 places a greater emphasis on cost analysis and cost effectiveness of educational programs. The perspectives of social cognition and social constructivism have been added to Chapter 3 as an update on the latest information about two increasingly popular orientations of cognitive learning theory. Chapter 4 addresses the Chronic Illness Model and the novice-to-expert concept. Chapter 5 offers new perspectives on andragogy and a discussion of the myths of ageism. Chapter 6 highlights Prochaska's Stages of Change Model. Chapter 7 includes a new emphasis on health literacy. Chapter 8 contains the latest neuroscience research on gender-related cognitive abilities in learning, an expansion on the teaching strategies specific to Black Americans as one of the four major cultural groups, ways to prepare nurses for diversity care, new terms related to cultural care, and the meaning and risks of stereotyping and ways to avoid it. Chapter 9 addresses the most current information on adaptive technologies for special populations and innovative teaching approaches to be used with clients with mental illness. Chapter 10 covers the concept of the learning curve, an old idea in business and industry with a new application to the achievement-of-learner outcomes in nursing practice. Chapters 11 and 12 have updated information on instructional methods and materials. Chapter 13 is completely new content as described previously, and Chapter 14 expands on the discussion of healthcare-related settings. Finally, Chapter 15 looks at pluralistic designs and the fourth-generation approach to evaluation.

An Instructor's Manual to accompany the second edition of this text is now available as a resource for faculty. It contains multiple choice and essay test items, learning activities, and instructional materials, including PowerPoint slides, for each chapter. In addition, a number of review questions appear at the end of every chapter to assist the student in focusing on the important content elements in each chapter. Also, many new terms have been added to the original glossary to correspond to the revisions and additions made throughout the text. The Instructor's Manual, the glossary, and the chapter review question sections are unique features of this book in comparison to other textbooks in the field of patient and staff education.

This second edition of *Nurse as Educator* is a comprehensive coverage, both in scope and depth, of the essential components of the education process and the principles of teaching and learning. It considers all the important attributes of the learner and the many aspects of the teaching role in nursing practice. Although this text focuses particularly on patient education, almost all of the chapters contain theory that is relevant, useful, and applicable to a diverse audience of learners. Thus, whoever the learner may be, this text serves as a resource for understanding the basics of teaching and learning to help nurses successfully implement their role as educators.

# Contributors

Susan B. Bastable, Ed.D., R.N.
Professor and Director of Nursing
Nursing Program
Le Moyne College
Syracuse, New York

Margaret M. Braungart, Ph.D.
Professor of Psychology
Center for Bioethics and Humanities
State University of New York
Upstate Medical University
Syracuse, New York

Richard G. Braungart, Ph.D.
Professor of Sociology and International Relations
Maxwell School
Syracuse University
Syracuse, New York

Kathleen Fitzgerald, M.S., R.N.
Patient Educator
St. Joseph's Hospital Health Center
Syracuse, New York

Diane S. Hainsworth, M.S., R.N., A.N.P.
Oncology Case Manager
State University of New York
Upstate Medical University
Syracuse, New York

Sharon Kitchie, M.S., R.N.C.S. (Doctoral Candidate)
Patient Education Coordinator and Nurse Educator at the
    Health Information Center
University Hospital
State University of New York
Upstate Medical University
Syracuse, New York

M. Janice Nelson, Ed.D, R.N.
Professor and Dean Emeritus
College of Nursing
State University of New York
Upstate Medical University
Syracuse, New York

Virginia E. O'Halloran, Ed.D, R.N.C.
Associate Professor (retired)
College of Mount St. Vincent
Bronx, New York
Nyack Hospital Home Care
Nyack, New York

Eleanor Richards, Ph.D., R.N.
Associate Professor
Department of Nursing
State University of New York at New Paltz
New Paltz, New York

Michelle A. Rinwalske, M.S., R.N.
Nurse Practitioner and Nurse Educator
Children's Diabetes Program
State University of New York
Upstate Medical University
Syracuse, New York

Deborah L. Sopczyk, M.S., R.N. (Doctoral Candidate)
Director of Graduate Program
School of Nursing
Excelsior College
Albany, New York

Kay Viggiani, M.S., R.N., C.N.S.
Associate Professor
Nursing Division
Keuka College
Keuka Park, New York

Priscilla Sandford Worral, Ph.D., R.N.
Coordinator of Nursing Research
University Hospital
State University of New York
Upstate Medical University
Syracuse, New York

# Acknowledgments

A special appreciation is given to my husband, Jeffrey, who demonstrated a great deal of patience, understanding, and encouragement during the many months of writing and editing. Without his support, this second edition text would never have been realized.

A sincere thanks to each and every one of my contributors, who have shared their professional expertise, been timely in responding to my requests, and remained loyal in their assistance with the completion of their respective chapters.

A special recognition of Rhonda Solomon, a master's student at the College of Nursing at Upstate Medical University, who spent countless hours researching and compiling current data to update the information and references in this text, particularly for the Developmental Stages of the Learner and Behavioral Objectives chapters.

To the staff and faculty at my College of Nursing, I wish to extend the utmost gratitude for their interest, flexibility, and support throughout every step of the publication process.

To the editorial staff at Jones and Bartlett Publishers, in particular Penny Glynn, Thomas Prindle, Karen Ferreira, and Amy Rose, for providing consistent guidance and expert advice.

And, it is so true that accomplishments can never be achieved without the constant love and support of family. My son, Garrett, my daughter, Leigh, and my parents, Robert and Dorrie Bacorn and Gerry Bastable, have always been and will always be the source of my inspiration.

# PART I

# Perspectives on Teaching and Learning

## CHAPTER 1

# Overview of Education in Health Care

*Susan B. Bastable*

## KEY TERMS

education process
teaching
instruction
learning

patient education
staff education
barriers to education
obstacles to learning

## OBJECTIVES

After completing this chapter, the reader will be
able to

1. Discuss the evolution of the teaching role of
   nurses.
2. Recognize trends affecting the healthcare
   system in general and nursing practice in
   particular.
3. Identify the purpose, benefits, and goals of
   patient and staff education.

4. Compare and contrast the education process to
   the nursing process.
5. Define the terms *teaching* and *learning*.
6. Identify reasons why patient and staff education
   is an important duty for professional nurses.
7. Discuss barriers to education and obstacles to
   learning.
8. Formulate questions that nurses in the role of
   educator should ask about the teaching–learning process.

Education in health care today—both patient education and nursing staff/student education—is a topic of utmost interest in every setting in which nurses practice. The current trends in health care are making it imperative that patients and their families be prepared to assume responsibility for self-care management. Also, these trends make it essential that nurses in the workplace be accountable for the delivery of high-quality care. The focus is on outcomes—whether it be that the patient and his or her family have learned essential knowledge and skills for independent care or that staff nurses and nursing students have acquired the up-to-date knowledge and skills needed to competently and confidently render care to the consumer in a variety of settings. The need for nurses to teach others and to help others learn will continue to increase in this era of healthcare reform. With changes rapidly forthcoming in the system of health care, nurses will find themselves in increasingly demanding, constantly fluctuating, and highly complex positions (Jorgensen, 1994). It is necessary for nurses in the role of educators to understand the forces, both historical and present-day, that have influenced and continue to influence their responsibilities in practice, with teaching being a major aspect of the nurse's professional role.

One purpose of this chapter is to shed light on the historical evolution of teaching as part of the professional nurse's role. Another purpose of this chapter is to offer a perspective on the current trends in health care making patient teaching a highly visible and required function of nursing care delivery. Also addressed are the continuing education efforts required to ensure ongoing practice competencies of nursing personnel. In addition, this chapter clarifies the broad purposes, benefits, and goals of the teaching–learning process, focuses on the philosophy of the nurse–patient partnership in teaching and learning, compares the education process to

the nursing process, identifies barriers to teaching and learning, and highlights the status of research in the field of patient as well as staff education. The focus is on the overall role of the nurse in teaching and learning, no matter who the audience of learners may be. Nurses must have a basic prerequisite understanding of the principles, practice, and process of teaching and learning to carry out their professional responsibilities with efficiency and effectiveness.

## ▣ HISTORICAL FOUNDATIONS FOR THE TEACHING ROLE OF NURSES

Patient education has long been considered a major component in the repertoire of standard care-giving by the nurse. The role of the nurse as educator is deeply entrenched in the heritage and development of the profession. Since the mid-1800s, when nursing was first acknowledged as a unique discipline, the responsibility for teaching has been recognized as an important healthcare initiative assumed by nurses. The focus of teaching efforts by nurses was not only on the care of the sick, but also on educating other nurses for professional practice.

Florence Nightingale, the founder of modern nursing, was the ultimate educator. Not only did she develop the first school of nursing, but she also devoted a large portion of her career to educating those involved in the delivery of health care. Nightingale taught nurses, physicians, and health officials about the importance of proper conditions in hospitals and homes to assist patients in maintaining adequate nutrition, fresh air, exercise, and personal hygiene to improve their well-being. By the early 1900s, public health nurses in this country clearly understood the significance of education in the prevention of disease and in the maintenance of health (Chachkes & Christ, 1996).

For decades, then, patient teaching has been recognized as an independent nursing function. Nurses have always educated others—patients, families, and colleagues—and it is from these roots that nurses have expanded their practice to include the broader concepts of health and illness (Glanville, 2000).

As early as 1918, the National League of Nursing Education (NLNE) in the United States [now the National League for Nursing (NLN)] observed the importance of health teaching as a function within the scope of nursing practice. This organization recognized the responsibility of nurses for the promotion of health and the prevention of illness in such settings as schools, homes, hospitals, and industries. Two decades later, the NLNE declared that a nurse was fundamentally a teacher and an agent of health regardless of the setting in which practice occurred (National League of Nursing Education, 1937). By 1950, the NLNE had identified course content dealing with teaching skills, developmental and educational psychology, and principles of the educational process of teaching and learning as areas in the curriculum common to all nursing schools (Redman, 1993). The implication was that nurses were to be prepared, upon graduation from their basic nursing program, to assume the role as teacher of others. The American Nurses Association has for years promulgated statements on the functions, standards, and qualifications for nursing practice, of which patient teaching is an integral aspect. In addition, the International Council of Nurses has long endorsed education for health as an essential requisite of nursing care delivery.

Today, state nurse practice acts (NPAs) universally include teaching within the scope of nursing practice responsibilities. Nurses are expected to provide instruction to consumers to assist them to maintain optimal levels of wellness, prevent disease, manage illness, and develop skills to give supportive care to family members. Nursing career ladders often incorporate teaching effectiveness as a measure of excellence in practice (Rifas et al., 1994). The more recent development of clinical pathways, also referred to as critical pathways, has led to a popular, multidisciplinary approach to delineating predetermined client outcomes that are used to measure patient adherence to pathway expectations. Nurses are in the forefront of innovative strategies for the delivery of patient care. The teaching of patients and families as well as healthcare personnel is the means to accomplish the professional goals of providing cost-effective, safe, and high-quality care.

In recognition of the importance of patient education by nurses, the Joint Commission on Accreditation of Healthcare Organizations (JCAHO) delineated nursing standards for patient education as early as 1993. These standards, which take the form of mandates, are based on descriptions of positive outcomes of patient care. They are to be met through teaching activities by nurses that must be patient- and family-oriented. Required accreditation standards have provided the impetus for nursing service managers to put greater emphasis on unit-based clinical education activities for staff to improve nursing interventions relating to patient education for the achievement of these client outcomes (McGoldrick et al.,1994).

More recently, JCAHO has expanded its expectations to include an interdisciplinary team approach in the provision of patient education as well as evidence that patients and their significant others understand what they have been taught. This requirement means that providers must consider the literacy level, educational background, language skills, and culture of every client during the education process (Davidhizar & Brownson, 1999). In addition, the Patient's Bill of Rights, first developed in the 1970s by the American Hospital Association and adopted by hospitals nationwide, has established the rights of patients to receive complete and current information concerning diagnosis, treatment, and prognosis in terms they can reasonably be expected to understand.

In 1995, the Pew Health Professions Commission, influenced by the dramatic changes currently surrounding health care, published a broad set of competencies that it believes will mark the success of the health professions in the twenty-first century. Most recently, the Commission (1998) released a fourth report as a follow-up on health professional practice in the new millennium. Numerous recommendations to the health professions have been proposed by the Commission. More than one-half of them pertain to the importance of patient and staff education and to the role of the nurse as educator. Among the recommendations, the Commission has addressed the need to:

- Provide clinically competent and coordinated care to the public
- Involve patients and their families in the decision-making process regarding health interventions
- Provide clients with education and counseling on ethical issues
- Expand public access to effective care
- Ensure cost-effective and appropriate care for the consumer
- Provide for prevention of illness and promotion of healthy lifestyles for all Americans

Accomplishing the goals and meeting the expectations of these organizations calls for a redirection of education efforts. Over time, the role of the nurse as educator has undergone a paradigm shift. In patient education, the provider teaching role has evolved from what once was a disease-oriented approach to a more prevention-oriented approach. Now and in the future, the focus will be on teaching for the promotion and maintenance of health. Since the 1980s, greater recognition has been given to client education as a healthcare activity. Once done as part of discharge plans at the end of hospitalization, patient education

efforts have expanded to become integrated into a comprehensive plan of care that occurs throughout the healthcare delivery process (Davidhizar & Brownson, 1999). As described by Grueninger (1995), this transition toward wellness has entailed a progression "from disease-oriented patient education (DOPE) to prevention-oriented patient education (POPE) to ultimately become health-oriented patient education (HOPE)" (p. 53). This metamorphosis has changed the role of educator from one of wise healer to expert advisor/teacher to facilitator of change. Instead of the traditional aim of simply imparting information, the emphasis is now on empowering patients to use their potentials, abilities, and resources to the fullest (Glanville, 2000). Presently, the demand for nurses in the role of educators of patients, their families, and the general public is rapidly accelerating.

Also, the role of today's educator is one of "training the trainer"—that is, preparing nursing staff through continuing education, in-service programs, and staff development to maintain and improve their clinical skills and teaching abilities. The key to the success of our profession is for nurses to teach other nurses. We are the primary educators of our fellow colleagues and other healthcare staff personnel. In addition, the demand for educators of nursing students is at an all-time high. It is essential that professional nurses be prepared to effectively perform teaching services that meet the needs of many individuals and groups in different circumstances across a variety of practice settings.

## SOCIAL, ECONOMIC, AND POLITICAL TRENDS AFFECTING HEALTH CARE

In addition to the professional and legal standards put forth by various organizations and agencies, there has arisen an increasing emphasis on nurses' potential role in teaching activities as a result of social, economic, and political trends nationwide affecting the public's health. The following are some of the significant forces affecting nursing practice in particular and the healthcare system in general (Jorgensen, 1994; McGinnis, 1993; Latter et al., 1992; Kellmer-Langan et al., 1992; DeSilets, 1995; Wilkinson, 1996; Glanville, 2000; Birchenall, 2000):

1. The federal government, through healthcare reform initiatives, has established national health goals and objectives for the future. *Healthy People 2010: National Promotion and Disease Prevention Objectives* (U.S. Department of Health and Human Services, 2000) is a document that describes national needs in relation to health promotion and disease prevention for the public. Objectives include the development of effective health education programs to assist individuals to recognize and change risk behaviors, to adopt or maintain protective health practices, and to make appropriate use of healthcare delivery systems. Achievement of these national objectives would dramatically cut healthcare costs, prevent the premature onset of disease and disability, and help all Americans lead healthier and more productive lives. Nurses, as the largest group of healthcare professionals, embody the professional philosophy of holistic care and are capable of making a real difference in educating people so that they can attain and maintain healthy lifestyles.

2. The growth of managed care, the shifts in payer coverage, and the issue of reimbursement for the provision of health care have placed an increasingly greater emphasis on outcome measures, achievable primarily through success of patient education efforts.

3. Health providers are beginning to recognize the economic and social values in practicing preventive medicine through health education initiatives.

4. Political emphasis is on productivity, competitiveness in the marketplace, and cost-containment measures to restrain health-service expenses. Politicians and healthcare administrators alike acknowledge the importance of health education as a requisite to accomplishing these economic goals in today's society.

5. The healthcare reform movement is opening up new avenues for expansion of preventive and promotion education efforts directed at communities, schools, and workplaces in addition to the traditional care settings.

6. There is concern on the part of healthcare professionals regarding the legal pressures associated with malpractice and disciplinary action for incompetency. In recent years, continuing education, either by legislative mandate or as a requirement of the employing institution, has come to the forefront as a potential answer to the challenge of ensuring the competency of practitioners. Continuing education has emerged as a response to the change and expansion of knowledge in the nursing profession. It is a means to transmit new knowledge and skills as well as to reinforce or refresh previously acquired knowledge and abilities, thereby guaranteeing the continuing growth of staff nurse competencies.

7. The interest that continues to be exhibited by nurses in defining their own role, body of knowledge, scope of practice, and professional expertise has focused on patient education as central to the practice of nursing.

8. Consumers are demanding increased knowledge and skills about how to care for themselves and how to prevent disease. A rise in consumerism in health-service provision is paralleling the interest exhibited in other aspects of consumer involvement in the marketplace. As people are becoming more aware of and more knowledgeable about healthcare matters, they are

questioning the nature of their impairments and needs and are demanding a greater understanding of treatments and goals. The healthcare trends of the 1990s, which emphasized consumer rights and responsibilities, will continue in the twenty-first century. Such trends have already increased the demand for patient and consumer information services, and these demands are expected to intensify in the future.

9. Demographic trends—namely, the aging of the population—are requiring an emphasis to be placed on self-reliance and maintenance of a healthy status over an extended lifespan. The percentage of the U.S. population older than 65 years will climb dramatically in the next 20 to 30 years as the baby boom generation of the post–World War II era reaches the late adulthood years. The baby boomers' health needs will become greater as they deal with degenerative illnesses and other effects of the aging process.

10. Among the major causes of morbidity and mortality are those diseases now recognized as being lifestyle-related and preventable through educational interventions.

11. The proportionate increase in the incidence of chronic and incurable conditions necessitates that individuals and families become informed participants to manage their own illnesses.

12. Advanced technology is increasing the complexity of care and treatment as well as diverting large numbers of patients from inpatient healthcare settings to community-based settings. Life support and maintenance technologies are enabling patients to carry on with their lives away from the acute, direct care-giving arenas. Patient education is necessary to assist them to independently follow through with self-management activities.

13. Earlier hospital discharge is forcing patients and their families to be more self-reliant while managing their own illnesses. Patient teaching can facilitate an individual's adaptive responses to illness.

14. There is a belief on the part of nurses and other healthcare providers, which is supported by research, that patient education improves compliance and, hence, health and well-being. Better understanding by clients of their treatment plans can lead to increased cooperation with therapeutic regimens. Patient education will enable them to independently solve problems encountered outside the protected care environments of hospitals, thereby increasing their independence.

15. There is an increased proliferation in the number of self-help groups established to support clients in meeting their physical and psychosocial needs. The success of these support groups and behavioral change programs has led to an upsurge in public interest as well as nurse involvement and advocacy for these educational endeavors.

These examples are indicative of the major trends operating in this country to create a climate of increased consumer and professional expectations. Nurses recognize the need to develop their expertise in teaching to keep pace with the demands of patient and staff education. In turn, nurses are in a key position to carry out health education. They are the healthcare providers who have the most continuous contact with patients and families, are usually the most accessible source of information for the consumer, and are the most highly trusted of all health professionals. In a recent Gallup poll, nurses were ranked first in honesty and ethics among 45 occupations (Mason,

2001). Patient teaching is becoming an increasingly important function within the scope of nursing practice.

## PURPOSE, BENEFITS, AND GOALS OF PATIENT AND STAFF EDUCATION

Current and continuously improving patient and staff education programs are an integral part of today's system of healthcare delivery to the public. The purpose of patient education is to increase the competence and confidence of clients for self-management. Our goal is to support patients through the transition from being invalids to being independent in care; from being dependent recipients to being involved participants in the care process; and from being passive listeners to active learners. The single most important action of nurses as caregivers is to prepare patients and their families for self-care. If clients cannot independently maintain or improve their health status when on their own, we have failed to help them reach their potential.

In light of cost-containment measures by healthcare agencies and despite the sometimes scarce resources available, nurses continue to pursue the goals of involving patients in exploring and expanding their self-care abilities through interactive patient education efforts (McGoldrick et al., 1994; Glanville, 2000). The benefits of effective patient education are many. Patient education has demonstrated its potential to:

- Increase consumer satisfaction
- Improve quality of life
- Ensure continuity of care
- Decrease patient anxiety
- Effectively reduce the incidence of complications of illness
- Promote adherence to healthcare treatment plans

- Maximize independence in the performance of activities of daily living
- Energize and empower consumers to become actively involved in the planning of their care

In turn, the educator role of nurses enhances their job satisfaction when they recognize that their teaching actions have the potential to forge therapeutic relationships with patients, allow for greater patient–nurse autonomy, increase their accountability for practice, and create change that really makes a difference in the lives of others.

Because an estimated 80% of all health needs and problems are handled at home, there truly does exist a need to educate people on how to care for themselves—both to get well and to stay well (Health Services Medical Corporation, 1993). Illness is a natural life process, but so is mankind's ability to learn. Along with the ability to learn comes a natural curiosity that allows people to view new and difficult situations as challenges rather than as defeats. As Robin Orr (1990) noted, "Illness can become an educational opportunity . .. a 'teachable moment' when ill health suddenly encourages [patients] to take a more active role in their care" (p. 47). Numerous studies have documented the fact that informed patients are more likely to comply with medical treatment plans and find innovative ways to cope with illness. Such individuals are also better able to manage symptoms of illness and are less likely to experience complications. Overall, patients are more satisfied with care when they receive adequate information about how to manage for themselves. One of the most frequently cited complaints by patients in litigation cases is that they were not adequately informed.

Just as the need exists for teaching clients to help them become participants and informed consumers to achieve independence in self-care, the need also exists for staff nurses to be exposed to up-to-date and ongoing information with the ultimate goal of enhancing their practice. The purpose of staff education is to increase the competence and confidence of nurses to function independently in providing quality care to the consumer. Nurses play a key role in improving the nation's health, and they recognize the importance of lifelong learning to keep their knowledge and skills current (DeSilets, 1995).

Our primary aims, then, as educators should be to nourish clients as well as mentor staff. We must value education and make it a priority for both our patients and our fellow colleagues.

## THE EDUCATION PROCESS DEFINED

The *education process* is a systematic, sequential, planned course of action consisting of two major interdependent operations, teaching and learning. This process forms a continuous cycle that also involves two interdependent players, the teacher and the learner. Together, they jointly perform teaching and learning activities, the outcome of which leads to mutually desired behavior changes. These changes foster growth in the learner and, it should be acknowledged, growth in the teacher as well. Thus, the education process should always be a participatory, shared approach to teaching and learning.

The education process has always been compared to the nursing process—rightly so, because the steps of each process run parallel to one another, although they have different goals and objectives. The education process, like the nursing process, consists of the basic elements of assessment, planning, implementation, and evaluation. The nursing process and the education process are logical, scientifically-based frameworks for nursing. Both processes provide a rational basis for nursing practice rather than an intuitive one. They are

methods for monitoring and judging the overall quality of nursing interventions based on objective data and scientific criteria. The two are different in that the nursing process focuses on the planning and implementation of care based on the assessment and diagnosis of the physical and psychosocial needs of the patient, whereas the education process identifies instructional content and methods based on an assessment and prioritization of the client's learning needs, readiness to learn, and learning styles. The outcomes of the nursing process are achieved when the physical and psychosocial needs of the client are met. The outcomes of the education process are achieved when changes in knowledge, attitudes, and skills occur. Both processes are ongoing, with assessment and evaluation perpetually redirecting the planning and implementation phases of the processes. If mutually agreed-on outcomes in either process are not achieved, as determined by evaluation, then the nursing process or the education process can and should begin again through reassessment, replanning, and reimplementation (Figure 1–1).

It should be noted that the actual act of teaching is merely one component of the education process. Education, as the broad umbrella process, includes the acts of teaching and instruction. *Teaching* is a deliberate intervention that involves the planning and implementation of instructional activities and experiences to meet intended learner outcomes according to a teaching plan. *Instruction*, a term often used interchangeably with teaching, is one aspect of teaching. It is a component of teaching that involves the communicating of information about a specific skill in the cognitive, psychomotor, or affective domain. Teaching and instruction are often formal, structured, organized activities prepared days in advance, but they can be performed informally on the spur of the moment during conversations or incidental encounters with the learner. Whether formal or informal,

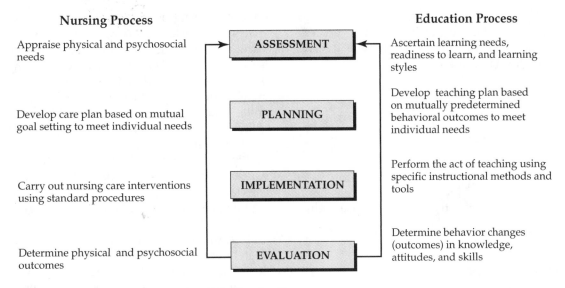

**Nursing Process**

Appraise physical and psychosocial needs

Develop care plan based on mutual goal setting to meet individual needs

Carry out nursing care interventions using standard procedures

Determine physical and psychosocial outcomes

**Education Process**

Ascertain learning needs, readiness to learn, and learning styles

Develop teaching plan based on mutually predetermined behavioral outcomes to meet individual needs

Perform the act of teaching using specific instructional methods and tools

Determine behavior changes (outcomes) in knowledge, attitudes, and skills

ASSESSMENT

PLANNING

IMPLEMENTATION

EVALUATION

**FIGURE 1–1    Education Process Parallels Nursing Process**

planned well in advance or spontaneous, teaching and instruction are nevertheless deliberate and conscious acts with the objective of producing learning.

The fact that teaching and instruction are intentional does not necessarily mean that they have to be lengthy and complex tasks, but it does mean that they comprise conscious actions on the part of the teacher in responding to an individual's need to learn. The cues that someone has a need to learn can be communicated in the form of a verbal request, a question, a puzzled or confused look, or a gesture of defeat or frustration. In the broadest sense, then, teaching is a highly versatile strategy that can be applied in preventing, promoting, maintaining, or modifying a wide variety of behaviors in a learner who is receptive, motivated, and adequately informed (Redman, 1971; Duffy, 1998).

*Learning* is defined as a change in behavior (knowledge, skills, and attitudes) that can occur at any time or in any place as a result of exposure to environmental stimuli. Learning is an action by which knowledge, skills, and attitudes are consciously or unconsciously acquired such

that behavior is altered in some way that can be observed or measured (see Chapter 3).

The success of the nurse educator's endeavors at teaching is measured not by how much content has been imparted, but rather by how much the person has learned. Specifically, *patient education* is a process of assisting people to learn health-related behaviors (knowledge, skills, attitudes, and values) so that they can incorporate those behaviors into everyday life. As stated previously, the purpose of patient education is to assist clients to achieve the goal of optimal health and independence in self-care. *Staff education,* by contrast, is the process of influencing the behavior of nurses by producing changes in their knowledge, attitudes, values, and skills. As stated previously, the purpose here is to help nurses maintain and improve their competencies as required for the delivery of quality care to the consumer. Both patient and staff education involve forging a relationship between learner and educator so that the learner's information needs (cognitive, psychomotor, and affective) can be met through the process of education.

A useful paradigm to assist nurses to organize and carry out the education process is the ASSURE model (Rega, 1993). The acronym stands for:

- **A**nalyze learner
- **S**tate objectives
- **S**elect instructional methods and tools
- **U**se teaching materials
- **R**equire learner performance
- **E**valuate/revise the teaching and learning process.

## ROLE OF THE NURSE AS EDUCATOR

For many years, organizations governing and influencing nurses have encouraged and supported the belief that nurses should play a major role in health education. Teaching has been seen as an essential component of nursing practice in caring for both well and ill clients. For nurses to fulfill the role of educator, no matter whether their audience consists of patients, family members, nursing students, nursing staff, or other agency personnel, they must have a solid foundation in the principles of teaching and learning. Educationalists have argued that teaching, and especially the teaching of adults, is a function involving complex concepts (Knowles et al., 1998). Teaching requires special training in instructional skills if education programs conducted by nurses are to be successful.

Luker and Caress (1989), in particular, have challenged the wisdom of involving all nurses in patient education as an unrealistic and undesirable goal of the profession. In their classic article, "Rethinking Patient Education," they suggested that it is unreasonable to expect every nurse to take responsibility for teaching patients when the majority of nursing practitioners have had only a basic nursing

education background from diploma or associate's degree–level programs. Patients, by virtue of their illnesses, may have special learning difficulties that require teaching interventions to be carried out by nurses who are well grounded in the principles of teaching and learning.

Luker and Caress (1989) also argued that the U.S. system of nursing education has a multiple-entry, unstandardized approach to educating nurses for practice. This strategy leaves little room in the diploma and associate's degree–level curriculum for including the breadth and depth of information on teaching and learning principles necessary to adequately prepare nurses to function in the role of educator. One solution, albeit a controversial one, is to make teaching the sole responsibility of, at minimum, baccalaureate-degree graduates. Ideally, these two authors contend, the educator role should be delegated to master's-prepared nurses—particularly the advanced practice nurses such as clinical nurse specialists and nurse practitioners—who have both the interest and the knowledge base to make them expert patient and staff educators.

Luker and Caress (1989) clearly distinguished between patient teaching and patient education. They noted that patient teaching "implies a didactic information giving approach," whereas patient education "implies something more comprehensive, for which specialist skills are required" (p. 714). Although all nurses are able to function as givers of information, they posed the following questions:

- Is every nurse adequately prepared to assess for learning needs?

- Can every nurse determine whether information given is received and understood?

- Are all nurses capable of taking appropriate action to revise the approach to educating the client if the information is not comprehended?

Because standardized teaching packages help to overcome these potential deficits in nurses' ability to function as teachers, there still remains the need for them to be able to assess the suitability of the standardized material for the learner and to adapt it accordingly if necessary. To ensure that patient education programs are clinically accurate and educationally sound, these two authors advocated that nurses with minimal basic education be excluded from the education process.

Despite Luker and Caress's arguments, legal and accreditation mandates as well as professional nursing standards of practice have made patient education an integral part of high-quality care to be delivered by all registered nurses licensed in the United States, regardless of their level of nursing school preparation. Given this fact, it is imperative to examine the present teaching role expectations of nurses, irrespective of their preparatory background.

The role of educator is not primarily to teach, but to promote learning and provide for an environment conducive to learning—to create the teachable moment rather than just waiting for it to happen (Wagner & Ash, 1998). Also, the role of the nurse as teacher of patients and families, nursing staff, and students certainly should stem from a partnership philosophy. The provision of information to the learner, whoever that learner may be, should stress the fact that teaching and learning are participatory processes. A learner cannot be made to learn, but an effective approach in educating others is to actively involve learners in the education process. A growing body of evidence suggests that effective education and learner participation go hand in hand. The nurse should act as a facilitator, creating an environment conducive to learning—one that motivates individuals to want to learn and makes it possible for them to learn. The assessment of learning needs, the planning and designing of a teaching program, the implementation of instructional methods and mate-

rials, and the evaluation of teaching and learning should involve both the educator and the learner. In the case of patient education, an approach that is more in keeping with ideals of self-care would be to transfer the responsibility for learning from the nurse to the patient. Thus the emphasis should be on the facilitation of learning from a nondirective rather than a didactic teaching approach (Knowles, 1989; Knowles et al., 1998).

No longer should teachers see themselves as simply transmitters of content and controllers of the learner. Indeed, the role of the educator has shifted from the traditional "giver of information" position to that of a process designer and manager. This role alteration requires skill in needs assessment as well as the ability to involve learners in planning, link learners to learning resources, and encourage learner initiative (Knowles et al., 1998). Instead of the teacher teaching, the new educational paradigm focuses on the learner learning. That is, the teacher becomes "the guide on the side," assisting the learner in his or her effort to determine objectives and goals for learning, with both parties being active partners in decision making throughout the learning process. If learners are to be able to comprehend, recall, and apply information, they must be actively involved in the learning experience (London, 1995). Glanville (2000) describes this move toward assisting learners to use their own abilities and resources as "a pivotal transfer of power" (p. 58).

Certainly patient education requires a collaborative effort among healthcare team members, all of whom play more or less important roles in teaching. Numerous authors, however, have cited documentation "that physicians are taught to treat, not to teach" (Gilroth, 1990, p. 30). Nurses, on the other hand, with their holistic approach to care delivery, should capture the educator role and make it part of their unique professional domain. The respect and trust traditionally bestowed on them by healthcare consumers provides the opportunity for nurses to position themselves as client advocates, clarifying confusing information and making "sense out of nonsense." Amidst a fragmented healthcare delivery system involving many providers, the nurse also needs to serve as coordinator of teaching efforts. By ensuring consistency of information, nurses can support the patients and family members in their efforts to achieve the goal of optimal health.

## BARRIERS TO EDUCATION AND OBSTACLES TO LEARNING

It has been said by many educators that adult learning takes place not by the teacher's initiating and motivating the learning process, but rather by the teacher's removing or reducing obstacles to learning and enhancing the process after it has begun. The educator should not limit learning to the information that is intended but should clearly make possible the potential for informal, unintended learning that can occur each and every day with each and every teacher–learner encounter (Redman, 1975).

Unfortunately, numerous barriers confront nurses in carrying out their responsibilities for educating clients and a variety of obstacles can potentially interfere with learning. *Barriers to education* are those factors impeding the nurse's ability to deliver educational services. *Obstacles to learning* are those factors that negatively affect the ability of the learner to attend to and process information.

### Barriers to Education

Numerous authors have addressed the major barriers interfering with the ability of nurses to carry out their roles as educators (Glanville, 2000; Casey, 1995; Chachkes & Christ, 1996; Gilroth, 1990; Lipetz et al., 1990; Honan et al., 1988; Duffy, 1998). The following are the key organizational, environmental, educational,

and clientele factors that serve as impediments to educating others:

1. Lack of time to teach is cited by nurses as the greatest barrier to being able to carry out their educator role effectively. Very ill patients are hospitalized for only short periods of time. Early discharge from inpatient settings and the movement toward community-based care often result in nurses and patients having fleeting contact with one another in emergency, outpatient, and other ambulatory care settings. In addition, nurses' schedules and responsibilities are very demanding. Finding time to allocate to teaching is very challenging in light of the competition from other work demands and expectations. The textbook approach to teaching has been the ideal but is no longer realistic. Nurses must know how to adopt an abbreviated, efficient, and expeditious approach to patient and staff education by first adequately assessing the learner and then by using appropriate instructional methods and tools at their disposal. Discharge planning will play an ever more important role in ensuring continuity of care across settings.

2. Many nurses and other healthcare personnel are traditionally ill prepared to teach. Studies have revealed that the principles of teaching and the concepts of learning are unclear to a large number of practicing nurses. Many nurses admit that they do not feel competent or confident with regard to their teaching skills. As cited previously, nursing education has for years failed to adequately prepare nurses for the role as educator, either during basic training or afterward. Although nurses are expected to teach, content in teaching and learning principles in nursing school curricula has been neglected, glossed over, or watered down. The concepts of patient education are usually integrated throughout nursing curricula rather than being

offered as a specific course of study. As early as the mid-1960s, Pohl (1965) found that one-third of 1500 nurses, when questioned, reported that they had no preparation for the teaching they were doing, while only one-fifth felt they had adequate preparation. More recently, Kruger (1991) surveyed 1230 nurses in staff, administrative, and education positions regarding their perceptions of the extent of nurses' responsibility for and level of achievement of patient education. Although all three groups strongly believed that patient education is a primary responsibility of nurses, the vast majority of them rated their ability to perform patient education activities as not being satisfactory. The findings of this research study indicate that the role of the nurse as patient educator needs to be strengthened.

3. Personal characteristics of the nurse educator play an important role in determining the outcome of a teaching–learning interaction. Motivation to teach is a prime factor in determining the success of any educational endeavor (see Chapter 11 on increasing effectiveness in teaching). Teaching by nurses sometimes is relegated to a low-priority status because of the physical, task-oriented nature of nursing care, the relatively minor importance assigned to teaching, and the lack of confidence on the part of practitioners in performing the teaching role.

4. Until recently, low priority was often assigned to patient and staff education by administration and supervisory personnel. With the new JCAHO mandates, the level of attention paid to the educational needs of consumers as well as healthcare personnel has changed significantly. However, budget allocations for educational programs remain tight and can interfere with the adoption of innovative and time-saving teaching strategies and techniques.

5. The lack of space and privacy in the various environmental settings where nurses are expected to teach and learners are expected to learn is not always conducive to carrying out the teaching–learning process. Noise, frequent interferences, treatment schedules, and the like serve to negatively affect concentration and effective interaction.

6. An absence of third-party reimbursement to support patient education programs relegates teaching and learning to less than high-priority status. Nursing services within healthcare facilities are subsumed under hospital room costs and, therefore, are not specifically reimbursed by insurance payers. In fact, patient education in some settings, such as home care, often cannot be incorporated as a legitimate aspect of routine nursing care delivery unless specifically ordered by a physician.

7. Some nurses and physicians question whether patient education is effective as a means to improve health outcomes. They view patients as impediments to teaching when patients do not display an interest in changing behavior, when they demonstrate an unwillingness to learn, or when their ability to learn is in question. Concerns about coercion and violation of free choice, based on the belief that patients have a right to choose and that they cannot be forced to comply, explain why some professionals choose not to invest time and effort in teaching. Unless all healthcare members buy into the "utility of patient education" (that is, they believe it can lead to significant behavioral changes and increased compliance to therapeutic regimens), then some professionals may continue to feel absolved from the responsibility to provide adequate and appropriate patient education.

8. There are a multitude of healthcare providers covering much of the same content, but not necessarily with consistency.

There seems to be a "malfunction" of the healthcare team as a result of inadequate coordination and delegation of responsibility so that health teaching can proceed in a timely, smooth, organized, and thorough fashion. Content needs to be standardized, teaching responsibilities need to be made clear, and lines of communication must be strengthened among a wide variety of healthcare providers.

9. The type of documentation system used by healthcare agencies has an effect on the quality and quantity of patient teaching recorded. Both formal and informal teaching are often done but not written down because of a lack of time as well as inattention to documentation and inadequate forms on which to record teaching activities. In addition, most nurses do not recognize the scope and depth of teaching that they perform on a daily basis. Inadequate recording of teaching efforts impedes communication among healthcare providers regarding what has been taught, diminishes the attention paid to the education efforts by nurses, and raises the very real possibility of legal liability of professionals.

## Obstacles to Learning

The following are some of the major obstacles interfering with a learner's ability to attend to and process information (Glanville, 2000; Lipetz et al., 1990; Gilroth, 1990; Seley, 1994):

1. The stress of acute and chronic illness, anxiety, sensory deficits, and low literacy in patients are just a few problems that can diminish learner motivation and interfere with the process of learning. However, it must be pointed out that illness alone seldom acts as an impediment to learning. Rather, illness is often the impetus for patients to make contact with the healthcare professional and to take positive action to improve their health status.

2. The negative influence of the hospital environment itself, resulting in loss of control, lack of privacy, and social isolation, can interfere with a client's active role in health decision making and involvement in the teaching–learning process.

3. Lack of time to learn due to rapid patient discharge from care can discourage and frustrate the learner, impeding the ability and willingness to learn.

4. Personal characteristics of the learner have major effects on the degree to which predetermined behavioral outcomes are achieved. Readiness to learn, motivation and compliance, developmental-stage characteristics, and learning styles are some of the prime factors influencing the success of educational endeavors.

5. The extent of behavioral changes needed, both in number and in complexity, can overwhelm learners and dissuade them from attending to and accomplishing learning objectives and goals.

6. Lack of support and ongoing positive reinforcement from the nurse and significant others serves to block the potential for learning.

7. Denial of learning needs, resentment of authority, and lack of willingness to take responsibility (locus of control) are some psychological obstacles to accomplishing behavioral change.

8. The inconvenience, complexity, inaccessibility, fragmentation, and dehumanization of the healthcare system often result in frustration and abandonment of efforts by the learner to participate in and comply with the goals and objectives for learning.

## PERSPECTIVES ON RESEARCH IN PATIENT AND STAFF EDUCATION

The literature on patient and staff education is extensive from both a research- and non-research-based perspective. A computer literature search in the library, for example, will reveal literally thousands of nursing and allied health articles on teaching and learning of patients and staff available from the general to the specific. The non-research literature on patient education is prescriptive in nature and tends to give tips on "how to do" patient teaching, promoting mainly individualized approaches to teaching and learning. In addition, the literature reveals that the psychological advantages of patient education are given more attention than the physiological outcomes.

An increasing number of articles report pertinent research on teaching specific population groups, but the focus is more on the needs of learners with short-term conditions as opposed to those suffering with long-term chronic illnesses. Much more research must be conducted on the benefits of patient education as it relates to the potential for increasing the quality of life, leading a disability-free life, decreasing the costs of health care, and managing independently at home through anticipatory teaching approaches. Studies from acute-care settings tend to focus on preparing a patient for a procedure, with emphasis on the benefits of information to alleviate anxiety and promote psychological coping. Evidence suggests that patients cope much more effectively when taught exactly what to expect (Smith, 1989; Duffy, 1998; Donovan & Ward, 2001; Mason, 2001).

More research is definitely needed on the benefits of teaching methods and tools using the new technologies of computer-assisted instruction, distance learning, video- and audiotapes for home use, cable television, and Internet access to health information for both patient and staff education. Given the significant incidence of low-literacy rates among patients and their family members, much more investigation needs to be done on learner comprehension of printed versus audiovisual materials as well as written versus verbal instruction. Gender issues, the

influence of socioeconomics on learning, and the strategies of teaching cultural groups and special populations need further exploration as well. This text attempts to address these subjects in much more detail than is typically found in other patient education resources. Unfortunately, primary sources of information from nursing literature on the issues of gender and socioeconomic attributes of the learner are scanty, to say the least, and the findings from interdisciplinary research on the influence of gender on learning remain inconclusive. Nevertheless, nurses are expected to teach diverse populations with complex needs and a range of abilities in both traditional and nontraditional, unstructured settings (Duffy, 1998). For more than 30 years, nurse researchers have been studying how best to teach patients, but much more research is required (Mason, 2001). We need to establish a stronger theoretical basis for intervening with clients throughout "all phases of the learning continuum, from information acquisition to behavioral change" (Donovan & Ward, 2001).

In addition, further investigation should be undertaken to document the cost-effectiveness of educational efforts in reducing hospital stays, decreasing readmissions, improving the personal quality of life, and minimizing complications of illness and therapies. Furthermore, given the number of variables that can potentially interfere with the teaching–learning process, additional studies must be conducted to examine the effects of environmental stimuli, the factors involved in readiness to learn, and the influences of learning styles on learner motivation, compliance, comprehension, and the ability to apply knowledge and skills once they are acquired. One particular void is the lack of information in the research database on how to assess motivation (Luker & Caress, 1989). The author of Chapter 6 proposes parameters to assess motivation but notes the paucity of information specifically addressing this issue.

Oberst (1989) delineated the major issues in patient education studies related to the evaluation of the existing research base and the design of future studies. The following four broad problem categories she identified remain pertinent today:

1. Selection and measurement of appropriate dependent variables (educational outcomes)

2. Design and control of independent variables (educational interventions)

3. Control of mediating and intervening variables

4. Development and refinement of the theoretical basis for research in education

## QUESTIONS TO BE ASKED REGARDING THE DELIVERY OF EDUCATIONAL SERVICES

In examining the elements of the education process and the role of the nurse as educator, many questions can be posed with respect to the principles of teaching and learning. Listed below are some of the important questions that the chapters in this textbook address:

- How can members of the healthcare team work together more effectively to coordinate educational efforts?

- What are the ethical, legal, and economic issues involved in patient and staff education?

- Which theories and principles support the education process?

- Which determinants influence learner behavior?

- How can teaching be tailored to specific clientele?

- Which factors negatively and positively influence patient and staff education efforts?

- What can be done about the inequities (in quantity and quality) in the delivery of education services?

- Which elements need to be taken into account when developing and implementing teaching plans?

- Which traditional as well as innovative instructional methods and materials are available to support teaching efforts?

- Under which conditions should certain teaching methods and materials be used?

- What are the common mistakes made in the teaching of others?

- Which resources are available for education in various healthcare settings?

- How are teaching and learning best evaluated?

## SUMMARY

Nurses are considered information brokers—educators who can make a significant difference in how patients and families cope with their illnesses, how the public benefits from education directed at prevention of disease and promotion of health, and how staff nurses gain competency and confidence in practice through continuing education activities. Many challenges and opportunities are ahead for nurse educators in the delivery of health care as this nation moves forward in the twenty-first century. The foremost challenge for nurses is to be able to demonstrate, through research and action, that a definite link exists between education and positive behavioral outcomes of the learner. In this era of cost containment, government regulations, and healthcare reform, the benefits of patient and staff education must be made clear to the public, to healthcare employers, to healthcare providers, and to payers of healthcare benefits. To be effective and efficient, nurses must be willing and able to work collaboratively with other members of the healthcare team to provide consistently high-quality care to the consumer. The responsibility and accountabil-ity of nurses for the delivery of care to the consumer can be accomplished, in part, through education based on solid principles of teaching and learning. The key to effective education for patients, families, and nursing staff is the nurse's understanding of and ongoing commitment to the role of educator.

## REVIEW QUESTIONS

1. How far back in history has teaching been a part of the professional nurse's role?

2. What is the overall outcome the nurse educator wants the learner to achieve as a result of the teaching-learning process?

3. Why is patient/staff education an important issue today in healthcare delivery?

4. Which nursing organization was the first to recognize health teaching as an important function within the scope of nursing practice?

5. What legal mandate universally includes teaching as a responsibility of nurses?

6. What influence do the JCAHO, ANA, NLN, ICN, AHA, and PEW Commission have on the role and responsibilities of the nurse as educator?

7. What current socioeconomic trends impacting health care are making it imperative that clients and nursing staff be adequately educated?

8. How does the education process parallel the nursing process?

9. How are the terms *education, teaching,* and *instruction* different from but interdependent with one another?

10. What is meant by the terms *teachable moment* and *training the trainer*?

11. How are *barriers to education* different from *obstacles to learning*?

12. What are six major barriers to education?

13. What are six obstacles to learning?

14. What common factor serves as both a barrier to education as well as an obstacle to learning?

15. What is the current status of research in patient and staff education?

## REFERENCES

Birchenall, P. (2000). Nurse education in the year 2000: Reflection, speculation and challenge. *Nurse Education Today, 20,* 1–2.

Casey, F. S. (1995). Documenting patient education: A literature review. *Journal of Continuing Education in Nursing, 26*(6), 257–260.

Chachkes, E. & Christ, G. (1996). Cross cultural issues in patient education. *Patient Education & Counseling, 27,* 13–21.

Davidhizar, R. E. & Brownson, K. (1999). Literacy, cultural diversity, and client education. *Health Care Manager, 18*(1), 39–47.

DeSilets, L. D. (1995). Assessing registered nurses' reasons for participating in continuing education. *Journal of Continuing Education in Nursing, 26*(5), 202–208.

Donovan, H. S. & Ward, S. (2001). A representational approach to patient education. *Journal of Nursing Scholarship,* Third Quarter, 211–216.

Duffy, B. (1998). Get ready—Get set—Go teach. *Home Healthcare Nurse, 16*(9), 596–602.

Gilroth, B. E. (1990). Promoting patient involvement: Educational, organizational, and environmental strategies. *Patient Education and Counseling, 15,* 29–38.

Glanville, I. K. (2000). Moving towards health oriented patient education (HOPE). *Holistic Nursing Practice, 14*(2), 57–66.

Grueninger, U. J. (1995). Arterial hypertension: Lessons from patient education. *Patient Education and Counseling, 26,* 37–55.

Health Services Medical Corporation, Inc. (1993). Wealth in wellness begins "Selfwise." *Worksite Wellnews, 1*(3), 1.

Honan, S., Krsnak, G., Petersen, D., & Torkelson, R. (1988). The nurse as patient educator: Perceived responsibilities and factors enhancing role development. *Journal of Continuing Education in Nursing, 19*(1), 33–37.

Jorgensen, C. (1994). Health education: What can it look like after health care reform? *Health Education Quarterly, 21*(1), 11–26.

Kellmer-Langan, D. M., Hunter, C., & Nottingham, J. P. (1992). Knowledge retention and clinical application after continuing education. *Journal of Nursing Staff Development, 8*(1), 5–10.

Knowles, M. S. (1989). *The Making of an Adult Educator: An Autobiographical Journey*, Chapter 4. San Francisco: Jossey-Bass.

Knowles, M. S., Holton, E. F., & Swanson, R. A. (1998). *The Adult Learner: The Definitive Classic in Adult Education and Human Resource Development*, 5th ed., Chapter 11. Houston, TX: Gulf Publishing.

Kruger, S. (1991). The patient educator role in nursing. *Applied Nursing Research, 4*(1), 19–24.

Latter, S., Clark, J. M., Wilson-Barnett, J., & Maben, J. (1992). Health education in nursing: Perceptions of practice in acute settings. *Journal of Advanced Nursing, 17*, 164–172.

Lipetz, M. J., Bussigel, M. N., Bannerman, J., & Risley, B. (1990). What is wrong with patient education programs? *Nursing Outlook, 38*(4), 184–189.

London, F. (1995). Teach your patients faster and better. *Nursing 95*, 68 and 70.

Luker, K. & Caress, A. L. (1989). Rethinking patient education. *Journal of Advanced Nursing, 14*, 711–718.

Mason, D. (2001). Promoting health literacy: Patient teaching is a vital nursing function. *American Journal of Nursing, 101*(2), 7.

McGinnis, J. M. (1993). The role of patient education in achieving national health objectives. *Patient Education and Counseling, 21*, 1–3.

McGoldrick, T. K., Jablonski, R. S., & Wolf, Z. R. (1994). Needs assessment for a patient education program in a nursing department: A delphi approach. *Journal of Nursing Staff Development, 10*(3), 123–130.

National League of Nursing Education. (1937). *A Curriculum Guide for Schools of Nursing*. New York: The League.

Oberst, M. T. (1989). Perspectives on research in patient teaching. *Nursing Clinics of North America, 24*(2), 621–627.

Orr, R. (1990). Illness as an educational opportunity. *Patient Education and Counseling, 15*, 47–48.

Pew Health Professions Commission. (1995). *Critical Challenges: Revitalizing the Health Professions for the Twenty-First Century. The Third Report of the Pew Health Professions Commission*. San Francisco: University of California.

Pew Health Professions Commission. (1998). *Recreating Health Professional Practice for a New Century. The Fourth Report of the Pew Health Professions Commission, Center for the Health Professions*. San Francisco: University of California.

Pohl, M. L. (1965). Teaching activities of the nursing practitioner. *Nursing Research, 14*(1), 4–11.

Redman, B. K. (1971). Patient education as a function of nursing practice. *Nursing Clinics of North America, 6*(4), 573–580.

Redman, B. K. (1975). Guidelines for quality of care in patient education. *Canadian Nurse, 71*(2), 19–21.

Redman, B. K. (1993). *The Process of Patient Education*, 7th ed. St. Louis: Mosby–Year Book.

Rega, M. D. (1993). A model approach for patient education. *MEDSURG Nursing, 2*(6), 477–479, 495.

Rifas, E., Morris, R., & Grady, R. (1994). Innovative approach to patient education. *Nursing Outlook, 42*(5), 214–216.

Seley, J. J. (1994). Ten strategies for successful patient teaching. *American Journal of Nursing, 94*(11), 63–65.

Smith, C. E. (1989). Overview of patient education: Opportunities and challenges for the twenty-first century. *Nursing Clinics of North America, 24*(3), 583–587.

U.S. Department of Health and Human Services. (2000). *Healthy People 2010: Objectives for Improving Health*. Volume II. Washington, DC: U.S. Government Printing Office.

Wagner, S. P. & Ash, K. L. (1998). Creating the teachable moment. *Journal of Nursing Education, 37*(6), 278–280.

Wilkinson, J. M. (1996). The C word: A curriculum for the future. *Nursing & Health Care, 17*(2), 72–77.

## CHAPTER 2

# Ethical, Legal, and Economic Foundations of the Educational Process

*M. Janice Nelson*

## OBJECTIVES

After completing this chapter, the reader will be able to

1. Identify the six major ethical principles.

2. Distinguish between ethical and legal dimensions of the healthcare delivery system, including patient education.

3. Describe the importance of nurse practice acts.

4. Describe the legal and financial implications of documentation.

5. Delineate the ethical, legal, and economic importance of federal, state, and accrediting body regulations and standards in the delivery of healthcare services.

6. Differentiate among financial terms associated with the development, implementation, and evaluation of patient education programs.

7. Identify trends in patient education.

Today as never before in the evolution of the healthcare field, there is a critical consciousness of individual rights stemming from both natural and constitutional law. Healthcare organizations are laden with laws and regulations ensuring clients' rights to a quality standard of care, to informed consent, and subsequently to self-determination. Consequently, it is crucial that the providers of care be equally proficient in both educating the public and educating students or staff who are or will be the practitioner educators of tomorrow. Although the physician is primarily held legally accountable for the medical regimen, it is a known fact that patient education generally falls to the nurse or some other appointed designee. Indeed, given the close relationship of the nurse to the client, the role of the nurse in this educational process is absolutely essential and mandated as such through a variety of state nurse practice acts.

We are indeed living in an age of an enlightened public that is not only aware, but also demands recognition of individual constitutional rights regarding freedom of choice and rights to self-determination. In fact, it may seem curious to some that federal and state governments, accrediting bodies, and professional organizations find it necessary to legislate, regulate, or provide standards and guidelines to ensure the protection of human rights when it comes to matters of health care. The answer, of course, is that the federal government has abandoned its historical "hands-off" policy toward physicians and other health professionals in the wake of serious breaches of public confidence and shocking revelations of abuses of human rights in the name of biomedical research.

These issues of human rights are fundamental to the delivery of quality healthcare services. They are equally fundamental to the education process, in that the intent of the educator should be to empower the client to make informed choices, and to be in control of the consequences of those choices regardless of the outcome. Thus, in explicating the role of the nurse in the teaching–learning process, it would be remiss to omit the ethical and legal foundations of that process. Also, in the interest of justice, which refers to the equal distribution of benefits and burdens, it is important to acknowledge the relationship of cost to the healthcare facility in the provision of such services.

Teaching and learning principles, with their inherent legal and ethical dimensions, apply to any situation where the educational process is occurring. The purpose of this chapter, however, is to provide the ethical, legal, and economic foundations that underpin the patient education initiative on the one hand and the rights and responsibilities of the provider on the other hand. This chapter explores the differences between and among ethical, moral, and legal concepts. It explores the ethical and legal foundations of human rights, and it reviews the ethical and legal dimensions of health care. Furthermore, this chapter examines the importance of documentation of patient teaching while analyzing the economic factors that must be considered in the delivery of patient education in healthcare settings.

## A DIFFERENTIATED VIEW OF ETHICS, MORALITY, AND THE LAW

Although ethics as a branch of classical philosophy has been studied throughout the centuries, by and large these studies were left to the domains of philosophical and religious thinkers. More recently, due to the complexities of modern-day living and the heightened awareness of an educated public, ethical issues related to health care have surfaced as a major concern of both healthcare providers and recipients of these services. In the end, the deontological posture of Kant—that is, the individual rights of clients—prevails. Thus the client has the right to know his or her medical diagnosis, the treatments available, and the expected outcomes. This information is necessary so that informed choices relative to their diagnosis can be made by clients in concert with advice offered by health professionals.

Ethical principles of human rights are rooted in natural laws, which, in the absence of any other guidelines, are binding on human society. Inherent in these natural laws are, for example, the principles of respect for parents, respect for others, truth telling, honesty, respect for life, and purity of heart. Ethics as a discipline interprets these basic principles of behavior in broader terms and assumes argumentative discourse in favor of particular postures. Although multiple perspectives on the rightness or wrongness of human acts exist, the most commonly referenced are the writings of the sixteenth-century philosopher Immanuel Kant, who promulgated the *deontological* notion of the "Golden Rule," and those of John Stuart Mill, who purported a *teleologi-*

*cal* approach to ethical decision making in the nineteenth century. That is, given the alternatives, choices should be made that result in the greatest good for the greatest number of people.

Likewise, the legal system and its laws are based on ethical and moral principles that, through experience and over time, society has accepted as behavioral norms (Lesnick and Anderson, 1962). This relationship accounts in part for the fact that the terms *ethical*, *moral*, and *legal* are so often used in synchrony.

It should be clear, however, that while these terms are certainly interrelated, they are not necessarily synonymous. *Ethics* refers to the guiding principles of behavior, and *ethical* refers to norms or standards of behavior. Although the terms *moral* or *morality* are generally used interchangeably with the terms *ethics* or *ethical*, one can differentiate the notion of *moral* rights and duties from the notion of *ethical* rights and duties. It could be posited that *moral* refers to an internal value system (the "moral fabric" of one's being). This value system, defined as *morality*, is expressed externally through ethical behavior. Ethical principles deal with intangible moral values, so they are not enforceable by law, nor are these principles laws in and of themselves. *Legal* rights and duties, on the other hand, refer to rules governing behavior or conduct that are enforceable under threat of punishment or penalty, such as a fine or imprisonment.

The intricate relationship between ethics and the law explains why ethics terminology, such as informed consent, confidentiality, nonmalfeasance, and justice, can be found within the language of the legal system. In keeping with this train of thought, nurses may cite professional commitment or moral obligation as the justification for education of clients as one dimension of their role. In reality, the legitimacy of this role stems from the nurse practice act in force in the particular state where the nurse resides, is licensed, and is employed. In essence, the nurse practice act is not only legally binding, but also protected by the police authority of the state in the interest of protecting the public (Brent, 2001).

## ▮ EVOLUTION OF ETHICAL AND LEGAL PRINCIPLES IN HEALTH CARE

In the past ethics was relegated almost exclusively to the philosophical and religious domains. Likewise, from a historical vantage point, medical and nursing care was considered a humanitarian, if not charitable, endeavor often provided by members of religious communities and others considered to be generous of spirit, caring in nature, and magnanimous, dedicated, and self-sacrificing in their service to others. Public sentiment was so strong in this regard that for many years healthcare organizations, which were considered to be charitable institutions, were largely immune from legal action "because it would compel the charity to divert its funds for a purpose never intended" (Lesnik and Anderson, 1962, p. 211). In the same manner, healthcare practitioners in the past—who were primarily physicians and nurses—were usually regarded as "Good Samaritans" who acted in "good faith."

Although there are numerous court records of lawsuits involving hospitals, physicians, and nurses dating back to the early 1900s, those numbers pale in comparison with the volumes being generated on a daily basis in today's world. Further, despite the horror stories that have been handed down through the years regarding inhumane and often torturous treatment of prisoners, the mentally infirm, the disabled, and the poor, there was limited focus in the past on ethical aspects of that "care." In turn, there was little thought of legal protection for the rights of such unfortunate people. Clearly, this situation has changed dramatically. Informed consent, for example, which is a basic tenet of ethical thought, was established in the courts as early

as 1914 by Justice Benjamin Cardozo. Cardozo determined that every adult of sound mind has a right to protect his or her own body and to determine how it shall be treated (Boyd, Graham, Gleit, & Whitman, 1998; Rankin & Stallings, 2001). Although the Cardozo decision was of considerable magnitude, governmental interest in the bioethical underpinnings of human rights in the delivery of healthcare services did not really surface until after World War II.

Over the years, legal authorities such as federal and state governments maintained a hands-off posture when it came to issues of biomedical research or physician–patient relationships. However, human atrocities committed by the Nazis in the name of biomedical research during World War II shocked the world into critical awareness of gross violations of human rights. Nor were such abuses confined to wartime Europe. On U.S. soil, for example, the nontreatment of syphilitic African Americans in Alabama, the injection of live cancer cells into uninformed, nonconsenting older adults at the Brooklyn Chronic Disease Hospital, and the use of institutionalized mentally retarded children to test hepatitis vaccines at Willowbrook Developmental Center on Long Island, New York, shocked the nation and raised a critical consciousness of disturbing breaches in the physician–patient relationship (Brent, 2001; Thomas & Quinn, 1991; Weisbard & Arras, 1984).

Stirred to action by these disturbing phenomena, in 1974 Congress moved with all due deliberation to create the *National Commission for the Protection of Human Subjects of Biomedical and Behavioral Research*. As an outcome of this unprecedented act, Institutional Review Boards for the Protection of Human Subjects (IRBPHS) were rapidly established at the local level. The primary emphasis of these review boards is on informed consent, confidentiality, and truth telling, with specific concern for vulnerable populations such as infants, children, prisoners, and the mentally ill. Every proposal for biomedical research today that involves human subjects must be submitted to a local IRBPHS for intensive review and approval before proceeding with a proposed study. Further, in response to its concern about the range of ethical issues associated with medical practice and a perceived need to regulate biomedical research, Congress established the *President's Commission for the Study of Ethical Problems in Medicine and Biomedical and Behavioral Research* (Brent, 2001; Thomas & Quinn, 1991; Weisbard & Arras, 1984).

Interestingly, as early as 1950, the American Nurses Association (ANA) developed and adopted a *Code for Nurses with Interpretative Statements*, which has since been revised and updated several times (ANA, 1976 and 1985). The latest revision of the ANA's *Code* (now entitled the *Code of Ethics for Nurses with Interpretive Statements*) was released in 2001 for implementation in the new millennium. This code represents an articulation of professional values and moral obligations in relation to the nurse–patient relationship and in support of the profession and its mission.

Whether coincidental or deliberate, in 1975 the American Hospital Association (AHA) followed suit by disseminating a document entitled *Patient's Bill of Rights* (Boyd et al., 1998; Aleksandrowicz & Norcross, 1984). A copy of these patient rights are framed and posted in a public place in every healthcare facility across the United States. In addition, federal standards developed by the Center for Medicare and Medicaid Services (CMMS)—an arm of the Health Care Financing Administration (HCFA)—require that the patient be provided with a personal copy of these rights either at the time of admission to the hospital or long-term care facility, or prior to the initiation of care or treatment when admitted to a surgicenter, an HMO, home care, or a hospice. As a matter of fact, many states have adopted the statement of patient rights as part of their state health code. Thus these rights fall under the jurisdiction of the law, rendering them legally enforceable under threat of penalty.

## APPLICATION OF ETHICAL AND LEGAL PRINCIPLES TO PATIENT EDUCATION

In considering the ethical and legal responsibilities inherent in the patient education process, the six major ethical principles intricately woven throughout the ANA's *Code of Ethics for Nurses with Interpretive Statements* (2001) and the AHA's *Patient's Bill of Rights* (1975) encompass the very issues that precipitated federal intervention into healthcare affairs. These principles are autonomy, veracity, confidentiality, nonmalfeasance, beneficence, and justice.

### Autonomy

In considering the principle of *autonomy*, the right to self-determination, laws have been enacted to protect the patient's right to make choices independently. Federal mandates regarding informed consent are evident in every application for federal funding to support biomedical research. The local IRBPHS assumes the role of judge and jury to ascertain adherence to these enforceable regulations. The *Patient Self-Determination Act* (PSDA), which was passed by Congress in 1991, is a second example of the principle of autonomy enacted into law. Any healthcare facility, such as acute- and long-term care institutions, surgicenters, HMOs, hospices, or home care, which receives Medicare and/or Medicaid funds must comply with the PSDA. The law requires, either at the time of hospital admission or prior to the initiation of care or treatment in a community health setting, "that every individual receiving health care be informed in writing of the right under state law to make decisions about his or her health care, including the right to refuse medical and surgical care and the right to initiate advance directives" (Mezey, Evans, Golub, Murphy, & White, 1994, p. 30). These authors readily acknowledge the nurse's responsibility to ensure informed decision making by patients, which includes but is certainly not limited to advance directives (e.g., living wills, durable power of attorney). Documentation of such instruction must appear in the patient record, which is the legal document validating that such instruction took place.

One principle worth noting in the ANA's *Code of Ethics for Nurses with Interpretive Statements* is addressing collaboration "with members of the health professions and other citizens in promoting community and national efforts to meet the health needs of the public" (*NYSNA Report*, 2001, p. 6). Although not specified in such detail in the ANA document, this principle certainly provides a justification for patient education both within and outside the healthcare organization. It provides an ethical rationale for health education classes open to the community, such as childbirth education courses, smoking cessation classes, weight reduction sessions, discussions of women's health issues, and positive interventions for child abuse. While health education per se is not an interpretive part of the principle of autonomy, it certainly lends credence to the ethical notion of assisting the public to attain greater autonomy when it comes to matters of health promotion and high-level wellness. In fact, consistent with the *Model Nurse Practice Act* published by the ANA in 1978, contemporary nurse practice acts contain a statement identifying health education as a legal duty or responsibility of the registered nurse.

## Veracity

*Veracity*, or truth telling, is closely linked with informed decision making and informed consent. The landmark Cardozo decision in 1994 (*Schloendorff* v. *Society of New York Hospitals*) specified an individual's fundamental right to make decisions about his or her own body. This ruling provided a basis in law for patient education or instruction regarding invasive medical procedures, including the truth regarding risks or benefits involved in these procedures (Boyd et al., 1998; Rankin & Stallings, 2001). Nurses are often confronted with issues of truth telling, as was exemplified in the *Tuma* case (Rankin & Stallings, 1990). In the interest of full disclosure of information, the nurse (Tuma) had advised a cancer patient of alternative treatments without consultation with the client's physician. She was sued by the physician for interfering with the medical regimen that he had prescribed for care of this particular patient. Although Tuma was eventually exonerated from professional misconduct charges, the case emphasized a significant point of law to be found in the *New York State Nurse Practice Act* (1972), which states, "A nursing regimen shall be consistent with and shall not vary from any existing medical regimen." In some instances, this creates a double bind for the nurse. Creighton (1986) emphatically explained that failure or omission to properly instruct the patient relative to invasive procedures is tantamount to battery.

Cisar and Bell (1995) addressed this concept of battery related to medical treatment exceedingly well. In addition to discussing Curtin's *Ethical Decision-Making Model*, which serves as a guide for healthcare providers facing an ethical dilemma, the authors offered an explanation of the four elements making up the notion of informed consent that is such a vital aspect of patient education.

The first element is competence, which refers to the capacity of the patient to make a reasonable decision. The second element is disclosure of information, which requires that sufficient information regarding risks and alternative treatments be provided to the patient to enable him or her to make a rational decision. The third element of informed consent is comprehension, which speaks to the individual's ability to understand or to grasp intellectually the information being provided. A child, for example, may not yet be of an age to understand any ramifications of medical treatment and must, therefore, depend on his or her parents to make a decision that will be in the child's best interest. The fourth element of informed consent relates to voluntariness, which indicates that the patient has made a decision without coercion or force from others.

While three of the four elements might be satisfied (for example, that the client is of sound mind, that sufficient information has been provided to enable the client to make an informed decision, and that he or she has the capacity to fully understand the information being explained) the client might still decide to reject the "treatment of choice." This decision could be due to the exorbitant cost of a treatment or to certain personal or religious beliefs. Whatever the case, it must be recognized by all concerned that a competent, informed client cannot be forced to accept treatment as long as he or she is aware of the alternatives as well as the consequences of any decision.

A final dimension of the legality of truth telling relates to the role of the nurse as expert witness. Professional nurses who are recognized for their skill or expertise in a particular area of nursing practice may be called on to testify in court on behalf of either the plaintiff (the one who initiates the litigation) or the defendant (the one being sued). In any case, the concept of expert testimony speaks for itself. Regardless of the situation, the nurse must always tell the truth and the client (or his or her health proxy) is always entitled to the truth.

## Nonmalfeasance

*Nonmalfeasance*, the principle of "do no harm," is the ethical fabric of legal determinations encompassing negligence and/or malpractice. According to Brent (2001), *negligence* is

defined as "conduct which falls below the standard established by law for the protection of others against unreasonable risk of harm" (p. 54). Brent further explains the concept of professional negligence, which, she asserts, "involves the conduct of professionals (e.g., nurses, physicians, dentists, and lawyers) that fall below a professional standard of due care" (p. 55). As clarified by Lesnick and Anderson in 1962, Brent (2001) reiterates that for negligence to exist, there must be a duty between the injured party and the person whose actions (or nonactions) caused the injury. A breach of that duty must have occurred, the breach of duty must have been the immediate cause of the injury, and the injured party must have experienced damages from the injury.

The term *malpractice*, by comparison, still holds as defined by Lesnick and Anderson (1962) so many years ago. Malpractice, they asserted, "refers to a limited class of negligent activities committed within the scope of performance by those pursuing a particular profession involving highly skilled and technical services" (p. 234). Thus malpractice is limited in scope to those whose life work requires special education and training as dictated by specific educational standards, whereas negligence embraces all improper and wrongful conduct by anyone arising out of any activity.

The concept of *duty* is closely tied to the concepts of malpractice and negligence. Nurses' duties are spelled out in job descriptions at their places of employment. Policy and procedure manuals of a particular facility exist certainly to protect the patient, but they also exist to protect the employee (the nurse) and the employer against litigation. Policies are more than guidelines. Policies and procedures determine standards of behavior (duties) expected of employees of a particular employing institution and can be used in court in the determination of negligence. Expectations of professional nursing performance are also measured against the nurse's level of education and concomitant skills, standing orders and protocols, standards of care promulgated by the profession (ANA), and standards of care promulgated by the various clinical specialty organizations of which the nurse may be a member (Yoder Wise, 1995). If the nurse is certified in a clinical specialty or is identified as a "specialist" although not certified, he or she will be held to the standards of that specialty (Smith, 1987).

In the instance of litigation, the key operational principle is that the nurse is not measured against the optimal or maximum of professional standards of performance; rather, the yardstick is laid against the prevailing practice of what a prudent and reasonable nurse would do under the same circumstances in a given community. Thus the nurse's duty of patient education (or lack thereof) is measured against not only prevailing policy of the employing institution, but also prevailing practice in the community. In the case of clinical nurse specialists (CNSs), nurse practitioners (NPs), or clinical education specialists (CESs), for example, the practice is measured against institutional policies for this level of worker as well as against the prevailing practice of nurses performing at the same level in the community or in the same geographic region.

## Confidentiality

*Confidentiality* refers to privileged information or to a social contract or covenant in legal terms. The nurse–patient relationship is considered to be privileged in most states. As a consequence, the nurse may not disclose information acquired in a professional capacity from a patient without the consent of the patient "unless the patient has been the victim or subject of a crime, the commission of which is the subject of legal proceeding in which the nurse is a witness" (Lesnik & Anderson, 1962, p. 48).

This discussion of confidentiality gives rise to the need to distinguish between the concepts of what is *private*, what is *privileged*, and what is *confidential.* The diagnosis of acquired immune deficiency syndrome (AIDS) readily lends itself to the clarification of these concepts. Despite its communicability, the person with a diagnosis of AIDS is protected by laws promulgated by federal and various state governments. Within this context, AIDS is considered to be *private* information. It need not be disclosed in the workplace, the home, or other social settings. By federal mandate (and in some states), this information is considered to be highly personal, the privacy of which is regarded as a fundamental right of the person. In essence, this right is protected by the U.S. Constitution (Brent, 2001). AIDS is further considered to be *privileged* information. Such information is "owned" by the patient alone and is subject to disclosure only at his or her individual discretion. Once this information is shared between the nurse and the client, it cannot be shared with other health professionals unless authorized by the client (Brent, 2001). The diagnosis of AIDS is also protected by law as *confidential.* Thus anyone not involved in a client's care has no right to private or privileged information regarding the health status of the client (Brent, 2001).

These protections are applicable despite the fact that AIDS is a communicable disease. According to Brent (2001), "this area of legislation concerned with health care privacy and disclosure reveals the tension between what is good for the individual and what is good for society" (p. 141). Interestingly, it is a fairly recent development in some states that under certain conditions, such as death or impending death, members of the family or a spouse can be apprised of the patient's condition if this information was previously unknown. Despite federal and state legislation, as the matter currently stands, the question of the ethical/moral obligation of the person with AIDS to disclose his or her condition remains largely unresolved.

## Beneficence

The principle of *beneficence* (doing good) is legalized through adherence to critical tasks and duties contained in job descriptions; in policies, procedures, and protocols set forth by the healthcare facility; and in standards and codes of ethical behaviors established and promulgated by professional nursing organizations. Adherence to these various professional performance criteria and principles, including adequate and current patient education, speaks to the nurse's commitment to acting in the best interest of the patient. Such behavior emphasizes patient welfare and deemphasizes the provision of quality care under threat of litigation.

## Justice

*Justice* speaks to fairness and equal distribution of goods and services. The law is the "Justice System." The focus of the law is the protection of society; the focus of health law is the protection of the consumer. As noted earlier, adherence to the *Patient's Bill of Rights* is legally enforced in most states. This means that the nurse or any other health professional can be subjected to penalty or to litigation for discrimination in provision of care. Regardless of his or her age, gender, physical disability, sexual orientation, or race, for example, the client has a right to proper instruction regarding risks and benefits of invasive medical procedures. He or she also has a right to proper instruction regarding self-care activities, such as home dialysis, that are beyond normal activities of daily living for most people.

Furthermore, when a nurse is employed by a particular healthcare facility, she or he enters into a contract, written or tacit, to provide nursing services in accordance with the policies of the facility. Failure to provide nursing care (including educational services) based on patient diagnosis or persistence in providing substandard care based on client age, diagnosis, culture, national origin, sexual preference, and the like can result in liability for breach of contract with the employing institution.

Most recently, the U.S. Congress has wrestled with another version of patients' rights within which every American carrying health insurance is guaranteed the right to emergency room care, the right to treatment by medical specialists, and the right of access to government-run clinical trials (Abood, 2001). Considerable argument among members of Congress has ensued over the extent to which health maintenance organizations (HMOs) can be sued for delay or denial of care, and what limits, if any, should be placed on the damages (Zuckerman, 2001).

This in-progress federal legislation adds an interesting dimension to the notion of justice as it applies to health care. The proposed patients' rights legislation is intended only for those covered by health insurance. This restriction raises serious questions for the uninsured regarding the right of access to health care and subsequently the right of access to health education. Emanuel (2000) raises a critical point in asserting that "the diffuseness of decision making in the American health care system precludes a coherent process for allocating health care resources" (p. 8). Emmanuel further contends that managed care organizations have systematically pursued drastic cost reductions by restructuring of delivery systems and investing in expensive and elaborate information systems. HMOs have bought out physician practices, and have become involved in a number of related activities with no substantial evidence that a high quality of health care will be achieved at lower prices.

To date, this incomplete enactment of a patient's bill of rights and the issues of just or unjust cost-cutting activities of HMOs as described by Emmanuel (2000) do, indeed, affect the role of the educator. These issues determine whether nurse educators can surmount the obstacles potentially blocking the patient education process. In the interest of cutting costs, HMOs have also succeeded in shortening lengths of hospital stays. This development, in turn, has had a tremendous effect on the delivery of education to the hospitalized patient. Lack of time serves as a barrier to the nurse in being able to provide sufficient information for self-care, and illness acuity level interferes with the patient's ability to process information necessary to meet his or her physical and emotional needs.

Clearly, professional nurses are mandated by organizational policy as well as by federal and state regulations to provide patient education. Thus great care must be taken to ensure that the education justly due to the client will be addressed post-discharge, either in the ambulatory care setting or at home.

## ▰▰▰ LEGALITY OF PATIENT EDUCATION AND INFORMATION

The patient's right to adequate information regarding his or her physical condition, medications, risks, and access to information regarding alternative treatments is specifically spelled out in the *Patient's Bill of Rights,* as put forth by the AHA in 1975. As noted earlier, many states have adopted these rights as part of their health code, thus rendering the rights legal and enforceable by law. Patients' rights to education and instruction are also regulated through standards promulgated by accrediting bodies such as the Joint Commission on Accreditation of Healthcare Organizations (JCAHO). Although these standards are not enforceable in the same manner as law, lack of organizational conformity can lead to loss of accreditation, which in turn jeopard-

izes the facility's eligibility for third-party reimbursement, as well as loss of Medicare and Medicaid reimbursement. Lack of organizational conformity can also lead to loss of public confidence.

In addition, state regulations pertaining to patient education are published and enforced under threat of penalty (fine, citation, or both) by the Department of Health in many states. Federal regulations, enforceable as laws, also mandate patient education in those healthcare facilities receiving Medicare and Medicaid funding. As discussed earlier, the federal government also mandates full patient disclosure in cases of participation in biomedical research in any setting or for any federally funded project or experimental research involving human subjects.

Federal authorities have generally tended to hold physicians responsible and accountable for proper patient education. This is particularly true as it pertains to issues of informed consent, such as those highlighted in *Scakia* v. *St. Paul Fire and Marine Ins. Co.,* 1975 (Smith, 1987). It is a well-known fact—at least in hospitals—that patient education usually is carried out by the nurse or some other facility- or physician-appointed designee. Physicians' responsibility notwithstanding, from a professional and legal vantage point, nurses are fully legitimized in their role as patient educators by virtue of their respective nurse practice acts. The issue regarding patient education is not necessarily one of omission on anyone's part. Rather, the heart of the matter may be proper documentation (or the lack thereof) that provides written testimony that client education has indeed occurred.

## ▰▰▰ DOCUMENTATION

The 89th Congress enacted the Comprehensive Health Planning Act in 1965 (Public Law 89-97, 1965). The entitlements of Medicare and

Medicaid—which revolutionized the provision of health care for the elderly and the poor—were established through this act. One acknowledgment in the act was the importance of the preventive and rehabilitative dimensions of health care. Thus, to qualify for Medicare and Medicaid reimbursement, "a hospital has to show evidence that patient education has been a part of patient care" (Boyd et al., 1998, p. 26). For at least the past 20 years, the JCAHO (formerly JCAH) has reinforced the federal mandate by requiring evidence (documentation) of patient and/or family education in the patient record. Pertinent to this point is the doctrine of *respondeat superior*, or the *master–servant* rule. *Respondeat superior* provides that the employer may be held liable for negligence, assault and battery, false imprisonment, slander, libel, or any other tort committed by an employee (Lesnik & Anderson, 1962). The landmark case supporting the doctrine of *respondeat superior* in the healthcare field was the 1965 case of *Darling* v. *Charleston Memorial Hospital*. Although the *Darling* case dealt with negligence in the performance of professional duties of the physician, it brought out—possibly for the first time—the professional obligations or duties of nurses to ensure the well-being of the patient.

Casey (1995) points out that of all omissions in documentation, patient teaching has been identified as "probably the most undocumented skilled service because nurses do not recognize the scope and depth of the teaching they do" (p. 257). Lack of documentation also reflects negligence in adhering to the mandates of the particular nurse practice act. This laxity is unfortunate, because patient records can be subpoenaed for court evidence. Appropriate documentation can be the determining factor in the outcome of litigation. Pure and simple, if the instruction isn't documented, it didn't occur!

Furthermore, documentation is a vehicle of communication that provides critical informa-

tion to other healthcare professionals involved with the patient's care. Failure to document not only renders other staff potentially liable, but also renders the facility liable and in jeopardy of losing its JCAHO accreditation. The institution is also in danger of losing its appropriate Medicare and Medicaid reimbursement.

In any litigation where the doctrine of *respondeat superior* is applied, outcomes can hold the organization liable for damages (monetary retribution). Thus it behooves the nurse as both employee and professional not only to provide patient education, but also to document it appropriately and to be critically conscious of the legal and financial ramifications to the healthcare facility in which he or she is employed.

Snyder (1996) presents an invaluable description of an interdisciplinary method to document patient education. The method involves use of a flowsheet that fits into the client's chart. The flowsheet includes identification of client and family educational needs based on a number of variables. These include the following: the client's "readiness to learn" (based on admission assessment of the client); "barriers to learning," which might include language, lack of vision, or other challenges; and "referrals," which might include a patient advocate, the library, or an ethics committee. The form provides documentation space for who was taught (e.g., client or family), what was taught (e.g., self-injection of insulin), when it was taught, what method of teaching was used, and how the client responded to instruction.

## A GRAPHIC SUMMATION

In consideration of the amount of material presented in this section, a visual representation of the linkages between ethical principles and the law is displayed in Table 2–1. It

**Table 2–1  Linkages between ethical principles and the law**

| Ethical Principles | Legal Actions/Decisions |
|---|---|
| Autonomy (self-determination) | Cardozo decision regarding informed consent<br>Institutional Review Boards<br>Patient Self-Determination Act<br>*Patient's Bill of Rights*<br>JCAHO/CMMS standards |
| Veracity (truth telling) | Cardozo decision regarding informed consent<br>*Patient's Bill of Rights*<br>*Tuma* decision<br>JCAHO/CMMS standards |
| Confidentiality (privileged information) | Privileged information<br>*Patient's Bill of Rights*<br>JCAHO/CMMS standards |
| Nonmalfeasance (do no harm) | Malpractice/negligence rights and duties<br>Nurse practice acts<br>*Patient's Bill of Rights*<br>*Darling* vs. *Charleston Memorial Hospital*<br>State health codes<br>JCAHO/CMMS standards |
| Beneficence (doing good) | *Patient's Bill of Rights*<br>State health codes<br>Job descriptions<br>Standards of practice<br>Policy and procedure manuals<br>JCAHO/CMMS standards |
| Justice (equal distribution of benefits and burdens) | *Patient's Bill of Rights*<br>Antidiscrimination/affirmative action laws<br>Americans with Disabilities Act<br>JCAHO/CMMS standards |

should be noted that the AHA's 1975 rendition of a *Patient's Bill of Rights* is linked to or associated with every ethical principle. The *Patient's Bill of Rights* (1975) is rooted in the conditions of participation in Medicare set forth under federal standards established by the Center for Medicare and Medicaid Services (CMMS). These standards are further emphasized by corresponding accreditation standards promulgated by JCAHO. All serve

to ensure the fundamental rights of every person as a consumer of healthcare services.

## ECONOMIC FACTORS OF PATIENT EDUCATION: JUSTICE AND DUTY REVISITED

Some might consider the parameters of healthcare economics and finances as objective information that can be used for any number of purposes. Fiscal solvency and forecasting of economic growth of an organization are good examples of this phenomenon. Others would agree that in addition to the legal considerations that mandate adherence to regulations in health care regardless of the economics involved, there is also an ethical dimension that speaks certainly to quality of care and also to justice. *Justice* refers to the equal distribution of goods and services. In the interest of patient care, the client as a human being has a right to quality care regardless of his or her economic status, national origin, race, and the like. Furthermore, health professionals have a duty to see to it that such services are provided. In like manner, the healthcare organization has the right to expect that it will receive its fair share of reimbursable revenues for services rendered. Thus, as an employee of the provider organization, the nurse has a duty to carry out organizational policies and mandates by acting in an accountable and responsible manner. This duty includes assuming fiscal accountability for patient education activities, whether these are offered on an inpatient or ambulatory care basis or as a service to the larger community.

The principle of justice is a critical consideration within the discourse on patient education. The rapid changes and trends so evident in the contemporary healthcare arena are described as chaotic by some and are, in many ways, defying the humanistic and charitable underpinnings that have characterized healthcare services in this country across the decades. Indeed, these organizations are caught between the proverbial horns of the dilemma. On the one hand, the realities of capitation and managed care mean shrinking revenues. This trend, in turn, dictates shorter patient stays in hospitals and "doing more with less." Despite severe shortages of healthcare personnel in most geographic areas of the country, healthcare facilities are concomitantly expanding their clinical expertise into satellite types of ambulatory and home care services.

On the other hand, these same organizations are held to the exact standards of care that are underwritten by the *Patient's Bill of Rights* (AHA, 1975), which are regulated as a contingency of Medicare and Medicaid participation by CMMS and for agency accreditation by JCAHO. In turn, although there are some exceptions (e.g., home healthcare agencies), hospital accreditation in particular dictates eligibility for third-party reimbursement in both the public and private sectors.

Over and above the financial facts, these same "charitable," not-for-profit organizations no longer enjoy the legal immunity that existed in yesteryear. The doctrine of *respondeat superior* is alive and well. In a Supreme Court decision stemming from *Abernathy* v. *Sisters of St. Mary's* in 1969, "the court held that a 'non-governmental charitable institution is liable for its own negligence and the negligence of its agents and employees acting within the scope of their employment'" (Strader, 1985, p. 364). The court further declared that this ruling would apply to all future cases as of November 10, 1969. Thus the regulated right of clients to health education carries a corresponding duty of healthcare organizations to provide that service.

In an environment of shrinking healthcare dollars, continuously shrinking nursing staffs, and shortened lengths of stay, the organization is challenged to ensure the competency of nursing staff to provide educational services and to do so in the most efficient and cost-effective manner possible. This is an interesting dilemma when considering the fact that patient education is invariably identified as a legal responsibility of registered nurses in the respective nurse practice acts of most states. Few, if any, pre-baccalaureate education programs adequately prepare nursing students for this critical function—if these programs prepare them at all. Consequently, it seems important here to provide an overview of fiscal terminology that directly affects both staff and patient education.

## Financial Terminology

No healthcare service (education or otherwise) is provided without an accompanying cost of human and material resources. Thus it is important to know that costs are essentially classified into two categories: direct and indirect.

## Direct Costs

*Direct costs* are tangible, predictable expenditures specifically associated with the actual delivery of an education program. A substantial portion of direct costs comprises personnel salaries and employment benefits. This portion of an organizational budget is almost always the largest of the total predictable expenditure of any healthcare facility.

Within this framework, because of its labor-intensive function, the division of nursing is generally apportioned the largest budgetary amount—usually 50% of the total facility budget or better. Of course, the higher the educational level of nursing staff, the higher the salaries and thus the higher the total direct costs.

Equipment is also classified as a direct cost. Regardless of their individual ingenuity, healthcare organizations obviously cannot function without equipment and its necessary replacement when indicated. In the same manner, educational functions cannot generally be carried out without proper audiovisual equipment, such as overhead projectors, slide projectors, copying machines, and computers. Although rental or leasing of educational tools and materials may sometimes be less expensive than purchasing them, rental and leasing costs are still categorized as direct costs.

Time is also considered to be a direct cost. Although in a technical sense the purpose of a salary is to buy an employee's time along with the benefit of his or her particular expertise, it is often difficult to predict the amount of time it will take to plan, implement, and evaluate various educational programs. If, for example, planning exceeds the allocated time allowed and the employee gets into "overtime," although the employee sees an increase in his or her paycheck, the extra cost may not have been anticipated or planned for in the budget planning process. Time then becomes one of the major factors considered in a cost-benefit analysis. In other words, if the cost of salaries and the time it takes to prepare and offer patient education programs is greater than the equivalent financial gain to the institution (e.g., no change in patient length of stay), the facility may seek other ways of providing the educational offering, such as programmed instruction via computer or a patient television channel.

Direct costs are also fixed or variable. *Fixed costs* are those costs that are predictable and remain the same over time. They are also controllable. Salaries, for example, are fixed costs. The facility usually makes an annual determination to give employee raises; by the same token, a decision can be made not only to freeze salaries but also to cut positions and thereby cut costs. Utilities such as heat, light, and air-conditioning are fixed costs, as are mortgages and loan repayments, as these relate to the overall operation of the facility.

*Variable costs* are those costs that, in the case of healthcare organizations, depend on volume. The number of meals prepared, for example, depends on the patient census. From an educational vantage point, the demand for diabetic instruction depends in large part on the volume of diabetic patients. If volume is low in a particular facility, cost may be high because instruction may need to be carried out on a one-to-one basis. Conversely, if volume is high, it is less costly to standardize programs of instruction or to conduct group teaching sessions for the diabetic clientele. Requirements for supplies can also vary depending on volume. Variable costs can become fixed costs when volume remains consistently high over time. This trend may warrant the addition of personnel and possibly volume purchasing.

## Indirect Costs

*Indirect costs* are those costs that may be fixed but are not directly related to the actual delivery of an educational program. These costs (which, coincidentally, are also categorized as fixed costs) include, but are certainly not limited to, institutional overhead such as heating or cooling, light, space, and support services of maintenance, housekeeping, security, and equipment. Such services are necessary and ongoing whether or not an educational session is in progress.

Hidden costs are those costs that can be neither anticipated nor accounted for until after the fact. Low employee productivity can produce hidden costs. Organizational budgets are prepared on the basis of what is known and predictable, with projections for variability included. Personnel budgets are based on a division of labor (e.g., × number of RNs, × number of LPNs, and × number of nursing assistants) to accommodate the predicted patient volume, as determined by the predicted number of patient-days and the number and classification of patient-care hours. There is an underlying assumption of employee productivity that is commensurate with the predicted workload. Low productivity of one person (or more) in a nursing unit, for example, can have a direct effect on the workload of others. This, in turn, can affect morale, which has the potential of precipitating turnover. Turnover has an inherent ripple effect of increasing recruitment and new-employee orientation costs. In this respect, the costs are appropriately identified as "hidden."

In her very pertinent article on "Understanding Costs," Gift (1994) makes a point of distinguishing between costs—direct or indirect—and charges. As discussed earlier, *costs* are those expenses incurred by the facility or provider of the service. *Charges* are set by the provider, but are billed to the recipient of the services. There may or may not be a relationship between costs and charges. In the retail business, for example, costs of raw materials could be very low, while charges for the completed items, goods, or services could far exceed the cost, thereby yielding a profit for the retailer. In the healthcare arena, not-for-profit healthcare organizations are limited by federal law in what they can charge the client in relation to the actual cost of the service. In many instances, particularly as it relates to pharmaceutical goods, the cost to the facility is the charge to the client. In such a case, the facility provides a service but realizes no financial gain (profit) (*Medicare & Medicaid Guide*, 1986).

## Cost Savings, Cost Benefit, and Cost Recovery

Although mandated by laws and standards, and required for participation in Medicare and Medicaid reimbursement programs, for all intents and purposes, patient education costs are generally not recoverable. Even though the cost of educational programs is a legitimate expense to the facility, unless specifically ordered by the physician, patient education is not recoverable under third-party reimbursement as a separate entity. Rather, the cost is subsumed under the room rate and is therefore technically absorbed by the healthcare organization.

Additionally, the *Balanced Budget Act of 1997* created a mélange of reimbursement methodologies dependent upon the type of healthcare facility (e.g., hospital, long-term care, home care) seeking payment for services rendered (*HCFA Legislative Summary*, 1997). Whether agency reimbursement is based on case mix, managed care methodologies, or episode-of-care formulae, the effectiveness of patient education becomes critical. To realize a cost savings, it is important that the client understand and carry out what is required of him or her so as to be discharged safely within the time frame allocated.

*Cost savings* are realized when hospital stays are shortened or fall within the DRG length of stay, when patients sustain fewer complications, and when utilization of expensive services decreases, thereby reducing hospital costs. In an ambulatory care setting such as an HMO, cost savings are realized when patient education keeps people healthy for a longer period of time, thereby controlling or preventing high utilization of expensive diagnostic testing or inpatient services. However, and perhaps most importantly, patient education becomes even more essential when a pattern of early discharge is detected, resulting in frequent readmissions to an agency. The facility comes under scrutiny by HCFA/CMMS and may be penalized either through citation or loss of payment—in which case, cost savings becomes a moot point.

*Cost benefit* is a result of increased patient satisfaction stemming from educational programs. In this era of "capturing" a patient population for lifetime coverage, patient satisfaction is critical to the individual's return for future healthcare services.

*Cost recovery* results when either the patient or insurer pays a fee for service for the educational services provided. Cost recovery is realized through the marketing of health education programs offered for a fee (fee for service). Also, under Medicare and Medicaid guidelines, reimbursement may be made for programs "furnished by providers of services to the extent that the programs are appropriate, integral parts in the rendition of covered services which are reasonable and necessary for the treatment of the individual's illness or injury" (*Medicare and Medicaid Guide*, 1986). The key to success in obtaining third-party reimbursement is the ability to demonstrate that as a result of education, patients can man-

age self-care at home and consequently experience fewer hospitalizations.

The final suggestion for cost recovery is the development and marketing of a cadre of health education programs that are open to all consumers in the community. These might include programs on childbirth education, smoking cessation, or weight control. The critical element, of course, is not only the recovery of costs but also revenue generation. *Revenue generation* refers to income realized over and above program costs. Revenue can also be regarded as profit.

To offset the dilemma of striving for cost containment and solvency in an environment of shrinking fiscal resources, healthcare organizations have developed alternative strategies for patient education to realize cost savings, cost benefit, cost recovery, or revenue generation. Kosik and Reynolds (1986) describe a preoperative teaching program for scheduled surgical patients prior to admission to the hospital. Reported outcomes, resulting in cost savings as well as cost benefit to the institution, include decreased patient anxiety, increased patient satisfaction, and decreased nursing hours. Wasson and Anderson (1993) describe other innovative programs designed for cost benefit, such as the "Teddy Bear Clinic" operated at Flint (Michigan) Osteopathic Hospital. Children were invited to bring their teddy bears in for a "checkup," which provided the opportunity for some health education for the children. The children subsequently toured the pediatric unit, with the overall goal of reducing their fears by acquainting them with common hospital equipment as well as the general design of the pediatric unit, should any of the children eventually require hospitalization.

## Program Planning and Implementation

The key elements to consider when planning a patient education offering intended for generation of revenue include an accurate assessment of material costs such as paper supplies, duplication or printing of program brochures, publicity, and rental space in which to offer the program, if necessary. It is essential that the time of professional personnel required to prepare and offer the program be included. If an hourly rate or annual salary is unknown, a simple rule of thumb is to divide the annual base salary by 2080, which is the standard number of hours worked by most people in the course of one year.

If the program is to be offered on the premises of the facility, there may be no need to plan for a space rental fee. However, indirect costs such as housekeeping and security should be prorated as a bona fide cost of the program. Such a practice not only is good fiscal management, but also provides an accounting of the contributions of other departments to the educational efforts of the facility.

Fees for a program should be set at a level high enough to cover the aggregate costs of program preparation and delivery. If the intent of an education program is that it be of cost benefit to the facility, such as provision of education classes for diabetics in the community to reduce the number of costly hospital admissions, then the goal may be to cover costs only. The fee is set by dividing the calculated cost by the number of anticipated attendees. If the intent is to offer a seven-week program for smoking cessation or a six-week childbirth education program in the interests of improving the wellness of the community and of generating revenue for the facility, then the fee is set higher than cost so as to realize a profit.

Over the course of a year, it is usually necessary to give an accounting of how the time of educational personnel was spent and whether such time allocation was of benefit to the institution. Cost benefit to the institution can be measured, for example, by increased patient satisfaction as determined via patient satisfaction questionnaires, decreased hospitalizations of the diabetic population, or an increase in utilization of obstetrical services.

## Cost-Effectiveness Analysis and Cost-Benefit Analysis

In the majority of healthcare organizations, the department of staff development bears the major responsibility for staff education and training and for patient education programs that exceed the boundaries of bedside instruction. Total budget preparation for these departments is best explained by the experts in the field (Abruzzese, 1992; Kelly, 1985; del Bueno & Kelly, 1980).

Fisher, Hume, and Emerick (1998) address the need for staff development departments to engage in responsibility-centered budgeting (RCB), also referred to as activity-based management (ABM). Given the shift away from providing at-will services and toward greater demand for cost accountability for educational programs, they propose a template for costing out programs that allows staff development departments to identify and recoup the true costs while responding to increased market competition.

There is no single best method for determining the effectiveness of patient education programs. Most experts in the field tend to differentiate between cost-benefit analysis and cost-effectiveness analysis (Kelly, 1985).

*Cost-benefit analysis* refers to the relationship between costs and outcomes. Outcomes can be actual revenue generated as a result of an educational offering, or they can be expressed in terms of shorter patient stays or reduced hospitalizations for particular diagnostic groupings of patients. Under DRGs or capitation methods of reimbursement, the facility realizes a cost savings that can be expressed in monetary terms. If the cost of an educational offering is less than the revenue generated, if costs are recoverable under third-party reimbursement, or if costs are less than savings to the facility, then the program is categorized as a cost benefit. The measurement of costs against monetary benefits is commonly referred to as cost-benefit analysis (often expressed as a cost-benefit ratio).

*Cost-effectiveness analysis* refers to the efficiency of an educational offering. If program objectives are achieved and there is a reliable measure of positive changes in behavior of the participants and reliable evidence of maintenance of these behaviors, the program is determined to be cost-effective. Although behavioral changes are highly desirable, they are in many respects less tangible. For example, reduction in patient anxiety cannot be measured in real dollars. Therefore, a comparative analysis of behavioral outcomes should be made between two or more programs to determine the one that is most cost-effective when an actual monetary value cannot be assigned. Changes in the philosophical posture of many healthcare organizations would dictate that those programs that realize a cost benefit are the most desirable.

As difficult as it may be from the standpoint of justice, it behooves the nurse educator to attempt to interpret behavioral changes in terms of cost savings to the institution by conducting a cost-effectiveness analysis between programs. This can be readily accomplished by first identifying and itemizing for each program all direct, indirect, and equipment costs in monetary terms and any identifiable hidden costs (e.g., employee turnover, orientation of new employees needed to conduct the educational program). Second, it is necessary to identify and itemize any benefits derived from the program offering (e.g., revenue generated or decreased readmission rates—converted into monetary values—among specific groups of patients, such as diabetics). Results of these findings can then be recorded on a grid so that each program's cost-effectiveness is visually apparent (see Figure 2–1)

| Program | I | II |
|---|---|---|
| **Costs** | | |
| Direct | $ | $ |
| Indirect | $ | $ |
| Hidden | $ | $ |
| **Benefits** | | |
| Decreased readmissions Revenue generated | $ | $ |
| Total | $ | $ |

FIGURE 2–1    **Cost-Effectiveness Grid**

## FUTURE DIRECTIONS IN PATIENT EDUCATION

Hospitals and other healthcare organizations have a long-standing commitment to patient education. This process as we have known it has usually occurred at the bedside, in clinic waiting rooms, or in groups on the hospital premises. Some aspects of this familiar educational process will certainly continue because it plays an important role in discharge planning for the patient and in the long run is cost-effective for the institution. At the same time, in the interest of conservation of time and resources, patient educators have used newer technologies to accomplish tasks associated with patient education. Closed-circuit television offers one good example. Although it has its limitations, this modality has become a common, useful tool to disseminate patient information. Patients can remain in their rooms during the presentation, and use of this technology releases nursing personnel for other duties when they might otherwise be involved with live demonstrations of baby baths or preparation of insulin for injection. Drawbacks of closed-circuit TV include the fact that it is usually fixed; that is, the programs are typically offered at a specified time of day or evening, which may not be conducive to a particular patient's learning. Also, if there is no follow-up, it is nearly impossible to determine whether the programmed instruction has been effective.

Meanwhile, many experts in the field (Wasson & Anderson, 1993; Abruzzese, 1992; Anderson, 1990) predict that patient education will take on new dimensions. These dimensions might include, but are not limited to, the following:

- Most teaching will occur in the ambulatory care setting.
- Use of computer-based instruction for hospitals, ambulatory care settings, physicians' offices, or homes will increase.

- Use of interactive video programs will increase.
- Wellness screening programs will increase.
- Emphasis on illness prevention and health promotion, such as nutrition, diet, and exercise, with various accompanying educational offerings, will increase.
- Interorganizational linkages to enhance cooperative endeavors in the patient education enterprise will increase.
- Third-party reimbursement will increase as cost-benefit ratios demonstrate the cost-effectiveness of consumer education.

## SUMMARY

Ethical and legal dimensions of human rights provide the justification for patient education, particularly as it relates to issues of self-determination and informed consent. These rights are enforced through federal and state regulations and through performance standards promulgated by accrediting bodies and professional organizations for implementation at the local level. The nurse's role as educator is legitimized through the definition of nursing practice as set forth by the prevailing nurse practice act in the state where the nurse is licensed and employed. In this respect, patient education is a nursing *duty* that is grounded in *justice*; that is, the nurse has a legal responsibility to provide patient education and, regardless of their culture, race, ethnicity, and so forth, all clients have a *right* to health education relevant to their physical and emotional needs. Justice also dictates that education programs should be designed to be consistent with organizational goals while meeting the needs of patients to be informed, self-directed, and in control of their own health.

## REVIEW QUESTIONS

1. What are the definitions of the terms: *ethical, moral, legal*?
2. How do the terms identified in Question 1 differ from one another?
3. Which national, state, professional, and private sector organizations legislate, regulate, and provide standards to ensure the protection of human rights in matters of health care?
4. Which ethical viewpoint, deontological or teleological, refers to the decision making approach that choices should be made for the common good of people?

5. With respect to ethical, moral, and legal obligations, how does the American Hospital Association's *Patient's Bill of Rights* compare to the American Nurses' Association's *Code of Ethics for Nurses with Interpretive Statements*?
6. What are the six ethical principles that dictate the actions of healthcare providers in delivering services to clients?
7. Why are nurse practice acts so important to nurses in carrying out their roles and responsibilities to the public?
8. What is the difference between the terms *negligence* and *malpractice*?

9. When was informed consent established as a basic tenet of ethics and what is the nurse's role in situations involving informed consent?

10. What is meant by the legal term *respondeat superior,* and how does this term apply to professional nursing practice?

11. Why is documentation of professional nursing duties, particularly patient education, so important in the provision of care by nurses?

12. What are the two categories of costs, and how are they defined?

13. What are the four examples of direct costs and the five examples of indirect costs in the provision of health education?

14. What are the definitions of these terms: *fixed direct costs, variable direct costs, indirect costs, cost savings, cost benefit, cost recovery, cost-effectiveness analysis,* and *cost benefit analysis?*

## REFERENCES

*Abernathy* v. *Sisters of St. Mary's,* 446 SW2d 559 (MO 1969).

Abood, S. (2001). The Bush regulatory agenda. *American Journal of Nursing, 101*(8), 22.

Abruzzese, R. S. (1992). *Nursing Staff Development: Strategies for Success.* St. Louis: Mosby.

Aleksandrowicz, L. I. & Norcross, S. (1984). *Nurse Administrator's Desk Reference.* Owings Mills, MD: Rynd Communications.

American Nurses Association. *Code for Nurses with Interpretative Statements* (1976, 1985). Kansas City, MO: American Nurses Association.

American Nurses Association. *Code of Ethics for Nurses with Interpretive Statements.* (2001). Washington, D.C.: American Nurses Association.

Anderson, C. (1990). *Patient Teaching and Communicating in an Information Age.* Albany, NY: Delmar.

Boyd, M. D., Gleit, C.J., Graham, B.A., & Whitman, N. I. (1998). *Health Teaching in Nursing Practice: A Professional Model.* 3rd ed. Stamford, CT: Appleton & Lange.

Brent, N. J. (2001). *Nurses and the Law.* 2nd ed. Philadelphia: Saunders.

Casey, F. S. (1995) Documenting patient education: A literature review. *Journal of Continuing Education in Nursing, 26*(6), 257–260.

Cisar, N. S. & Bell, S. K. (1995). Informed consent: An ethical dilemma. *Nursing Forum, 30*(3), 20–28.

Creighton, H. (1986). Informed consent. *Nursing Management, 17*(10), 11–13.

*Darling* v. *Charleston Memorial Hospital,* 211 NE2d 253 (IL 1965).

del Bueno, D. & Kelly, K. (1980). How cost-effective is your staff development program? *Journal of Nursing Administration, 10*(4), 31.

Emanuel, E. J. (May–June 2000). Justice and managed care: Four principles for the just allocation of health care resources. *Hastings Center Report, 30*(3), 8–16.

Fisher, M. L., Hume, R., & Emerick, R. (1998). Costing nursing education programs: It's as easy as 1-2-3. *Journal for Nurses in Staff Development, 14*(5), 227–285.

Gift, A. G. (1994). Understanding costs. *Clinical Nurse Specialist, 8*(2), 90.

*HCFA Legislative Summary. (1997).* The balanced budget act of 1997. (P.L.105-33). Washington, DC: Office of Legislation, August 5, 1997.

Kelly, K. J. (1985). Cost-benefit and cost-effectiveness analysis: Tools for the staff development manager. *Journal of Nursing Staff Development, 6*(2), 9–15.

Kosik, S. L. & Reynolds, P. J. (1986). A nursing contribution to cost containment: A group preoperative teaching program that shortens hospital stay. *Journal of Nursing Staff Development, 5*(1), 18–22.

Lesnick, M. J. & Anderson, B. E. (1962). *Nursing Practice and the Law.* Philadelphia: Lippincott.

*Medicare and Medicaid Guide* (1986). Washington, DC: U.S. Government Printing Office, 9023.

Mezey, M., Evans, L. K., Golub, Z. D., Murphy, E., & White, G. B. (1994).The patient self-determination act: Sources of concern for nurses. *Nursing Outlook, 42*(1), 30–38.

*Model Nurse Practice Act.* (1978). Kansas City, MO: American Nurses' Association.

*New York State Nurse Practice Act.* (1972). Albany, NY: New York State Nurses Association.

*Patient's Bill of Rights.* (1975). Chicago: American Hospital Association.

NYSA Report (2001). The official newsletter of the New York State Nurses Association. 32(7).

Rankin, S. H. & Stallings, K. D. (1990). *Patient Education: Issues, Principles, Practices.* Philadelphia: Lippincott.

Rankin, S. H. & Stallings, K. D. (2001). *Patient Education: Principles and Practices.* 4th ed. Philadelphia: Lippincott.

Smith, C. E. (1987). *Patient education: Nurses in Partnership with other Health Professionals.* Philadelphia: Saunders.

Snyder, B. (1996). An easy way to document patient ed. *RN*, March, 43–45.

Strader, M. K. (1985). Malpractice and nurse educators: Defining legal responsibilities. *Journal of Nursing Education, 24*(9), 363–367.

Thomas, S. B. & Quinn, S. C. (1991). Public health then and now. The Tuskegee syphilis study, 1932 to 1972: Implications for HIV education programs in the black community. *American Journal of Public Health, 81*(11), 1498–1505.

Wasson, D. & Anderson, M. A. (1993). Hospital-patient education: Current status and future trends. *Journal of Nursing Staff Development, 10*(3), 147–151.

Weisbard, A. J. & Arras, J. D. (1984). Commissioning morality: An introduction to the symposium. *Cardozo Law Review, 6*(4), 223–241.

Yoder Wise, P. S. (1995). *Leading and Managing in Nursing.* St. Louis: Mosby.

Zuckerman, J. (2001). "Patients Bill of Rights." *New York Times,* August 3, 1.

## CHAPTER 3

# Applying Learning Theories to Healthcare Practice

*Margaret M. Braungart*
*Richard G. Braungart*

## CHAPTER HIGHLIGHTS

## KEY TERMS

learning
learning theory
behaviorist learning
respondent conditioning
stimulus generalization
discrimination learning
spontaneous recovery
operant conditioning
escape conditioning
avoidance conditioning

cognitive learning
gestalt perspective
information-processing perspective
cognitive development perspective
social constructivist perspective
social cognition perspective
social learning
psychodynamic learning
humanistic learning

## OBJECTIVES

After completing this chapter, the reader will be able to

1. Differentiate among the basic approaches to learning for each of the five learning theories.

2. Define the principal constructs of each learning theory.

3. Give an example applying each theory to changing the attitudes and behaviors of learners in a specific situation.

4. Outline alternative strategies for learning in a given situation using at least two different learning theories.

5. Identify the differences and similarities in the learning theories specific to (a) the basic procedures of learning, (b) the assumptions made about the learning, (c) the task of the educator, (d) the sources of motivation, and (e) the way in which the transfer of learning is facilitated.

*Learning* is defined in this chapter as a relatively permanent change in mental processing, emotional functioning, and/or behavior as a result of experience. It is the lifelong, dynamic process by which individuals acquire new knowledge or skills and alter their thoughts, feelings, attitudes, and actions. Despite the significance of learning to human development, it has long been debated how learning occurs, what kinds of experiences facilitate or hinder the learning process, and what ensures that learning becomes relatively permanent.

Until the late nineteenth century, most of the discussions and debates about learning were grounded in philosophy, public and normal school administration, and conventional wisdom (Hilgard, 1996). Around the dawn of the twentieth century, the new field of educational psychology emerged and became a defining force for the scientific study of learning, teaching, and assessment (Berliner & Calfee, 1996; Gage & Berliner, 1998; Woolfolk, 2001). As a science, educational psychology rests on the systematic gathering of evidence or data to test theories and hypotheses about learning. A *learning theory* is a coherent framework and set of integrated constructs and principles that describe, explain, or predict how people learn. Rather than offering a single theory of learning, educational psychology provides alternative theories and perspectives on how learning occurs and what motivates people to learn and change (Bigge & Shermis, 1992; Hilgard & Bower, 1966; Hill, 1990).

The development and testing of learning theories over the past century have contributed much to our understanding of how individuals acquire knowledge and change their ways of thinking, feeling, and behaving. The accumulated body of research information can be used to guide the teaching and learning processes and has challenged a number of popular notions and myths about learning (e.g., "Spare the rod and spoil the child," "Males are more intelligent than females," "You can't teach an old dog new tricks"). In addition, the major learning theories have wide applicability and form the foundation of not only the field of education but also psychological counseling, workplace organization and human resource management, and marketing and advertising.

Whether used singly or in combination, learning theories have much to offer the practice of health care. Increasingly, health professionals must demonstrate that they regularly employ sound methods and a clear rationale in their education efforts, patient and client interactions, staff management and training, and continuing education and health promotion programs. Given the current structure of health care in the United States, nurses, in particular, are often responsible for designing and implementing plans and procedures for improving health education and encouraging wellness. Beyond one's profession, however, knowledge of the learning process relates to nearly every aspect of daily life. Learning theories can be applied at the individual, group, and community levels not only to comprehend and teach new material, but also to solve problems, change unhealthy habits, build constructive relationships, manage emotions, and develop effective behavior.

This chapter reviews the principal learning theories. Behaviorist, cognitive, and social learning theories are most often applied to patient education and healthcare practice (Redman, 2001). It is argued in this chapter that emotions and feelings also need explicit focus in relation to learning in general (Goleman, 1995) and to health care in particular. Why? Emotional reactions are often learned as a result of experience, they play a significant role in the learning process, and they are a vital consideration when dealing with health, disease, prevention, wellness, medical treatment, recovery, healing, and relapse prevention. While not always treated as learning theories in psychology (Hilgard & Bower, 1966), psychodynamic and humanistic perspectives are included in this review because they add much to our understanding of human motivation, emotions, and the learning process.

The chapter is organized as follows. First, the basic principles of learning advocated by behaviorist, cognitive, social learning, psychodynamic, and humanistic theories are summarized and illustrated with examples from health care. Next, these theories are compared with regard to (1) their fundamental procedures for changing behavior, (2) the assumptions made about the learner, (3) the role of the educator in encouraging learning, (4) sources of motivation, and (5) ways in which learning is transferred to new situations and problems. Finally, some common features of learning are identified in relation to the issues raised earlier about ways that learning occurs, the kinds of experiences that promote the learning process, and ways to ensure that learning is relatively permanent.

The goals of this chapter are to provide a conceptual framework for subsequent chapters in this book and to offer a toolbox of approaches that can be used to enhance learning and change in patients, clients, staff, and oneself. Physiological and neuropsychological perspectives on learning (Baker, 1998; Gluck & Myers, 1997; Sprenger, 1999) are not included in the chapter, because the emphasis here is on teaching and social interaction in the healthcare setting rather than on the underlying biological mechanisms of learning. After completing the chapter, readers should be able to identify the essential principles of learning, describe various ways in

which the learning process can be approached, and develop alternative strategies to change attitudes and behaviors in different settings.

## LEARNING THEORIES

This section summarizes the basic principles and related concepts of the behaviorist, cognitive, social learning, psychodynamic, and humanistic learning theories. While reviewing each theory, readers are asked to consider the following questions:

- How do the environment and the internal dynamics of the individual influence learning?
- Is the learner viewed as relatively passive or more active?
- What is the educator's task in the learning process?
- What motivates individuals to learn?
- What encourages the transfer of learning to new situations?

### Behaviorist Learning Theory

Focusing mainly on what is directly observable, behaviorists view learning as the product of the stimulus conditions (S) and the responses (R) that follow—sometimes termed the S-R model of learning. Whether dealing with animals or people, the learning process is relatively simple. Generally ignoring what goes on inside the individual—which, of course, is always difficult to ascertain—behaviorists closely observe responses and then manipulate the environment to bring about the intended change (Bigge & Shermis, 1992; Hilgard & Bower, 1966).

To modify people's attitudes and responses, behaviorists recommend either altering the stimulus conditions in the environment or changing what happens after a response occurs. Motivation is explained as the desire to reduce some drive (drive-reduction); hence, satisfied, complacent, or satiated individuals have little motivation to learn and change. Getting behavior to transfer from the initial learning situation to other settings is largely a matter of practice (strengthening habits) and a similarity in the stimuli and responses between the learning situation and future situations where the response is to be performed. Much of behaviorist learning is based on respondent conditioning and operant conditioning procedures.

*Respondent conditioning* (also termed classical or Pavlovian conditioning) emphasizes the importance of stimulus conditions and the associations formed in the learning process (Hilgard & Bower, 1966; Klein & Mowrer, 1989). In this basic model of learning, a neutral stimulus (NS)—a stimulus that has no particular value or meaning to the learner—is paired with a naturally occurring unconditioned or unlearned stimulus (UCS) and unconditioned response (UCR) (Figure 3–1). After a few such pairings, the neutral stimulus alone, without the unconditioned stimulus, elicits the same response. Often occurring without thought or awareness, learning takes place when the newly conditioned stimulus (CS) becomes associated with the conditioned response (CR).

Consider an example from health care. Someone without much experience with hospitals (NS) may visit a sick relative (see Figure 3–1). While in the relative's room, the visitor may smell offensive odors (UCS) and feel queasy and light-headed (UCR). After this initial visit and later repeated visits, hospitals (now the CS) may become associated with feeling anxious and nauseated (CR), especially if the visitor smells odors similar to

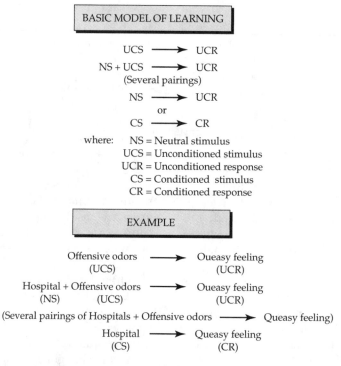

FIGURE 3–1   **Respondent Conditioning Model of Learning**

those encountered during the first experience. Respondent conditioning highlights the importance of the "atmosphere" and staff morale in health care. Often without thinking or reflection, patients and visitors formulate these associations as a result of their hospital experiences, providing the basis for long-lasting attitudes toward medicine, healthcare facilities, and health professionals.

Besides influencing the acquisition of new responses to environmental stimuli, principles of respondent conditioning may be used to extinguish a previously learned response. Responses decrease if the presentation of the conditioned stimulus is not accompanied by the unconditioned stimulus over time. Thus, if the visitor who became dizzy in one hospital subsequently goes to other hospitals to see relatives or friends without smelling offensive odors, then her discomfort and anxiety about hospitals may lessen after several such experiences.

Systematic desensitization is a technique based on respondent conditioning that is used by psychologists to reduce fear and anxiety in their clients (Wolpe, 1982). The assumption is that fear of a particular stimulus or situation is learned, so it can, therefore, be "unlearned" or extinguished. Fearful individuals are first taught relaxation techniques. While they are in a state of relaxation, the fear-producing stimulus is gradually introduced at a nonthreatening level so that anxiety and emotions are not aroused. After repeated pairings of the stimulus under relaxed, nonfrightening conditions, the individual learns that no harm will come to him or her from the once-fear-inducing stimulus. Finally, the client is able to confront the stimulus without being anxious and afraid.

In health care, systematic desensitization has been used to treat drug addiction (Piane, 2000), phobias (McCullough & Andrews, 2001), and tension headaches (Deyl & Kaliappan, 1997), and to help bone-marrow transplant patients (DuHamel, Ostroff, Bovbjerg, Pfeffer, Morasco, Papadopoulos, & Redd, 2000). Taking the time to help patients relax

and reduce their stress when applying some medical intervention—even a painful procedure—lessens the likelihood that patients will build up negative and anxious associations about medicine and health care.

Certain respondent conditioning concepts are especially useful in the healthcare setting. *Stimulus generalization* is the tendency of initial learning experiences to be easily applied to other similar stimuli. For example, when listening to friends and relatives describe a hospital experience, it becomes apparent that a highly positive or negative personal encounter may color patients' evaluations of their hospital stays as well as their subsequent feelings about having to be hospitalized again. With more and varied experiences, individuals learn to differentiate among similar stimuli, and *discrimination learning* occurs. Much of professional education and clinical practice involves discrimination learning.

*Spontaneous recovery* is another useful concept to know and needs to be given careful consideration in relapse prevention programs. The principle operates as follows: Although a response may appear to be extinguished, it may "recover" and reappear at any time (even years later), especially when stimulus conditions are similar to those in the initial learning experience. Spontaneous recovery helps us understand why it is so difficult to completely eliminate unhealthy habits and addictive behaviors such as smoking, alcoholism, or drug abuse.

*Operant conditioning*, developed largely by B. F. Skinner (1974, 1989), focuses on the behavior of the organism and the reinforcement that occurs after the response (Alberto & Troutman, 1990). A reinforcer is a stimulus or event applied after a response that strengthens the probability that the response will be performed again. When specific responses are reinforced on the proper schedule, behaviors can be either increased or decreased.

Table 3–1 summarizes the principal ways to increase and decrease responses using the

**TABLE 3–1    Operant conditioning model: Contingencies to increase and decrease the probability of an organism's response**

I.  To *increase* the probability of a response:

    A. *Positive reinforcement:* application of a pleasant stimulus

    *Reward conditioning:* a pleasant stimulus is applied following an organism's response

    B. *Negative reinforcement:* removal of an aversive or unpleasant stimulus

    *Escape conditioning:* as an aversive stimulus is applied, the organism makes a response that causes the unpleasant stimulus to cease

    *Avoidance conditioning:* an aversive stimulus is anticipated by the organism, who makes a response to avoid the unpleasant event

II. To *decrease* or extinguish the probability of a response:

    A. *Nonreinforcement:* an organism's conditioned response is not followed by any kind of reinforcement (positive, negative, or punishment)

    B. *Punishment:* following a response, an aversive stimulus is applied which the organism cannot escape or avoid

---

contingencies of operant conditioning. Two methods to increase the probability of a response are to apply positive or negative reinforcement after a response occurs. According to Skinner (1974), using positive reinforcement (i.e., reward) greatly enhances the likelihood that a response will be repeated in similar circumstances. As an illustration, although a patient moans and groans as he attempts to get up and walk for the first time after an operation, praise and encouragement (reward) for his efforts at walking (response) will improve the chances that he will continue struggling toward independence.

A second way to increase a behavior is by applying negative reinforcement after a response is made. This form of reinforcement involves the removal of an unpleasant stimulus through either escape conditioning or avoidance conditioning. The difference between the two types of negative reinforcement relates to timing.

In *escape conditioning,* as an unpleasant stimulus is being applied, the individual responds in some way that causes the uncom-

fortable stimulation to cease. For example, suppose as a member of the healthcare team is being chastised in front of the group for being late and missing meetings, she says something humorous. The head of the team stops criticizing her and laughs. Because the use of humor has allowed the team member to escape an unpleasant situation, chances are that she will employ humor again to alleviate a stressful encounter and thereby deflect attention from her problem behavior.

In *avoidance conditioning,* the unpleasant stimulus is anticipated rather than being applied directly. Avoidance conditioning has been used to explain some people's tendency to become ill so as to avoid doing something they do not want to do. For example, a child fearing a teacher or test may tell his mother that he has a stomachache. If allowed to stay home from school, the child increasingly may complain of sickness to avoid unpleasant situations. If a person becomes truly ill when fearful events are anticipated, sickness is the behavior that has been increased through negative reinforcement.

According to operant conditioning principles, behaviors may be decreased through either nonreinforcement or punishment. Skinner (1974) maintained that the simplest way to extinguish a response is not to provide any kind of reinforcement for some action. For example, offensive jokes in the workplace may be handled by showing no reaction; after several such experiences, the joke teller, who more than likely wants attention—and negative attention is preferable to no attention—may curtail his or her use of abrasive humor. Keep in mind, too, that desirable behavior that is ignored may lessen as well.

If nonreinforcement proves ineffective, then punishment may be employed as a way to decrease responses, although there are risks in using this approach. Under punishment conditions, the individual cannot escape or avoid an unpleasant stimulus. Suppose, for example, the healthcare team member's attempt at humor is met by the leader's curt remark, "You are continually a source of difficulty in this group, and if this continues, your job is in jeopardy," embarrassing her in front of her peers. The problem with using punishment as a technique for teaching is that the learner may become highly emotional and may well divert attention away from the behavior that needs to be changed. Some people who are being punished become so emotional (sad or angry) that they do not remember the behavior for which they are being punished. One of the cardinal rules of operant conditioning is to "punish the behavior, not the person."

If punishment is employed, it should be administered immediately after the response with no distractions or means of escape. Punishment must also be consistent and at the highest "reasonable" level (e.g., health professionals who apologize and smile as they admonish the behavior of a staff member or client are sending out mixed messages and are not likely to be taken seriously or to

decrease the behavior they intend). Moreover, punishment should not be prolonged (bringing up old grievances or complaining about a misbehavior at every opportunity), but there should be a "time-out" following punishment to eliminate the opportunity for positive reinforcement. The purpose of punishment is not to do harm or to serve as a release for anger; rather, the goal is to decrease a specific behavior and to instill self-discipline.

The use of reinforcement is central to the success of operant conditioning procedures. For operant conditioning to be effective, it is necessary to assess what kinds of reinforcement are likely to increase or decrease behaviors for each individual. Not every client, for example, finds health practitioner's terms of endearment rewarding. Comments such as "Very nice job, dear," may be presumptuous or offensive to some clients. A second issue involves the timing of reinforcement. Through experimentation with animals and humans, it has been demonstrated that the success of operant conditioning procedures partially depends on the schedule of reinforcement (Hill, 1990). Initial learning requires a continuous schedule, reinforcing the behavior quickly every time it occurs. If the desired behavior does not occur, then responses that approximate or resemble it can be reinforced, gradually shaping behavior in the direction of the goal for learning. As an illustration, for geriatric patients who appear lethargic and unresponsive, nurses or physicians might begin by rewarding small gestures such as eye contact or a hand that reaches out, then build on these friendly behaviors toward greater human contact and connection with reality. Once a response is well established, however, it becomes ineffective and inefficient to continually reinforce the behavior; reinforcement then can be administered on a fixed (predictable) or variable (unpredictable) schedule after a given number of responses have been emitted or after the passage of time.

Operant conditioning techniques provide relatively quick and effective ways to change behavior. Carefully planned programs using behavior modification procedures can readily be applied to health care (Bootzin, 1975; De Grandpre, 2000; Taylor, 1999). For example, the families of chronic back pain patients have been taught to minimize their attention to the patients whenever they complain and behave in dependent, helpless ways, but to pay a lot of attention when the patients attempt to function independently, express a positive attitude, and try to live as normal a life as possible. Some patients respond so well to operant conditioning that they report experiencing less pain as they become more active and involved. Operant conditioning and behavior modification techniques also have been found to work well with some nursing home and long-term care residents (Proctor, Burns, Powell, & Tarrier, 1999).

The behaviorist theory is simple and easy to use, and it encourages clear, objective analysis of observable environmental stimulus conditions, learner responses, and the effects of reinforcements. There are, however, some criticisms and cautions to consider. Under this model, learners are assumed to be relatively passive and easily manipulated, which raises the crucial issue of ethics: "Who" is to decide "what" the "desirable" behavior should be? Too often the desired response is conformity and cooperation to make someone's job easier or more profitable. In addition, the theory's emphasis on extrinsic rewards and external incentives reinforces and promotes materialism rather than self-initiative, a love of learning, and intrinsic satisfaction. Another shortcoming of behavior modification programs is that clients' changed behavior may deteriorate over time, especially once they are back in their former environment—an environment with a system of rewards and punishments that may have fostered their problems in the first place.

We now move from focusing on responses and behavior to the role of mental processes in learning.

## Cognitive Learning Theory

While behaviorists generally ignore the internal dynamics of learning, cognitive learning theorists stress the importance of what goes on "inside" the learner (Brien & Eastmond, 1994; Lambert & McCombs, 1998; Palincsar, 1998). The key to learning and changing is the individual's cognition (perception, thought, memory, and ways of processing and structuring information). According to this perspective, to learn, individuals must change their cognitions. A highly active process largely directed by the individual, learning involves perceiving the information, interpreting it based on what is already known, and then reorganizing the information into new insights or understanding. Cognitive theory currently is enjoying considerable popularity in psychology (Bandura, 2001; Tatman & Gilgen, 1999).

Cognitive theorists, unlike behaviorists, maintain that reward is not necessary for learning. More important are learners' goals and expectations, which create disequilibrium, imbalance, and tension that motivate them to act. Educators and those trying to influence the learning process must recognize the variety of past experiences, perceptions, ways of incorporating and thinking about information, and diverse aspirations, expectations, and social influences affecting any learning situation. To promote transfer of learning, the learner must mediate or "act on" the information in some way. Similar patterns in the initial learning situation and subsequent situations also facilitate this transfer.

Cognitive learning theory includes several well-known perspectives, such as gestalt, information processing, human development, social constructivism, and social cognition theory. Each of these perspectives emphasizes a particular feature of cognition, which when pieced together, indicates much about what goes on inside the learner. As the various cognitive perspectives are briefly summarized here, readers are encouraged to think of their potential applications in the healthcare setting. In keeping with cognitive principles of learning, being mentally active with information encourages memory and retention.

The *gestalt perspective* emphasizes the importance of perception in learning (Garcia, Baker, & deMayo, 1999; Hilgard & Bower, 1966; Kohler, 1947, 1969). Rather than focusing on discrete stimuli, gestalt refers to the configuration or patterned organization of cognitive elements, reflecting the maxim that "the whole is greater than the sum of the parts." A principal assumption is that each person perceives, interprets, and responds to any situation in his or her own way. While there are many gestalt principles worth knowing (Hilgard & Bower, 1966), several will be discussed here as they relate to health care.

A basic principle is that psychological organization is directed toward simplicity, equilibrium, and regularity. For example, study the bewildered faces of some patients listening to a detailed, evasive explanation about their disease, when what they desire most is a simple, clear explanation that settles their uncertainty and relates directly to them and their familiar experiences.

Another central gestalt principle is that perception is selective, which has several ramifications. First, because no one can attend to all the surrounding stimuli at any given time, individuals orient themselves to certain features of an experience while screening out or habituating to other features. Patients in severe pain or worried about their hospital bills may not attend to well-intentioned patient education information. Second, what individuals pay attention to and what they ignore are influenced by a host of factors: past experiences, needs, personal motives and attitudes, reference groups, and the particular structure of the stimulus or situation (Sherif &

Sherif, 1969; Sherif, 1976). Assessing these internal and external dynamics has a direct bearing on how a health educator approaches any learning situation with an individual or group. Moreover, because individuals vary widely with regard to these and other characteristics, they will perceive, interpret, and respond to the same event in different ways, perhaps distorting reality to fit their goals and expectations. This tendency helps explain why an approach that is effective with one client may not work with another client. The gestalt perspective is one of the oldest schools of psychology and has strongly influenced a number of more recent cognitive perspectives.

*Information processing* is a cognitive perspective that emphasizes thinking processes: thought, reasoning, the way information is encountered and stored, and memory functioning (Bigge & Shermis, 1992; Gagné, 1985; Sternberg, 1991, 1996). How information is incorporated and retrieved is useful for health professionals to know, especially in relation to older people's learning (Hooyman & Kiyak, 1999).

An information-processing model of memory functioning is illustrated in Figure 3–2. The first stage in the memory process involves paying attention to environmental stimuli; attention, then, is the key to learning. Thus, if a client is not attending to what a nurse educator is saying, perhaps because the client is weary or distracted, it would be prudent to try the explanation at another time when he is more receptive and attentive.

In the second stage, the information is processed by the senses. Here it becomes important to consider the client's preferred mode of sensory processing (visual, auditory, or motor manipulation) and to ascertain whether there are sensory deficits.

In the third stage, the information is transformed and incorporated (encoded) briefly into short-term memory, after which it is either disregarded and forgotten or stored in long-term memory. Long-term memory involves

FIGURE 3–2   Information-Processing Model of Memory

the organization of information by using a preferred strategy for storage (e.g., imagery, association, rehearsal, breaking the information into units). While long-term memories are enduring, a central problem is retrieving the stored information at a later time.

The last stage involves the action or response that the individual makes on the basis of how information was processed and stored.

Education involves assessing how a learner attends to, processes, and stores the information that is presented as well as finding ways to encourage the retention and retrieval processes. Errors are corrected by helping learners "reprocess" what needs to be learned. Neuropsychologists have contributed to understanding the physiological mechanisms underlying memory and information processing (Gluck & Myers, 1997; Sprenger, 1999).

In general, cognitive psychologists note that memory processing and the retrieval of information are enhanced by organizing information and making it meaningful. A widely used descriptive model has been provided by Robert Gagné (1985). Subsequently, Gagné and his colleagues outlined nine events and their corresponding cognitive processes

that activate effective learning (Gagné, Briggs, & Wagner, 1992):

- Gain the learner's attention (reception)
- Inform the learner of the objectives and expectations (expectancy)
- Stimulate the learner's recall of prior learning (retrieval)
- Present information (selective perception)
- Provide guidance to facilitate the learner's understanding (semantic encoding)
- Have the learner demonstrate the information or skill (responding)
- Give feedback to the learner (reinforcement)
- Assess the learner's performance (retrieval)
- Work to enhance retention and transfer through application and varied practice (generalization)

In employing this model, instructors must carefully analyze the requirements of the activity, design and sequence the instructional events, and select appropriate media to achieve the outcomes.

Within the information-processing perspective, Sternberg (1996) reminds us to consider styles of thinking, which he defined as "a preference for using abilities in certain ways." Thinking styles concern differences, he noted, and not judgments of "better" or "worse." In education, the instructor's task is to get in touch with the learner's way of processing information and thinking. Some implications for health care are the need to carefully match jobs with styles of thinking, to recognize that people may shift from preferring one style of thinking to another, and, most important, to appreciate and respect the different styles of thinking reflected among the many players in the healthcare setting (see Chapter 4 on learning styles).

The information-processing perspective is particularly helpful for assessing problems in acquiring, remembering, and recalling information. Some strategies include the following: (1) have learners indicate how they believe they learn (metacognition), (2) ask them to describe what they are thinking as they are learning, (3) evaluate learners' mistakes, and (4) give close attention to their inability to remember or demonstrate information. For example, forgetting or having difficulty in retrieving information from long-term memory is a major stumbling block in learning. This problem may occur because the information has faded from lack of use, other information interferes with its retrieval (what comes before or after a learning session may well confound storage and retrieval), or individuals are motivated to forget for a variety of conscious and unconscious reasons. This material on memory processing and functioning is highly pertinent to healthcare practice—whether developing health education brochures, engaging in one-to-one patient education, delivering a staff development workshop, preparing community health lectures, or studying for one's courses and examinations.

*Cognitive development* is a third perspective that focuses on qualitative changes in perceiving, thinking, and reasoning as individuals grow and mature (Baltes, Staudinger, & Lindenberger, 1999; Vander Zanden, Crandell, & Crandell, 2000). Cognitions are based on how external events are conceptualized, organized, and represented within each person's mental framework or *schema*—a framework that is partially dependent on the individual's stage of cognitive development and readiness to learn.

Much of the theory and research in this area has been concerned with identifying the thought processes of children and adolescents. A principal assumption is that learning is a developmental, sequential, and active process that transpires as the child interacts with the environment, makes "discoveries" about how the world operates, and interprets these discoveries in keeping with what she knows (schema).

Jean Piaget is the best-known cognitive developmental theorist, and his observations of children's perception and thought processes at different ages have contributed much to our recognition of the unique ways that youngsters reason, the changes in their ability to conceptualize, and their limitations in understanding, communicating, and performing (Piaget & Inhelder, 1969). By watching, asking questions, and listening to children, Piaget identified and described four sequential stages of cognitive development (sensorimotor, preoperational, concrete operations, and formal operations) that become evident over the course of infancy, early childhood, middle childhood, and adolescence.[1]

---

[1] Piaget (Piaget & Inhelder, 1969) identified four sequential stages of cognitive development: (1) the sensorimotor stage during infancy, where infants explore their environments and attempt to coordinate sensory information with motor skills; (2) the preoperational stage during early childhood, where youngsters are able to mentally represent the environment, regard the world from their own egocentric perspective, and come to grips with symbolization; (3) the concrete operations stage during the elementary school years, where children are able to attend to more than one dimension at a time, conceptualize relationships, and operate on the environment; and (4) the formal operations stage during adolescence, where teenagers begin to think abstractly, are able to deal with the future, and can see alternatives and criticize.

(See Chapter 5 on developmental stages.) According to this view, children take in information as they interact with people and the environment and either make their experiences fit with what they already know (assimilation) or change their perceptions and interpretations in keeping with the new information (accommodation). Health professionals and family members need to determine what children are thinking about themselves and a given situation. As an illustration, young children usually do not comprehend fully that death is final. They respond to the experience in their own way, perhaps asking God to give back the dead person or believing that if they act like a good person, the deceased loved one will return to them (Gardner, 1978).

Within the cognitive development perspective are some differences worth considering. For example, while Piaget stressed the importance of perception in learning and viewed children as little scientists exploring and interacting with the world in a relative solitary manner, Lev Vygotsky (1986) emphasized the significance of language, social interaction, and adult guidance in the learning process. One implication is that some children may learn more effectively by discovering and putting pieces together on their own, whereas other children benefit from a more social and directive approach. It is the health educator's responsibility to identify the child's or teenager's stage of thinking, to provide experiences at an appropriate level for children to actively discover and participate in the learning process, and to determine whether a child learns best through language and social interaction or through perceiving and experimenting in his or her own way. Research suggests that young children's learning is often more solitary, whereas older children may learn more readily through social interaction (Palincsar, 1998).

What do cognitive developmental theorists say about adult learning? First, although the cognitive stages develop sequentially, some adults never reach the formal operations stage. These adults may learn better from explicitly concrete approaches to health education. Second, adult developmental psychologists and gerontologists have proposed advanced stages of reasoning in adulthood beyond formal operations. For example, not until early middle age may adults become able to deal with contradictions, synthesize information, and more effectively integrate what they have learned—characteristics that differentiate adult thought from adolescent thinking (Kramer, 1983). Third, older adults may demonstrate an advanced level of reasoning derived from their wisdom and life experiences, or they may reflect lower stages of thinking due to lack of education, disease, depression, extraordinary stress, or medications (Hooyman & Kiyak, 1999; Quadagno, 1999).

Whether dealing with children or adults, assessing each person's level of cognitive functioning is a first step in communicating effectively and accomplishing health education. It also should be noted that moral reasoning depends on a person's stage of cognitive development (Kohlberg, 1984), which is useful information in understanding patient, family, and healthcare providers' responses to the many ethical dilemmas that arise in medicine. Gender differences in reactions to caring, morality, and healthcare ethics need to be recognized as well (Gilligan, 1982).

Because cognitive theory was criticized for neglecting the social context, the effects of social factors on perception, thought, and motivation are receiving increased attention. *Social constructivism* and *social cognition* are two increasingly popular orientations. Drawing heavily from gestalt psychology and developmental psychology, social constructivists take issue with some of the highly rational assumptions of the information-processing view and build on the works of Piaget and Vygotsky (Palincsar, 1998). Reflecting the influence of postmodernism, social constructivists posit that learning and human development are richly colored by the ever-fluid social and cultural context in which people find themselves. Central tenets of this perspective are that (1) the learning process is influenced strongly by the culture and (2) effective learning occurs through social interaction, collaboration, and negotiation (Berliner & Calfee, 1996).

According to this view, the players in any healthcare setting may have differing perceptions of external reality. Every person operates on the basis of her or his unique representations and interpretations of a situation, all of which have been heavily influenced by that individual's social and cultural experiences. Learning is facilitated by sharing beliefs, by acknowledging and challenging differing conceptions, and by negotiating new levels of conceptual understanding (Marshall, 1998). Cooperative learning and self-help groups are examples of social constructivism in action. With America's rapidly changing age and ethnic composition, the social constructivist perspective has much to contribute to health education and health promotion efforts.

Rooted in social psychology, the social cognition perspective highlights the influence of social factors on perception, thought, and motivation. A host of scattered explanations can be found under the rubric of social cognition (Fiske & Taylor, 1991), which, when applied to learning, emphasize the need for instructors to consider the dynamics of the social environment and groups on both interpersonal and intrapersonal behavior. As an illustration, attribution theory concerns the cause–effect relationships and explanations that individuals formulate to account for their own and others' behavior and the way in which the world operates. Many of these explanations are unique to the individual and tend to be strongly colored by cultural values and beliefs. For example, patients with certain religious views or a particular parental upbringing may believe that their disease is a punishment for their sins (internalizing blame); other patients may attribute their disease to the actions of others (externalizing blame). From this perspective, patients' attri-

butions may or may not promote wellness and well-being. The route to changing health behaviors is to change distorted attributions. The medical staff's attributions need to be considered as well in the healing process.

A significant benefit of the cognitive theory to health care is its encouragement of a recognition and appreciation of the individuality and rich diversity in how people learn and process experiences (Farnham-Diggory, 1992; Lewis & Daltroy, 1990). Consider, for example, the wide variations in how learners actively structure their perceptions, confront a learning situation, and encode-process-store-retrieve information. The challenge to educators is to identify a learner's level of cognitive development and the social influences that affect learning, and then find ways to foster insight, creativity, and problem solving. Difficulties lie in ascertaining exactly what is transpiring inside the mind of each individual and in designing learning activities that encourage people to restructure their perceptions, reorganize their thinking and behavior, and originate solutions.

The next learning theory to be discussed combines principles from both the behaviorist and cognitive theories.

## Social Learning Theory

Most learning theories assume that the individual must have direct experiences to learn. According to early social learning theory, much of learning occurs by observation—watching other people and discerning what happens to them. Learning is often a social process, and other individuals, especially "significant others," provide compelling examples or role models for how to think, feel, and act. While Miller and Dollard (1941) viewed social learning as a mixture of behaviorist and psychodynamic influences, Bandura (1977, 1986, 2001) is credited with outlining the behaviorist, cognitive, and, more recently, social cognition dimensions of the theory. Figure 3–3 illustrates the dynamics of social learning based on Bandura's work.

FIGURE 3–3    **Social Learning Theory**  SOURCE: Based on Bandura (1977).

Role modeling is a central concept of the theory. As an example, a more experienced nurse who demonstrates desirable professional attitudes and behaviors sometimes is used as a mentor for a less experienced nurse, while medical students, interns, and residents are mentored by attending physicians. Vicarious reinforcement is another concept from the social learning theory and involves viewing other people's emotions and determining whether role models are rewarded or punished for their behavior. The behavior of a role model may be imitated, even when no reward is involved for either the role model or the learner. In many cases, however, whether the model is perceived by the observer to be rewarded or punished may have a direct influence on learning. This relationship may be one reason why it is difficult to attract health professionals to geriatric care. Although some highly impressive role models work in the field, geriatric health care is often accorded low status within the health

professions and may pay less than other specialty areas.

While social learning theory is based partially on behaviorist principles, the self-regulation and the control that the individual exhibits in the learning process are critical and reflect cognitive principles. Bandura (1977) outlined a four-step, largely internal process that directs social learning. As seen in Figure 3–3, the first phase is the attentional phase, a necessary condition for any learning to occur. Research indicates that role models with high status and competence are more likely to be observed, although the learner's own characteristics (needs, self-esteem, competence) may be the more significant determiner of attention. Second is the retention phase, which involves the storage and retrieval of what was observed. Third is the reproduction phase, where the learner copies the observed behavior. Mental rehearsal, immediate enactment, and corrective feedback strengthen the reproduction of behavior. Fourth is the motivational phase, which focuses on whether the learner is motivated to perform a certain type of behavior. Reinforcement or punishment for a role model's behavior, the learning situation, and the appropriateness of subsequent situations where the behavior is to be displayed all affect a learner's performance (Bandura, 1977; Gage & Berliner, 1998). Well suited to conducting health education and staff development training, this organized approach to learning requires attention to the social environment, the behavior to be performed, and the individual learner (Bahn, 2001).

More recently, Bandura (2001) has shifted his focus to sociocultural influences, viewing the learner as the agent through which learning experiences are filtered. As he argues, the human mind is not just reactive; it is "generative, creative, and reflective." Essentially, the individual engages in a transactional relationship between the social environment and the self, where sociocultural factors are mediated by "psychological mechanisms of the self-system to produce behavioral effects" (p. 4). In his model, Bandura stressed the internal dynamics of personal selection, intentionality, self-regulation, self-efficacy, and self-evaluation in the learning process. This perspective applies particularly well to health behaviors and partially explains why some people select positive role models and effectively regulate their attitudes, emotions, and actions, whereas other people choose negative role models and engage in unhealthy and destructive behaviors. One of Bandura's principal research findings is that self-efficacy contributes to productive human functioning. The implication is that healthcare professionals need to find ways to encourage patients' feelings of competency and to promote wellness rather than fostering dependency, helplessness, and feelings of low self-worth.

The social learning theory extends the learning process beyond the educator–learner relationship and the learner's direct experiences to the larger social world. The theory helps explain the socialization process as well as the breakdown of behavior in society. Responsibility is placed on the educator or leader to act as an exemplary role model and to choose socially healthy experiences for individuals to observe and repeat (requiring the careful evaluation of learning materials for stereotypes, mixed or hidden messages, and negative effects). However, simple exposure to competent role models correctly performing a behavior that is rewarded (or performing some undesirable behavior that is punished) does not ensure learning. Attention to the learner's "self-system" and the dynamics of self-regulation may help sort out the varying effects of the social learning experience.

In health care, social learning theory has been applied to staff training and to interventions that address public health problems such as teenage smoking and alcoholism among the elderly (Akers, 1989, 1996). The major difficulty is that this theory is complex and not easily operationalized, measured, and assessed.

The final two theories to be reviewed in this chapter focus on the importance of emotions and feelings in the learning process.

## Psychodynamic Learning Theory

Although not usually treated as a learning theory, some of the constructs from the psychodynamic theory (based on the work of Sigmund Freud and his followers) have significant implications for learning and changing behavior (Bracher, 1999; Hilgard & Bower, 1966; Notterman & Drewry, 1993). Largely a theory of motivation stressing emotions rather than cognition and responses, the psychodynamic perspective emphasizes the importance of conscious and unconscious forces in guiding behavior, personality conflicts, and the enduring effects of childhood experiences.

A central principle of the theory is that behavior may be conscious or unconscious—that is, individuals may or may not be aware of their motivations and why they feel, think, and act as they do. According to the psycho-dynamic view, the most primitive source of motivation comes from the id and is based on libidinal energy (the basic instincts, impulses, and desires we are born with), which includes eros (the desire for pleasure and sex, some-times called the "life force") and thanatos (aggressive and destructive impulses, or "death wish"). Patients who survive or die, despite all predictions to the contrary, provide illustrations of such primitive motivations. The id, according to Freud, operates on the basis of the pleasure principle—to seek pleasure and avoid pain. Dry, dull lectures given by health professionals who go through the motions of the presentation without much enthusiasm or emotion inspire few patients to listen or heed the advice. This does not mean, however, that only pleasurable presentations will be acceptable.

The id (primitive drives) and superego (internalized societal values and standards, or the "conscience") are mediated by the ego, which operates on the basis of the reality prin-ciple—rather than insisting on immediate gratification, people learn to take the long road to pleasure and to weigh the choices or dilemmas in the conflict between the id and superego. Healthy ego (self) development, as emphasized by Freud's followers, is an impor-tant consideration in the health fields. For example, patients with ego strength can cope with painful medical treatments because they recognize the long-term value of enduring discomfort and pain to achieve a positive out-come. Patients with weak ego development, in contrast, may miss their appointments and treatments or engage in short-term pleasura-ble activities that work against their healing and recovery. Helping patients develop ego strength and adjust realistically to a changed body image or lifestyle brought about by dis-ease and medical interventions is a significant aspect of the learning and healing process. Health professionals, too, require personal

ego strength to cope with the numerous predicaments in the everyday practice of med-icine, as they face conflicting values, ethics, and demands. Professional burnout, for exam-ple, is rooted in an overly idealized concept of the healthcare role and unrealistic expecta-tions for the self in performing the role.

When the ego is threatened, as can easily occur in the healthcare setting, defense mechanisms may be employed to protect the self. The short-term use of defense mecha-nisms is a way of coming to grips with real-ity. The danger comes in the overuse or long-term reliance on defense mechanisms, which allows individuals to avoid reality and may act as a barrier to learning and transfer. Table 3–2 describes some of the more com-monly used defense mechanisms. Use of defense mechanisms is not limited to patients, however; medical staff may employ them as well. Because providing health care and working in hospitals and long-term care facilities are likely to be stressful experi-ences, knowledge of defense mechanisms is essential.

As an example of defense mechanisms in health care, Elizabeth Kübler Ross (1969) pointed out that many terminally ill patients' initial reaction to being told they have a serious illness is to employ the defense mechanism of denial. It is too overwhelming for patients to process the information that they are likely to die. While most patients gradually accept the reality of their illness, the dangers are that if they remain in a state of denial, they may not seek treatment and care, and if their illness is contagious, they may not protect others against infection. A common defense mechanism employed by medical staff is to intellectualize rather than deal realistically at an emotional level with the significance of disease and death. Dehumanization and treating patients as body parts rather than as whole individuals (with spiritual, emotional, and physical needs) are occupational hazards in the health professions.

| TABLE 3–2  Ego defense mechanisms: Ways of protecting the self from perceived threat | |
|---|---|
| *Denial:* ignoring or refusing to acknowledge the reality of a threat<br>*Rationalization:* excusing or explaining away a threat<br>*Displacement:* taking out hostility and aggression on other individuals rather than directing anger at the source of the threat<br>*Repression:* keeping unacceptable thoughts, feelings, or actions from conscious awareness<br>*Regression:* returning to an earlier (less mature, more primitive) stage of behavior as a way of coping with a threat | *Intellectualization:* minimizing anxiety by responding to a threat in a detached, abstract manner without feeling or emotion<br>*Projection:* seeing one's own unacceptable characteristics or desires in other people<br>*Reaction formation:* expressing or behaving the opposite of what is really felt<br>*Sublimation:* converting repressed feelings into socially acceptable action<br>*Compensation:* making up for weaknesses by excelling in other areas |

Another central assumption of the psychodynamic theory is that personality development occurs in stages, with much of adult behavior derived from earlier childhood experiences and conflicts. One of the most widely used models of personality development is Erikson's (1968) eight stages of life, organized around a psychosocial "crisis" to be resolved at each stage.[2] Treatment regimens, communication, and health education need to include considerations of the patient's stage of personality development. For example, in working with four- and five-year-old patients, where the crisis is "initiative versus guilt," health professionals should encourage these children to offer their ideas and to make and do things themselves. Staff also must be careful not to make these children feel guilty for their illness or misfortune. As a second example, the adolescent's desire to have friends and to find an identity requires special attention in health care. Adolescent patients may need help and support adjusting to a changed body image and addressing their fears of weakness, lack of activity, and social isolation. One danger is that they may treat their illness or impairment as a significant dimension of their identity and self-concept.

According to the psychodynamic view, personal difficulties arise and learning is limited when individuals become fixated or stuck at an earlier stage of personality development. They then must work through their previously unresolved crises to develop and mature emotionally. For example, some staff members and patients feel an inordinate need to control the self, other people, and certain social situations. This behavior may be rooted in their inability to resolve the crisis between "trust versus mistrust" at the earliest stage of life. In working with these individuals, it is

---

[2] Erikson's (1968) eight stages in life and their respective crises are outlined as follows: During infancy, the psychosocial crisis to be resolved is trust versus mistrust. The early childhood years involve issues of autonomy versus doubt, followed by initiative versus guilt. The school-aged child comes to terms with industry versus inferiority. Adolescence involves the crisis of identity versus identity diffusion or confusion. Young adults attempt to resolve the crisis of intimacy versus isolation. Middle-aged adults focus on generativity versus stagnation. Older adults struggle with integrity versus despair. Erikson noted that the two most significant periods of personality growth occur during adolescence and older adulthood—an important observation for health professionals to consider when working with members of these two age groups.

essential to build a trusting relationship and to encourage them gradually to relinquish some control.

Past conflicts, especially during childhood, may interfere with the ability to learn or to transfer learning. What people resist talking about or learning, termed *resistance*, is an indicator of underlying emotional difficulties, which must be dealt with for them to move ahead emotionally and behaviorally. For instance, a young, pregnant teenager who refuses to engage in a serious conversation about sexuality (e.g., changes the subject, giggles, looks out into space, expresses anger) indicates underlying emotional conflicts that need to be addressed.

Serious problems in miscommunication can occur in health care as a result of childhood learning experiences. For example, some physicians and nurses may have had the experience as a child of standing helplessly by watching someone they love and once depended on endure disease, suffering, and death. Although they could do little as children to improve the situation, they may be compensating for their childhood feelings of helplessness and dependency as adults by devoting their careers to fending off and fighting disease and death. These motivations, however, may not serve them well as they attempt to cope, communicate, and educate dying patients and their families.

Emotional conflicts are not always due to internal forces; society exerts pressures on individuals that promote emotional difficulties as well. The reluctance of health professionals to be open and honest with a terminally ill patient partially may be derived from American culture, which encourages medical personnel to "fix" their patients and extend life. Staff members may or may not be conscious of these pressures, but either way they are likely to feel guilty and "a failure" when dealing with a dying patient.

The concept of transfer has special meaning to psychodynamic theorists. Transference occurs when individuals project their feelings, conflicts, and reactions—especially those developed during childhood with significant others such as parents—onto authority figures and other individuals in their lives. The danger is that the relationship between the health professional and the patient may become distorted and unrealistic because of the biases inherent in the transference reaction. For example, because patients are sick, they may feel helpless and dependent and then regress to an earlier stage in life when they relied on their parents for help and support. Their childhood feelings and relationship with a parent—for better or worse—may be transferred to a nurse or physician taking care of them. While sometimes flattering, the "love" and dependency that patients feel may operate against the autonomy and independence needed to "get back on their feet." A particular patient may also remind a staff member of someone from her or his past, creating a situation of countertransference.

The psychodynamic approach reminds health professionals to pay attention to emotions, unconscious motivations, and the psychological growth and development of all those involved in health care and learning. This theory is well suited to understanding patient and family noncompliance (Menahern & Halasz, 2000), trauma and loss (Duberstein & Masling, 2000), palliative care and the deeply emotional issues of terminal illness (Chochinov & Breitbart, 2000), and the stresses of working with long-term care residents (Goodwin & Gore, 2000).

One problem with the psychodynamic approach is that much of the analysis is speculative and subjective. Health professionals' biases, emotional conflicts, and needs may distort their evaluation of other persons and situations. Another caution is that the psychodynamic theory may be used inappropriately; it is not the job of health professionals with little clinical psychology or psychiatric training to probe into the private lives and feelings of patients so as to uncover deep, unconscious conflicts. A third danger is that health professionals may use the many psychodynamic principles as a way of explaining away, rather than dealing with, people as individuals who need emotional care. As an illustration, researchers found that rather than using Kübler Ross's (1969) model of death and dying to help terminally ill patients and their families discuss their fears and emotions, some health professionals used it to categorize, label, and dismiss dying patients (Dunkel-Schetter & Wortman, 1982; Pattison, 1977).

## Humanistic Learning Theory

Underlying the humanistic perspective on learning is the assumption that each individual is unique and that all individuals have a desire to grow in a positive way. Unfortunately, positive psychological growth may be damaged by some of society's values and expectations (e.g., males are less emotional than females, some ethnic groups are "inferior" to others, making money is more important than caring for people) and by adults' mistreatment of their children and each other (e.g., inconsistent or harsh discipline, humiliation and belittling, abuse and neglect). Spontaneity, the importance of emotions and feelings, the right of individuals to make their own choices, and human creativity are the cornerstones of a humanistic approach to learning (Gage & Berliner, 1998; Pine, 1977; Rogers, 1994).

Like the psychodynamic theory, the humanistic perspective is largely a motivational theory. From a humanistic perspective, motivation is derived from each person's needs, subjective feelings about the self, and the desire to grow. The transfer of learning is facilitated by curiosity, a positive self-concept, and open situations where people respect individuality and promote freedom of choice. Under such conditions, transfer is likely to be widespread, enhancing flexibility and creativity.

Maslow (1954, 1987), a major contributor to humanistic theory, is perhaps best known for identifying the hierarchy of needs (Figure 3–4), which he says play an important role in human motivation. At the bottom of the hierarchy are physiological needs (food, warmth, sleep); then come safety needs; then the need for belonging and love; followed by self-esteem. At the top of the hierarchy are self-actualization needs (maximizing one's potential). Additional considerations include cognitive needs (to know and understand) and, for some individuals, aesthetic needs (the desire for beauty). An assumption is that basic-level needs must be met before individuals can be concerned with learning and self-actualizing. Thus, clients who are hungry, tired, and in pain will be motivated to get these biological needs met before being interested in learning about their medications, rules for self-care, and health education. While intuitively appealing, research has not been able to support Maslow's hierarchy of needs with much consistency. For example, although some people's basic needs may not be met, they may nonetheless engage in creative activities, extend themselves to other people, and enjoy learning (Pfeffer, 1985).

Besides personal needs, humanists contend that self-concept and self-esteem are necessary considerations in any learning situation. The therapist Carl Rogers (1961, 1994) argued that what people want is unconditional positive self-regard (the feeling of being loved without strings attached). Experiences that are threatening, coercive, and judgmental undermine the ability and enthusiasm of individuals to learn. It is essential that those in positions of authority convey a fundamental respect for the people with whom they work. If a health professional is prejudiced against AIDS patients, then little will be healing or therapeutic in her relationship with them until she is genuinely able to feel respect for the patient as an individual.

Rather than acting as an authority, say humanists, the role of any educator or leader is to be a facilitator (Buscaglia, 1982; Rogers,

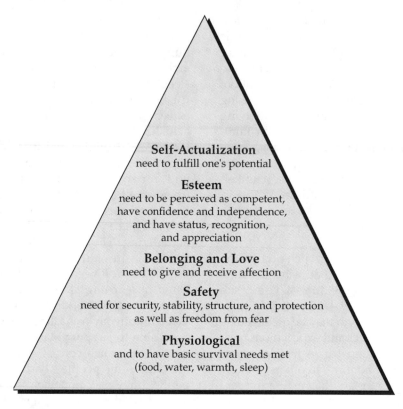

**FIGURE 3–4   Maslow's Hierarchy of Needs** SOURCE: Adapted from Maslow (1987).

1994). Listening—rather than talking—is the skill needed. Because the uniqueness of the individual is fundamental to the humanistic perspective, much of the learning experience requires a direct relationship between the educator and the learner, with instruction tailored to the needs, self-esteem, and positive growth of each learner. Learners, not educators, choose what is to be learned, and within this framework educators serve as resource persons whose job is to help guide learners to make wise choices. Mastering information and facts is not the central purpose of learning. Instead, fostering curiosity, enthusiasm, initiative, and responsibility is much more important and enduring and should be the primary goal of any educator. Rather than inserting health education videos into televi-

sion sets for hospital patients to view or routinely distributing lots of pamphlets and pages of small-print instructions, the humanist perspective would suggest establishing rapport and becoming emotionally attuned to patients and their family members.

Humanistic psychology contends that feelings and emotions are the keys to learning, communication, and understanding. Humanists worry that in today's stressful society people can easily lose touch with their feelings, which sets the stage for emotional problems and difficulties in learning (Rogers, 1961). "Tell me how you feel" is a much more important statement to humanists than "tell me what you think," as thoughts and admonitions (the latter of which Rogers calls "the shoulds") may be at odds with true feelings.

Consider the implications of the following statements: (1) a young person who says, "I know I should go to medical school and become a doctor because I am smart and that is what my parents want, but I don't feel comfortable with sick people—I don't even like them!" or (2) the dying patient who says, "I realize that I am going to die and should be brave, but I feel so sad that I am losing my family, my friends, and my self; frankly, I am afraid of dying—all the pain and suffering, being a burden—I'm scared!" In both cases, humanists would argue, the overriding factor that will affect the behavior of the young person and the dying patient is their feelings, not their cognitions.

The humanistic learning theory has modified the approach to education and changing behavior by giving primary focus to the subjective needs and feelings of the learner and by redefining the role of the educator. One study reported that medical students who selected primary care specialties had higher "humanism scores" compared to those drawn to surgery or support areas (Coutts-van Dijk, Bray, Moore, & Rogers, 1997). Humanistic principles have been a cornerstone of self-help groups, wellness programs, and palliative care. Humanistic theory has also been found to be well suited to working with children and young patients undergoing separation anxiety due to illness, surgery, and recovery (Holyoake, 1998). Within this perspective, a principal emphasis is on client-centered medicine and the need for health professionals to learn and grow from their healthcare experiences (Block & Billings, 1998).

The theory has its weaknesses as well. Research has not been able to substantiate some of its strongest claims, and the theory has been criticized for promoting self-centered learners who cannot take criticism or compromise their deeply felt positions. Charged with being more of a philosophy—or a cult—than a science, the "touchy-feely" approach of humanists makes some learners and educators feel truly uncomfortable. More-

over, information, facts, memorization, drill, practice, and the tedious work sometimes required to master knowledge, which humanists minimize and sometimes disdain, have been found to contribute to significant learning, knowledge building, and skill development (Gage & Berliner, 1992).

## COMPARISON OF LEARNING THEORIES

Table 3–3 provides a comparative summary of the five learning theories outlined in this chapter. Generalizations can be made about both the differences and the similarities in what the theories say about acquiring knowledge and changing feelings, attitudes, and behavior. With regard to some of the differences among the theories, each theory has its own assumptions, vocabulary, and way of conceptualizing the learning process. The theories differ in their emphasis on the relative influence of external or internal factors in learning, the view of the learner as more passive or active, the task of the educator, the explanation of motivation, and the way in which the transfer of learning is accomplished. A logical question is which of these five theories "best" describes or explains learning—which theory, in other words, would be the most helpful to health professionals interested in increasing knowledge or changing the behavior of patients, staff, or themselves? The answer to this question is that each theory contributes to understanding various aspects of the learning process and can be used singly and in combination to help practitioners acquire new information and alter existing thoughts, feelings, and behavior.

Each theory also gives focus to important considerations in any learning situation. For example, behaviorists urge us to pay attention to and change stimulus conditions and to provide reinforcement to alter behavior. While

**TABLE 3–3    Summary of learning theories**

| Learning Procedures | Assumptions About Learner | Educator's Task | Sources of Motivation | Transfer of Learning |
|---|---|---|---|---|
| **BEHAVIORIST** | | | | |
| Environmental stimulus conditions and reinforcement promote changes in responses. <br><br> To change behavior, change the environment. | Passive, reactive learner responds to environmental conditions (stimuli and reinforcement). | Active educator manipulates stimuli and reinforcement to direct learning and change. | Drive reduction. | Practice; similarity in stimulus conditions and responses between learning and new situations. |
| **COGNITIVE** | | | | |
| Internal perception and thought processing within context of human development promote learning and change. <br><br> To change behavior, change cognitions. | Active learner determines patterning of experiences; is strongly influenced by attributions. | Active educator structures experiences (through organization and meaningfulness) to encourage the reorganization of cognitions. | Goals. <br> Expectations. <br> Disequilibrium. | Mental and physical activity. <br> Common patterns. <br> Understanding. <br> Learning to learn. |
| **SOCIAL LEARNING** | | | | |
| External role models and their perceived reinforcement along with learner's internal influences. <br><br> To change behavior, change role models, perceived reinforcement, and the learner's self-regulating mechanisms. | Active learner observes others and regulates decision to reproduce behavior. | Active educator models behavior, encourages perception of reinforcement, carefully evaluates learning materials for social messages, and attempts to influence learner's self-regulation. | Socialization experiences, role models, and self-reactive influences (observe self, set goals, and reinforce performance). | Similarity of setting and role models' behavior. |

**TABLE 3–3 (continued)**

| Learning Procedures | Assumptions About Learner | Educator's Task | Sources of Motivation | Transfer of Learning |
|---|---|---|---|---|
| **PSYCHODYNAMIC** | | | | |
| Internal forces such as developmental stage, childhood experiences, emotional conflicts, and ego strength influence learning and change.<br><br>To change behavior, change interpretations and make unconscious motivations conscious. | Active learner's lifestyle, past experiences, and current emotional conflicts influence what is learned and how it is remembered and performed. | Educator as a reflective interpreter makes sense of learner's personality and motivation by listening and posing questions to stimulate conscious awareness, insight, and ego strength. | Pleasure principle and reality principle.<br><br>Imbalance.<br><br>Conscious and unconscious influence of conflict, development, and defense mechanisms. | Personality conflict, resistance, and transference associated with learning situations may act as barrier. |
| **HUMANISTIC** | | | | |
| Internal feelings about self, ability to make wise choices, and needs affect learning and change.<br><br>To change behavior, change feelings, self-concept, and needs. | Active learner attempts to actualize potential for positive self-growth and confirm self-concept; is spontaneous, creative, and playful. | Facilitative educator encourages positive self-growth, listens empathetically, allows freedom of choice, and respects learner. | Needs, desire for positive self-growth, and confirmation of self-concept. | Positive or negative feelings about self and freedom to learn promote or inhibit transfer. |

criticized for being reductionistic, behaviorists' emphasis on manipulating the environment and reinforcements is admittedly simpler and easier than trying to undertake a massive overhaul of an individual's internal dynamics (perceptions, cognition, memory, feelings, and personality history and conflicts). Moreover, getting someone first to behave in a more appropriate way (abstaining from bad habits and engaging in healthy behavior) may not be as threatening or daunting to the learner as it would be to suggest the need for internal personality changes. Desired responses are modified and strengthened through practice; the new learned responses, in turn, may lead to more fundamental changes in attitudes and emotions. The social learning perspective is another relatively simple theory to use, stressing the importance of effective role models, who by their example demonstrate exactly what behavior is expected.

In one way or another, the theories indicate that all the players in any learning situation are strongly influenced by the environment, society, and culture. A clash of cultures in the healthcare setting is thoroughly described in Anne Fadiman's (1997) book, *The Spirit Catches You and You Fall Down*, where a Vietnamese family with entirely different conceptions of health and illness becomes caught up in the American system of health care in California.

Cognitive, social learning, psychodynamic, and humanistic theories remind us to consider internal factors—perceptions, thoughts, ways of processing information, feelings, and emotions. These factors cannot be ignored because, ultimately, it is the learner who controls and regulates learning: how information is perceived, interpreted, and remembered, and whether the new knowledge is expressed or performed. In practice, learning theories should not be considered to be mutually exclusive but rather to operate together to change attitudes and behavior. For example, patients undergoing painful procedures are first taught systematic desensitization (behaviorist) and while experiencing pain or discomfort are encouraged to employ imagery, such as thinking about a favorite, beautiful place or imagining the healthy cells "gobbling up" the unhealthy cells (cognitive). Staff members are highly respectful, upbeat, and emotionally supportive of each patient (humanistic) and create the time and opportunity to listen to patients discuss some of their deepest fears and concerns (psychodynamic). Waiting rooms and lounge areas for patients and their families are designed to be comfortable, friendly, and pleasant to facilitate conversation and interaction (social learning).

Another generalization from this discussion is that some learning theories are better suited to certain kinds of individuals than to others. While theoretical assumptions about the learner range from passive to highly active, passive individuals may learn more effectively from behaviorist techniques, whereas curious, highly active, and self-directed persons may do better with cognitive and humanistic approaches. Also, keep in mind that some learners require external reinforcement and incentives, whereas other learners do not seem to need—and may even resent—attempts to manipulate and reinforce them. Individuals who are well educated, verbal, and reflective may be better candidates for cognitive and psychodynamic approaches, whereas behaviorist approaches may be more suitable for persons whose cognitive processes are impaired or who are uncomfortable dealing with abstractions or scrutinizing and communicating their thoughts and emotions. In addition, each individual's preferred modes of learning and processing may help determine the selection of suitable theoretical approaches. That is, while some individuals learn by acting and responding (behaviorist), the route to learning for others may be through perceptions and thoughts (cognitive) or through feelings and emotions (humanistic and psychodynamic). Most people appear to benefit from demonstration and example (social learning).

## ◼ COMMON PRINCIPLES OF LEARNING

Taken together, the theories discussed in this chapter indicate that learning is a more complicated process than any one theory implies. Besides the distinct considerations for learning suggested by each theory, these perspectives' similarities point to some core features of learning. The issues raised at the beginning of the chapter can be addressed by synthesizing the learning theories and identifying their common principles.

### How Does Learning Occur?

Learning takes place as individuals interact with their environment and incorporate new information or experiences with what they already know or have learned. Factors in the environment that affect learning include the society and culture, the structure or pattern of stimuli, the effectiveness of role models and reinforcements, feedback for correct and incorrect responses, and opportunities to process and apply learning to new situations. The individual exerts significant control over learning, often involving considerations of his or her developmental stage, past history (habits, cultural conditioning, socialization, childhood experiences and conflicts), cognitive style, dynamics of self-regulation, conscious and unconscious motivations, personality (stage, conflicts, self-concept), and emotions. Learners often have a preferred mode for taking in information (visual, motor, auditory, or symbolic) and, while some individuals may learn best on their own, others will benefit from expert guidance, social interaction, and cooperative learning.

A critical influence on whether learning occurs is motivation (see Chapter 6 on motivation). The learning theories reviewed here suggest that to learn, the individual must want to gain something (receive rewards and pleasure, meet goals and needs, confirm expectations, grow in positive ways, resolve conflicts), which in turn arouses the learner by creating tension (drives to be reduced, disequilibrium and imbalance) and the propensity to act or change behavior. The relative success or failure of the learner's performance may affect subsequent learning experiences. In some cases, an inappropriate, maladaptive, or harmful previously learned behavior may need to be extinguished and then replaced with a more positive response. It is, of course, easier to instill new learning than to correct faulty learning.

### What Kinds of Experiences Facilitate or Hinder the Learning Process?

The educator's selection of learning theories and structuring of the learning experience become important in this realm. To be effective, educators must have knowledge (of the material to be learned, the learner, the social context, and educational psychology), and they must be competent (be imaginative, flexible, and able to employ teaching methods; display solid communication skills; and have the ability to motivate others). All the learning theories discussed in this chapter acknowledge the need to recognize and relate the new information to the learner's past experiences (old habits, culture, familiar patterns, childhood memories, feelings about the self, and what is valued, normative, and perceived as successful or rewarded in society).

Ignoring these considerations, of course, may hinder learning. Other impediments to learning may involve a lack of clarity and meaningfulness in what is to be learned, neglect or harsh punishment, fear, negative or ineffective role models, and rewards for unhealthy behavior, confusing reinforcement, and inappropriate materials for the individual's ability, readiness to learn, or stage of life-cycle development. Moreover, individuals are unlikely to want to learn who have had detrimental socialization experiences, are deprived of stimulating environments, and are without goals and realistic expectations for themselves.

## What Helps Ensure That Learning Becomes Relatively Permanent?

First, the likelihood of learning is enhanced by organizing the learning experience, making it meaningful and pleasurable, and by pacing the presentation in keeping with the learner's ability to process information. Second, practicing (mentally and physically) new knowledge

or skills under varied conditions strengthens learning.

The third issue concerns reinforcement. Although reinforcement may or may not be necessary, some theorists have argued that it may be helpful because it serves as a signal to the individual that learning has occurred (Hill, 1990).

A fourth consideration involves whether learning transfers beyond the initial educational setting. Learning cannot be assumed to be relatively lasting or permanent; it must be assessed and evaluated soon after the learning experience as well as by follow-up measurements at later times. Research skills, knowledge of evaluation procedures, and the willingness and resources to engage in educational assessment are now considered essential aspects of the learning process. Evaluation feedback can then be used to revamp and revitalize learning experiences.

## SUMMARY

This chapter demonstrates that learning is complex. Readers may feel overwhelmed by the diverse theories, sets of learning principles, and cautions associated with employing the various approaches. Yet, like the blind men exploring the elephant, each theory highlights an important dimension that affects the overall learning process, and together the theories provide a wealth of complementary strategies and alternative options. There is, of course, no single best way to approach learn-

ing, although all the theories indicate the need to be sensitive to the unique characteristics and motivations of each learner. Health professionals and educators cannot be expected to know everything about the learning process. More important, perhaps, is that they can determine what needs to be known, where to find the necessary information, and how to help others benefit directly from a learning experience.

## REVIEW QUESTIONS

1. What are the five (5) major learning theories discussed in this chapter?
2. What are the principal constructs of each of the five learning theories?
3. According to the Operant Conditioning Model, what are three (3) techniques to increase the probability of a response, and what are two (2)

    techniques to decrease or extinguish the probability of a response?

4. Each cognitive perspective discussed in the chapter focuses on a particular feature of cognition in the learning process. What contribution does each of the following perspectives make to help us understand the cognitive learning

process: gestalt, information-processing, developmental, social constructivist, and social cognition? Write one sentence describing the contribution of each perspective.

5. How do the major learning theories compare to one another with regard to their similarities and differences? Give examples of the ways that various learning theories are similar and how they differ.

6. How does motivation serve as the critical influence on whether learning occurs or not?

7. What kinds of experiences facilitate learning, and what sorts of experiences hinder the learning process?

8. What factors help ensure that learning becomes relatively permanent? Give examples.

## REFERENCES

Akers, R. L. (1989). Social learning theory and alcohol behavior among the elderly. *Sociological Quarterly, 30*, 625–638.

Akers, R. L. (1996). A longitudinal test of social learning theory: Adolescent smoking. *Journal of Drug Issues, 26*, 317–343.

Alberto, P. & Troutman, A. C. (1990). *Applied Behavior Analysis for Teachers: Influencing Student Performance*, 3rd ed. Columbus, OH: Merrill.

Bahn, D. (2001). Social learning theory: Its application to the context of nurse education. *Nurse Education Today, 21*, 110–117.

Baker, J. C. (1998). *A Neural Network Guide to Teaching.* Bloomington, IN: Phi Delta Kappa Foundation.

Baltes, P. B., Staudinger, U. M., & Lindenberger, U. (1999). Lifespan psychology: Theory and application to intellectual functioning. *Annual Review of Psychology, 50*, 471–507.

Bandura, A. (1977). *Social Learning Theory.* Englewood Cliffs, NJ: Prentice-Hall.

Bandura, A. (1986). *Foundations of Thought and Action: A Social-Cognitive Theory.* Englewood Cliffs, NJ: Prentice-Hall.

Bandura, A. (2001). Social cognitive theory: An agentic perspective. *Annual Review of Psychology, 52*, 1–26.

Berliner, D. C. & Calfee, R. C. (eds.) (1996). *Handbook of Educational Psychology.* New York: Simon & Schuster Macmillan.

Bigge, M. L. & Shermis, S. S. (1992). *Learning Theories for Teachers*, 5th ed. New York: HarperCollins.

Block, S. & Billings, J. A. (1998). Nurturing humanism through teaching palliative care. *Academic Medicine, 73*, 763–765.

Bootzin, R. R. (1975). *Behavior Modification and Therapy.* Cambridge, MA: Winthrop.

Bracher, M. (1999). Psychoanalysis and education. *Journal for the Psychoanalysis of Culture and Society, 4*, 175–192.

Brien, R. & Eastmond, N. (1994). *Cognitive Science and Instruction.* Englewood Cliffs, NJ: Educational Technology Publications.

Buscaglia, L. (1982). *Living, Loving and Learning.* New York: Fawcett Columbine.

Chochinov, H. M. & Breitbart, W. (eds.). (2000). *Handbook of Psychiatry in Palliative Medicine.* New York: Oxford University Press.

Coutts-van Dijk, L. C., Bray, J. H., Moore, S., & Rogers, J. (1997). Prospective study of how students' humanism and psycholocial beliefs relate to specialty matching. *Academic Medicine, 72*, 1106–1108.

DeGrandpre, R. J. (2000). A science of meaning: Can behaviorism bring meaning to psychological science? *American Psychologist, 55*, 721–739.

Deyl, S. G. & Kaliappan, K. V. (1997). Improvement of psychosomatic disorders among tension headache subjects using behaviour therapy and Somatic Inkblot Series. *Journal of Projective Psychology and Mental Health 4*, 113–120.

Duberstein, P. R. & Masling, J. M. (eds.). (2000). *Psychodynamic Perspectives on Sickness and Health.* Washington, DC: American Psychological Association.

DuHamel, K. N., Ostroff, J. S., Bovbjerg, D. H., Pfeffer, M., Morasco, B. J., Papadopoulos, E., & Redd, W. H. (2000). Trauma-focused intervention after bone marrow transplantation: A case study. *Behavior Therapy, 31*, 175–186.

Dunkel-Schetter, C. & Wortman, C. B. (1982). The interpersonal dynamics of career: Problems in social relationships and their impact on the patient. In H. Freeman (ed.), *Interpersonal Issues in Health Care* (pp. 69–100). New York: Academic Press.

Erikson, E. (1968). *Identity: Youth and Crisis*. New York: Norton.

Fadiman, A. (1997). *The Spirit Catches You and You Fall Down*. New York: Farrar Straus & Giroux.

Farnham-Diggory, S. (1992). *Cognitive Processes in Education*, 2nd ed. New York: HarperCollins.

Fiske, S. T. & Taylor, S. E. (1991). *Social Cognition*. New York: McGraw-Hill.

Gage, N. L. & Berliner, D. C. (1992). *Educational Psychology*, 5th ed. Boston: Houghton Mifflin.

Gage, N. L. & Berliner, D. C. (1998). *Educational Psychology*, 6th ed. Boston: Houghton Mifflin.

Gagné, R. M. (1985). *The Conditions of Learning*, 4th ed. New York: Holt, Rinehart & Winston.

Gagné, R. M., Briggs, L. J., & Wagner, W. W. (1992). *Principles of Instructional Design*, 4th ed. Fort Worth, TX: HBJ College Publishers.

Garcia, C., Baker, S., & deMayo, R. (1999). Academic anxieties: A gestalt approach. *Gestalt Review*, 3, 239–250.

Gardner, H. (1978). *Developmental Psychology: An Introduction*. Boston: Little, Brown.

Gilligan, C. (1982). *In a Different Voice: Psychological Theory and Women's Development*. Cambridge, MA: Harvard University Press.

Gluck, M. A. & Myers, C. E. (1997). Psychobiological models of hippocampal function in learning and memory. *Annual Review of Psychology, 48*, 481–514.

Goleman, D. (1995). *Emotional Intelligence*. New York: Bantum Books.

Goodwin, A. M. & Gore, V. (2000). Managing the stresses of nursing people with severe and enduring mental illness: A psychodynamic observation study of a long-stay psychiatric ward. *British Journal of Medical Psychology, 73*, 311–325.

Hilgard, E. R. (1996). History of educational psychology. In D. C. Berliner & R. C. Calfee (eds.), *Handbook of Educational Psychology* (pp. 990–1004). New York: Simon & Schuster Macmillan.

Hilgard, E. R. & Bower, G. H. (1966). *Theories of Learning*, 3rd ed. New York: Appleton-Century-Crofts.

Hill, W. F. (1990). *Learning: A Survey of Psychological Interpretations*, 5th ed. New York: Harper & Row.

Holyoake, D. D. (1998). A little lady called Pandora: An exploration of philosophical traditions of humanism and existentialism in nursing ill children. *Child Care, Health and Development, 24*, 325–336.

Hooyman, N. & Kiyak, H. A. (1999). *Social Gerontology*, 5th ed. Boston: Allyn & Bacon.

Klein, S. B. & Mowrer, R. R. (eds.). (1989). *Contemporary Learning Theories: Pavlovian Conditioning and the Status of Traditional Learning Theory*. Hillsdale, NJ: Lawrence Erlbaum.

Kohlberg, L. (1984). *The Psychology of Moral Development: The Nature and Validity of Moral Stages*. San Francisco: Harper & Row.

Kohler, W. (1947). *Gestalt Psychology*. New York: Mentor Books.

Kohler, W. (1969). *The Task of Gestalt Psychology*. Princeton, NJ: Princeton University Press.

Kramer, D. A. (1983). Post-formal operations? A need for further conceptualization. *Human Development, 26*, 91–105.

Kübler Ross, E. (1969). *On Death and Dying*. New York: Macmillan.

Lambert, P. A. & McCombs, B. L. (1998). Introduction: Learner-centered schools and classrooms as a direction for school reform. In N. M. Lambert & B. L. McCombs (eds.), *How Students Learn: Reforming Schools Through Learner-Centered Education* (pp. 1–22). Washington, DC: American Psychological Association.

Lewis, F. M. & Daltroy, L. H. (1990). How causal explanations influence health behavior: Attribution theory. In K. Glanz, F. M. Lewis, & B. K. Rimer (eds.), *Health Education and Health Behavior: Theory, Research and Practice*. San Francisco: Jossey-Bass.

Marshall, H. H. (1998). Teaching educational psychology: Learner-centered constructivist perspectives. In N. M. Lambert & B. L. McCombs (eds.), *How Students Learn: Reforming Schools Through Learner-Centered Education* (pp. 449–473). Washington, DC: American Psychological Association.

Maslow, A. (1954). *Motivation and Personality*. New York: Harper & Row.

Maslow, A. (1987). *Motivation and Personality*, 3rd ed. New York: Harper & Row.

McCullough, L. & Andrews, S. (2001). Assimilative integration: Short-term dynamic psychotherapy for treating affect phobias. *Clinical Psychology Science and Practice, 8*, 82–97.

Menahern, S. & Halasz, G. (2000). Parental noncompliance—a paediatric dilemma: A medical and psychodynamic perspective. *Child Care, Health and Development, 26,* 61–72.

Miller, N. E. & Dollard, J. (1941). *Social Learning and Imitation.* New Haven, CT: Yale University Press.

Notterman, J. M. & Drewry, H. N. (1993). *Psychology and Education.* New York: Plenum.

Palincsar, A. S. (1998). Social constructivist perspectives on teaching and learning. *Annual Review of Psychology, 49,* 345–375.

Pattison, E. M. (1977). *The Experience of Dying.* Englewood Cliffs, NJ: Prentice-Hall.

Pfeffer, J. (1985). Organizations and organizational theory. In G. Lindzey & E. Aronson (eds.), *Handbook of Social Psychology,* 3rd ed., vol. 1, *Theory and Method* (pp. 379–440). New York: Random House.

Piaget, J. & Inhelder, B. (1969). *The Psychology of the Child* (H. Weaver, trans.). New York: Basic Books.

Piane, G. (2000). Contingency contracting and systematic desensitization for heroin addicts in methadone maintenance programs. *Journal of Psychoactive Drugs, 32,* 311–319.

Pine, G. J. (1977). *Learner-Centered Teaching: A Humanistic View.* Denver, CO: Love.

Proctor, R., Burns, A., Powell, H. S., & Tarrier, N. (1999). Behavioural management in nursing and residential homes: A randomized controlled trial. *Lancet, 354,* 26–29.

Quadagno, J. (1999). *Aging and the Life Course: An Introduction to Social Gerontology.* Boston: McGraw-Hill.

Redman, B. L. (2001). *The Practice of Patient Education,* 9th ed. St. Louis: Mosby.

Rogers, C. (1961). *On Becoming a Person.* Boston: Houghton Mifflin.

Rogers, C. (1994). *Freedom to Learn,* 3rd ed. New York: Merrill.

Sherif, C. W. (1976). *Orientation in Social Psychology.* New York: Harper & Row.

Sherif, M. & Sherif, C. W. (1969). *Social Psychology.* New York: Harper & Row.

Skinner, B. F. (1974). *About Behaviorism.* New York: Vintage Books.

Skinner, B. F. (1989). *Recent Issues in the Analysis of Behavior.* Columbus, OH: Merrill.

Sprenger, M. (1999). *Learning and Memory: The Brain in Action.* Alexandria, VA: Association for Supervision and Curriculum Development.

Sternberg, R. J. (1991). A triarchic model for teaching intellectual skills. In A. McKeough & J. L. Lupart (eds.), *Toward the Practice of Theory-Based Instruction* (pp. 92–116). Hillsdale, NJ: Lawrence Erlbaum.

Sternberg, R. J. (1996). Styles of thinking. In P. B. Baltes & U. M. Staudinger (eds.), *Interactive Minds: Life-Span Perspectives on the Social Foundation of Cognition* (pp. 347–365). New York: Cambridge University Press.

Tatman, A. W. & Gilgen, A. R. (1999). Authorities and research emphasized in the Annual Review of Psychology, 1975–1998. *Psychological Reports, 85,* 89–100.

Taylor, S. E. (1999). *Health Psychology,* 4th ed. Boston: McGraw-Hill.

Vander Zanden, J. W., Crandell, T. L., & Crandell, C. H. (2000). *Human Development,* 7th ed. Boston: McGraw-Hill.

Vygotsky, L. S. (1986). *Thought and Language.* Cambridge, MA: MIT Press.

Wolpe, J. (1982). *The Practice of Behavior Therapy,* 3rd ed. New York: Pergamon.

Woolfolk, A. E. (2001). *Educational Psychology.* Boston: Allyn & Bacon.

# PART II

# Characteristics of the Learner

# Determinants of Learning

*Sharon Kitchie*

## KEY TERMS

determinants of learning
learning needs

readiness to learn
learning styles

## OBJECTIVES

After completing this chapter, the reader will be able to

1. State the nurse educator's role in the learning process.
2. Identify the three components of what is known as "determinants of learning."
3. Describe the steps involved in the assessment of learning needs.

4. Explain methods that can be used to assess learner needs.
5. Discuss the factors that need to be assessed in each of the four types of readiness to learn.
6. Describe what is meant by learning styles.
7. Discriminate between the major learning styles identified.
8. Discuss ways to assess learning styles.

In a variety of settings, nurses are responsible for the education of patients, families, nursing staff, other healthcare staff, and nursing students. Several factors have made using principles of learning particularly challenging for the nurse educator to meet learners' needs for information. For example, same-day surgery has compressed patient and family contact with the nurse. Often the teachable moment is hard to capture because of shortened hospital stays. In the case of staff, many times the difficulty with meeting learners' needs arises because of the various educational and experiential levels of staff and time constraints in the practice arena.

To meet these challenges, the nurse educator must know what determines how well a person learns. The determinants are (a) assessing the needs of the learner, (b) recognizing factors involved in the readiness to learn, and (c) being able to correlate teaching interventions with learning styles to maximize opportunities for learning. This chapter will address the determinants of learning in relation to the patient teaching and staff education component of the practice of nursing.

## THE EDUCATOR'S ROLE IN LEARNING

The role of educating can be one of the most challenging and essential interventions that a nurse performs. To do it well, the nurse must identify the information learners need as well as consider their readiness to learn and their styles of learning. Nevertheless, the learner remains the single most important person in the education process. Learning can actually occur without an educator, but it is enhanced by the addition of an educator who can serve as a facilitator. Just providing information to the learner, however, does not ensure that learning will occur. There is no guarantee that the learner will learn the information given, although there is more of an opportunity to learn if the educator assesses the determinants of learning.

Assessment permits the nurse, as an educator, to facilitate the process of learning by arranging experiences within the environment so as to help the learner find meaning and purpose for learning. That is, an assessment of the determinants of learning enables the educator to present information in a variety of ways, which a learner cannot do alone. The educator manipulates the environment so that learners experience meaningful parts and wholes to reach their unique potential. This strategy helps the learner to incorporate the information into his or her behavior. The educator plays a crucial role in the learning process by (a) assessing problems or deficits, (b) providing appropriate information and presenting it in unique ways, (c) identifying progress being made, (d) giving feedback and follow-up, (e) reinforcing learning in the acquisition of knowledge, the performance of a skill, or a change in attitude, and (f) evaluating learners' abilities.

The educator is vital in giving support, encouragement, and direction during the process of learning. Learners may make self-choices without the assistance of an educator, but these choices may be limited or inappropriate. The educator can help to identify optimal learning approaches and then provide assistance in choosing learning activities that can both support and challenge the learner based on his or her individual learning needs, readiness to learn, and learning style.

## ASSESSMENT OF THE LEARNER

The importance of assessment of the learner may seem self-evident, but often only lip service is given to this phase of the educational process. Often patients with the same condition are taught with the same materials in the same way (Haggard, 1989). The result is that information given to the patient is neither individualized nor based on the educational assessment. Frequently, the nurse delves into teaching before addressing all of the *determinants of learning*. Nursing assessment of needs, readiness, and styles of learning is the first and most important step in instructional design—but it is also the step most often neglected. For years nurses have been taught that any nursing intervention should be preceded by an assessment. Few would deny that this is the correct approach, no matter whether planning for giving direct physical care, meeting the psychosocial needs of a patient, or teaching someone to be independent in self-care or the delivery of care. The effectiveness of nursing interventions clearly depends on the scope, accuracy, and comprehensiveness of assessment prior to interventions. What is it about assessment that is so significant and fundamental to the educational process, and why is it often overlooked or only partially carried out?

This initial step in the educational process helps validate the need for learning and the approach to be used in designing learning experiences. Persons who desire or require information to maintain optimal health as well as staff nurses who must have a greater scope or depth of knowledge to deliver quality care to patients deserve to have an assessment done by the educator so that the needs of the learner are appropriately addressed. Many factors must be considered with respect to the three determinants of learning, and assessments of all three should be based on theories, concepts, and principles. Assessments do more than simply identify and prioritize information for purposes of setting behavioral goals and objectives, planning instructional interventions, and being able to evaluate in the long run whether the learner has achieved the desired goals and objectives. Good assessments ensure that optimal learning will occur with the least amount of stress and anxiety for the learner. Assessment prevents needless repetition of known material,

saves time and energy on the part of both the learner and the educator, and helps to establish rapport between the two parties (Haggard, 1989). Furthermore, it increases the motivation to learn by focusing on what the patient or staff member feels is most important to know or to be able to do.

Lack of time—the result of such factors as shortened hospital stays and limited contact in other settings with patients and families as well as tighter schedules of nursing staff as a result of increased practice demands—has often led nurse educators to shortchange the assessment phase. In addition, many nurses, although expected and required to instruct others, are unfamiliar with the concepts and techniques of teaching. The nurse in the role of educator must become more familiar and comfortable with all the elements of instructional design, but particularly with the assessment phase, because it provides the foundation for the rest of the educational process. Because of time constraints, which are major concerns when having to teach, nurses must become skilled in accurately carrying out assessments so as to have reserve time left for actual teaching.

Assessment of the learner includes attending to the three determinants (Haggard, 1989):

1. Learning needs (*what* the learner needs to learn)

2. Readiness to learn (*when* the learner is receptive to learning)

3. Learning style (*how* the learner best learns)

## ASSESSING LEARNING NEEDS

Of the three determinants, learning needs must be examined first because there may be no reason to assess readiness to learn or learning styles if, by chance, learning needs are nonexistent. Assessment is essential to determine learning needs so that an instructional plan can be designed to address deficits in any of the cognitive, affective, or psychomotor domains (Gessner, 1989). The purposes of assessing learning needs are to discover what has to be taught and to determine the extent of instruction or if instruction is necessary at all.

Not every individual perceives a need for education. Consequently, an assessment is used to identify and prioritize the needs and interests of the learner. This information, in turn, is used to set objectives and plan appropriate and effective teaching methodologies whereby education can begin at a point suitable to the learner rather than from an unknown or inappropriate place. Significant differences have been found between the perception of needs identified by patients versus the needs identified by nurses caring for them. In one study, there was only a 20% nurse–patient agreement score with respect to congruency on problems identified (Roberts, 1982).

*Learning needs* are defined as gaps in knowledge that exist between a desired level of performance and the actual level of performance (Healthcare Education Association, 1985). A learning need is the gap between what someone knows and what someone needs to know. Such gaps exist because of a lack of knowledge, attitude, or skill.

Most learners—90% to 95% of them, according to the estimates of many educators in educational psychology (Bloom, 1968; Carroll, 1963; Bruner, 1966; Skinner, 1954)—can master a subject with a high degree of success if given sufficient time and appropriate types of help. It is the task of the educator to determine exactly what needs to be learned and to identify an approach for presenting the material that will be best understood by the learner. That is, the teacher must first discover the needs of the learner and then find the most appropriate means of instruction that will enable the learner to master the subject under consideration.

The following are important steps in the assessment of learning needs:

1. *Identify the learner.* Who is the audience? If the audience is one individual, is there a single need or do many needs have to be fulfilled? Is there more than one learner? If so, are their needs congruent or diverse? The development of formal and informal education programs for patients and their families, nursing staff, or students must be based on accurate identification of the learner. For example, an educator may believe that all postpartum mothers need a formal class on safety issues for the newborn. This perception may be based on the educator's interaction with one patient and may not be true of all postpartum mothers. The manager of a healthcare agency might request an in-service workshop for all staff on documentation of infection control because of an isolated incident involving one staff member's failing to report the time at which isolation techniques were begun. This break in protocol may or may not indicate that everyone needs to have an update.

2. *Choose the right setting.* Establishing a trusting environment will help learners feel a sense of security in confiding information, believe their concerns are taken seriously and considered important, and feel respected. Assuring privacy and confidentiality is essential to establishing a trusting relationship (Rankin & Stallings, 2001).

3. *Collect data on the learner.* Once the learner is identified, the educator can determine characteristic needs of the population by exploring typical health problems or issues of interest to that population. Subsequently, a literature search can assist in identifying the type and extent of content to be included in teaching sessions as well as the educational strategies for teaching a specific population based on the analysis of needs.

4. *Include the learner as a source of information.* Learners themselves are usually the most important source of needs assessment data. Allow the patient and/or family members to

identify what is important to them, what types of social support systems are available or perceived to be available, and how their social support system can help. If the audience for teaching consists of staff members or students, solicit them for information as to those areas of practice in which they feel they need new or additional information. Actively engaging learners in defining their own problems and needs allows them to learn in the process and also motivates them to learn because they have an investment in planning for a program specifically tailored to their unique circumstances.

**5.** *Involve members of the healthcare team.* Other healthcare professionals may have insight into patient or family needs or the educational needs of the nursing staff or stu-

dents as a result of their frequent contacts with consumers as well as caregivers. Nurses are not the sole teachers, and they must remember to collaborate with other members of the healthcare team for a richer assessment of learning needs. In addition, associations such as the American Heart Association, March of Dimes, American Diabetes Association, and Muscular Dystrophy Association are examples of organizations within the healthcare field that are also excellent sources of information.

**6.** *Prioritize needs.* A list of needs can become endless and seemingly impossible to accomplish. Maslow's (1970) hierarchy of human needs may help the educator prioritize identified learning needs (Figure 4–1). The educator can then assist the learner to meet the most

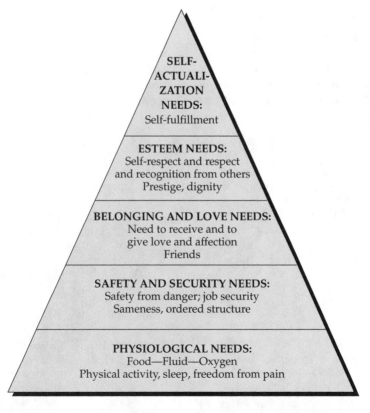

FIGURE 4–1  **Maslow's Hierarchy of Needs**  SOURCE: Reprinted from M. Lafleur-Brooks, *Health Unit Coordinating.* p. 48, Philadelphia: W.B. Saunders, 1979.

basic needs first. Learning of other needs will be delayed if basic needs are not attended to first and foremost. For example, learning about a low-sodium diet will not occur if a patient faces problems with basic physiological needs such as pain and discomfort; the latter needs must be addressed before any other learning can occur.

Setting priorities for learning is often difficult when faced with many learning needs in several areas. An effort to prioritize the identified needs will help the patient or nursing staff to set realistic and achievable learning goals. Choosing what information to cover is imperative, and choices must be made deliberately. Learning needs must be prioritized based on the criteria in Table 4–1 (Healthcare Education Association, 1985, p. 23) to foster maximum learning. Not all learners need to know everything, and assessment can help to discriminate the "need to know" from the "nice to know" information. If patients want to know the pathophysiology of their disease, that curiosity is fine, but it is not fundamental to learning how to carry out self-care activities that are essential for discharge from the hospital. A good analogy to remember is that one does not have to know how an engine works to be able to drive a car. Often, highly technical information will serve only to confuse and distract patients from learning what they need to know to comply with their regimen (Ruzicki, 1989; Hansen & Fisher, 1998). Some needs may not be amenable to education. It is important to sort out types of learning needs from nonlearning needs. This will help the educator know when action other than education would be more appropriate.

Education in and of itself is not always the answer to a problem. Often, healthcare providers believe that more education is necessary when something goes wrong, when something is not being done, when a patient is not following a prescribed regimen, or when a staff member does not adhere to a protocol. In such instances, always look for other needs that are nonlearning. For example, the nurse may discover that the patient is not taking his medication and may begin a teaching plan without adequate assessment. The patient may already understand the importance of taking a prescribed medication, know how to administer it, and be willing to follow regimen but may

---

**TABLE 4–1    Criteria for prioritizing learning needs**

*Mandatory:* Needs that must be learned for survival or situations in which the learner's life or safety is threatened. Learning needs in this category must be met immediately. For example, a patient who has experienced a recent heart attack needs to know the signs and symptoms and when to get immediate help. The nurse who works in a hospital must learn how to do cardiopulmonary resuscitation or be able to carry out correct isolation techniques for self-protection.

*Desirable:* Needs that are not life-dependent but are related to well-being or the overall ability to provide quality care in situations involving changes in institutional procedure. For example, it is important for patients who have cardiovascular disease to understand the effects of a high-fat diet on their condition. It is desirable for nurses to update their knowledge by attending an in-service program when hospital management decides to focus more attention on the appropriateness of patient education materials in relation to the patient populations being served.

*Possible:* Needs for information that are "nice to know" but not essential or required or situations in which the learning need is not directly related to daily activities. The patient who is newly diagnosed as having diabetes mellitus most likely does not need to know about traveling across time zones or staying in a foreign country because this information does not relate to the patient's everyday activities.

not have the finances necessary to purchase the medication. In this case, the patient does not have a learning need but rather requires help in exploring financing options or mechanisms to be able to obtain the medication.

**7.** *Determine availability of educational resources.* A need may be identified, but it may be useless to proceed with interventions if the proper educational resources are not available, are unrealistic to obtain, or do not match the learner's needs. In this case, it may be better to focus on other identified needs. For example, a patient who has asthma needs to learn how to use an inhaler and peak-flow meter. The nurse educator may determine that this patient learns best if the nurse first gives a demonstration on the use of the inhaler and peak-flow meter and then allows the patient the opportunity to do a return demonstration. If the proper equipment is not available for demonstration/return demonstration at that moment, it might be better for the nurse educator to concentrate on teaching the signs and symptoms the patient might experience when having poor air exchange than to cancel the encounter altogether. Thereafter, the educator would work immediately on obtaining the necessary equipment for future encounters.

**8.** *Assess demands of the organization.* This assessment will yield information that reflects the climate of the organization. What is the organization's philosophy, mission, strategic plan, and goals? The educator should be familiar with standards of performance required in various employee categories, along with job descriptions and hospital, professional, and agency regulations. If, for example, the organization is focused on health promotion versus trauma care, then there likely will be a different educational focus or emphasis that dictates learning needs of both consumers and employees.

**9.** *Take time-management issues into account.* Because time constraints are a major impediment to the assessment process,

Rankin and Stallings (2001) suggest the educator should emphasize some important points with respect to time-management issues:

- Although close observation and active listening take time, it is much more efficient and effective to do a good initial assessment than to have to waste time going back to discover the obstacles to learning that prevented progress in the first place.

- Learners must be given time to offer their own perceptions of their learning needs if the educator expects them to take charge and become actively involved in the learning process.

- Assessment can be made anytime and anywhere the educator has formal or informal contact with learners. Data collection does not have to be restricted to a specific, predetermined schedule. With patients, many potential opportunities arise, such as when giving a bath, serving a meal, making rounds, distributing medications, and so forth. For staff, assessments can be made when stopping to talk in the hallway or while enjoying lunch or break time together.

- Informing someone ahead of time that the educator wishes to spend time discussing problems or needs gives the person advanced notice to sort out his or her thoughts and feelings.

- Minimizing interruptions and distractions during planned assessment interviews maximizes productivity such that the educator might accomplish in 15 minutes what otherwise might have taken the educator an hour in less directed, more frequently interrupted circumstances.

## METHODS TO ASSESS LEARNING NEEDS

The nurse in the role of educator must obtain objective data about the learner as well as subjective data from the learner. The following are various methods that can be used to assess learner needs and should be used in conjunction with one another to yield the most reliable information (Haggard, 1989).

## Informal Conversations

Often learning needs will be discovered during informal conversations that take place with other healthcare team members involved in the care of the client, and between the nurse and the patient or his or her family. The nurse educator must rely on active listening. Other staff can provide valuable input about what they perceive to be the needs of the client. Open-ended questions posed to the client will encourage learners to reveal information about what they perceive their learning needs to be.

## Structured Interviews

The structured interview is perhaps the most common form of needs assessment to solicit the learner's point of view. The nurse asks the learner direct and often predetermined questions to gather information about learning needs. As with the gathering of any information from a learner in the assessment phase, the nurse should strive to establish a trusting environment, use open-ended questions, choose a setting that is free of distractions, and allow the learner to state what is believed to be the learning needs. It is important to remain nonjudgmental when collecting information about the learner's strengths, beliefs, and motivations. Notes should be taken with the learner's permission, so important information is not lost. The telephone is a good tool to use for an interview if it is impossible to ask questions in person. The major drawback of a telephone interview, however, is the inability on the part of the nurse educator to perceive nonverbal cues from the learner.

Interviews yield answers that may reveal uncertainties, conflicts, inconsistencies, unex-

pected problems, anxieties, fears, and present knowledge base. Examples of questions that could be asked of a patient as learner are as follows:

- What do you think caused your problem?
- How severe is your illness?
- What does your illness/health mean to you?
- What do you do to stay healthy?
- What results do you hope to obtain from treatments?
- What are your strengths and weaknesses?

If the learner is a staff member or student, the following questions could be asked:

- What do you think you will have the most problem in learning?
- Is there any skill that you have doubts you can perform?
- What problems have you encountered in the past when you had to deal with a patient who had this illness?
- What do you see as your strengths and weaknesses?

These types of questions help to determine the needs of the learner and serve as a foundation for beginning to plan for the education of the learner.

## Focus Groups

Focus groups involve getting together a small number (4 to 12) of potential learners (Breitrose, 1988) to determine areas of educational need by using group discussion to identify points of view or knowledge about a certain topic. A facilitator leads the discussion by asking questions. The questions are open-ended, and detailed discussion of each question is encouraged by the facilitator. These groups of potential learners should be homogeneous with similar characteristics such as age, gender, and past experience with the topic under discussion. However, if the purpose of the focus group is to solicit attitudes about a particular subject or to discuss ethical issues, for example, it may not be necessary to have a homogeneous group.

## Self-Administered Questionnaires

The learner's written responses to questions about learning needs can be obtained by self-administered questionnaires. Checklists are one of the most common forms of question-naires. They are easy to administer, provide more privacy than interviews, and yield easy-to-tabulate data. Learners seldom object to this method of obtaining information about their learning needs. Because checklists usu-ally reflect what the nurse educator perceives as needs, there should also be a space for the learner to add any other items of interest or concern.

## Tests

Written pretests given before teaching is planned can help identify the knowledge level of the potential learner regarding a particular subject and assist in identifying specific needs of the learner. This approach also prevents the educator from repeating already known material in the teaching plan. Furthermore, pretest results are useful to the educator after the completion of teaching to determine whether learning has taken place by comparing pretest scores to post-test scores.

## Observations

Observations can provide useful data related to needs. Observing health behaviors in sev-eral different time periods can help to deter-mine established patterns of behavior. It must be remembered that conclusions cannot be drawn from a single observation. Actually watching the learner perform a skill more than once is an excellent way of assessing a psychomotor need. Are all steps performed correctly? Is there any difficulty with manipu-lating various equipment? Does the learner require prompting? Learners may believe they can accurately perform a skill or task (e.g., walking with crutches, changing a dress-ing, giving an injection), but the educator can best determine what additional learning may be needed by observing the skill performance.

## Patient Charts

Often documentation in patient charts will create patterns that reveal learning needs. Physicians' progress notes, nursing care plans, nurses' notes, and discharge planning forms can also provide information on learn-ing needs. Remember not to disregard the valuable insights other members of the health-care team, such as physical therapists, social workers, respiratory therapists, and nutrition-ists, can provide with respect to the needs of the learner.

## Assessing Learning Needs of Nursing Staff

Williams (1998) specifically addresses the importance of identifying the learning needs of staff nurses. He evaluates the assumptions of learning needs assessments, provides practical advice about designing a survey needs assess-ment (SNA), and outlines implementation issues that must be considered prior to carrying out an assessment of the learning needs of staff.

The following are methods that can be used specifically to determine the learning needs of nursing staff.

**Written Job Descriptions**  A written de-scription of what is required to effectively carry out job responsibilities is a source to determine potential learning needs of staff. It can be the basis of establishing content in an orientation program for new staff or of designing continuing education opportunities for seasoned nurses.

**Formal and Informal Requests**    Many times staff will be asked for ideas for educational programs, which reflect what they perceive as needs. When doing a formalized educational program, the educator must verify that these requests are congruent with the needs of other staff members.

**Quality Assurance Reports**    Trends found in incident reports indicating safety violations or errors in procedures are a source for establishing learning needs of staff that education could adequately address.

**Chart Audits**    Audits of charts help identify trends in practice. Does the staff have a learning need in terms of the actual charting? Is an intervention being newly implemented that was not done before? Does the record indicate some inconsistency with implementation?

**Rules and Regulations**    A thorough knowledge of hospital, professional, and healthcare requirements helps to identify possible learning needs of staff. It is important for the educator to monitor new rules of practice that may arise from changes occurring within an institution or external to the organization that have implications for the delivery of care.

**Four-Step Appraisal of Needs**    Panno (1992) described a systematic approach for assessing learning needs of caregivers and the organizations in which they practice. Panno expanded on Alan Knox's (1974, 1977, 1986) interest in teaching related to adult development and learning. Knox's interpretation of how adults learn has led to information on how to develop and coordinate education programs that would be responsive to the backgrounds and aspirations of various adult learners.

The four steps in assessing learning needs are (a) defining the target population, (b) analyzing learner and organizational needs, (c) analyzing the perceived needs of the learner and comparing these to the actual needs, and

(d) using data to prioritize learning needs identified (Panno, 1992). This organizing framework can be used to assess multiple caregiver levels, from registered nurse to the nursing assistant, which is typically the target audiences for in-service programs within an institution. Panno (1992) pointed out that often plans for educational activities are based on personal preference, mandates from administration, intuition, or trends in the profession, which may meet the sponsor's needs but not the needs of the learner. A systematic approach, as described by Panno (1992), is useful because it benefits all involved and is a process that justifies the resources required for the assessment process.

## READINESS TO LEARN

Once the learning needs have been identified, the next step is to determine the learner's readiness to receive information. *Readiness to learn* can be defined as the time when the learner demonstrates an interest in learning the type or degree of information necessary to maintain optimal health or to become more skillful in a job. Often, educators have noted that when a patient or staff member asks a question, the time is prime for learning. Readiness to learn occurs when the learner is receptive to learning and is willing and able to participate in the learning process. The educator must never overuse the expression "The patient is not ready to learn." It is the responsibility of the educator to discover through assessment exactly when patients are ready to learn and what they want to learn. For example, the educator needs to adapt the content to be learned to fit with what the learner is ready to learn. In preparing to teach a patient, the educator must determine what must be known about the illness to assist the patient in moving toward independence in self-care.

Assessing readiness to learn requires the educator to first understand what needs to be taught and to be competent in collecting and validating information. The same methods that were used to assess learning needs can also be used for assessing readiness to learn, such as making observations, conducting interviews, gathering information from the learner as well as other healthcare team members, and reviewing written data in charts.

An assessment of readiness to learn must be done prior to the time when actual learning is to occur. No matter how important the information is or how much the educator feels the recipient of teaching needs the information, if the learner is not ready, the information will not be absorbed. If educational objectives are set by the educator prior to assessing readiness to learn, then both the educator's and the learner's time could very well be wasted, because the established objectives may be beyond the readiness of the learner. The educator must give thought as to what is required of the learner—that is, what needs to be learned, what the learning objectives should be, and in which domain and at what level of learning these objectives should be classified. The educator will then have an idea about what to focus on in the assessment of the learner's abilities.

Timing—that is, the point at which teaching should take place—is very important, because anything that affects physical or psychological comfort can affect a learner's ability and willingness to learn. A learner who is unreceptive to information at one time may be more receptive to the same information at another time. Within the healthcare system, the nurse often has limited contact with patients and family members. This contact may occur during a two-day stay in the hospital or a one-hour visit in the outpatient setting. The patient's readiness to learn is confined to that particular time and is based on learning being brief and basic. Timing is also an important factor with the nursing staff, because readiness to learn is based on current demands of practice and needs to correspond to the ever constant changes in practice. Adults, whether patient, family, nursing staff, or students, are eager to learn when the sub-

ject of teaching is relevant and applicable to their everyday concerns.

Before teaching can begin, the educator must find the time to first take a PEEK (Lichtenthal, 1990) at the four types of readiness to learn. Readiness to learn can be determined by the learner's characteristics as follows: **P**hysical readiness, **E**motional readiness, **E**xperiential readiness, and **K**nowledge readiness.

These four types of readiness to learn may or may not prove to be obstacles to learning. Nevertheless, the few minutes the educator spends assessing learning readiness can help overcome these possible obstacles. The following factors must be taken into consideration (Table 4–2).

**TABLE 4–2   Take time to take a PEEK at the four types of readiness to learn**

**P = PHYSICAL READINESS**

- Measures of ability
- Complexity of task
- Environmental effects
- Health status
- Gender

**E = EMOTIONAL READINESS**

- Anxiety level
- Support system
- Motivation
- Risk-taking behavior
- Frame of mind
- Developmental stage

**E = EXPERIENTIAL READINESS**

- Level of aspiration
- Past coping mechanisms
- Cultural background
- Locus of control
- Orientation

**K = KNOWLEDGE READINESS**

- Present knowledge base
- Cognitive ability
- Learning disabilities
- Learning styles

SOURCE: From C. Lichtenthal, *A Self-Study Model on Readiness to Learn*, August 1990. Reprinted with permission from Cheryl Lichtenthal.

## Physical Readiness

Several physical factors related to readiness need to be considered by the educator because they may have an adverse effect on the degree to which learning will occur (Singer, 1972). There are five major components to physical readiness: measures of ability, complexity of task, environmental effects, health status, and gender.

**Measures of Ability**   If the task requires gross movements using the large muscles of the body, then adequate strength, flexibility, and endurance must be present. Walking on crutches is a good example of a psychomotor skill for which a patient must have the physical ability to be ready to learn. If the educator is conducting an in-service workshop for staff on the subject of lifting and transfer activities of patients, the nurse as educator must be cognizant of the endurance level required of the staff for them to be able to return demonstrate this skill. In addition, for information to be accurately processed, sense organs and receptors must be functioning adequately. For example, if a person has a visual deficit, are eyeglasses available to allow the patient to see the lines on an insulin syringe? If not, then the individual is not physically ready to learn. Measures involving visual and auditory acuity as well as the capacity to perform adequate movements affect the ability to learn. Creating a stimulating and accepting environment by using instructional tools to match learners' sensory abilities will help to pique their interest in learning.

**Complexity of Task**   In learning to perform a skill, the nurse educator must take into account the difficulty level of the subject or task to be mastered by the learner. Variations in the complexity of the task will affect the extent to which behavioral changes are necessary in the cognitive, affective, and psychomotor domains. Psychomotor skills, in particular, require different degrees of manual

dexterity and physical energy output. Once acquired, however, they are usually retained better and longer than learning in the other domains (Greer, Hitt, Sitterly, & Slebodnick, 1972). Once ingrained, psychomotor skills become habitual and may be difficult to alter. For example, if the learner has been performing a psychomotor skill over a long period of time and then the procedural steps of the task change, the learner will need to unlearn those steps and relearn a new way. This requirement may increase the complexity of the task and put additional physical demands on the learner as a result of lengthening the time needed to adjust to doing something in a new way. Older adults or those with low literacy skills will likely find the effort particularly difficult and time-consuming, and they may even refuse to make a change.

**Environmental Effects**   An environment conducive to learning will help to keep the learner's attention and stimulate interest in learning. For example, extremely high levels of noise can interfere with the accuracy and precision in performing manual dexterity tasks. Noise induces vibration of body parts and negatively affects concentration levels. Intermittent noise tends to have greater disruptive effects than the more rapidly habituated steady-state noise. Intermittent use of a jackhammer in the street outside the patient's room, for instance, is more disruptive to a nurse's ability to perform skills than a constant roar of traffic coming from the same street.

The older adult, in particular, needs more time to react and respond to stimuli. The increased inability to receive and transmit information is a symptom of older age. Thus, tasks requiring large amounts of strength, endurance, speed, or flexibility can be difficult for the older person. Complex motor tasks, with too much information given during demonstration by the educator, may result in the older learner becoming overwhelmed and can contribute to a tendency for an older person to focus on irrelevant information rather than on cues critical to accomplishing the task at hand. When an activity is self-paced, the older learner will respond more favorably. Breaking down complex learning material into more simplified steps is helpful for all learners in improving their retention of information, reducing inattention and confusion, and decreasing energy demands, thereby increasing physical readiness to learn.

**Health Status** Assessment of the learner's health status is important to determine the amount of energy available as well as present comfort level—both of these factors heavily influence one's readiness to learn. Energy-reducing demands caused by the body's response to illness require the learner to expend large amounts of physical and psychic energy, with little reserve left for actual learning. A person's health status, which can be classified as well, acutely ill, or chronically ill, must be taken into serious consideration when assessing for readiness.

Healthy learners have energy available for learning. Readiness to learn about health-promoting behaviors is based on their perception of self-responsibility. The extent to which an illness is perceived to potentially affect future well-being influences someone's desire to learn both preventive and promotion measures. If learners perceive a threat to their quality of life, more information will be sought in an attempt to control the negative effects of an illness (Bubela & Galloway, 1990). This type of response behavior can be best understood by examining the Health Belief Model and the Health Promotion Model described in Chapter 6.

Learners who are acutely ill tend to focus their energies on the physiological and psychological demands of their illness. Learning is at a minimum because most of these individuals' energy is needed for the demands of the illness and gaining immediate relief. Any learning that may occur should be related to

treatments, tests, and minimizing pain or other discomforts. As these patients improve and the acute phase of illness diminishes, they can then focus on learning follow-up management and the avoidance of complications. The educator must assess an acutely ill person's readiness to learn by observing his or her energy levels and comfort status. One observation that can signify increased energy and comfort levels is the ability to move more readily without becoming easily fatigued. Improvement in physical status usually results in more receptivity to learning. Note, however, that medications that induce side effects such as drowsiness, mental depression, impaired depth perception, decreased ability to concentrate, and learner fatigue will also reduce task-handling capacity. Giving a patient a sedative prior to a learning experience may result in less apprehension, but cognitive and psychomotor abilities will be impaired, thus requiring a longer time, more physical output, and more frustration for the learner to master a skill (Greer et al., 1972).

Chronic illness, on the other hand, has no time limits and is of long-term duration. Models of how people deal with chronic illness also are useful as frameworks for understanding readiness to learn. A patient with a chronic condition, however, may experience acute episodes either as an exacerbation of the chronic disease or as a separate event, such as a motor vehicle accident. The physiological and psychological demands vary in chronic illness and are not always predictable. Patients go through different stages in adjusting to their illness.

Boyd, Gleit, Graham, and Whitman (1998) have suggested that these stages are similar to the adjustment stages that a person experiences with a loss. These states are initial avoidance, beginning approach, and then repetitious approach/avoidance cycles. If the learner is in the avoidance stage, readiness to learn will be limited to simple explanations, because the patient's energy is sapped by the stress involved in emotionally attempting to deny the illness. Energy levels will become more stable as the patient becomes aware of the realities of the situation or symptoms become too obvious to avoid. Readiness to learn may be indicated by the questions asked by the patient. It must never be assumed, but rather must be assessed during each encounter with the chronically ill patient.

Corbin and Strauss (1991) proposed a nursing model for chronic illness management based on Strauss and Glaser's (1975) trajectory framework. For patients, this course represents the cumulative effects of illness, including physical symptoms. It encompasses eight phases, which are linear in nature. The preventive phase is the first phase, when no signs or symptoms are present. The phases of chronic illness continue until downward or progressive deterioration in physical/mental status occurs and eventually death ensues. This dynamism reflects the continual nature of adaptation that occurs with people living with chronic illness (Burton, 2000).

Unlike the Corbin and Strauss model, the shifting perspectives model of chronic illness (Patterson, 2001) suggests that living with chronic illness is an ongoing and continually shifting process. The model provides an explanation of chronically ill persons' variations in their attention to symptoms over time. Chronically ill individuals experience a complex dialectic between themselves and their world that is continually changing. As the reality of the illness experience changes, the individual's perspectives shift in the degree to which illness is in the foreground or background of their world. Individuals with chronic illness shift between illness and wellness being in the foreground, with the other being in the background. Understanding this cycle is important when assessing readiness to learn, as the nurse educator cannot assume that an approach that worked before will be just as effective again. Learners' perspectives about learning self-care are not static, and there may be periods of time when learners are more receptive to learning than at other times.

**Gender**   Research has indicated that women are generally more receptive to medical care and take fewer risks to their health than men (Ashton, 1999; Stein & Nyamathi, 2000; Bertakis, Rahman, Helms, Callahan, & Robbins, 2000). This difference may arise because women traditionally have taken the role of caregivers and therefore are more open to health promotion teaching. In addition, they have more frequent contacts with health providers while bearing and raising children. Men, on the other hand, tend to be less receptive to healthcare interventions and are more likely to be risk takers. As a good deal of this behavior is thought to be socially induced, changes are beginning to be seen in the health-seeking behavior of men and women because of the increased attention paid to healthier lifestyles and because of the blending of gender roles in the home and workplace.

## Emotional Readiness

The learner must be emotionally ready to learn. Like physical readiness, emotional readiness includes several factors that need to be assessed.

**Anxiety Level**   Anxiety is a factor that influences the ability to perform at a cognitive, affective, and psychomotor level. Depending on the level of anxiety, it may or may not be a hindrance to the learning of new skills. Fear is a major contributor to anxiety and thus negatively affects readiness to learn in any of the learning domains. The performance of a task in and of itself may be fear-inducing to a patient because of its very nature or meaning. For example, having to learn self-administration of a medication by injection may produce fear for the patient because of the necessity of inflicting pain on oneself and the perceived danger of the needle breaking off into the skin.

A staff member or nursing student, on the other hand, may have real difficulty mastering a skill because of the fear of harming a patient or of failing to do a procedure correctly.

Fear may also lead patients to deny their illness, which interferes with their ability to learn. If a situation is life-threatening or overwhelming, anxiety will be high, and readiness to learn will be diminished. While teaching may be imperative for survival, learning usually can take place only if instructions are repeated over and over again. In such circumstances, families and support persons should be educated instead. In later stages of adaptation, acceptance of illness will allow the individual to be more receptive to learning because anxiety levels will be less acute.

Some degree of anxiety is a motivator to learn, but low or high anxiety will interfere with readiness to learn. On either end of the continuum, mild or severe anxiety may lead to inaction on the part of the learner, whereas moderate anxiety may drive someone to take action. As the level of anxiety begins to increase, emotional readiness peaks and then begins to decrease (Figure 4–2). A moderate level of anxiety is best for success in learning and is considered the optimal time for learning. Discovering what stressful events or major life changes the learner is experiencing will give the educator clues as to that person's emotional readiness to learn.

**Support System**   The availability and strength of a support system also influence emotional readiness and are closely tied to how anxious someone might feel. If persons in the patient's support system are available to assist with self-care activities at home, then they should be present during at least some of the teaching sessions to learn how to help the patient if the need arises. A strong support system decreases anxiety, while the lack of one increases anxiety levels.

Beddoe (1999) describes the unique opportunity that nurses have to provide emotional support to patients. She labels this opportunity as the "reachable moment"—the time when a nurse truly connects with clients by directly meeting them on mutual terms. The reachable moment allows for the mutual exchange of concerns and a sharing of possible intervention options without the nurse being inhibited by prejudice or bias. This time, when the client feels emotionally supported, sets the stage for the "teachable moment," when the client will be most receptive to learning.

**Motivation**   The motivation and interest on the part of the learner to achieve a task also lead to more meaningful teaching–learning experiences. Emotional readiness is strongly associated with motivation. Knowing the motivational level of the learner assists the educator in determining when someone is ready to learn. The learner must have intentions of improving performance. Otherwise, merely going through the motions in a haphazard or mechanical manner, disregarding important learning cues, and demonstrating purposeless activity will not result in task mastery.

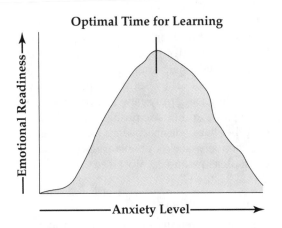

**Optimal Time for Learning**

*Emotional Readiness →*

*← Anxiety Level →*

FIGURE 4–2   **Effect of Anxiety on Emotional Readiness to Learn**

Assessment of emotional readiness involves ascertaining the level of motivation, not necessarily the reasons for the motivation. There are many reasons why a learner may be motivated to learn, and almost any reason to learn is a valid one. The level of motivation is related to what learners perceive as an expectation of themselves or others. Interest in informal or formal educator–learner interactions is a cue to motivation. The learner who is ready to learn shows an interest in what the nurse educator is doing by demonstrating a willingness to participate or to ask questions. Prior learning experiences, whether they be past accomplishments or failures, will be reflected in the current level of motivation demonstrated by the learner for accomplishing the task at hand (see Chapter 6).

**Risk-Taking Behavior**    Taking risks is intrinsic in the activities people perform daily. Many activities are done without thinking about the outcome. According to Joseph (1993), some patients, by the very nature of their personalities, will take more risks than others. The educator can help patients develop strategies to help reduce the risk of their choices. If patients prefer to participate in activities that may shorten their life spans, rather than complying with a rigid treatment plan, the educator must be willing to teach these patients how to recognize certain body symptoms and then what to do.

Healthcare providers also have risk-taking behavior. Understanding how much individual risk taking nurses have or do not have will help the educator understand why some learners may be hesitant to try new approaches to delivering care. Wolfe (1994) stated that taking risks can be threatening when the outcomes are not guaranteed.

Educators can, however, help nurses and other healthcare providers learn how to take risks. First, the decision has to be made to take the risk. The next step is to develop strategies to minimize the risk. The learner then needs to develop a worst, best, and most probable case scenario. Lastly, the learner must decide whether the worst-case scenario developed is acceptable.

**Frame of Mind**    Frame of mind involves concern about the here and now. If survival is of primary concern, then readiness to learn will be focused on meeting basic human needs. Physical needs such as food, warmth, comfort, and safety as well as psychosocial needs of feeling accepted and secure must be met before someone can focus on higher learning. People from lower socioeconomic levels tend to have an immediate orientation to present-day concerns because they are trying to satisfy everyday needs. Children also regard life in the here and now because they are developmentally focused on what makes them happy and satisfied. In addition, their thinking is concrete rather than abstract. Adults who have reached self-actualization and whose basic needs are met are more ready to learn health promotion tasks and are said to have a more futuristic orientation.

**Developmental Stage**    Each task associated with human development produces a peak time for readiness to learn, known as a "teachable moment" (Tanner, 1989; Wagner & Ash, 1998; Hansen & Fisher, 1998). Unlike children, adults can build on meaningful past experiences and are strongly driven to learn information that will help them to cope better with real-life tasks. They see learning as relevant when they can apply new knowledge to help them solve immediate problems. Children, on the other hand, desire to learn for learning sake and actively seek out experiences that give them pleasure and comfort (see Chapter 5).

## Experiential Readiness

Experiential readiness refers to the learner's past experiences with learning. Before starting to teach, the educator should assess whether previous learning experiences have been positive or negative in overcoming problems or accomplishing new tasks. Someone who has had negative experiences with learning is not likely to be motivated or willing to take a risk in trying to change behavior or acquire new behaviors.

**Level of Aspiration** The extent to which someone is driven to achieve is related to the type of short- and long-term goals established, not by the educator, but by the learner. Previous failures and past successes influence what goals learners set for themselves. Early successes are important motivators in learning subsequent skills. Satisfaction, once achieved, elevates the level of aspiration, which in turn increases the probability of continued performance output in undertaking future endeavors to change behavior.

**Past Coping Mechanisms** The coping mechanisms someone has been using must be explored to understand how the learner has dealt with previous problems. Once these mechanisms are identified, the educator must determine if past coping strategies have been effective and, if so, whether they work well under the present learning situation.

**Cultural Background** Knowledge on the part of the educator about other cultures and being sensitive to behavioral differences between cultures are important to avoid teaching in opposition to cultural beliefs (see Chapter 8). Assessment of what an illness means to the patient from the patient's cultural perspective is imperative in determining readiness to learn. Remaining sensitive to cultural influences allows the teacher to bridge the gap, when necessary, between the medical healthcare culture and the patient's culture. Building on the learner's knowledge base or belief system (unless it is dangerous to well-being), rather than attempting to change it or claim it is wrong, will encourage rather than dampen readiness to learn.

Language is also a part of culture and may prove to be a significant obstacle to learning if the educator and the learner do not fluently speak the same language. Assessing whether the learner understands English well enough is the first step. A qualified interpreter will be necessary if the learner and caregiver do not fluently speak the same language. A trained interpreter may not always be available, and the nurse may need to call upon a relative, a friend, or another healthcare person to act as an interpreter. Sometimes, enlisting the help of someone else, other than a trained interpreter, to bridge cultural differences may negatively influence learning. This effect will depend on such issues as the sensitivity of the topic and the need for privacy. In some instances, the patient may not want family members or associates to know about a health concern or illness.

Remember, also, that medical terminology in and of itself may be a foreign language to many patients, whether or not they are from another culture. In addition, sometimes a native language does not have an equivalent word to describe the terms that are being used in the teaching situation. Differences in language compound the cultural barrier. Teaching should not be started unless you have determined that the learner understands you and that you have an understanding of the learner's culture (see Chapter 8).

**Locus of Control** Whether readiness to learn comes from internal or external stimuli can be determined by ascertaining the learner's previous life patterns of responsibility and assertiveness. When patients are internally motivated to learn, they have what is known as an *internal locus of control*. They are ready to learn when they feel a need to know about something. This drive to learn comes from within the learner. Usually, this type of learner will indicate a need to know by asking questions. Remember that when someone asks a question, the time is prime for learning.

If patients have an *external locus of control*—that is, they are externally motivated—then someone other than themselves must encourage a feeling of wanting to know something. The responsibility often falls on the educator's shoulders to motivate them to want to learn.

**Orientation**  The tendency to adhere to a parochial or cosmopolitan point of view is known as orientation. Patients with a parochial orientation tend to be more close-minded in their thinking, are more conservative in their approach to situations, are less willing to learn new material, and place the most trust in traditional authority figures such as the physician. This type of orientation is seen most often in people who have been raised in a small-town atmosphere or who come from cohesive neighborhoods or protective family environments. Conversely, people who exhibit a cosmopolitan orientation most likely have a more worldly perspective on life due to broader experiences outside their immediate spheres of influence. These individuals are more likely to be receptive to new ideas and to opportunities to learn new ways of doing things. One must be careful not to unfairly stereotype individuals, but learners usually possess representative characteristics of one or the other of these two opposing types of orientation.

## Knowledge Readiness

Knowledge readiness refers to the learner's present knowledge base, the level of learning capability, and the preferred style of learning. These components must be assessed to determine readiness to learn, and teaching should be planned accordingly.

**Present Knowledge Base**  How much someone already knows about a particular subject or how proficient that person is at performing a task is an important factor to determine before designing and implementing instruction. If the

educator makes the mistake of teaching subject material that has already been learned, then he or she risks, at the very least, creating boredom and disinterest in the learner, or, at the extreme, causing insult to the learner, which could produce resistance to further learning. Always find out what the patient knows prior to teaching, and build on this knowledge base to encourage readiness to learn.

**Cognitive Ability**  The extent to which information can be processed is indicative of the level at which the learner is capable of learning. The educator must match behavioral objectives to the cognitive ability of the learner, or failure to achieve learning will result. The learner who is capable of understanding, memorizing, recalling, or recognizing subject material is functioning at a lower level than the learner who demonstrates problem solving, concept formation, or application of information. For example, the educator can assume that nursing staff or students who are able to answer questions about cardiopulmonary resuscitation (CPR) on a written test understand the subject. This does not mean, however, that the staff member or student can perform CPR in the clinical setting. Patients who can identify the risk factors of hypertension are functioning at the lower level in the cognitive domain and may have difficulty generalizing the information to find ways of incorporating a low-salt diet into their lifestyle. Thus, the level at which the learner is able to learn is of major importance when designing instruction.

Individuals with cognitive impairment due to mental retardation present a special challenge to the educator and will require simple explanations and step-by-step progression of instruction with frequent repetition. Be sure to make information meaningful to those with cognitive impairments by teaching at their level and communicating in ways that the learner will be able to understand (see Chapter 9 on special populations). Enlisting the help of members of the patient's support system by teaching them requisite skills will allow them to positively contribute to the reinforcement of self-care activities.

**Learning Disabilities** Other than those deficits caused by mental retardation, learning disabilities and low-level reading skills are not necessarily indicative of an individual's intellectual abilities but will require special or innovative approaches to instruction to sustain or bolster readiness to learn. It is easy for low-literacy and learning-disabled persons to become easily discouraged unless the teacher recognizes their special needs and seeks ways to help them accommodate or overcome their problems with processing information (see Chapters 7 and 9).

**Learning Styles** A variety of preferred styles of learning exist, and assessing how someone learns best will help the educator to select teaching approaches accordingly. Knowing the teaching methods and materials with which a learner is most comfortable or, conversely, does not tolerate well will help the educator to tailor teaching to meet the needs of individuals with different styles of learning, thereby increasing their readiness to learn. For more information, see the following discussion on learning styles.

## ◼ LEARNING STYLES

*Learning style* refers to the ways individuals process information (Guild & Garger, 1998). Each learner is unique and complex, with a distinct learning style preference that distinguishes one learner from another. The learning style models are based on the premise that certain characteristics of style are biological in origin, whereas others are sociologically developed as a result of environmental influences. Recognizing that people have different approaches to learning helps the nurse educator to understand the various educational interests and needs of diverse populations. Accepting diversity of style can help educa-

tors create an atmosphere for learning that offers experiences that encourage each individual to reach his or her full potential. Understanding learning style can also help educators to make deliberate decisions about program development and instructional design (Arndt & Underwood, 1990). In addition, consideration given to matching the learning style of nursing staff orientees with the training style of clinical nurse preceptors may provide the opportunity to maximize learning outcomes during staff orientation to clinical sites (Anderson, 1998).

No learning style is either better or worse than another. Given the same content, most learners can assimilate information with equal success, but how they go about mastering the content is determined by their individual style. The more flexible the educator is in using teaching methodologies related to individual learning styles, the greater the likelihood that learning will occur.

## Six Learning Style Principles

Six principles have emerged from research about learning styles. To develop these six principles, Friedman and Alley (1984) reviewed an enormous volume of literature, which included more than 30 different learning style instruments. The six principles are described next (the reference to "student" can be interpreted as any learner who is the recipient of teaching):

1. *Both the style by which the teacher prefers to teach and the style by which the student prefers to learn can be identified.* Identification of different styles offers specific clues as to the way a person learns. By understanding one's own learning style, the educator can appreciate why it may be easier to help one style of learner to master information but more difficult to work with another learner who needs an entirely different approach to learning.

2. *Teachers need to guard against overteaching by their own preferred learning styles.* Nurse educators need to realize that just because they gravitate to learning a certain way, it does not mean that everyone else can or wants to learn this way. It is much easier for the educator to change the teaching approach than for the learner to adapt to the teacher's style.

3. *Teachers are most helpful when they assist students in identifying and learning through their own style preferences.* Making learners aware of their individual style preferences will lead to an understanding of which teaching–learning approaches work best for them. Also, an awareness of their preference for a particular learning style sensitizes learners to the fact that whatever style is most comfortable for them may not be the best approach for others.

4. *Students should have the opportunity to learn through their preferred style.* The nurse educator can provide the means by which each learner can experience successful learning. Visual learners, for example, should be given movies, computer simulations, and videos from which to learn rather than insisting that they read. Concrete and abstract thinkers need to capitalize on their strengths; concrete thinkers need facts, whereas abstract thinkers need theories.

5. *Students should be encouraged to diversify their style preferences.* Today, learners are constantly faced with learning situations where one approach to learning will not suffice if they are to reach their fullest potential. Without encouragement, learners tend to automatically gravitate to using their preferred style of learning. The more frequently learners are exposed to different methods of learning, the less stressful those methods will be in future learning situations.

6. *Teachers can develop specific learning activities that reinforce each modality or style.* Nurse educators must become aware of various methods and materials available to address and augment the different learning styles. To be effective, educational strategies should be geared toward different learning styles, because using only a limited number of approaches will selectively exclude many learners.

Three mechanisms to determine learning style are observation, interviews, and administration of learning style instruments. By observing the learner in action, the educator can determine how the learner problem solves. When doing a math calculation, does the learner write every step down or only the answer? In an interview, the educator can ask the learner about preferred ways of learning as well as the environment most comfortable for learning. Is a warm or cold room more conducive to concentration? Is group discussion or self-instruction more preferable? Finally, the educator can determine learning style by administering learning style instruments, like those described in the next section.

All three techniques should be used to determine learning style. This determination can be looked at as occurring parallel to the nursing process. Once data are gathered through interview, observation, and instrument administration, then learning style can be validated by the educator, and methods and materials for instruction can be chosen to match the preferred style of the learner. Nurse educators can also use the learning style approach in directing patients, nursing students, or the nursing staff toward those ways they best can learn.

The implications of using the learning style approach to instruction are enormous and exciting. If learning styles of the nurses participating in the clinical or academic setting have been assessed and identified, then educational experiences to complement those styles can be designed. Adapting educational experiences to coincide with learning styles thus increases the likelihood that learning will take place. Understanding and recognizing various styles are especially useful when making decisions about planning, implementing, and evaluating educational programs.

### ◼ LEARNING STYLE INSTRUMENTS

A word of caution: Before using any learning style instrument, it is important to determine its reliability and validity. Another factor to consider is that an all-inclusive instrument does not exist that can measure all domains of learning—cognitive, affective, and psychomotor—and, therefore, it is best to use more than one measurement tool for assessment. Also, the educator should not rely heavily on these instruments because they are intended not for diagnosis but rather to validate what the learner perceives in comparison to what the educator perceives. These instruments will help the nurse in developing a more personalized form of instruction. This chapter does not attempt to review all the instruments that are available, but rather highlights those instruments that are the most useful to nurse educators for assessment purposes.

The identification and application of learning styles remains an emerging movement and is just beginning to be applied to the health education field. To date, researchers have defined learning styles differently, but often the concepts are overlapping. The remainder of this chapter looks at some of the better-known theories on learning styles. These do not offer any single framework for instructional design but do provide the educator with a more profound view of the learner than known previously (Villejo & Meyers, 1991).

### Right-Brain/Left-Brain and Whole-Brain Thinking

Twenty-five years ago, Dr. Roger Sperry and his research team established that the brain functions in many ways as two brains (Sperry, 1977; Herrman, 1988). The brain is composed of two hemispheres that have separate and complementary functions. Studies were conducted on people whose hemispheres were separated to observe how each hemisphere functions. The left hemisphere of the brain was found to be the vocal and analytical side, which is used for verbalization and for reality-based and logical thinking. The right hemisphere was found to be the emotional, visual-spatial, nonverbal hemisphere. Thinking processes using the right brain are intuitive, subjective, relational, holistic, and time-free. Sperry and his colleagues discovered that learners are able to use both sides of the brain because of a connector between the two hemispheres called the corpus callosum.

There is no "correct" or "wrong" side of the brain. Each hemisphere gathers in the same sensory information but handles the information in different ways. One hemisphere may take over and inhibit the other in processing information, or the task may be divided between the two sides, with each handling the part best suited to its way of processing information. Educators need to know which side of the brain is better equipped for certain kinds of tasks and, thus, what is the most effective way to present information to learners who may have a dominant brain hemisphere (Table 4–3). These findings are important for instructional design because educators have limited time and contact with the learner and need to meaningfully present the material to be learned. Brain hemisphericity is linked to cognitive learning style or the way individuals perceive and gather information to problem solve, complete assigned tasks, relate to others, and meet the daily challenges of life.

Recent advances in brain research, mainly due to neuroimaging methods such as positron emission tomography (PET) and magnetic resonance imaging (MRI), provide the educator with new knowledge on how the brain works. This information adds to the relevance of

| TABLE 4–3   Examples of hemisphere functions | |
|---|---|
| **LEFT-HEMISPHERE FUNCTIONS** | **RIGHT-HEMISPHERE FUNCTIONS** |
| Thinking is critical, logical, convergent, focal | Thinking is creative, intuitive, divergent, diffuse |
| Analytical | Synthesizing |
| Prefers talking and writing | Prefers drawing and manipulating objects |
| Responds to verbal instructions and explanations | Responds to written instructions and explanations |
| Recognizes/remembers names | Recognizes/remembers faces |
| Relies on language in thinking and remembering | Relies on images in thinking and remembering |
| Solves problems by breaking them into parts, then approaches the problem sequentially, using logic | Solves problems by looking at the whole, the configurations, then approaches the problem through patterns, using hunches |
| Good organizational skills, neat | Loose organizational skills, sloppy |
| Likes stability, willing to adhere to rules | Likes change, uncertainty |
| Conscious of time and schedules | Frequently loses contact with time and schedules |
| Algebra is the preferred math | Geometry is the preferred math |
| Not as good at interpreting body language | Good at interpreting body language |
| Controls emotions | Free with emotions |

learning styles and brain hemispherical performance. McIntoch (1998) proposed a general hypothesis that learning and memory are emergent properties of network interactions. Sylvester (1995, 1998) reported on the research that has led to a better understanding of the functions of the brain and individual learning differences. Iaccino (1993) provided more detailed accounts of the clinical evidence that has contributed to the left–right dichotomy of the brain. These advances in technology have confirmed many of the assumptions about the functioning of the brain. Educators can apply these advances to learning style assessment and education techniques (Stover, 2001; Caulfield, Kidd, & Kocher, 2000).

Knowledge of one's own brain hemispherical performance can aid educators in identifying strengths and weaknesses in their teaching methods. The Brain Preference Indicator (BPI) is a set of questions used to determine hemispheric dominance. The BPI instrument can reveal a general style of thought that results in a consistent pattern of behavior in all areas of the individual's life. More information about the BPI can be found in *Whole-Brain Thinking* by Wonder and Donovan (1984).

Statistics show that most learners have left-brain dominance and that only approximately 30% have right-brain dominance (Gondringer, 1989). This may be because the Western world is geared toward rewarding left-brain skills to the extent that right-brain skills go undeveloped. Teaching methods need to be employed that enable the learner to use both sides of the brain, however. For example, to stimulate the development of left-brain thinking, the nurse educator might use objectives and a course outline. To stimulate the development of the right brain, the nurse educator might play soft music in the background at a slow, even rhythm. By employing teaching strategies aimed at helping the learner use both brain hemispheres, the educator will facilitate more effective and efficient learning. Whole-brain thinking allows the learner to get the best of both worlds, in terms of thought processes. Duality of thinking is what educators should strive to teach to encourage learners to reach their full learning potential.

Also, the educator must realize that the brain does not exist in isolation but rather within a body (Gardner, 1999). The nurse must, therefore, take into account many other variables that may affect a learner's style of learning. Gardner (1999) argues that for a brain to be more than an organ, consideration must be given to a number of variables. First, the educator must think of the brain from the perspective of such things as mental processes, feelings, and desires. Second, the culture in which one lives is important in the development and expression of one's learning style. Lastly, educators bring a set of values when teaching and learners bring a set of values when learning, both of which determine what learners chose to learn.

## Field-Independent/Field-Dependent Embedded Figures Test

An extensive series of studies by H. Witkin and associates (1971a) identified two styles of learning in the cognitive domain. These two cognitive styles are based on the bipolar distribution of characteristics of learners affecting the manner in which learners process and structure information in the environment. Learners have preference styles for certain environmental cues: A field-independent person perceives items as separate or differentiated from the surrounding field; a field-dependent person's perception is influenced by or immersed in the surrounding field.

Witkin and associates (1971b) devised a tool called the Embedded Figures Test (EFT) to measure field independence/dependence. This tool measures how a person's perception of an item is influenced by the context in which it appears. Bonham (1988) noted that the EFT is designed to measure a person's ability to find simple geometric figures within complex drawings. This tool takes approximately 30 minutes to complete. Witkin's work is based on 35 years of psychological research on more than 2000 subjects. Educators must keep in mind that the EFT is based on psycho-logical research when they attempt to broadly apply findings to the educational setting (Witkin, Moore, & Oltman, 1977).

Field-independent individuals have internalized frames of reference and experience themselves as separate or differentiated from others and the environment. They are less sensitive to social cues, are not affected by criticism, favor an active participant role, and are eager to test out their ideas or opinions in a group.

Field-dependent individuals are more socially oriented, more aware of social cues, and able to reveal their feelings. They are more dependent on others for reinforcement. They have a need for extrinsic motivation and externally defined objectives. Field-dependent individuals learn better if the material to be learned has a social context. They are more easily affected by criticism, take a passive, spectator role, and change their opinions in the face of peer pressure.

Garity (1985) stated that these individual differences in characteristics and interpersonal behavior can be used as a basis for looking at different learning styles. Understanding these differences can facilitate the way educators work with learners and structure the learning task and environment (Table 4–4).

Bonham (1988) pointed out in her analysis of learning style instruments that the EFT measures the ability to do something, not the manner (style) in which it is done. There is no way to tell whether a person is good at both approaches and could choose which style is most effective in a given situation (Shipman & Shipman, 1985; Witkin & Goodenough, 1981). Adults generally do not do well on tests in which speed is important (Botwinick, 1978), but speed is important in this assessment tool. Field independence/dependence might be related to hemispheric brain processes (Chall & Mirsky, 1978). The studies in *Sex and the Brain* (Durden-Smith & deSimone, 1983) show that the males' right hemisphere tends to be stronger than their left hemisphere; the opposite is true for females.

| TABLE 4–4    Characteristics of field-independent and field-dependent learners | |
| --- | --- |
| **FIELD-INDEPENDENT** | **FIELD-DEPENDENT** |
| Are not affected by criticism | Are easily affected by criticism |
| Will not conform to peer pressure | Will conform to peer pressure |
| Are less influenced by external feedback | Are influenced by feedback (grades and evaluations) |
| Learn best by organizing their own material | Learn best when material is organized |
| Have an impersonal orientation to the world | Have a social orientation to the world |
| Place emphasis on applying principles | Place emphasis on facts |
| Are interested in new ideas or concepts for own sake | Prefer learning to be relevant to own experience |
| Provide self-directed goals, objectives, and reinforcement | Need external goals, objectives, and reinforcements |
| Prefer lecture method | Prefer discussion method |

Scientists continue to research gender differences in brain activities (Speck, Ernst, Braun, Koch, Miller, and Chang, 2000). To date, sex-related differences in behavior have been documented in the literature, but their neuroanatomic substates remain unclear (Gur et al., 1999). The significance of the research findings for the educator is difficult to gauge. Males have better visual-spatial abilities, and females have better linguistic skills. Thus, females generally do not do as well as males on tests of spatial ability. Men should be measured only against other men, and women against women, to reduce the differential effect of the test on the sexes.

The best time to use the EFT seems to be when the educator wants to measure field independence, not field dependence, in a context in which the educator wants to test the extent to which learners are able to ignore distractions from other persons who may offer incorrect information or ideas. The results should be used to help individuals determine why they may have trouble with a particular learning experience (Bonham, 1988). Flynn, Barker, Gibson, Pearson, Berger, and Smith (1999) found a significant association between the amount of interruptions and distractions in an ambulatory care pharmacy and dispensing errors (incorrect label information). As the distractions increased, more errors occurred.

Field-dependent pharmacists tended to be more likely to be distracted and fill prescriptions inaccurately. It was also more difficult for field-dependent persons to overcome the effects of distracting background elements (the field). Consideration of field-independence/dependence can be useful for the educator who is involved with teaching in a clinical setting characterized by constant distractions.

The educator can also use this instrument to determine whether a learner sees the whole first (global, field-independent) and then the individual parts (specific, field-dependent), or vice versa. This consideration is important when selecting the approach the educator uses to facilitate learning. The field-independent person will want to know the end result of teaching and learning prior to concentrating on the individual parts of the process, whereas the field-dependent person will want to know the individual parts in sequence prior to looking at the expected overall outcome of teaching–learning efforts.

## Dunn and Dunn Learning Style Inventory

In 1967, Rita and Kenneth Dunn set out to develop an instrument that would assist educators in identifying those characteristics that allow individuals to learn in different ways.

Stimuli                                                    Elements

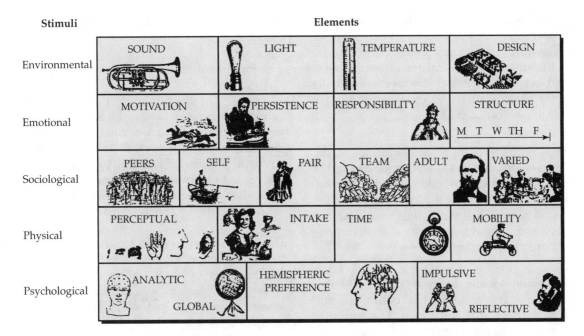

FIGURE 4–3   **Dunn and Dunn's Learning Style Elements**  SOURCE: R. Dunn, "Can Students Identify Their Own Learning Styles." *Educational Leadership,* 40, 5:61. Reprinted by permission of the Association for Supervision and Curriculum Development. Copyright © 1983 by ASCD. All rights reserved.

What has evolved since then is a highly tested and continuously revised instrument that has proved to be both valid and reliable. The Dunn and Dunn Learning Style Inventory is a self-reporting instrument that is widely used in the identification of how individuals prefer to function, learn, concentrate, and perform in their educational activities. It is available in three different forms: for grades 3–5; for grades 6–12; and in an adult version, called the Productivity Environmental Preference Survey (PEPS). Dunn and Dunn (1978) identified five basic stimuli (Figure 4–3) that affect a person's ability to learn:

1. Environmental elements (such as sound, light, temperature, and design), which are biological in nature

2. Emotional elements (such as motivation, persistence, responsibility, and structure), which are developmental and emerge over time as

an outgrowth of experiences that have happened at home, school, and play or work

3. Sociological patterns, which are indicative of the desire to work alone or in groups or a combination of these two approaches

4. Physical elements (such as perceptual strength, intake, time of day, and mobility), which are also biological in nature and relate to the way learners function physically

5. Psychological elements, which are indicative of the way learners process and react to information

### The Environmental Elements

*Sound*  Individuals react to sound in different ways. Some need complete silence, others are able to block out sounds around them, and still others require sound in their environment for learning. Cognizant of the effect of sound on learning, the educator should permit learners to study either in silent areas for those who need quiet or, for those who need noise, with music from headsets to prevent interfering with those who need quiet.

*Light*  Some learners work best under bright lights, whereas others need dim or low lighting. The educator should provide lighting conducive to learning by moving furniture around to establish both well- and dimly lit areas and permitting learners to sit where they are most comfortable.

*Temperature*  Some learners have difficulty thinking or concentrating if a room is too hot or, conversely, if it is too cold. The educator needs to make learners aware of the temperature of the environment and encourage them to wear lighter or heavier clothing. If windows are available, they should be opened to permit variable degrees of temperature in the room to accommodate different comfort levels.

*Design*  Dunn and Dunn established that when learners are seated on wooden, steel, or plastic chairs, 75% of the total body weight is supported on only four square inches of bone. This results in stress on the tissues of the buttocks, which causes fatigue, discomfort, and the need for frequent body changes. Hard surfaces are especially disturbing for those learners who are not well padded (Dunn & Dunn, 1987). Also, some learners are more relaxed and can learn better in an informal environment by being able to position themselves in a lounge chair, on the floor, on pillows, or on carpeting. Others cannot learn in an informal environment because it makes them drowsy and unable to achieve. If possible, the educator should vary the furniture in the classroom

to allow some to sit more informally while learning.

## The Emotional Elements

*Motivation*  Motivation, or the desire to achieve, increases when learning success increases. Unmotivated learners need short learning assignments that enhance their strengths. Motivated learners, by comparison, are eager to learn and should be told exactly what they are required to do, with resources available so they can self-pace their learning.

*Persistence*  Learners differ in their preference to want either to complete tasks that are begun in one sitting or to take periodic breaks and return to the task at a later time. By giving learners objectives and a time interval for completion of a task ahead of time, those with long attention spans can get the job done in a block of time, while those whose attention span is short can take the opportunity for breaks without feeling guilty or rushed.

*Responsibility*  Responsibility involves the desire to do what the learner thinks is expected. It is related to the concept of conformity or following through on what an educator asks or tells the learner to do. Learners with low responsibility scores usually are nonconforming. They do not like to do something because someone asks them to do it. Knowing this, the educator should give them choices and allow learners to select different ways to complete the assignment. When given appropriate choices, the nonconformist will likely be more willing to meet expectations set forth.

*Structure*  Structure refers to either the preference for specific directions, guidance, or rules prior to carrying out an assignment or the preference for doing an assignment without structure in the learner's own way. Structure should vary in the amount and kind that is provided, depending on the learner's ability to make responsible decisions.

## The Sociological Elements

*Learning alone*    Some learners prefer to study by themselves, whereas others prefer to learn with a friend or colleague. When learners prefer to be with others, group discussion and role-playing may facilitate learning. For learners who do not do well learning with others because they tend to socialize or are unable to concentrate, self-instruction, one-to-one interaction, or lecture-type methods are the best approaches.

*Presence of an authority figure*    Some learners feel more comfortable when someone with authority or recognized expertise is present during learning. Others become fearful, are embarrassed to show inability, and often become too tense to concentrate. Depending on the style of the learner, either one-to-one interaction or self-study may be the appropriate approach.

*Variety of ways*    Some learners can learn as well alone as they can with authority figures and with peer groups; that is, these learners are versatile in their style of learning and would benefit from variety as opposed to routine approaches.

## The Physical Elements

*Perceptual strengths*    Four types of learners are distinguished in this category: those with auditory preferences, who learn best while listening to verbal instruction; those with visual preferences, who learn best from reading or observation; those with tactile preferences, who learn best when they can underline as they read, take notes when they listen, and

otherwise keep their hands busy; and those with kinesthetic preferences, who absorb and retain information best when allowed to perform whole-body movement or participate in simulated or real-life experiences.

Auditory learners should be introduced to new information first by hearing about it, followed by verbal feedback for reinforcement of the information. Lecture and group discussion are instructional methods best suited to their style. Visual learners learn more easily by viewing, watching, and observing; simulation and demonstration methods of instruction are therefore most beneficial to their learning. Tactile learners learn through touching, manipulating, and handling objects, so they remember more when they write, doodle, draw, or move their fingers. The use of models and computer-assisted instruction is most suitable for their learning style. Kinesthetic learners learn more easily by doing and experiencing; they profit from opportunities for field trips, role-playing, interviewing, and participating in return demonstration.

*Intake*    Some learners need to eat, drink, chew, or bite objects while concentrating. Others prefer no intake until after they have finished studying. A list of rules needs to be established to satisfy the oral needs of those who prefer intake while learning as long as it is not offensive to others or does not interfere with building rules and regulations of the agency.

*Time of day*    Some learners perform better at one time of day than another. The four time-of-day preferences are on a continuum, and the educator needs to identify these preferences with an effort toward structuring teaching and learning to occur during the times that are most suitable for the learner:

Early-morning learners—The ability to concentrate and focus energies on learning are oriented to this time of day.

Late-morning learners—The energy curve peaks before noontime, when their ability to perform is at its height.

Afternoon learners—The energy curve is highest in the mid to late afternoon, and they perform best during this time of day.

Evening learners—The ability to concentrate and focus energies on learning is oriented to this time of day.

Dunn (1995) contends that among adults, 55% are "morning people" and 28% work best in the evening. Many adults experience energy lows in the afternoon. School-aged children, on the other hand, have high energy levels in the late morning and early afternoon. About 13% of high school students work best in the evening. This time sensitivity means that it may be more difficult for a person to learn a new skill or behavior at certain times of the day than at other times. To increase learning, the educator should group the most important topics at the learner's best time of day (Dunn, 1995).

*Mobility*    Mobility refers to how still the learner can sit and for how long a period of time. Some learners need to move about, whereas others can sit for hours engaged in learning. For those who require mobility, it is necessary to provide opportunity for movement by assigning them to less restrictive sections of the room. During workshops or any type of group learning, give frequent 30-to 60-second breaks during which participants can stand. This is a good time to have the participants turn to another and tell one thing that they have learned during that time.

**The Psychological Elements**

*Global versus analytic*    Some learners are global in their thinking and learn best by obtaining meaning from a broad, overall concept before focusing on the details in the surrounding environment. Other learners are

analytic in their thinking and learn sequentially in a step-by-step process.

*Hemispheric preference*    Learners who possess right-brain preference tend to learn best in environments that have low illumination, background music, casual seating, and tactile instructional resources. Learners with left-brain preference require an opposite environment of bright lighting, quiet environment, formal seating, and visual or auditory instructional resources.

*Impulsivity versus reflectivity*    Impulsive learners prefer opportunities to participate verbally in groups and tend to answer questions spontaneously and without consciously processing their thinking. Reflective learners seldom volunteer information unless they are asked to do so, prefer to contemplate information, and tend to be uncomfortable participating in group discussions (Dunn, 1984).

Dunn and Dunn stress that the PEPS is not intended to be used as an indicator of underlying psychological factors, value systems, or the quality of attitudes. This instrument yields information concerned with the patterns through which learning occurs but does not assess the finer aspects of an individual's skills, such as the ability to outline procedures and to organize, classify, or analyze new material. It indicates how people prefer to learn, not the abilities they possess.

## Myers-Briggs Type Indicator

The Myers-Briggs Type Indicator (MBTI) is a forced choice, self-report inventory based on the Jungian theory of personality type. Since its development in the 1920s, this instrument has undergone several revisions, and its reliability and validity are well established. C. G. Jung, a Swiss psychiatrist, developed a theory that explains personality similarities and differences by identifying the ways people prefer to take in and make use of data from the world around them. Jung proposed that peo-

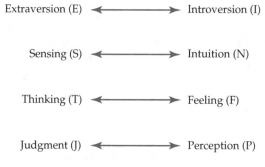

**FIGURE 4–4  Myers-Briggs Dichotomous Dimensions or Preferences**

ple are likely to operate in a variety of ways depending on the circumstances. Despite these situational adaptations, each individual will tend to develop comfortable patterns, which dictate behavior in certain predictable ways. Jung used the word "types" to identify these styles of personality.

Katherine Briggs and her daughter Isabel Briggs Myers became convinced that Jung's theories had an application for increasing human understanding (Myers, 1980). They developed an instrument based on Jung's theories that would permit people to learn about their own type of behavior and thus understand themselves better with respect to the way in which they interact with others. Although the MBTI is not a learning style instrument per se, it does measure differences in personality types that affect how individuals behave and how people tend to interact with one another. The instrument uses forced-choice questions and word pairs to measure four dimensions of behavior as indicated by the following dichotomous preferences (Figure 4–4):

**1.** *Extraversion-Introversion (EI)* reflects an orientation to either the outside world of people and things or to the inner world of concepts and ideas. This dimension describes

the extent to which our behavior is determined by our attitudes toward the world. Jung invented the terms from Latin words meaning *outward turning* (extraversion) or *inward turning* (introversion). Jung said extraverts operate comfortably and successfully by interacting with things external to themselves, such as other people, experiences, and situations. Extraverts like to clarify thoughts and ideas through talking and doing. Those who operate more comfortably in an extraverted way think aloud. Introverts, on the other hand, are more interested in the internal world of their minds, hearts, and souls. They like to brew over thoughts and actions, reflecting on them until they become more personally meaningful. Those who operate more comfortably in an introverted way are often thoughtful, reflective, and slow to act because they need time to translate internal thoughts to the external world. Introverts have their thoughts well formulated before they are willing to share them with others.

**2.** *Sensing-Intuition (SN)* describes perception as coming directly through the five senses or indirectly by way of the unconscious. This dimension explains how people understand what is experienced. People who fall into the sensing category view the world through their senses—vision, hearing, touch, taste, and smell. They observe what is real, what is factual, and what is actually happening. Seeing (or other sense experiences) is believing. These sensory functions allow the individual to observe carefully, gather facts, and focus on practical actions. Conversely, those people who are associated with the intuition category tend to read between the lines, focus on meaning, and attend to what is and what might be. Intuitives view the world through possibilities and relationships, and are tuned into subtleties of body language and tones of voice. This kind of perception leads them to examine problems and issues in creative and original ways.

**3.** *Thinking-Feeling (TF)* is the approach used by individuals to arrive at judgments through impersonal, logical, or subjective processes. Thinkers analyze information, data, situations, and people and make decisions based on logic. They are careful and slow in the analysis of the data, because accuracy and thoroughness are important to them. They trust objectivity and put faith in logical predictions and rational arguments. Thinkers explore and weigh all alternatives, and the final decision is reached unemotionally and carefully. In the feeling dimension, on the other hand, the approach to decision making takes place through a subjective, perceptive, empathetic, and emotional perspective. Feeling people search for the effect of a decision on themselves and others. They consider alternatives and examine evidence to develop a personal reaction and commitment. They believe the decision-making process is complex and not totally objective. Circumstantial evidence is extremely important, and these individuals see the world as gray rather than black and white.

Jung said that everyone uses these opposing perceptions to some degree in each of the three dimensions (EI, SN, TF) when dealing with people and situations, but each person has a preference for one way of looking at the world. Individuals become more skilled in arriving at a decision in either a thinking or feeling way and can function as extraverts at one time and as introverts at another time, but they tend to develop patterns that are most typical and comfortable.

**4.** *Judgment-Perception (JP)* In addition to Jung's dimensions, Myers and Briggs discovered another dimension, whereby an individual comes to a conclusion about something or becomes aware of something. Each individual has a preference for either the judging function or the perceptive function. The desire to regulate and bring closure to circumstances

| ISTJ | ISFJ | INFJ | INTJ |
|------|------|------|------|
| ISTP | ISFP | INFP | INTP |
| ESTP | ESFP | ENFP | ENTP |
| ESTJ | ESFJ | ENFJ | ENTJ |

FIGURE 4–5   **Myers-Briggs Types** SOURCE: Modified and reproduced by special permission of the Publisher. Consulting Psychologists Press, Inc., Palo Alto, CA 94303 from *Introduction to Type*® 6th *Edition* by Isabel Briggs Myers. Copyright 1998 by Consulting Psychologists Press, Inc. All rights reserved. Further reproduction is prohibited without the Publisher's written consent.

in life is called judgment, and the desire to be open-minded and understanding is known as perception.

By combining the different dimensions, Myers and Briggs identified 16 personality types, each with its own strengths and interests (Figure 4–5). The Myers-Briggs Type Indicator can be useful for the educator to understand the many different ways in which learners perceive and judge information when learning (Table 4–5). These preferences can be reflected in how the educator teaches based on how the learner learns. The logical, detailed educator (sensing-thinking) may have difficulty communicating with a learner who is more holistically oriented (intuitive-feeling). What each party values and believes most important to be learned or discussed may be different and can lead to misunderstanding and conflicts (Bargar & Hoover, 1984) unless the educator recognizes this potential and adapts teaching to meet the style of the learner. Another example of how the dimensions function together is that the sensing-thinking learner's preferred learning style emphasizes hands-on experience, demon-

**TABLE 4-5 Myers-Briggs types: Examples of learning**

| EXTRAVERT | INTROVERT |
|---|---|
| Likes group work | Likes quiet space |
| Dislikes slow-paced learning | Dislikes interruptions |
| Likes action and to experience things so as to learn | Likes learning that deals with thoughts, ideas |
| Offers opinions without being asked | Offers opinions only when asked |
| Asks questions to check on the expectations of educator | Asks questions to allow understanding of learning activity |

| SENSING | INTUITION |
|---|---|
| Practical | Always likes something new |
| Realistic | Imaginative |
| Observant | Sees possibilities |
| Learns from orderly sequence of details | Prefers the whole concept versus details |

| THINKING | FEELING |
|---|---|
| Low need for harmony | Values harmony |
| Finds ideas and things more interesting than people | More interested in people than things or ideas |
| Analytical | Sympathetic |
| Fair | Accepting |

| JUDGMENT | PERCEPTION |
|---|---|
| Organized | Open-ended |
| Methodical | Flexible |
| Work-oriented | Play-oriented |
| Controls the environment | Adapts to the environment |

stration, and application of concepts, whereas intuitive-thinking learners prefer emphasis on the theoretical concerns before they can concentrate on the practical applications.

Schoessler, Conedera, Bell, Marshall, and Gilson (1993) discuss the use of the MBTI to develop a continuing education department for nursing. Costello (1993) demonstrates the application of the MBTI by nurse managers as a tool to meet the needs of the staff they supervise.

## Kolb's Learning Style Inventory

David Kolb (1984), a management expert from Case Western Reserve University, developed an experiential learning model in the early 1970s. Kolb believes knowledge is a transformational process that is continuously created

and recreated. Learning is a continuous process grounded in the reality that the learner is not a blank slate. Every learner approaches a topic to be learned with preconceived ideas. Kolb's theory on learning style is that learning is a cumulative result of past experiences, heredity, and the demands of the present environment. These factors combine to produce different individual orientations to learning. By knowing each learner's preferred style, the nurse educator is better equipped to assist learners in refining or modifying these preconceived ideas so that real learning can occur.

Kolb's model, known as the Cycle of Learning, includes four modes of learning, which reflect two major dimensions of perception and processing. He hypothesized that learning results from the way learners perceive as well as how they process what they perceive. The dimension of perception involves two opposite perceptual viewpoints. Some learners perceive through concrete experience (CE mode), whereas others perceive through abstract conceptualization (AC mode). At the CE stage of the learning cycle, learners tend to rely more on feelings than on a systematic approach to problems and situations. Learners who fall into this category like relating with people, benefit from specific experiences, and are sensitive to others. They learn from feeling. At the AC stage, on the other hand, learners rely on logic and ideas rather than on feelings to deal with problems or situations. People who fall into this category use systematic planning and logical analysis to solve problems. They learn by thinking.

The process dimension also has two opposing orientations. Some learners process information through active experimentation (AE mode), whereas others process information through reflective observation (RO mode). At the AE stage of the learning cycle, learning is active, and learners like to experiment to get things done. They prefer to influence or change situations and see the results of their actions. They enjoy involvement and are risk takers. They learn by doing. At the RO stage of the learning cycle, learners rely on objectivity, careful judgment, personal thoughts, and feelings to form opinions. People who fall into this category look for meaning of things by viewing them from different perspectives. They learn by watching and listening.

Kolb described each learning style as a combination of the four basic learning modes (CE, AC, AE, and RO), identifying separate learning style types that best define the strengths and weaknesses of a learner. The learner predominantly demonstrates characteristics of one of four style types: (1) diverger, (2) assimilator, (3) converger, or (4) accommodator (Figure 4–6).

The *diverger* combines the learning modes of CE and RO. People with this learning style are good at viewing concrete situations from many points of view. They like to observe, gather information, and gain insights rather than take action. Working in groups to generate ideas appeals to them. They place a high value on understanding for knowledge's sake and like to personalize learning by connecting information with something familiar in their experiences. They have active imaginations, enjoy being involved, and are sensitive to feelings. Divergent thinkers learn best, for example, through group discussions and participating in brainstorming sessions.

The *assimilator* combines the learning modes of RO and AC. People with this learning style demonstrate the ability to understand large amounts of information by putting it into concise and logical form. They are less interested in people and more focused on abstract ideas and concepts. They are good at inductive reasoning, value theory over practical application of ideas, and need time to reflect on what has been learned and how information can be integrated into their past experiences. They rely on knowledge from experts. Assimilative thinkers learn best, for example, through lecture, one-to-one instruction, and self-instruction methods with ample reading materials to support their learning.

The *converger* combines the learning modes of AC and AE. People with this learning style type find practical application for ideas and theories and have the ability to use deductive reasoning to solve problems. They like structure and factual information, and they look for specific solutions to problems. Learners with this style prefer technical tasks rather than dealing with social and interpersonal issues. Kolb postulates that individuals with this learning style have skills that are important for specialist and technology careers. The convergent thinker

Concrete Experience (CE)
"Feeling"

Active Experimentation (AE)
"Doing"

| Accommodator | Diverger |
|---|---|
| Converger | Assimilator |

Reflective Observation (RO)
"Watching"

Abstract Conceptualization (AC)
"Thinking"

**FIGURE 4–6   Kolb's Learning Style Inventory** SOURCE: Kolb, D. *Experiental Learning: Experience as a Source of Learning and Development* © 1984, Figures 3.1, 4.2. Reprinted by permission of Prentice-Hall, Inc., Upper Saddle River, NJ.

learns best, for example, through demonstration–return demonstration methods of teaching accompanied by handouts and diagrams.

The *accommodator* combines the learning modes of AE and CE. People with this learning style learn best by hands-on experience and enjoy new and challenging situations. They act on intuition and "gut feelings" rather than on logic. These risk takers like to explore all possibilities and learn by experimenting with materials and objects. Accommodative thinkers are perhaps the most challenging to educators because they demand new and exciting experiences and are willing to take risks that might endanger their safety. Role-playing, gaming, and computer simulations, for example, are methods of teaching most preferred by this style of learner.

Kolb's Learning Style Inventory is a self-report instrument that measures learning style types and is based on Piaget's and Guilford's theories of thinking, creativity, and intellect. The instrument rank-orders four word phrases in a list of sets. Each word phrase represents one of the four learning modes. A scoring process reduces the ranking evidence to four mode scores (CE, RO, AC, and AE) and then further reduces these down into two dimension scores (concrete-abstract and reflective-active). The predominant score indicates the learner's style (diverger, assimilator, converger, or accommodator).

Knowledge of learning style differences enables the educator to enhance individuals' strengths and to assist learners in developing additional ways of learning. Kolb believes that understanding a person's learning style, including its strengths and weaknesses, represents a major step toward increasing learning power and helping learners to get the most from their learning experiences. By using different teaching strategies to address these four learning styles, particular modes of learning can be matched, at least some of the time, with the educator's methods of teaching. For every group of learners, about 25% will fall into each of the four categories. If the educator predominantly uses only one method of teaching, such as the lecture to promote learning, then 75% of all learners will be selectively excluded.

When teaching groups of learners, instruction should begin with activities best suited to the divergent thinker and progress sequentially to include activities for the assimilator, converger, and accommodator, respectively (Arndt & Underwood, 1990). This pattern works because learners must first have foundational knowledge of a subject before they can test out information. Otherwise, they will be operating from a level of ignorance. They must first have familiarity with facts and ideas before they can explore and test concepts.

## Gregorc Style Delineator

Anthony Gregorc's extensive research on learning style (1982) identifies four sets of dualities: perception, ordering, processing, and relating. Thus this model has more depth than do the other theories. Based on his research, Gregorc developed an instrument called the Gregorc Style Delineator. This self-analysis instrument is designed to assess a person's learning style. Sets of words are ranked, a numerical score is derived from each of the four patterns, and the scores are then plotted on a grid (Figure 4–7).

Gregorc states that a learning style consists of distinctive and observable behavior that provides cues about the mediation abilities of individuals. According to him, the human mind has channels through which it receives and expresses information most efficiently and effectively. The power, capacity, and dexterity to utilize these channels are collectively termed *mediation abilities*. Two mediation abilities of the mind are how people perceive and how they order knowledge. Perception is seen as a continuum with two opposite tendencies—concrete and abstract. Ordering also exists on a continuum, with sequential and

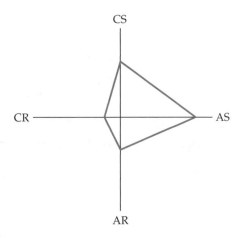

FIGURE 4–7   **Gregorc Style Delineator**
SOURCE: Adapted from Gregorc, A. *An Adult's Guide to Style.* Columbia, CT: Gregorc Associates, Inc., 1982.

random tendencies. The other two mediation abilities of processing and relating are still being refined.

Learners vary in their particular balance of these four qualities of perception and ordering. Four learning patterns are identified: concrete sequential (CS), abstract sequential (AS), abstract random (AR), and concrete random (CR). In each of these patterns, learners demonstrate perceived attitudes, motivations, and reasoned thought toward the learning environment.

*Concrete sequential* learners tend to operate in a highly structured, conservative manner in which specific details and time schedules are critical. Objectives are important to CS learners as well as a clear beginning and a clear end to the task. These learners do not tolerate being interrupted during the performance of a skill because questioning throws the learning sequence off and causes the CS learner to have difficulty completing the skill. External distractions should be eliminated because the CS individual learns better in a quiet environment than in a noisy environment. If more than one educator is involved in an interaction with such a learner, it is important that they all provide the same information in the same sequence. Consistency is important because CS learners can detect a minute flaw or variance in details. A CS learner likes recognition or a compliment on a job well done in learning: "Thank you" and "good" are terms the CS learner likes to hear. Standards that CS individuals set for themselves are extremely high. The educator must be aware that concise words should be used and that the CS learner will interpret words and labels literally. With this type of individual, learning can be enhanced by using handouts, demonstration teaching, hands-on opportunities with guided practice, lectures with visual aids, and computer-aided instruction.

*Abstract sequential* learners are global thinkers and surround themselves with language and other symbols of knowledge. They also like to deal with abstract ideas, and their style of learning continually leads to further understanding. These types of learners also do not learn well when sequence is interrupted. The AS learner needs facts and written documentation to refer to, such as statistics and resource references. When learning, the AS individual typically does not display emotion and has difficulty picking up subtle verbal and nonverbal cues. The AS learner also needs a quiet environment to concentrate and learn. Learning can be enhanced by audiotapes, lectures, and supplemental reading.

*Abstract random* learners value relationships over time-bound structures. They think in global terms, and their thinking processes are anchored in feelings. Often AR learners will direct attention to information that has personal meaning to them. Learning can be enhanced with color, music, pictures, drawings, symbols, poetry, and humor. Educators need to know that the AR learner will ask questions randomly during teaching episodes and likes a busy environment for learning. Learning is best achieved in groups, with the opportunity for discussion and question-and-answer sessions.

Finally, *concrete random* learners tend to seek alternatives and create choices where none existed before. The CR learner is very inquisitive and will question motives. Attention is focused on the process, and the CR individual will make intuitive leaps or insights. The "why" is more important than the "how." The CR learner does not like detail and has difficulty with step-by-step learning. Learning for the CR individual is enhanced with simulations, computer and board games, case studies, and brainstorming sessions.

Gregorc believes that most people have the ability to operate to some extent in all four styles, although 90% of learners are better able to operate in only one or possibly two learning styles. In a new or stressful learning situation, the learner will exhibit stronger characteristics of one particular style. The Gregorc Style Delineator instrument is designed to measure the extent to which a learner's pattern of thinking reflects the four modes. A higher score in a mode indicates a stronger orientation to that mode. With an understanding of these modes, the educator can design teaching methods based on the individual styles of learners.

## 4MAT System

McCarthy (1981) developed a model based on previous research on learning styles and brain functioning. In particular, she used Kolb's model combined with right/left-brain research findings to create the 4MAT System (Figure 4–8). McCarthy's model describes four types of learners and defines the learning process as a natural sequence from type 1 to type 4. Educators can address all four learning styles by teaching sequentially, thus attending to all types of learners. Learners are then able to work with their own strongest learning style, while at the same time developing the ability through exposure to work in the other quadrants.

To use this sequence, learners begin in the first quadrant, known as type 1, and

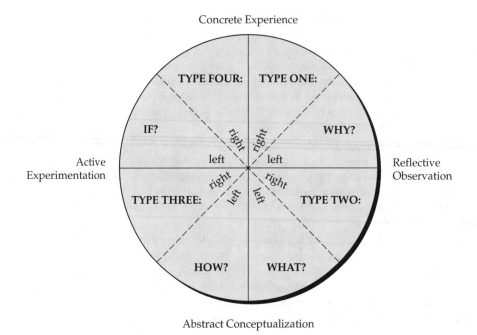

Concrete Experience

**FIGURE 4–8    McCarthy's 4MAT System**  SOURCE: From P. B. Guild and S. Garger, *Marching to Different Drummers.* Alexandria, VA: Association for Supervision and Curriculum Development, 1998.

engage the right brain by sensing and feeling their way through an experience. Eventually, they move to the left brain to analyze what they have experienced. They ask, "Why is this important? Why should I try to learn this?"

The next quadrant is type 2, in which learning also begins with the right brain to make observations and integrate data with present knowledge. Learners then engage the left brain to think about new theories and concepts relative to these observations. They ask, "What is it I am supposed to be learning? What is the relationship?"

Type 3 learners (third quadrant) begin with the left brain by working with defined concepts, then shifting to the right brain to experiment with what has to be learned. They ask, "How does this work? How can I figure this out?"

Finally, type 4 learners also begin with the left brain by analyzing the practicality of what has been learned. They then move to the right brain to show mastery through application and the sharing of findings with others. They ask, "If I learn this, what can I do with it? Can I apply it?"

The learning sequence is circular and cyclic, beginning at type 1 and moving to type 4, which is characteristic of a higher level and greater complexity of learning. Based on this model, it is important for the educator to begin type 1 learning by including personal meaning for the learner to make the learning experience relevant and to answer the "why" question. Next, it is essential to introduce new knowledge based on accurate information to answer the "what" question. The third step in sequential learning is to deal with reality in a practical manner through application of knowledge to enable learners to answer the "how" question. Finally, in the fourth step, the learning experience must allow the learner to be innovative and inspiring and to create new possibilities so the "if" question is answered.

The educator needs to determine cognitive skill and attitude changes to be attained by all learners to be certain teaching matches expected outcomes. By using this sequential approach to learning, the educator can instill personal meaning and motivation for what is to be learned (type 1), assist the learner in the acquisition of the new knowledge and concepts (type 2), allow for active experimentation (type 3), and provide the opportunity for more complex synthesis and extension through practical application (type 4). Through use of the 4MAT System, each learning style will then have an opportunity to exert itself at least part of the time.

## Gardner's Seven Types of Intelligence

Most theories and measurement instruments on learning style focus on the adult as learner. However, children also have their own way of learning. Learning styles of children can be assessed from the standpoint of growth and each individual's unique pattern of neurological functioning. Psychologist Howard Gardner (1983) developed a theory focused on seven kinds of intelligence, which is useful in looking at styles of learning in children. Gardner based his theory on findings from brain research, developmental work with children, and psychological testing. He identified seven kinds of intelligence located in different parts of the brain: linguistic, logical-mathematical, spatial, musical, bodily kinesthetic, interpersonal, and intrapersonal. All learners have all the seven kinds of intelligence but in different proportions.

*Linguistic* intelligence seems to be in the Broca's area of the left side of the brain for most people. Children with a preference for this type of intelligence have highly developed auditory skills and think in words. They like to write, tell stories, spell words accurately, enjoy reading, and can recall names, places, and dates. These children learn best by verbalizing, hearing, or seeing words. Word games or crossword puzzles are an excellent method for helping these children learn new material.

*Logical-mathematical* intelligence involves both sides of the brain. The right side deals with concepts, and the left side remembers the symbols. The children who are strong in this intelligence explore patterns, categories, and relationships. In the adolescent years, they have the ability for logical thinking with a high degree of abstraction. As learners, they question many things and ask where, what, and when. A question such a learner could ask is, "If people are always supposed to be good to each other, then why do people always say they are sorry?" They can do arithmetic problems quickly in their heads, like to learn by computers, and do experiments to test concepts they do not understand. They enjoy strategy board games such as chess or checkers.

*Spatial* intelligence is related to the right side of the brain. These children learn by images and pictures. They enjoy such things as building blocks, jigsaw puzzles, and daydreaming. They like to draw or do other art activities, can read charts and diagrams, and learn with visual methods such as videos or photographs.

*Musical* intelligence is also related to the right side of the brain. These children can be found singing a tune, telling you when a note is off-key, playing musical instruments with ease, dancing to music, and keeping time rhythmically. They are also sensitive to sounds in the environment, such as the sound of walking on snow on a cold winter morning. Often musically intelligent children learn best with music playing in the background.

*Bodily kinesthetic* intelligence includes the basal ganglia and cerebellum of the brain in addition to other brain structures. These children learn by processing knowledge through bodily sensations. They need to learn by moving or acting things out. It is difficult for these learners to sit still for long periods of time. They are good at athletic sports and have highly developed fine-motor coordination. Use of body language to communicate and copying people's behaviors or movements come easily for this group of learners.

*Interpersonal* intelligence involves the prefrontal lobes of the brain. These children understand people, are able to notice others' feelings, tend to have many friends, and are gifted in the social skills. They learn best in groups and gravitate toward activities that involve others.

*Intrapersonal* intelligence, like interpersonal intelligence, involves the prefrontal lobes of the brain. These children have strong personalities and prefer the inner world of feelings and ideas and like being alone. They are very private individuals, like a quiet area to learn, and many times need to be by themselves to learn. They tend to be self-directed and self-confident. They learn well with independent, self-paced instruction.

Educators should always approach a child's learning using concepts from the perspective of the seven intelligences (Armstrong, 1987). Often it can be difficult to assess the preferred learning style of a child when the child is facing an illness or surgery. Asking some key questions of the child or parents may give the educator some clues as to the preferred style of learning. What does the child already know how to do? What subjects does the child excel in or like best? What kinds of hobbies does the child have? What excites this child? What kinds of toys does the child play with? What inner qualities does the child possess, such as courage, playfulness, curiosity, friendliness, or creativity? What talents does the child have? Does the child like to take things apart and put them back together?

By using the theory of the seven intelligences, the educator can assess each child's style of learning and tailor teaching accordingly. For example, if the educator wants to assist a child in learning about a kidney disorder, then one of seven different approaches can be used, depending on the child's style of learning:

*Linguistic*—Practice quizzing the child orally on the different parts of the kidney, the disease itself, and ways to take care of oneself.

*Spatial*—Have a diagram or chart that allows the child to associate different colors or shapes with concepts. Storytelling can be used illustrating a child with the same chronic illness.

*Kinesthetic*—Have a kidney model available that can be felt, taken apart, and manipulated. Have the child identify tactile features of the kidney or "act out" appropriate behavior.

*Logical-mathematical*—Group concepts into categories, starting with simple generalizations or health behaviors. Reasoning works well in showing the child the consequences of actions.

*Musical*—Teach self-care or the material to be learned by putting information into a song. Soft music also serves as a relaxing influence on the child.

*Interpersonal*—Have a group of children play a card game such as a version of Old Maid that matches information with medical pictures or pictures of healthcare activities and procedures. Use group work for problem-solving activities.

*Intrapersonal*—Suggest that the child become active by writing to friends, family, or local and state government officials to advocate for kidney disease. Such learners need to research the facts and then convey these findings to others. These children learn best by one-to-one teaching and through use of self-learning modules.

## NOVICE-TO-EXPERT CONCEPT

Recent theories on learning style have addressed the novice-to-expert concept. These theories are particularly applicable when assessing learning of professional nursing staff and students. Benner (1994) is well known for applying the concept of novice-to-expert in nursing practice. How one proceeds from a novice to an expert learner in each learning domain is described in an article entitled "The Mind's Journey from Novice to Expert," by John Bruer (1993). Bruer discusses how progress made by cognitive scientists in understanding the learning process can help educators promote subjects' optimal learning. Cognitive scientists have determined how expertise in a particular subject matter requires mastery of a distinct knowledge base in a specific domain.

Newell and Simon (1972) argued that to understand learning in a particular domain, the educator must begin with a detailed analysis of how people solve problems in that domain. By analyzing chess players, Chase and Simon (1973) found that experts see chunks whereas novices see individual pieces. The experts envision potential moves, and this approach permits them to choose the best strategies because they operate using information-rich chunks. Chunking, rather than concentrating on each move, accounts for the experts' superiority.

In this classic example of chess players, Bruer (1993) acknowledged that novices see the chessboard in terms of individual pieces. They can store the positions of only five or six pieces in their short-term memory. This number saturation is consistent with what research has shown to be our working memory span capacity. Therefore, if each chunk contains four or five pieces and experts are able to hold five such chunks in their working memory, then the experts can reproduce accurately the positions of 20 to 25 individual pieces. In addition, Simon and Chase (1973) found that when experts reproduce the positions of chess pieces on the board, they did so in chunks. Thus, if an educator knows how a novice solves a particular problem in a domain, compared with the way an expert thinks, then learning can be traced to changes that occur in mental processes in moving from novice to expert. Learning is the process by which novices become experts.

## INTERPRETATION OF THE USE OF STYLE INSTRUMENTS

Learning style is an important consideration in the teaching–learning process. Nevertheless, caution must be exercised in assessing styles so as not to ignore other factors that are equally important in learning, such as readiness and capabilities to learn, educational background, and rates of learning. Styles, which vary from person to person, also differ from capabilities in that the style by which someone learns describes how that individual processes stimuli as opposed to defining how much and how well the information is processed (Thompson & Crutchlow, 1993). Many learning theorists advocate that learning style be matched with a similar teaching style for learners to attain an optimal level of achievement. However, research in this area is clouded by inconsistent findings. Some studies have found that learning styles have no significant effect on achievement of learning. It may be that learning occurs not so much as a result of matching teacher and learner styles, but that when the educator uses a variety of teaching approaches rather than relying on just one, learners feel less stressed. As a result, learners will be more satisfied overall with the learning experience and hence more motivated to learn. Nevertheless, using teaching methods that coincide with the dominant learning style of individuals is usually considered the best way to effect the greatest learning achievement (deTornay & Thompson, 1987). Application of learning style theory to facilitate education allows the educator to approach each learner holistically by recognizing that not all learners process information in the same way (Arndt & Underwood, 1990).

Much of the research implies that individuals have a certain learning style that prevails over time, although the use of certain styles may depend on the context in which learners are operating at any given moment. The concept of matching styles implies that individuals are static, which contradicts the purpose of education. Learners need to experience some discomfort before they can grow. Educators need to generate "dynamic disequilibrium" rather than creating an environment that is too harmonious (Joyce, 1984).

When selecting a learning style instrument, the educator must first evaluate the instrument for validity, reliability, and the population for which it is to be used. In addition, the ease of administering the instrument and the ease of analyzing the results need to be taken into consideration. Also, copyright laws must be adhered to, which means that the instrument must be bought or the author's permission must be obtained before the tool is used.

When considering using a learning style instrument for purposes of assessment, the nurse educator is encouraged to use more than one such tool. If the educator focuses on only one model, then the possibility arises of trying to make the learner fit an unsuitable style. By using more than one model, given the learning situation, the educator may find that one learning style is more appropriate than another. The educator will also have more strategies for dealing with problems or unique situations.

Of course, it may not always be practical to use learning style instruments because of cost, time, or appropriateness of the instrument fit for a specific population. Educators should therefore follow some general guidelines when assessing individual learning styles:

- Become familiar with the different instruments available and the ways in which styles are classified so that it becomes easier to recognize various learning styles.

- Identify key elements of an individual's learning style by observing and asking questions to verify observations and then matching instructional methods and materials to those unique qualities. For example, such questions could include the following: Do you prefer to attend lectures or group discussions? Which do you like to do better, read or view a film? Would you like me to demonstrate this skill first, or would you rather learn by doing while I talk you through the procedure?

- Always allow learners the opportunity to say when the teaching method is not working for them.

- Place emphasis on assessing learning styles as a way to increase understanding both from the educator's and the learner's perspectives. No one style is better than another, and everyone should realize that a variety of learning modalities exist.

- Be cautious about saying that certain instructional methods are always more effective for certain styles. Remember that everyone is unique, and there are many different ways to influence learning.

- Encourage learners to expand their style ranges rather than to seek only comfortable experiences.

- Provide structured learning choices that enable learners to recognize and choose the style in which they prefer to learn.

- Use a team of educators, who have different teaching styles, to introduce new and complex information. This technique may be useful for helping learners, all of whom have varied learning styles, to master information.

Caution must be exercised when using any of these instruments to assess learning style. The educator must remember not to place too much emphasis or reliance on these tools to categorize learners. The educator's goal should not be to stereotype learners as to style but rather to ensure that each individual learner is given an equal opportunity to learn the best or most comfortable way. The learning style instruments may help the educator to understand how someone prefers to learn so that diverse teaching methods and materials can be chosen to meet the needs of all learners.

## SUMMARY

This chapter stressed the importance of the assessment phase of learning, because the educator must be aware of as well as know how to determine learning needs, the learner's readiness to learn, and the learner's individual learning style prior to planning for any educational encounter.

Learning is a complex concept that is not directly seen but can be inferred from permanent changes that occur in the learner's behavior. Learning takes place in all three of the cognitive, psychomotor, and affective domains. Behavioral objectives for these three domains should not be set until the educator establishes what the needs of the learner are, when the learner is ready to learn, and how the learner best learns. Learning by the patient, family member, or nurses and other healthcare professionals requires that the educator identify learning approaches and activities based on the determinants of learning for each individual.

Identifying and prioritizing the learning needs requires finding out what the learner feels is important. Once these needs are established, the educator must assess the learner's readiness to learn based on the physical, emotional, experiential, and knowledge components particular to each learner so that teaching interventions can be adjusted to facilitate the learning process.

The last determinant of learning is assessing the learner's learning style. Assessment of learning style by way of interviewing, observing, and instrument measurement can reveal how individuals best learn as well as how they prefer to learn. By accepting the diversity of style among learners, the educator can create a versatile atmosphere and provide optimal experiences that encourage all learners to reach their full potential. Whoever the audience may be, the nurse educator should be able to identify and select approaches and activities most beneficial for the learner based on the three determinants of learning.

## REVIEW QUESTIONS

1. How would you define the term *determinants of learning*?
2. What are four of the seven methods to assess learning needs?
3. What is meant by the term readiness to learn?
4. What are the four types of readiness to learn?
5. What are the components of each type of readiness to learn?

6. What are the six learning style principles that should guide the nurse educator in teaching any audience of learners?
7. Which is the most reliable and valid method to determine someone's learning style?
8. What do each of the eight learning style instruments measure?

## REFERENCES

Anderson, J. K. (1998). Orientation with style: Matching teaching/learning style. *Journal for Nurses in Staff Development, 14*(4), 192–197.

Armstrong, T. (1987). *In Their Own Way.* New York: St. Martin's Press.

Arndt, M. J. & Underwood, B. (1990). Learning style theory and patient understanding. *Journal of Continuing Education in Nursing, 21*(1), 28–31.

Ashton, K. C. (1999). How men and women with heart disease seek care: The delay experience. *Progress in Cardiovascular Nursing, 14*(2), 53–60.

Bargar, R. & Hoover, R. (1984). Psychological type and the matching of cognitive styles. *Theory into Practice, 23*(1), 56–63.

Beddoe, S. S. (1999). Reachable moment. *Image: Journal of Nursing Scholarship, 31*(3), 248.

Benner, P. (1994). *Interpretive Phenomenology.* Thousand Oaks, CA: Sage Publications.

Bertakis, K. D., Rahman, A., Helms, L. J., Callahan, E. J., & Robbins, J. A. (2000). *Journal of Family Practice, 49,*(2), 147–152.

Bloom, B. (1968). *Learning for Mastery.* Instruction and Curriculum, Topical Papers and Reprints No. 1 (Durham, NC: National Laboratory for Higher Education.)

Bonham, L. A. (1988). Learning style instruments: Let the buyer beware. *Lifelong Learning, 11*(6),14–17.

Botwinick, J. (1978). *Aging and Behavior,* 2nd ed. New York: Springer.

Boyd, M. D., Gleit, C. J., Graham, B. A., & Whitman, N. I. (1998). *Health Teaching in Nursing Practice: A Professional Model,* 3rd ed. Stamford, CT: Appleton & Lange.

Breitrose, P. (1988). *Focus Groups—When and How to Use Them: A Practical Guide.* Palo Alto, CA: Health Promotion Resource.

Bruer, J. (1993). The mind's journey from novice to expert. *American Educator, 17*(2), 6–15, 38–46.

Bruner, J. (1966). *Toward a Theory of Instruction.* Cambridge, MA: Harvard University Press.

Bubela, N. & Galloway, S. (1990). Factors influencing patients' informational needs at time of hospital discharge. *Patient Education and Counseling, 16,* 21–28.

Burton, C. (2000). Re-thinking stroke rehabilitation: The Corbin and Strauss chronic illness trajectory framework. *Journal of Advanced Nursing, 32*(3), 595–602.

Carroll, I. (1963). A model of school learning. *Teachers College Record, 64,* 723–733.

Caulfield, J., Kidd, S., & Kocher, T. (2000). Brain-based instruction in action. *Educational Leadership, 58*(3),62–65.

Chall, J. & Mirsky, A. (eds.). (1978). *Education and the Brain. Seventy-seventh Yearbook of the National Society for the Study of Education, Part 2.* Chicago: University of Chicago Press.

Chase, W. G. & Simon, H. A. (1973). Perception in chess. *Cognitive Psychology, 4,* 55–81.

Corbin, J. M. & Strauss, A. (1991). A nursing model for chronic illness management based upon the trajectory framework. *Scholarly Inquiry for Nursing Practice: An International Journal, 5*(3), 155–174.

Costello, K. (1993). The Myers-Briggs Type Indicator—A management tool. *Nursing Management, 24*(5), 46–47, 50–51.

deTornay, R. & Thompson, M.A. (1987). *Strategies for Teaching Nursing,* 3rd ed. Albany, NY: Delmar.

Dunn, R. (1984). Learning Style: State of the Science. *Theory into Practice, 23*(1), 10–19.

Dunn, K. & Dunn, R. (1987). Dispelling outmoded beliefs about student learning. *Educational Leadership, 44*(6), 55–62.

Dunn, R. (1995). *Strategies for Educating Diverse Learners.* Bloomington, IN: Phi Delta Kappa Educational Foundation.

Dunn, R. & Dunn, K. (1978). *Teaching Students Through Their Individual Learning Styles: A Practical Approach.* Reston, VA: National Association of Secondary School Principals.

Durden-Smith, J. & deSimone, D. (1983). *Sex and the Brain.* New York: Arbor House.

Flynn, E. A., Barker, K. N., Gibson, J. T., Pearson, R. E., Berger, B. A., & Smith, L. A. (1999). Impact of interruptions and distractions on dispensing errors in an ambulatory care pharmacy. *American Journal of Health-System Pharmacy, 56*(13), 1319–1325.

Friedman, P. & Alley, R. (1984). Learning/teaching styles: Applying the principles. *Theory into Practice, 23*(1), 77–81.

Gardner, H. (1999). *The Disciplined Mind: What All Students should Understand.* New York: Simon and Schuster.

Gardner, H. (1983). *Frames of Mind.* New York: Basic Books.

Garity, J. (1985). Learning styles: Basis for creative teaching and learning. *Nurse Educator, 10*(2), 12–16.

Gessner, B. (1989). Adult education: The cornerstone of patient education. *Nursing Clinics of North America, 24*(3), 589–595.

Gondringer, N. (1989). Whole brain thinking: A potential link to successful learning. *Journal of the American Association of Nurse Anesthetists, 57*(3), 217–219.

Greer, G., Hitt, J. D, Sitterly, T. E., & Slebodnick, E. B. (1972). An examination of four factors impacting on psychomotor performance effectiveness. In D. P. Ely (ed.), *Psychomotor Domain: A Resource Book for Media Specialists.* Washington, DC: Gryphon House.

Gregorc, A. F. (1982). *An Adult's Guide to Style.* Maynard, MA: Gabriel Systems.

Guild, P. B. & Garger, S. (1998) *Marching to Different Drummers,* 2nd ed. Alexandria, VA: Association for Supervision and Curriculum Development.

Gur, R. C, Turetsky, B. I., Matsui, M., Yan, M., Bilker, W., Hughett, P., & Gur, R. E. (1999). Sex differences in brain gray and white matter in healthy young adults: Correlations with cognitive performance. *Journal of Neuroscience, 19*(10), 4065–4072.

Haggard, A. (1989). *Handbook of Patient Education.* Rockland, MD: Aspen.

Hansen, M. & Fisher, J. C. (1998). Patient-centered teaching: From theory to practice. *American Journal of Nursing, 98*(1), 56–60.

Healthcare Education Association. (1985). *Managing Hospital Education.* Laquana Niquel, CA: Healthcare Education Associates.

Herrman, N. (1988). *The Creative Brain.* Lake Lure, NC: Brain Books.

Iaccino, J. F. (1993). *Left-brain–Right brain Differences: Inquiries, Evidence and New Approaches.* Hillsdale, NJ: Lawrence Erlbaum Associates.

Joseph, D. H. (1993). Risk: A concept worthy of attention. *Nursing Forum, 28*(1), 12–16.

Joyce, B. (1984). Dynamic disequilibrium: The intelligence of growth. *Theory into Practice, 23*(1), 26–34.

Knox, A. B. (1977). *Adult Development and Learning.* San Francisco: Jossey-Bass.

Knox, A. B. (1986). *Helping Adults Learn.* San Francisco: Jossey-Bass.

Knox, A. B. (1974). *Life-long Self-directed Education.* San Francisco: Jossey-Bass.

Kolb, D. A. (1984). *Experiential Learning: Experience as the Source of Learning and Development.* Englewood Cliffs, NJ: Prentice-Hall.

Lichtenthal, C. (1990). *A Self-study Model on Readiness to Learn.* Unpublished.

Maslow, A. (1970). *Motivation and Personality.* New York: Harper & Row.

McCarthy, B. (1981). *The 4Mat System: Teaching to Learning Styles with Right/Left Mode Techniques.* Barrington, IL: Excel.

McIntosh, A. R. (1998). Understanding neural interactions in learning and memory using functional neuroimaging. *Annals of the New York Academy of Sciences. Olfaction and Taste Xll: An International Symposium, 855,* 556–571.

Myers, I. B. (1980). *Gifts Differing.* Palo Alto, CA: Consulting Psychologists Press.

Meyers, I. B. (1987). *Introduction to Type.* Palo Alto, CA: Consulting Psychologists Press, Inc.

Newell, A. & Simon, H. A. (1972). *Human Problem Solving.* Englewood Cliffs, NJ: Prentice-Hall.

Panno, J. M. (1992). A systematic approach for assessing learning needs. *Journal of Nursing Staff Development, 8*(6), 267–273.

Patterson, B. L. (2001). The shifting perspectives model of chronic illness. *Journal of Nursing Scholarship, 33*(1), 21–26.

Rankin, S. H. & Stallings, L. D. (2001). *Patient Education: Principles and Practice,* 4th ed. Philadelphia: Lippincott.

Roberts, C. (1982). Identifying the real patient problems. *Nursing Clinics of North America, 17*(3), 484–485.

Ruzicki, D. A. (1989). Realistically meeting the educational needs of hospitalized acute and short-stay patients. *Nursing Clinics of North America, 24*(3), 629–636.

Schoessler, M., Conedara, F., Bell, L. F., Marshall, D., & Gilson, M. (1993). Use of the Myers-Briggs Type Indicator to develop a continuing education department. *Journal of Nursing Staff Development, 9*(1), 8–13.

Shipman, S. & Shipman, V. C. (1985). Cognitive styles: Some conceptual, methodological, and applied issues. In E. W. Gordon (ed.), *Review of*

*Research in Education, vol. 12.* Washington, DC: American Educational Research Associates.

Simon, H. A. & Chase, W. G. (1973). Skill in chess. *American Scientist, 61*, 394–403.

Singer, R. N. (1972). The psychomotor domain: General considerations. In D. P. Ely (ed.), *Psychomotor Domain: A Resource Book for Media Specialists.* Washington, DC: Gryphon House.

Skinner, B. F. (1954). The science of learning and the art of teaching. *Harvard Educational Review, 24*, 86–97.

Speck, O., Ernst, T., Braun, J., Koch, C., Miller, E., & Chang, L. (2000). Gender differences in the functional organization of the brain for working memory. *Neuroreport, 11*(11), 2581–2585.

Sperry, R. W. (1977). Bridging science and values: A unifying view of mind and brain. *American Psychologist, 32*(4), 237–245.

Stein, J. A. & Nyamathi, A. (2000). Gender differences in behavioural and psychosocial predictors of HIV testing and return for test results in a high-risk population. *AIDS Care, 12*(3), 343–356.

Stover, D. (2001). Applying brain research in the classroom is not a no-brainer. *Education Digest, 66*(8), 26–29.

Strauss, A. & Glaser, B. (1975) *Chronic Illness and the Quality of Life.* St. Louis: Mosby.

Sylvester, R. (1998). The brain revolution. *School Administrator, 55*(1), 6.

Sylvester, R. (1995). *A Celebration of Neurons: An Educator's Guide to the Human Brain.* Alexandria, VA: Association for Supervision and Curriculum Development.

Tanner, G. (1989). A need to know. *Nursing Times, 85*(31), 54–56.

Thompson, C. & Crutchlow, E. (1993). Learning style research: A critical review of the literature and implications for nursing education. *Journal of Professional Nursing, 9*(1), 34–40.

Villejo, L. & Myers, C. (1991). Brain function, learning styles, and cancer patient education. *Seminars in Oncology Nursing, 7*(2), 97–104.

Wagner, P.S. & Ash, K. L. (1998). Creating the teachable moment. *Journal of Nursing Education, 37*(6), 278–280.

Williams, M. L. (1998). Making the most of learning needs assessments. *Journal for Nurses in Staff Development, 14*(3), 137–142.

Witkin, H. & Goodenough, D. R. (1981). *Cognitive Styles: Essence and Origins.* New York: International Universities Press.

Witkin, H., Moore, C. A., & Oltman, P. K. (1977). Cognitive styles and their educational implications. *Review of Educational Research, 47*, 1–64.

Witkin, H., Oltman, P. K., Raskin, E., & Karp, S. (1971a). *A Manual for the Embedded Figures Tests.* Palo Alto, CA: Consulting Psychologists Press.

Witkin, H., Otlman, P. K., Raskin, E., & Karp, S. (1971b). *Group Embedded Figures Test.* Palo Alto, CA: Consulting Psychologists Press.

Wolfe, P. (1994). Risk taking: Nursing's comfort zone. *Holistic Nurse Practice, 8*(2), 43–52.

Wonder, J. & Donovan, M. (1984). *Whole-brain Thinking.* New York: Ballantine.

## CHAPTER 5

# Developmental Stages of the Learner

*Susan B. Bastable*
*Michelle A. Rinwalske*

## CHAPTER HIGHLIGHTS

Developmental Characteristics

The Developmental Stages of Childhood

    Infancy (0–12 Months of Age) and Toddlerhood
    (1–3 Years of Age)

    Preschooler (3–6 Years of Age)

    School-Aged Childhood (6–12 Years of Age)

    Adolescence (12–18 Years of Age)

The Developmental Stages of Adulthood

    Young Adulthood (18–40 Years of Age)

    Middle-Aged Adulthood (40–65 Years of Age)

    Older Adulthood (65 Years of Age and Older)

The Role of the Family in Patient Education

## KEY TERMS

pedagogy

physical maturation

cognitive development

psychosocial development

andragogy

gerogogy

crystallized intelligence

fluid intelligence

## OBJECTIVES

After completing this chapter, the reader will be able to

1. Identify the physical, cognitive, and psychosocial characteristics of learners that influence learning at various stages of growth and development.

2. Recognize the role of the nurse as educator in assessing stage-specific learner needs according to maturational levels.

3. Determine the role of the family in patient education.

4. Discuss appropriate teaching strategies effective for learners at different developmental stages.

When planning, designing, and implementing an educational program, the nurse as educator must carefully consider the characteristics of learners with respect to their developmental stage in life. The more heterogeneous the target audience, the more complex the development of an educational program to meet the diverse needs of the population. Conversely, the more homogeneous the population of learners, the more straightforward the approach to teaching.

An individual's developmental stage significantly influences the ability to learn. Pedagogy, andragogy, and gerogy are three different orientations to learning. To meet the health-related educational needs of learners, a developmental approach must be used. Three major stage-range factors associated with learner readiness—physical, cognitive, and psychosocial maturation—must be taken into account at each developmental period throughout the life cycle. Developmental psychologists have for years explored the various patterns of behavior particular to stages of development. Educators, more than ever before, acknowledge the effects of growth and development on an individual's willingness and ability to make use of instruction.

This chapter has specific implications for staff nurses and staff development and in-service nurse educators because of the recent mandates by the Joint Commission on Accreditation of Healthcare Organizations (JCAHO). For healthcare agencies to meet JCAHO accreditation requirements, teaching plans must address stage-specific competencies of the learner. In this chapter, the distinct life stages of learners are examined from the perspective of physical, cognitive, and psychosocial development; the role of the nurse in assessment of stage-specific learner needs; the role of the family in the teaching–learning process; and teaching strategies specific to meeting the needs of learners at various developmental stages of life.

A deliberate attempt has been made to minimize reference to age as the criterion for categorization of learners. Research shows that chronological age per se is not a good predictor of learning ability (Whitener, Cox, & Maglich, 1998). At any given age, one finds a wide variation in the acquisition of abilities related to physical, cognitive, and psychosocial maturation. Age ranges, included after each developmental stage heading in this chapter, are intended only to be used as general guidelines; they do not imply that chronological ages necessarily correspond to the various stages of development. Thus, the term *developmental stage* will be used based on the confirmation by psychologists that human growth and development are sequential but not always specifically age-related.

Although this chapter focuses on the patient as the learner throughout the life span, the stage-specific characteristics of adulthood and the associated teaching principles of adult learning presented can be applied to any audience of older learners, whether the nurse is instructing the general public in the community or teaching continuing education to staff nurses. Emphasis is placed on the learning needs of the adult learner because middle-aged and older adults account for the largest percentage of the patient population. Furthermore, all nurses have studied content in developmental psychology and pediatrics in their basic nursing education programs, which thoroughly cover the specifics of childhood development.

## DEVELOPMENTAL CHARACTERISTICS

Actual chronological age is only a relative indicator of someone's physical, cognitive, and psychosocial stage of development. Unique as each individual is, however, some typical developmental trends have been identified as milestones of normal progression through the life cycle. When dealing with the teaching–learning process, it is imperative to examine the developmental phases as an individual progresses from infancy to senescence so as to fully appreciate the behavioral changes that occur in the cognitive, affective, and psychomotor domains. As influential as age can be to learning readiness, it should never be examined in isolation. Growth and development interact with experiential background, physical and emotional health status, and personal motivation, as well as numerous environmental factors such as stress, the surrounding conditions, and the available support systems, to affect a person's ability and readiness to learn.

If the nurse as educator is to encourage learners to take responsibility for their own health, then learners must be recognized as an important source of data regarding their health status. Before any learning can occur, the nurse must assess how much knowledge the learner already possesses with respect to the topic to be taught. With the child as client, for example, new content should be introduced at appropriate stages of development and should build on the child's previous knowledge base and experiences.

The major question underlying the planning for educational experiences is, When is the most appropriate or best time to teach the learner? The answer is when the learner is ready—the "teachable moment" as defined by Havighurst (1976)—that point in time when the learner is most receptive to a teaching situation. It is important to remember that the nurse as educator does not always have to wait for teachable moments to occur; the teacher can create these opportunities by taking an interest in and attending to the needs of the learner. When assessing readiness to learn, the nurse educator must determine not only if an interpersonal relationship has been established, if prerequisite knowledge and skills have been mastered, and if the learner

exhibits motivation, but also if the plan for teaching matches the developmental level of the learner (Hussey & Hirsh, 1983).

## ▨ THE DEVELOPMENTAL STAGES OF CHILDHOOD

*Pedagogy* is the art and science of helping children to learn. The different stages of childhood are divided according to what developmental theorists and educational psychologists define as specific patterns of behavior seen in particular phases of growth and development. Remember always that, throughout all of childhood, learning is subject centered. The following is a review of the teaching strategies to be used in the four stages of childhood in relation to the physical, cognitive, and psychosocial maturational levels indicative of learner readiness (Table 5–1).

### Infancy (0–12 Months of Age) and Toddlerhood (1–3 Years of Age)

The field of growth and development is highly complex, and at no other time is physical, cognitive, and psychosocial maturation so changeable as during the very early years of childhood. Because of the dependency of this age group, the main focus of instruction is geared toward the parents, who are considered to be the primary learners rather than the very young child. However, the older toddler should not be excluded from healthcare teaching and can participate to some extent in the education process (Hussey & Hirsh, 1983).

**Physical, Cognitive, and Psychosocial Development** At no other time in life is *physical maturation* so rapid as during the period of development from infancy to toddlerhood. Exploration of self and the environment becomes paramount and a stimulant for further physical development. Patient education must focus on teaching the parents of very young children the importance of stimulation,

## TABLE 5-1  Stage-appropriate teaching strategies

| Learner | General Characteristics | Teaching Strategies | Nursing Interventions |
|---|---|---|---|
| **INFANCY–TODDLERHOOD** | | | |
| Approximate age: Birth–3 yr<br>Cognitive stage: Sensorimotor<br>Psychosocial stage: Trust vs. mistrust (Birth–12 mo)<br>Autonomy vs. shame and doubt (1–3 yr) | Dependent on environment<br>Needs security<br>Explores self and environment<br>Natural curiosity | Orient teaching to caregiver<br>Use repetition and imitation of information<br>Stimulate all senses<br>Provide physical safety and emotional security<br>Allow play and manipulation of objects | Welcome active involvement<br>Forge alliances<br>Encourage physical closeness<br>Provide detailed information<br>Answer questions and concerns<br>Ask for information on child's strengths/limitations and likes/dislikes |
| **PRESCHOOLER** | | | |
| Approximate age: 3–6 yr<br>Cognitive stage: Preoperational<br>Psychosocial stage: Initiative vs. guilt | Egocentric<br>Thinking precausal, concrete, literal<br>Believes illness self-caused and punitive<br>Limited sense of time<br>Fears bodily injury<br>Cannot generalize<br>Animistic thinking (objects possess life or human characteristics)<br>Centration (focus is on one characteristic of an object)<br>Separation anxiety<br>Motivated by curiosity<br>Active imagination, prone to fears<br>Play is his/her work | Use warm, calm approach<br>Build trust<br>Use repetition of information<br>Allow manipulation of objects and equipment<br>Give care with explanation<br>Reassure not to blame self<br>Explain procedures simply and briefly<br>Provide safe, secure environment<br>Use positive reinforcement<br>Encourage questions to reveal perceptions/feelings<br>Use simple drawings and stories<br>Use play therapy, with dolls and puppets<br>Stimulate senses: visual, auditory, tactile, motor | Welcome active involvement<br>Forge alliances<br>Encourage physical closeness<br>Provide detailed information<br>Answer questions and concerns<br>Ask for information on child's strengths/limitations and likes/dislikes |

| Learner | General Characteristics | Teaching Strategies | Nursing Interventions |
|---|---|---|---|
| **SCHOOL-AGED CHILDHOOD** | | | |
| Approximate age: 6–12 yr<br>Cognitive stage: Concrete operations<br>Psychosocial stage: Industry vs. inferiority | More realistic and objective<br>Understands cause and effect<br>Deductive/inductive reasoning<br>Wants concrete information<br>Able to compare objects and events<br>Variable rates of physical growth<br>Reasons syllogistically<br>Understands seriousness and consequences of actions<br>Subject-centered focus<br>Immediate orientation | Encourage independence and active participation<br>Be honest, allay fears<br>Use logical explanation<br>Allow time to ask questions<br>Use analogies to make invisible processes real<br>Establish role models<br>Relate care to other children's experiences; compare procedures<br>Use subject-centered focus<br>Use play therapy<br>Provide group activities<br>Use drawings, models, dolls, painting, audio- and video-tapes | Welcome active involvement<br>Forge affiances<br>Encourage physical closeness<br>Provide detailed information<br>Answer questions and concerns<br>Ask for information on child's strengths/limitations and likes/dislikes |
| **ADOLESCENCE** | | | |
| Approximate age: 12–18 yr<br>Cognitive stage: Formal operations<br>Psychosocial stage: Identity vs. role confusion | Abstract, hypothetical thinking<br>Can build on past learning<br>Reasons by logic and understands scientific principles<br>Future orientation<br>Motivated by desire for social acceptance<br>Peer group important<br>Intense personal preoccupation, appearance extremely important (imaginary audience)<br>Feels invulnerable, invincible/immune to natural laws (personal fable) | Establish trust, authenticity<br>Know their agenda<br>Address fears/concerns about outcomes of illness<br>Identify control focus<br>Include in plan of care<br>Use peers for support and influence<br>Negotiate changes<br>Focus on details<br>Make information meaningful to life<br>Ensure confidentiality and privacy<br>Arrange group sessions<br>Use audiovisuals, role-play, contracts, reading materials<br>Provide for experimentation and flexibility | Explore emotional and financial support<br>Determine goals and expectations<br>Assess stress levels<br>Respect values and norms<br>Determine role responsibilities and relationships<br>Allow for 1:1 teaching without parents present, but with adolescent's permission; inform family of content covered |

| Learner | General Characteristics | Teaching Strategies | Nursing Interventions |
|---|---|---|---|
| **TABLE 5-1** Stage-appropriate teaching strategies | | | |
| **YOUNG ADULTHOOD** | | | |
| Approximate age: 18–40 yr<br>Cognitive stage: Formal operations<br>Psychosocial stage: Intimacy vs. isolation | Autonomous<br>Self-directed<br>Uses personal experiences to enhance or interfere with learning<br>Intrinsic motivation<br>Able to analyze critically<br>Makes decisions about personal, occupational, and social roles<br>Competency-based learner | Use problem-centered focus<br>Draw on meaningful experiences<br>Focus on immediacy of application<br>Encourage active participation<br>Allow to set own pace, be self-directed<br>Organize material<br>Recognize social role<br>Apply new knowledge through role-playing and hands-on practice | Explore emotional, financial, and physical support system<br>Assess motivational level for involvement<br>Identify potential obstacles and stressors |
| **MIDDLE-AGED ADULTHOOD** | | | |
| Approximate age: 40–65 yr<br>Cognitive stage: Formal operations<br>Psychosocial stage: Generativity vs. self-absorption and stagnation | Sense of self well-developed<br>Concerned with physical changes<br>At peak in career<br>Explores alternative lifestyles<br>Reflects on contributions to family and society<br>Reexamines goals and values<br>Questions achievements and successes<br>Has confidence in abilities<br>Desires to modify unsatisfactory aspects of life | Focus on maintaining independence and reestablishing normal life patterns<br>Assess positive and negative past experiences with learning<br>Assess potential sources of stress due to midlife crisis issues<br>Provide information to coincide with life concerns and problems | Explore emotional, financial, and physical support system<br>Assess motivational level for involvement<br>Identify potential obstacles and stressors |

| Learner | General Characteristics | Teaching Strategies | Nursing Interventions |
|---|---|---|---|
| **OLDER ADULTHOOD**<br><br>Approximate age: 65 yr and over<br>Cognitive stage: Formal operations<br>Psychosocial stage: Ego integrity vs. despair | Cognitive changes<br>Decreased ability to think abstractly, process information<br>Decreased short-term memory<br>Increased reaction time<br>Increased test anxiety<br>Stimulus persistence (afterimage)<br>Focuses on past life experiences | Use concrete examples<br>Build on past life experiences<br>Make information relevant and meaningful<br>Present one concept at a time<br>Allow time for processing/response (slow pace)<br>Use repetition and reinforcement of information<br>Avoid written exams<br>Use verbal exchange and coaching<br>Establish retrieval plan (use one or several clues)<br>Encourage active involvement<br>Keep explanations brief<br>Use analogies to illustrate abstract information | Involve principal caregivers<br>Encourage participation<br>Provide resources for support (respite care)<br>Assess coping mechanisms<br>Provide written instructions for reinforcement<br>Provide anticipatory problem solving (what happens if . . .) |
| | Sensory/motor deficits<br>Auditory changes<br>Hearing loss, especially high-pitched tones, consonants (*S, Z, T, F,* and *G*), and rapid speech<br>Visual changes<br>Farsighted (needs glasses to read)<br>Lenses become opaque (glare problem)<br>Smaller pupil size (decreased visual adaptation to darkness)<br>Decreased peripheral perception | Speak slowly, distinctly<br>Use low-pitched tones<br>Face client when speaking<br>Minimize distractions<br>Avoid shouting<br>Use visual aids to supplement verbal instruction<br>Avoid glares, use soft white light<br>Provide sufficient light<br>Use white backgrounds and black print<br>Use large letters and well-spaced print<br>Avoid color coding with blues, greens, purples, and yellows<br>Increase safety precautions/provide safe environment | |

**TABLE 5-1** Stage-appropriate teaching strategies

| Learner | General Characteristics | Teaching Strategies | Nursing Interventions |
|---|---|---|---|
| **OLDER ADULTHOOD (CONTINUED)** | Yellowing of lenses (distorts low-tone colors: blue, green, violet)<br>Distorted depth perception<br>Fatigue/decreased energy levels<br>Pathophysiology (chronic illness) | Ensure accessibility and fit of prostheses (i.e., glasses, hearing aid)<br>Keep sessions short<br>Provide for frequent rest periods<br>Allow for extra time to perform<br>Establish realistic short-term goals | |
| | Psychosocial changes<br>Decreased risk taking<br>Selective learning<br>Intimidated by formal learning | Give time to reminisce<br>Identify and present pertinent material<br>Use informal teaching sessions<br>Demonstrate relevance of information to daily life<br>Assess resources<br>Make learning positive<br>Identify past positive experiences<br>Integrate new behaviors with formerly established ones | |

nutrition, and the practice of safety measures to prevent illness and injury.

Piaget (1951, 1952, 1976), the noted expert in defining the key milestones in the *cognitive development* of children, labeled the stage of infancy to toddlerhood as the *sensorimotor* period. As children mature from infancy to toddlerhood, learning is enhanced through sensory experiences and through movement and manipulation of objects in the environment. Motor activities promote their understanding of the world and an awareness of themselves as well as others' reactions in response to their own actions. Encouraging parents to create a safe environment will allow their child to develop with a decreased risk for injury.

The toddler has the rudimentary capacity for basic reasoning, understands object permanence, has the beginnings of memory, and begins to develop an elementary concept of causality. With limited ability to recall past happenings or anticipate future events, the toddler is oriented primarily to the "here and now" and has little tolerance for delayed gratification. The child who has lived with strict routines and plenty of structure will have more of a grasp of time than the child who lives in an unstructured environment. Children at this stage have short attention spans,

are easily distracted, are egocentric in their thinking, and are not amenable to correction of their own ideas. Unquestionably, they believe their own perceptions to be reality. Asking questions is the hallmark of this age group, and curiosity abounds as they explore places and things. They can respond to simple, step-by-step commands and obey such directives as "kiss Daddy goodnight" or "put your hat on" (Petrillo & Sanger, 1980; Levine, 1983). Language skills are acquired rapidly during this period, and parents should be encouraged to foster this aspect of development by talking with and listening to their child. As they progress through this phase, children begin to engage in fantasizing and "make-believe" play. Because they are unable to distinguish fact from fiction and have limited cognitive capacity for understanding cause and effect, a child may feel that illness and hospitalization are a punishment for something done wrong.

According to Erikson (1963), the noted authority on *psychosocial development*, the period of infancy is one of *trust versus mistrust*. During this time, children must work through their first major dilemma of developing a sense of trust with their primary caretaker (see Table 5–2). As the infant matures into toddlerhood, *autonomy versus shame and*

| TABLE 5–2. Erickson's eight stages of psychosocial development | | |
|---|---|---|
| **Developmental Stages** | **Psychosocial Crises** | **Strengths** |
| Infancy | Trust vs. mistrust | Hope |
| Toddlerhood | Autonomy vs. shame and doubt | Will |
| Preschooler | Initiative vs. guilt | Purpose |
| School-aged childhood | Industry vs. inferiority | Competence |
| Adolescence | Identity vs. role confusion | Fidelity |
| Young adulthood | Intimacy vs. isolation | Love |
| Middle-aged adulthood | Generativity vs. self-absorption and stagnation | Care |
| Older adulthood | Ego integrity vs. despair | Wisdom |

SOURCE: Adapted from Ahroni, J. H. (1996). Strategies for teaching elders from a human development perspective. *Diabetes Educator, 22*(1), 48.

*doubt* emerges as the central issue. During this period of psychosocial growth, toddlers must learn to balance feelings of love and hate and learn to cooperate and control willful desires (Table 5–2). Children progress sequentially through accomplishing the tasks of developing basic trust in their environment to reaching increasing levels of independence and self-assertion. Their newly discovered sense of independence often is expressed by demonstrations of negativism. Children may have difficulty in making up their minds, and, aggravated by personal and external limits, their level of frustration and feelings of ambivalence may be expressed in words and behaviors, such as in exhibiting temper tantrums to release tensions (Falvo, 1994). With peers, play is a parallel activity, and it is not unusual for them to end up in tears because they have not yet learned about tact, fairness, or rules of sharing (Babcock & Miller, 1994).

Toddlers like routines because they give these children a sense of security, and they gravitate toward ritualistic ceremonial-like exercises when carrying out activities of daily living. Separation anxiety is also characteristic of this stage of development and is particularly apparent when children are hospitalized and feel insecure in an unfamiliar environment. This anxiety is often compounded when they are subjected to medical procedures and other healthcare interventions performed by people who are strangers to them.

**Teaching Strategies** Patient education for infancy through toddlerhood need not be illness related. Usually less time is devoted to teaching parents about illness care, and considerably more time is spent teaching aspects of normal development, safety, health promotion, and disease prevention. When the child is ill, the first priority for teaching interventions would be to assess the parent's and child's anx-

iety levels and help them cope with their feelings of stress related to uncertainty and guilt. Anxiety on the part of the child and parent can adversely affect their readiness to learn.

Although teaching activities primarily are directed to the main caregiver(s), children at this developmental stage in life have a great capacity for learning. Toddlers are capable of some degree of understanding procedures that they may experience. Because of the child's natural tendency to be intimidated by unfamiliar people, it is imperative that a primary nurse be assigned to establish a relationship with the child and parents. This approach will not only provide consistency in the teaching–learning process but also help to reduce the child's fear of strangers. Parents should be present whenever possible during learning activities to allay stress, which could be compounded by separation anxiety.

Ideally, health teaching should take place in an environment familiar to the child, such as the home or day-care center. When the child is hospitalized, the environment selected for teaching and learning sessions should be as safe and secure as possible, such as the child's bed or the playroom, to increase the child's sense of feeling protected.

Movement is an important mechanism by which toddlers communicate. Immobility due to illness or hospital confinement tends to increase children's anxiety by restricting activity. Nursing interventions should be chosen that promote children's use of gross motor abilities and that stimulate their visual, auditory, and tactile senses. Developing a rapport with children through simple teaching will help to elicit their cooperation and active involvement. The approach to children should be warm, honest, calm, accepting, and matter-of-fact. A smile, a warm tone of voice, a gesture of encouragement, or a word of praise goes a long way in attracting their attention and helping children adjust to new circumstances. Fundamental to the child's response is how the parents respond to health-care personnel and medical interventions.

The following teaching strategies are suggested to convey information to members of this age group. These strategies feed into children's natural tendency for play and their need for active participation and sensory experiences:

## For Short-Term Learning

- Read simple stories from books with lots of pictures.
- Use dolls and puppets to act out feelings and behaviors.
- Use simple audiotapes with music and videotapes with cartoon characters.
- Role-play to bring the child's imagination closer to reality.
- Give simple, concrete, nonthreatening explanations to accompany visual and tactile experiences.
- Perform procedures on a teddy bear or doll first to help the child comprehend what an experience will be like.
- Allow the child something to do—squeeze your hand, hold a Band-Aid, cry if it hurts—to channel their responses to an unpleasant experience.
- Keep teaching sessions brief (no longer than about five minutes each) because of the child's short attention span.
- Cluster teaching sessions close together so that children can remember what they learned from one instructional encounter to another.
- Avoid analogies and explain things in straightforward and simple terms because children take their world literally and concretely.
- Individualize the pace of teaching according to the child's responses and level of attention.

## For Long-Term Learning

- Focus on rituals, imitation, and repetition of information in the form of words and actions to hold the child's attention.
- Use reinforcement as an opportunity for children to achieve permanence of learning through practice.
- Employ the teaching methods of gaming and modeling as a means by which children can learn about the world and test their ideas over time.
- Encourage parents to act as role models because their values and beliefs serve to reinforce healthy behaviors and significantly influence the child's development of attitudes and behaviors.

## Preschooler (3–6 Years of Age)

Preschool children continue with development of skills learned in the earlier years of growth. Their sense of identity becomes clearer, and their world expands to encompass involvement with others external to the family unit. Children in this developmental category acquire new behaviors that give them more independence from their parents and allow them to care for themselves more autonomously. Learning during this time period occurs through interactions with others and through mimicking or modeling the behaviors of playmates and adults (Whitener et al., 1998).

**Physical, Cognitive, and Psychosocial Development** The physical maturation of preschoolers is an extension of their prior growth. Fine and gross motor skills become increasingly more refined and coordinated so that they are able to carry out activities of daily living with greater independence. Although their efforts are more coordinated, supervision of activities is still required because they lack judgment in carrying out the skills they have developed.

The preschooler's stage of cognitive development is labeled by Piaget (1951, 1952, 1976) as the *preoperational* period. The young child continues to be egocentric and is essentially unaware of others' thoughts or the existence of others' points of view. Preschoolers can recall past experiences and anticipate future events. They can classify objects into groups and categories, but have only a vague understanding of their relationships. Thinking remains literal and concrete—they believe what is seen and heard. Reasoning is transductive—that is, from the particular to the particular—rather than inductive or deductive. Precausal thinking allows preschoolers to understand that people can make things happen, but they are unaware of causation as the result of invisible physical and mechanical forces. They often believe that they can influence natural phenomena, and their beliefs reflect animistic thinking—the tendency to endow inanimate objects with life and consciousness (Pidgeon, 1977).

Preschoolers are very curious, can think intuitively, and pose questions about almost anything. They want to know the reasons, cause, and purpose for everything (the *why*) but are unconcerned at this point with the process (the *how*). Fantasy and reality are not well differentiated. Children in this cognitive stage mix fact and fiction, tend to generalize, think magically, develop imaginary playmates, and believe they can control events with their thoughts. At the same time, they do possess self-awareness and realize that they are vulnerable to outside influences.

The preschooler also continues to have a limited sense of time. For children of this age, being made to wait 15 minutes before they can do something can feel like an eternity. They do, however, understand the timing of familiar events in their daily lives, such as when breakfast or dinner is eaten and when they can play or watch their favorite television program. Their attention span begins to lengthen such that they can usually remain quiet long enough to listen to a song or hear a short story read.

In the preschool stage, children begin to develop sexual identity and curiosity, an interest that may cause considerable discomfort for their parents. Cognitive understanding of their bodies related to structure, function, health, and illness becomes more specific and differentiated. They can name external body parts but have only an ill-defined concept of the size and shape of internal organs and the function of body parts (Kotchabhakdi, 1985). Explanations of the purpose of and reasons for a procedure remain beyond their level of reasoning, so explanations have to be kept very simple and matter-of-fact (Pidgeon, 1985). Preschoolers have a fear of body mutilation and pain, which not only stems from their lack of understanding of the body but also is compounded by their active imagination. Their ideas regarding illness also are primitive with respect to cause and effect; illness is seen as a punishment for something they did wrong, either through omission or commission. Health, on the other hand, may be identified with doing things right. Health allows them to play with friends and participate in desired activities; illness prevents them from doing so (Hussey & Hirsh, 1983).

Erikson (1963) has labeled the preschooler's psychosocial maturation level as the period of *initiative versus guilt*. Children take on tasks for the sake of being involved and on the move (Table 5–2). Excess energy and a desire to dominate may lead to frustration and anger on their part. They show evidence of expanding imagination and creativity, are impulsive in their actions, and are curious about almost everything they see and do. Their growing imagination can lead to many fears—of separation, disapproval, pain, punishment, and aggression from others. Loss of body integrity is the preschooler's greatest threat, which significantly affects his or her willingness to interact with healthcare personnel (Poster, 1983; Vulcan, 1984).

In this phase of development, children begin interacting with playmates rather than just playing alongside one another. Appropriate social behaviors demand that they learn to wait for others, give others a turn, and recognize the needs of others. Play in the mind of a child is equivalent to the work performed by adults. Play can be as equally productive as adult work and is a means for self-education of the physical and social world (Whitener et al., 1998). It helps the child act out feelings and experiences to master fears, develop role skills, and express joys, sorrows, and hostilities. Through play, the preschooler also begins to share ideas and imitate parents of the same sex. Role-playing is typical of this age as the child attempts to learn the responsibilities of family members and others in society.

**Teaching Strategies** The nurse's interactions with preschool children and their parents are often sporadic, usually occurring during occasional well-child visits to the pediatrician's office or when minor medical problems arise. During these interactions, the nurse should take every opportunity to teach parents about health promotion and disease prevention measures, to provide guidance regarding normal growth and development, and to offer instruction about medical recommendations when illnesses do arise. Parents can be a great asset to the nurse in working with children in this developmental phase, and they should be included in all aspects of the educational plan and the actual teaching experience (Ryberg & Merrifield, 1984; Woodring, 2000). Parents can serve as the primary resource to answer questions about children's disabilities, their idiosyncrasies, their favorite toys—all of which may affect their ability to learn (Hussey & Hirsh, 1983).

Children's fear of pain and bodily harm is uppermost in their minds, whether they are well or ill. Because of preschoolers' fantasies and active imaginations, it is most important for the nurse to reassure them and allow them to express themselves openly about their fears (Heiney, 1991). Choose your words carefully when describing procedures. Preschoolers are familiar with many words,

but using terms like "cut" or "knife" is frightening to them. Instead, use less threatening words like "fix," "sew," or "cover up the hole." "Band-Aids" rather than "dressings" is a much more understandable term, and bandages are often thought by children to have magical healing powers (Babcock & Miller, 1994).

Although still dependent on family, the preschooler has begun to have increasing contact with the outside world and is usually able to interact more comfortably with others. Nevertheless, significant adults in a child's life should be included as participants during teaching sessions. They can provide support to the child, substitute as the teacher if the child is reluctant to interact with the nurse, and reinforce teaching at a later point in time. The primary caretakers, usually the mother and father, are the recipients of the majority of the nurse's teaching efforts. They will be the learners to assist the child in achieving desired health outcomes (Hussey & Hirsh, 1983; Kennedy & Riddle, 1989; Whitener et al., 1998).

The following specific teaching strategies are recommended:

For Short-Term Learning

- Provide physical and visual stimuli because language ability is still limited, both for expressing ideas and for comprehending verbal instructions.

- Keep teaching sessions short (no more than 15 minutes) and scheduled sequentially at close intervals so that information is not forgotten.

- Relate information needs to activities and experiences familiar to the child.

- Encourage the child to participate in selecting between a limited number of teaching–learning options, such as playing with dolls or reading a story, which promotes active involvement and helps to establish nurse–client rapport.

- Arrange small group sessions with peers as a way to make teaching less threatening and more fun.

- Give praise and approval, through both verbal expressions and nonverbal gestures, which are real motivators for learning.

- Give tangible rewards, such as badges or small toys, immediately following a successful learning experience as reinforcers in the mastery of cognitive and psychomotor skills.

- Allow the child to manipulate equipment and play with replicas or dolls to learn about body parts. Special kidney dolls, ostomy dolls with stomas, or orthopedic dolls with splints and tractions provide opportunity for hands-on experience.

- Use storybooks to emphasize the humanity of healthcare personnel; to depict relationships between child, parents, and others; and to assist with helping the child identify with particular situations.

### For Long-Term Learning

- Enlist the help of parents, who can play a vital role in modeling a variety of healthy habits, such as practicing safety measures and eating a balanced diet.

- Reinforce positive health behaviors and the acquisition of specific skills.

## School-Aged Childhood (6–12 Years of Age)

School-aged children have progressed in their physical, cognitive, and psychosocial skills to the point where most begin formal training in structured school systems. They approach learning with enthusiastic anticipation, and their minds are open to new and varied ideas. Children at this developmental level are motivated to learn because of their natural curiosity and their desire to understand more about themselves, their bodies, their world, and the

influence that different things in the world have on them (Hussey & Hirsh, 1983; Whitener et al., 1998). This stage is a period of great change for them, when attitudes, values, and perceptions of themselves, their society, and the world are shaped and expanded. Visions of their own environment and the cultures of others take on more depth and breadth.

**Physical, Cognitive, and Psychosocial Development**  The gross- and fine-motor abilities of school-aged children are increasingly more coordinated so that they are able to control their movements with much greater dexterity than ever before. Involvement in all kinds of curricular and extracurricular activities helps them to fine-tune their psychomotor skills. Physical growth during this phase is highly variable, with the rate of development differing from child to child. Toward the end of this developmental period, girls more so than boys on the average begin to experience prepubescent bodily changes and tend to exceed the boys in physical maturation. Growth charts, which monitor the rate of growth, are a more sensitive indicator of health or disability than actual size (Burkett, 1989).

Piaget (1951, 1952, 1976) has labeled the cognitive development in the school-aged child as the period of *concrete operations*. During this time, logical thought processes and the ability to reason inductively and deductively develop. School-aged children are able to think more objectively, are willing to listen to others, and will selectively use questioning to find answers to the unknown. At this stage, they begin to reason syllogistically—that is, they can consider two premises and draw a logical conclusion from them (Elkind, 1984). They are intellectually able to understand cause and effect in a concrete way. Concepts are beginning to be mastered (Babcock & Miller, 1994), such as conservation (a piece of clay weighs the same no matter whether it changes shape), reversibility (liquid is the same amount whether it is poured into a tall glass or into a short wide cup), and inferred reality (an object remains its original color even when a black filter is put in front of it). Fiction and fantasy are separate from fact and reality. The skills of memory, decision making, insight, and problem solving are all more fully developed.

Children in this phase of development are capable of engaging in systematic thought through inductive reasoning. They are able to classify objects and systems, express concrete ideas about relationships and people, and carry out mathematical operations (Lambert, 1984). Also, they begin to understand and use sarcasm as well as to employ well-developed language skills for telling jokes, conveying complex stories, and communicating increasingly more sophisticated thoughts. Nevertheless, thinking remains quite literal, with only a vague understanding of abstractions. Early on in this phase, children are reluctant to do away with magical thinking in exchange for reality thinking. Cherished beliefs, such as the existence of Santa Claus or the tooth fairy, are clung to for the fun and excitement that the fantasy provides them, even when they have information that proves contrary to their beliefs.

School-aged children have developed the ability to concentrate for extended periods, can tolerate delayed gratification, are responsible for independently carrying out activities of daily living, have a good understanding of the environment as a whole, and can generalize from experience. They understand time, can predict time intervals, are oriented to the past and present, have some grasp and interest in the future, and have a vague appreciation for how immediate actions can have implications over the course of time. Special interests in topics of their choice begin to emerge, and they can pursue subjects and activities with devotion to increase their talents in particular areas.

Children at this cognitive stage can make decisions and act in accordance with how events are interpreted, but they understand only to a limited extent the seriousness or con-

sequences of their choices. Children in the early period of this developmental phase know the functions and names of many common body parts, whereas older children have a more specific knowledge of anatomy and can differentiate between external and internal organs with a beginning understanding of their complex functions (Kotchabhakdi, 1985).

In the shift from precausal to causal thinking, the child begins to incorporate the idea that illness is related to cause and effect and can recognize that germs create disease. Illness is thought of in terms of social consequences and role alterations, such as the realization that they will miss school and outside activities, people will feel sorry for them, and they will be unable to maintain their usual routines (Banks, 1990). Research indicates, however, that systematic differences exist in children's reasoning skills with respect to understanding body functioning and the cause of illness as a result of their experiences with illness. Children suffering from chronic diseases have been found to have more sophisticated conceptualization of illness causality and body functioning than do their healthy peers. Piaget (1976) postulated that experience with a phenomenon catalyzes a better understanding of it. On the other hand, the stress and anxiety resulting from having to live with a chronic illness can interfere with a child's general cognitive performance. Chronically ill children have a less refined understanding of the physical world than healthy children do, and the former often are unable to generalize what they learned about a specific illness to a broader understanding of illness causality (Perrin, Sayer, and Willet, 1991). Thus, illness may act as an intrusive factor in overall cognitive development.

Erikson (1963) characterizes school-aged children's psychosocial stage of life as *industry versus inferiority*. During this period, children begin to gain an awareness of their unique talents and special qualities that distinguish them from one another (Table 5–2). They begin to establish their self-concept as members of a social group larger than their own nuclear family and start to compare family values with those of the outside world. The school environment, in particular, facilitates their gaining a sense of responsibility and reliability. With less dependency on family, they extend their intimacy to include special friends and social groups. Relationships with peers and adults external to the home environment become important influences in their development of self-esteem and their susceptibility to social forces outside the family unit. School-aged children fear failure and being left out of groups. They worry about their inabilities and become self-critical as they compare their own accomplishments to those of their peers. They also fear illness and disability that could significantly disrupt their academic progress, interfere with social contacts, decrease their independence, and result in loss of control over body functioning.

**Teaching Strategies**  In today's healthcare environment, school-aged children and their families must be taught in an efficient, cost-effective manner how to maintain health and manage illness. Woodring (2000) emphasizes the importance of following sound educational principles with the child and family, such as identifying individual learning styles, determining readiness to learn, and accommodating particular learning needs and abilities to achieve positive health outcomes.

With their increased ability to comprehend information and their desire for active involvement and control of their lives, it is very important to include school-aged children in patient education efforts. The nurse in the role of educator should explain illness, treatment plans, and procedures in simple, logical terms in accordance with the child's level of understanding and reasoning. Although school-aged children are able to think logically, their ability for abstract thought remains limited. Therefore, teaching

should be presented in concrete terms with step-by-step instructions (Pidgeon, 1985). It is imperative that you observe children's reactions and listen to their verbal feedback to confirm that information shared has not been misinterpreted or confused.

To the extent feasible, parents should be informed of what their child is being taught. Teaching parents directly is encouraged so that they may be involved in fostering their child's independence, providing emotional support and physical assistance, and giving guidance regarding the correct techniques or regimens in self-care management. Siblings and peers should also be considered as sources of support (Hussey & Hirsh, 1983). In attempting to master self-care skills, children thrive on praise from others important in their lives as rewards for their accomplishments and successes.

Education for health promotion and health maintenance is most likely to occur in the school system through the school nurse, but the parents as well as the nurse outside the school setting should be told what content is being addressed. Information then can be reinforced and expanded on when in contact with the child in other care settings. Numerous opportunities for nurses to teach the individual child or groups of school-aged children about health promotion and disease and injury prevention are available in schools, physicians' offices, community centers, outpatient clinics, or hospitals. Health education for children of this age can be very fragmented because of the many encounters they have with nurses in a variety of settings. The school nurse, in particular, is in an excellent position to coordinate the efforts of all other providers so as to avoid duplication of teaching content or the giving of conflicting information as well as to provide reinforcement of learning.

The specific conditions that may come to the attention of the nurse in caring for children at this phase of development include problems such as behavioral disorders, hyperactivity, learning disorders, diabetes, asthma, and enuresis. Extensive teaching may be needed to help children and parents understand a particular condition and learn how to overcome or deal with it. The need to sustain or bolster their self-image and self-esteem requires that children be invited to participate, to the extent possible, in planning for and carrying out learning activities. For children newly diagnosed with diabetes, for example, it is beneficial to allow them to administer an injection to a stuffed animal or another person. This strategy allows them to participate and will decrease their fear. Because of children's fears of falling behind in school, being separated from peer groups, and being left out of social activities, teaching must be geared toward fostering normal development despite any limitations that may be imposed by illness (Falvo, 1994).

Because school-aged children are used to the structured, direct, and formal learning in the school environment, they are receptive to a similar teaching–learning approach when hospitalized or confined at home. The following teaching strategies are suggested when caring for children in this developmental stage of life:

### For Short-Term Learning

- Allow school-aged children to take responsibility for their own health care because they are not only willing but also capable of manipulating equipment with accuracy. Because of their adeptness in relation to manual dexterity, mathematical operations, and logical thought processes, they can be taught, for example, to calculate and administer their own insulin or use an asthma inhaler as prescribed.

- Teaching sessions can be extended to last as long as 30 minutes each because the increased cognitive abilities of school-aged children aids in the retention of information. However, lessons should be spread apart to allow for comprehension of large amounts of content and to provide opportunity for the practice of newly acquired skills between sessions.

- Use diagrams, models, pictures, videotapes, and printed materials as adjuncts to various teaching methods because an increased facility with language (both spoken and written) as well as with mathematical concepts allows for these children to work with more complex instructional tools.

- Choose audiovisual and printed materials that show peers undergoing similar procedures or facing similar situations.

- Clarify any scientific terminology and medical jargon used.

- Use analogies as an effective means of providing information in meaningful terms, such as "A chest x-ray is like having your picture taken" or "White blood cells are like police cells that can attack and destroy infection."

- Use one-to-one teaching sessions as a method to individualize learning relevant to the child's own experiences and as a means to interpret the results of nursing interventions particular to the child's own condition.

- Provide time for clarification, validation, and reinforcement of what is being learned.

- Select individual instructional techniques that provide opportunity for privacy, an increasingly important concern for this group of learners, who often feel quite self-conscious and modest when learning about bodily functions.

- Employ group teaching sessions with others of similar age and with similar problems or needs to help children avoid feelings of isolation and to assist them in identifying with their own peers.

- Prepare children for a procedure well in advance to allow them time to cope with their feelings and fears, to anticipate events, and to understand what the purpose of a procedure is, how it relates to their condition, and how much time it will take.

- Encourage participation in planning for procedures and events because active involvement will help the child to assimilate information more readily.

- Provide much needed nurturance and support, always keeping in mind that young children are not just small adults.

## For Long-Term Learning

- Help school-aged children acquire skills that they can use to assume self-care responsibility for carrying out therapeutic treatment regimens on an ongoing basis with minimal assistance.

- Assist them in learning to maintain their own well-being and prevent illnesses from occurring.

Research suggests that lifelong health attitudes and behaviors begin in the early childhood phase of development and remain intrapersonally consistent throughout the stage of middle childhood. The development of cognitive understanding of health and illness has been shown to follow a systematic progression parallel to the stage of general cognitive development. As the child matures, beliefs about health and illness become less concrete and more abstract, less egocentric, and increasingly differentiated and consistent. Motivation, self-esteem, and positive self-perception are personal characteristics that influence health behavior. Research has shown that the higher the grade level of the child, the greater the understanding of illness and an awareness of body cues. Thus, children become more actively involved in their own health care as they progress developmentally (Farrand & Cox, 1993; Whitener et al., 1998). Teaching should be directed at assisting them to incorporate positive health actions into

their daily lives. Because of the importance of peer influence, group activities are an effective method of teaching health behaviors, attitudes, and values.

## Adolescence (12–18 Years of Age)

The stage of adolescence marks the transition from childhood to adulthood. During this prolonged and very changeable period of time, many adolescents and their families experience much turmoil. How adolescents think about themselves and the world significantly influences many healthcare issues facing them, from anorexia to diabetes. Teenage thought and behavior give insight into the etiology of some of the major health problems of this group of learners (Elkind, 1984). Adolescents are known to be among the nation's most at-risk populations (American Association of Colleges of Nursing, 1994). For patient education to be effective, an understanding of the characteristics of the adolescent phase of development is crucial.

**Physical, Cognitive, and Psychosocial Development**   Adolescents vary greatly in their biological, psychological, social, and cognitive development. From a physical maturation standpoint, they must adapt to rapid and significant bodily changes, which can temporarily result in clumsiness and poorly coordinated movement. Alterations in physical size, shape, and function of their bodies, along with the appearance and development of secondary sex characteristics, bring about a significant preoccupation with their appearance and a strong desire to express sexual urges (Falvo, 1994).

Piaget (1951, 1952, 1976) termed this stage of cognitive development as the period of *formal operations*. Adolescents have attained a new, higher-order level of reasoning superior to earlier childhood thoughts. They are capable of abstract thought and complex logical reasoning described as propositional as opposed to syllogistic. Their reasoning is both inductive and deductive, and they are able to hypothesize and apply the principles of logic to situations never encountered before. Adolescents can conceptualize and internalize ideas, debate various points of view, understand cause and effect, comprehend complex explanations, and respond appropriately to multiple-step directions (Heiney, 1991; Day, 1981).

Formal operational thought enables adolescents to conceptualize invisible processes and make determinations about what others say and how they behave. With this capacity, teenagers can become obsessed with what others are thinking and begin to believe that everyone is focusing on the same things they are—namely, themselves and their activities. Elkind (1984) labeled this belief as the *imaginary audience*, which has considerable influence over an adolescent's behavior. The imaginary audience explains the pervasive self-consciousness of adolescents, who, on the one hand, may feel embarrassed because they believe everyone is looking at them and, on the other hand, desire to be looked at and thought about because this attention confirms their sense of specialness and uniqueness.

Adolescents are able to understand the concept of health and illness, the multiple causes of diseases, the influence of variables on health status, and the ideas associated with health promotion and disease prevention. They recognize that illness is a process resulting from a dysfunction or nonfunction of a part or parts of the body and can comprehend the outcomes or prognosis of an illness. They can also identify health behaviors but may reject practicing them or begin to engage in risk-taking behaviors because of the social pressures they receive from peers as well as their feelings of invincibility. Elkind (1984) has called this belief of invulnerability the *personal fable*. The personal fable leads the adolescent to believe that *other* people grow old and die, but not *them*; *other* people may not realize their personal ambitions, but *they* will. This fable has value in that it allows individuals to carry on with their lives even in the face of all kinds of dangers. Unfortunately, it also leads teenagers to believe they are cloaked in an invisible shield that will protect them from bodily harm despite any risks to which they may subject themselves. They can understand implications of future outcomes, but their immediate concern is with the present. Recent research, however, reveals that adolescents 15 years of age and older are not as susceptible to the personal fable as once thought (Cauffman & Steinberg, 2000). Although children in the mid-to-late adolescent period appear to be aware of the risks they take, it is important, nevertheless, to recognize that this population continues to need support and guidance.

Erikson (1968) has labeled the psychosocial dilemma adolescents face as one of *identity versus role confusion*. These children indulge in comparing their self-image with an ideal image (Table 5–2). Adolescents find themselves in a struggle to establish their own identity, match their skills with career choices, and determine their "self." They work to emancipate themselves from their parents, seeking independence and autonomy so that they can emerge as more distinct individual personalities. Teenagers have a strong need for belonging to a group, friendship, peer acceptance, and peer support. They tend to rebel against any actions or recommendations by adults whom they consider authoritarian. Their concern over personal appearance and their need to look and act like their peers drive them to conform to the dress and behavior of this age group, which is usually contradictory and nonconformist in relation to the models, codes, and values of their parents' generation. Conflict, toleration, or alienation characterizes the relationship between adolescents and their parents and other authority figures. Adolescents seek to develop new and trusting relationships outside the home but remain vulnerable to the opinions of those they emulate.

Adolescents demand personal space, control, privacy, and confidentiality. To them, illness, injury, and hospitalization means dependency, loss of identity, a change in body image and functioning, bodily embarrassment, confinement, separation from peers, and possible death. The provision of knowledge alone is, therefore, not sufficient for this population. Due to the many issues apparent during the adolescent period, the need for coping skills is profound and can influence the successful completion of this stage of development (Grey, Kanner, & Lacey, 1999).

**Teaching Strategies**  Although the majority of individuals at this phase of development remain relatively healthy, an estimated 20% of the United States' 31 million teenagers have at least one serious health problem, such as asthma, diabetes, a range of disabilities as a result of injury, or psychological problems as a result of depression or physical and/or emotional maltreatment. In addition, adolescents are considered at high risk for teen pregnancy, the effects of poverty, drug or alcohol abuse, suicide, and sexually transmitted diseases such as venereal disease and AIDS. More than 30% of all adolescent deaths result from motor vehicle accidents.

Despite all of these potential threats to their well-being, adolescents use medical services the least frequently of all age groups. Compounding this problem is the realization that adolescent health has not been a national priority and their health issues have been largely ignored by the healthcare system (American Association of Colleges of Nursing, 1994). Thus, the educational needs of adolescents are broad and varied. The potential topics for teaching are numerous, ranging from sexual adjustment, contraception, and venereal disease to accident prevention, nutrition, and substance abuse.

Healthy teens have difficulty imagining themselves as sick or injured. Those with an illness or disability often comply poorly with medical regimens and continue to indulge in risk-taking behaviors. Because of their preoccupation with body image and functioning and the perceived importance of peer acceptance and support, they view health recommendations as a threat to their autonomy and sense of control. Probably the greatest challenge to the nurse responsible for teaching the adolescent, whether healthy or ill, is to be able to develop a mutually respectful, trusting relationship. Adolescents, because of their well-developed cognitive and language abilities, are able to participate fully in all aspects of learning, but they need privacy, understanding, an honest and straightforward approach, and unqualified acceptance in the face of their fears of losing independence, identity, and self-control.

The existence of an imaginary audience and personal fable can contribute to the exacerbation of existing problems or cause new ones. Adolescents with disfiguring handicaps, who as young children exhibited a great deal of spirit and strength, may now show signs of depression and lack of will. For the first time, they look at themselves from the standpoint of others and reinterpret behavior once seen as friendly as actually condescending. Teenagers may fail to use contraceptives because the fable tells them that *other* people will get pregnant or get venereal disease, but not *them*. Teenagers with chronic illnesses may stop taking prescribed medications because they feel they can manage without them to prove to others that they are well and free of medical constraints; *other* people with similar diseases need to follow therapeutic regimens, but not *them*.

Adolescents' language skills and ability to conceptualize and think abstractly give the nurse as educator a wide range of teaching methods and instructional tools from which to choose. The following teaching strategies are suggested when caring for adolescents:

## For Short-Term Learning

- Use one-to-one instruction to ensure confidentiality of sensitive information.

- Choose peer group discussion sessions as an effective approach to deal with health topics as smoking, alcohol and drug use, safety measures, and teenage sexuality. Adolescents benefit from being exposed to others who have the same concerns or who have successfully dealt with problems similar to theirs.

- Use group discussion, role-playing, and gaming as methods to clarify values and problem-solve, which feed into the teenager's need to belong and to be actively involved. Getting groups of peers together can be very effective in helping teens confront health challenges and learn how to significantly change behavior (Fey & Deyes, 1989).

- Employ adjunct instructional tools, such as complex models, diagrams, and specific, detailed written materials, which can be used competently by many adolescents. Audiovisual materials in the form of audiotapes, videotapes, simulated games, and interactive discs using the hardware of TV, audiocassette players, and computers usually are a comfortable approach to learning for adolescents, who generally have facility with technological equipment after years of academic and personal experience with telecommunications in the home and at school.

- Clarify any scientific terminology and medical jargon used.

- Share decision making whenever possible because control is an important issue for adolescents.

- Include them in formulating teaching plans related to teaching strategies, expected outcomes, and determining what needs to be learned and how it can best be achieved to meet their needs for autonomy.

- Suggest options so that they feel they have a choice about courses of action.

- Give a rationale for all that is said and done to help adolescents feel a sense of control.

- Approach them with respect, tact, openness, and flexibility to elicit their attention and encourage their responsiveness to teaching–learning situations.

- Expect negative responses, which are common when their self-image and self-integrity are threatened.

- Avoid confrontation and acting like an authority figure. Instead of directly contradicting their opinions and beliefs, acknowledge their thoughts and then casually suggest an alternative viewpoint, such as "Yes, I can see your point, but what about the possibility of . . . ?"

## For Long-Term Learning

- Accept adolescents' personal fable and imaginary audience as valid, rather than challenging their feelings of uniqueness and invincibility.

- Acknowledge that their feelings are very real because denying them their opinions simply will not work.

- Allow them the opportunity to test their own convictions. Let them know, for example, that while some other special people may get away without taking medication, others cannot. Suggest, if medically feasible, setting up a trial period with medications scheduled farther apart or in lowered dosages to determine how they can manage.

Although much of patient education should be done directly with adolescents to respect their right to individuality, privacy, and confidentiality, teaching effectiveness may be enhanced by including their families to some extent. The nurse as educator can give guidance and support to families, helping them to better understand adolescent behavior. Parents should be taught how to set realistic limits while at the same time foster the adolescent's sense of independence. Through prior assessment of potential sources of stress, teaching both the parents and the adolescent (as well as siblings) can be enhanced. Because of the ambivalence the adolescent feels while in this transition stage from childhood to adulthood, healthcare teaching, to be effective, must consider the learning needs of the adolescent as well as the parents (Falvo, 1994).

## THE DEVELOPMENTAL STAGES OF ADULTHOOD

*Andragogy*, the term coined by Knowles (1990) to describe his theory of adult learning, is the art and science of helping adults learn. Education within this framework is more learner-centered and less teacher-centered; that is, instead of one party imparting knowledge on another, the power relationship between the educator and the adult learner is much more horizontal (Milligan, 1997). The concept of andragogy has served for years as a useful framework in guiding instruction for patient teaching and for continuing education of staff. Recently, Knowles and associates (1998) discussed new perspectives on andragogy, emerging from research and theory in a variety of disciplines, that have refined and strengthened the core adult learning principles he originally proposed.

The following basic assumptions about Knowles's framework have major implications for planning, implementing, and evaluating teaching programs for adults as the individual matures:

1. His or her self-concept moves from one of being a dependent personality to being an independent, self-directed human being.

2. He or she accumulates a growing reservoir of previous experience that serves as a rich resource for learning.

3. Readiness to learn becomes increasingly oriented to the developmental tasks of social roles.

4. The perspective of time changes from one of postponed application of knowledge to one of immediate application; there is a shift in orientation of learning from being subject centered to problem centered.

A limitation of Knowles's assumptions about child versus adult learners is that they are derived from studies done on healthy people. It is important to keep in mind, however, that illness and injury have the potential for significantly changing cognitive and psychological processes used for learning (Bille, 1980).

The period of adulthood constitutes three major developmental stages—that of the young adult, the middle-aged adult, and the older adult (see Table 5–1). Although adulthood, like childhood, can be divided into various developmental phases, the focus for learning is quite different. Whereas readiness to learn in the child depends on physical, cognitive, and psychosocial development, adults have essentially reached the peak of their physical and cognitive capacities. Piaget's (1951, 1952, and 1976) cognitive stage of formal operations begins in adolescence and carries through the three periods of adulthood. Erickson (1963), on the other hand, continues to delineate psychosocial characteristics of the different stages of adulthood.

The emphasis for adult learning revolves around differentiation of life tasks and social roles with respect to employment, family, and other activities beyond the responsibilities of home and career (Boyd et al., 1998). In contrast to childhood learning, which is subject centered, adult learning is problem centered. The prime motivator to learn in adulthood is to be able to apply knowledge and skills for the solution of immediate problems. Unlike children, who enjoy learning for the sake of gaining an understanding of themselves and the world, adults must clearly perceive the relevancy in acquiring new behaviors or changing old ones for them to be willing and eager to learn. In the beginning of any teaching–learning encounter, therefore, adults want to know the benefit they will derive from their efforts at learning.

Unlike the child learner, who is dependent on authority figures for learning, the adult is much more self-directed and independent in seeking information. For adults, past experiences are internalized and form the basis for further learning. Adults already have a rich resource of stored information on which to build a further understanding of relationships between ideas and concepts. They are quicker than children at grasping relationships, and they do not tolerate learning isolated facts as well as children do (Table 5–3). Because they already have established ideas, values, and attitudes, they tend to be more resistant to change. In addition, adults must overcome obstacles to learning to a greater extent than children are subjected. They have the burden of family, work, and social responsibilities, which can diminish their time, energy, and concentration for learning. Their need for self-direction also may present problems because various stages of illness, as well as the health-care setting in which they may find themselves, can force dependency. Anxiety, too, may negatively affect their motivation to learn. They may feel too old or too out of touch with the formal learning of the school years, and if past experiences with learning were not positive, they may shy away from assuming the role of learner for fear of the risk of failure (Boyd et al., 1998). Although we accept the adult learner as autonomous, self-directed, and independent, these individuals often really want and need structure, clear and concise specifics, and direct guidance. As

| TABLE 5–3 Summary of adult learning principles | |
|---|---|
| **ADULTS LEARN BEST WHEN:** | |
| Principle #1 | Learning is related to an immediate need, problem, or deficit. |
| Principle #2 | Learning is voluntary and self-initiated. |
| Principle #3 | Learning is person centered and problem centered. |
| Principle #4 | Learning is self-controlled and self-directed. |
| Principle #5 | The role of the teacher is one of facilitator. |
| Principle #6 | Information and assignments are pertinent. |
| Principle #7 | New material draws on past experiences and is related to something the learner already knows. |
| Principle #8 | The threat to self is reduced to a minimum in the educational situation. |
| Principle #9 | The learner is able to participate actively in the learning process. |
| Principle #10 | The learner is able to learn in a group. |
| Principle #11 | The nature of the learning activity changes frequently. |
| Principle #12 | Learning is reinforced by application and prompt feedback. |

SOURCE: Adapted from Burgireno, J. (1985). Maximizing learning in the adult with SCI. *Rehabilitation Nursing, 10*(5), 20–21.

such, Taylor, Marienau, and Fiddler (2000) label adults as *paradoxical learners*.

A variety of reasons explain why adults pursue learning throughout their lives. Basically, three categories describe the general orientation of adults toward continuing education (Babcock & Miller, 1994):

1. *Goal-oriented learners* engage in educational endeavors to accomplish clear and identifiable objectives. Continuing education for them is episodic and occurs as a recurring

pattern throughout their lives as they realize the need for or identify an interest in expanding their knowledge and skills. Adults who attend night courses or professional workshops do so to build their expertise in a particular subject or for advancement in their professional or personal lives.

2. *Activity-oriented learners* select educational activities primarily to meet social needs. The learning of content is secondary to their need for human contact. While they may choose to attend support groups, special-interest groups, self-help groups, or academic classes because of an interest in a particular topic being offered, they join essentially out of their desire to be with and talk to other people in similar circumstances—retirement, parenting, divorce, or widowhood. Their drive is to alleviate social isolation or loneliness.

3. *Learning-oriented learners* view themselves as perpetual students who seek knowledge for knowledge sake. They are active learners all of their lives and tend to join groups, classes, or organizations with the anticipation that the experience will be educational and personally rewarding.

In most cases, all three types of learners initiate the learning experience for themselves. In planning educational activities for adults, it is important to know their motives for wanting to be involved. In caring for clients with various needs and problems, it is advantageous for the nurse as educator to understand the purpose and expectations of different continuing education groups to best serve as a referral or resource person for the learners.

Only recently has it been recognized that learning is a lifelong process that begins at birth and does not cease until the end of life. Growth and development are a process of becoming, and learning is inextricably a part of that process. As a person matures, learning

is a significant and continuous task to maintain and enhance oneself.

Obviously, there are many differences between child and adult learners (Table 5–1). As the following discussion will clearly reveal, there also are differences in the characteristics of adult learners within the three developmental stages of adulthood.

## Young Adulthood (18–40 Years of Age)

Early adulthood is a time for establishing long-term, intimate relationships with other people, choosing a lifestyle and adjusting to it, deciding on an occupation, and managing a home and family. All of these decisions lead to changes in the lives of young adults that can be a potential source of stress for them. It is a time when intimacy and courtship are pursued and spousal and/or parental roles are developed.

**Physical, Cognitive, and Psychosocial Development**   During this period, physical abilities for most young adults are at their peak, and the body is at its optimal functioning capacity. The vast majority of individuals at this stage can master, if they so desire, almost any psychomotor skill they undertake to accomplish.

The cognitive capacity of young adults is fully developed, but with maturation, they continue to accumulate new knowledge and skills from an expanding reservoir of formal and informal experiences. Young adults continue in the formal operations stage of cognitive development (Piaget 1951, 1952, 1976). These experiences add to their perceptions, allow them to generalize to new situations, and improve their abilities to critically analyze, problem-solve, and make decisions about their personal, occupational, and social roles. Their interests for learning are oriented toward those experiences that are relevant for immediate application to problems and tasks in their daily lives. Young adults are motivated to learn about the possible implications of various lifestyle choices.

Erikson (1963) describes the young adult's stage of psychosocial development as the period of *intimacy versus isolation*. During this time, individuals work to establish a trusting, satisfying, and permanent relationship with others (Table 5–2). They strive to establish commitment to others in their personal, occupational, and social lives. The independence and self-sufficiency they worked to obtain in adolescence they are now working to maintain.

Young adults face many challenges as they take steps to control their lives. Many of the events they experience are happy and growth-promoting from an emotional and social perspective, but they also can prove disappointing and psychologically draining. The new experiences and multiple decisions they must make regarding choices for a career, marriage, parenthood, and higher education can be quite stressful. Young adults realize that the avenues they pursue will affect their lives for years to come.

**Teaching Strategies**  At this developmental stage, prior to the emergence of the chronic diseases that characterize the middle-age and older years, young adults are generally very healthy and tend to have limited exposure to health professionals. Their contact with the healthcare system is usually for preemployment, college, or pre-sport physicals; for a minor episodic complaint; or for pregnancy and contraceptive care. At the same time, young adulthood is a crucial period for the establishment of behaviors that help individuals to lead healthy lives, both physically and emotionally. Many of the choices young adults make, if not positive ones, will be difficult to modify later. As Havighurst pointed out, this stage is full of "teachable moment" opportunities, but it is the most devoid of efforts by health providers to teach (Johnson-Saylor, 1980).

Health promotion is the most neglected aspect of healthcare teaching at this stage of life. Yet, many of the health issues related to risk factors and stress management are important to deal with to help young adults establish positive health practices for preventing problems with illness in the future. The major factors associated with increased risk of death in later life, such as high blood pressure, elevated cholesterol, obesity, smoking, overuse of alcohol and drugs, and pertinent family history of major illnesses such as cancer and heart disease all need to be addressed.

The nurse as educator must find a way of reaching and communicating with this audience about health promotion and disease prevention measures. Readiness to learn does not always require the nurse educator to wait for it to develop. Rather, such readiness can be fostered through experiences the nurse creates. Knowledge of the individual's lifestyle can provide cues to concentrate on when determining specific aspects of education for the young adult. For example, if the individual is planning marriage, then teaching about family planning, contraception, and parenthood are potential topics to address. The motivation for adults to learn comes in response to internal drives, such as need for self-esteem, a better quality of life, or job satisfaction, or in response to external motivators, such as job promotion, more money, or more time to pursue outside activities (Babcock & Miller, 1994).

When young adults are faced with acute or chronic illnesses, many of which may significantly alter their lifestyles, they are stimulated to learn so as to maintain their independence and return to normal life patterns. It is likely they will view an illness or disability as a serious setback to achieving their immediate or future life goals. Because adults typically desire active participation in the educational process, it is important for the nurse as educator to allow them the opportunity for mutual collaboration in health education decision making.

They should be encouraged to select what to learn (objectives), how they want material to be presented (instructional methods and tools), and which indicators will be used to determine the achievement of learning goals (evaluation) (Gessner, 1989). Also, it must be remembered that adults bring to the teaching–learning situation a variety of experiences that can serve as a foundation on which to build new learning. Consequently, it is important to draw on their experiences to make learning relevant, useful, and motivating. Young adults tend to be reluctant to expend the resources of time, money, and energy to learn new information, skills, and attitudes if they do not see the content of instruction as relevant to their current lives or anticipated problems (Babcock & Miller, 1994).

Teaching strategies must be directed at encouraging young adults to seek information that expands their knowledge base, helps them control their lives, and bolsters their self-esteem. Whether they are well or ill, young adults need to know about the opportunities available for learning. Making them aware of health issues and learning opportunities can occur in a variety of settings, such as physicians' offices, community clinics, outpatient departments, or hospitals. In all cases, these educational opportunities must be convenient and accessible to them in terms of their lifestyle with respect to work and family responsibilities.

Because they tend to be very self-directed in their approach to learning, young adults do well with written patient education materials and audiovisual tools that allow them to independently self-pace their learning. Group discussion is an attractive method for teaching and learning because it provides young adults with the opportunity to interact with others of similar age and situation, such as parenting groups, prenatal classes, or marital adjustment sessions. Although assessment prior to teaching will help to determine the level at which to begin teaching, no matter what the content, the enduring axiom to make learning easier and more relevant is to present con-

cepts logically from simple to complex and to establish conceptual relationships through specific application of information.

## Middle-Aged Adulthood (40–65 Years of Age)

Just as adolescence is the link between childhood and adulthood, midlife is the transition period between young adulthood and older adulthood. During middle age, many individuals have reached the peak in their careers, their sense of who they are is well developed, their children are grown, and they have time to pursue other interests. It is a time for them to reflect on the contributions they have made to family and society and to reexamine their goals and values.

**Physical, Cognitive, and Psychosocial Development**    At this stage of maturation, a number of physiological changes begin to take place. Skin and muscle tone decreases, metabolism slows down, body weight tends to increase, endurance and energy levels lessen, hormonal changes bring about a variety of symptoms, and hearing and visual acuity begin to diminish. All these physical changes and others affect middle-aged adults' self-image, ability to learn, and motivation for learning about health promotion, disease prevention, and maintenance of health.

The ability to learn from a cognitive standpoint remains at a steady state throughout middle age as they continue in the formal operations stage of cognitive development (Piaget, 1951, 1952, 1976). For many adults, the accumulation of life experiences and their proven record of accomplishments often allow them to come to the teaching–learning situation with confidence in their abilities as learners. However, if their past experiences with learning were minimal or not positive, their motivation likely will not be at a high enough level to facilitate learning. Physical changes, especially with respect to hearing and vision, may impede learning as well.

Erikson (1963) labeled this psychosocial stage of adulthood as *generativity versus self-absorption and stagnation*. Midlife marks a point at which adults realize that half of their life has been spent. This realization may cause them to question their level of achievement and success. Middle-aged adults, in fact, may choose to modify aspects of their lives that they perceive as unsatisfactory or adopt a new lifestyle as a solution to dissatisfaction. Developing concern for the lives of their grown children, recognizing the physical changes in themselves, dealing with the new role of being a grandparent, and taking responsibility for their own parents whose health may be failing—all are factors that may cause them to become aware of their own mortality (Table 5–2). At this time, middle-aged adults may either feel greater motivation to follow health recommendations more closely or, just the opposite, may deny illnesses or abandon healthy practices altogether (Falvo, 1994).

The later years of middle adulthood are the phase in which productivity and contributions to society are valued. They offer an opportunity to feel a real sense of accomplishment from having cared for others—children, spouse, friends, parents, and colleagues for whom they have served as mentor. During this time, individuals often become oriented away from self and family to the larger community. New social interests and leisure activities are pursued as they find more free time from family responsibilities and career demands. As they move toward their retirement years, individuals begin to plan for what they want to do after culminating their career. This transition sparks their interest in learning about financial planning, alternative lifestyles, and ways to remain healthy as they approach the later years.

**Teaching Strategies** Depending on individual situations, middle-aged adults may be facing either a more relaxed lifestyle or an increase in stress level due to midlife crisis issues such as menopause, obvious physical changes in their bodies, responsibility for their own parents' declining health status, or concern about how finite their life really is. They may have regrets and feel they did not achieve the goals or live up to the values they had set for themselves in young adulthood or the expectations others had of them as young adults.

When teaching members of this age group, the nurse must be aware of their potential sources of stress, the health risk factors associated with this stage of life, and the concerns typical of midlife. Misconceptions regarding physical changes such as menopause are common. Stress may interfere with their ability to learn or may stimulate them to seek the help of healthcare providers. Those who have lived healthy and productive lives are often motivated to make contact with health professionals to ensure maintenance of their healthy status. It is an opportune time on the part of the nurse educator to reach out to assist these middle-aged adults in coping with stress and maintaining optimal health status. Many need and want information related to chronic illnesses that can arise at this phase of life.

Adult learners need to be reassured or complimented on their learning competencies. Reinforcement for learning is internalized and serves to reward them for their efforts. Teaching strategies for learning are similar to those instructional methods and tools used for the young adult learner, but the content is different to coincide with the concerns and problems specific to this group of learners.

## Older Adulthood (65 Years of Age and Older)

Older persons constitute approximately 12% of the U.S. population, and those aged 85 and older make up the fastest-growing segment of the population in our country today. By 2020, 16.5% (or 52 million) of the population is expected to be aged 65 years and older (Gollop, 1997). Of the total amount of healthcare expenditures, 36% are incurred by those older than 65 years of age (Pearson & Wessman, 1996). Most older persons suffer from at least one chronic condition, and many have multiple conditions. On the average, they are hospitalized longer than persons in other age categories and require more teaching overall to broaden their knowledge of self-care.

Because many older persons did not have the educational opportunities that are available to the young today, one-third of them have completed only eight years or less of formal schooling, and 45% of them have less than a high school education (Pearson & Wessman, 1996). Low educational levels in the older adult population may contribute to these individuals' decreased ability to read and comprehend written materials (Jackson et al., 1994). For these reasons, their educational needs are generally greater and more complex than those for persons in any of the other developmental stages. Numerous studies have documented that older adults can benefit from health education programs. Their compliance, if they are given specific health directions, can be quite high. In light of considerable healthcare cost expenditures for older people, education programs to improve their health status would be a cost-effective measure (Weinrich et al., 1989; Pearson & Wessman, 1996).

*Ageism* describes prejudice against the older adult. This term perpetuates the negative stereotype of aging as a period of decline. Ahroni (1996) suggests that ageism, in many respects, is similar to the discriminatory attitudes of racism and sexism. Because our society values physical strength, beauty, social networking, productivity, and integrity of body and mind, we fear the natural losses that accompany the aging process. Growing older is a normal event, yet the inevitable continua-

tion of human development that results in biological, psychological, and social changes with the passage of time is, as Ahroni (1996) asserts, a reminder of our own mortality. We must recognize that many older persons respond to these changes as challenges rather than defeats. Many aspects of older adulthood can be pleasurable, such as becoming a grandparent and experiencing retirement that gives one time to pursue lifelong interests, as well as freedom to explore new avenues of endeavor. Ageism, which interferes with interactions between the older adult and younger age groups, must be counteracted because it "prevents older people from living lives as actively and happily as they might" (Ahroni, 1996, p. 48). Given that the aging process is universal, eventually everyone is potentially subjected to this type of prejudice. New research that focuses on healthy development and positive lifestyle adaptations, rather than on illnesses and impairments, in the older adult can serve to reverse the stereotypical images of aging. Education to inform people of the significant variations that occur in the way that individuals age and education to help the older adult learn to cope with irreversible losses can combat the prejudice of ageism as well.

The teaching of older persons, known as *gerogogy*, is different from teaching adults (andragogy) and children (pedagogy). For teaching to be effective, gerogogy must accommodate the normal physical, cognitive, and psychosocial changes that occur at this phase of growth and development (Weinrich & Boyd, 1992). Until recently, little has been written about the special learning needs of older adults that acknowledges the physiological and psychological aging changes that affect their ability to learn. Age changes, which begin in the second decade of life, can create barriers to learning unless nurses understand these changes and adapt appropriate teaching interventions to meet the older person's needs (Weinrich et al., 1989; Ahroni, 1996). The following discussion of physical, cognitive, and psychosocial maturation is based on findings reported by numerous authors (Ellison, 1985; Weinrich et al., 1989; Culbert & Kos, 1971; Alford, 1982; Weinrich & Boyd, 1992; Ahroni, 1996; Palmore, 1977; Pearson & Wessman, 1996).

**Physical, Cognitive, and Psychosocial Development** With advancing age, so many physical changes occur that it becomes difficult to establish normal boundaries. As a person grows older, normal physiological changes in all systems of the body are universal, progressive, decremental, and intrinsic. The senses of sight, hearing, touch, taste, and smell are usually the first areas of decreased functioning noticed by older persons. Alterations in physiological functioning can lead secondarily to changes in learning ability.

The sensory perceptive abilities that relate most closely to learning capacity are visual and auditory changes. Hearing loss, which is very common beginning in the late forties and fifties, includes diminished ability to discriminate high-pitched sounds. Visual changes such as cataracts, reduced pupil size, and presbyopia prevent older persons from being able to see small print, read words printed on glossy paper, or drive a car. Yellowing of the ocular lens produces color distortions and diminished color perceptions.

Other physiological changes affect organ functioning, which result in decreased cardiac output, lung performance, and metabolic rate; these changes reduce energy levels and lessen the ability to cope with stress. Nerve conduction velocity also is thought to decline by as much as 15%, influencing reflex times and muscle response rates. The interrelatedness of each body system has a total negative cumulative effect on individuals as they grow older.

Aging affects the mind as well as the body. According to Piaget (1951, 1952, 1976), this population remains in the stage of formal operations. *Cognitive ability* changes with age as permanent cellular alterations invariably occur in the brain itself, resulting in an actual loss of neurons, which have no regenerative powers. Physiological research has demonstrated that people have two kinds of intellectual ability—crystallized and fluid intelligence. *Crystallized intelligence* is the intelligence absorbed over a lifetime, such as vocabulary, general information, understanding social interactions, arithmetic reasoning, and ability to evaluate experiences. This kind of intelligence actually increases with experience as people age (Theis & Merritt, 1994). It is important to understand that crystallized intelligence can be impaired by disease states, such as Alzheimer's dementia (Matsuda & Saito, 1998). *Fluid intelligence* is the capacity to perceive relationships, to reason, and to perform abstract thinking. This kind of intelligence declines as degenerative changes occur.

The decline in fluid intelligence results in the following specific changes:

1. *Slower processing time:* Older persons need more time to process and react to information, especially as measured in terms of relationships between actions and results. However, if the factor of speed is removed from IQ tests, for example, older people can perform as well as younger ones. Research suggests that this decline in fluid intelligence relates to the decreased speed at which older persons process information (Kray & Lindenberger, 2000).

2. *Persistence of stimulus (afterimage):* Older people can confuse a previous symbol or word with a new word or symbol just introduced.

3. *Decreased short-term memory:* Older people sometimes have difficulty remembering events or conversations that occurred just hours or days before.

4. *Increased test anxiety:* Older people are especially anxious about making mistakes when performing; when they do make an error, they become easily frustrated. Because of their anxiety, they may take an inordinate amount of time to respond to questions, particularly on tests that are written rather than verbal.

5. *Altered time perception:* For older persons, life becomes more finite, issues of the here and now are more important, and many adhere to the philosophy of Scarlett O'Hara, "I'll worry about that tomorrow." This philosophy can be detrimental when applied to health issues because it serves as a vehicle for denial.

Despite the changes in cognition as a result of aging, most research supports the premise that the ability of older adults to learn and remember is virtually as good as ever if special care is taken to slow the pace of presenting information, to ensure relevance of material, and to give appropriate feedback when teaching (Figure 5–1).

Erikson (1963) labeled the major psychosocial developmental task at this stage in life as *ego integrity versus despair.* This phase of older adulthood includes dealing with the reality of aging, the acceptance of the inevitability that we all will die, the reconciling of past failures with present and future concerns, and developing a sense of growth and purpose for those years remaining (Table 5–2). The most common psychosocial tasks of aging involve changes in lifestyle and social status as a result of

- Retirement (often mandatory at 70 years in this country)
- Illness or death of spouse, relatives, and friends
- The moving away of children, grandchildren, and friends
- Relocation to an unfamiliar environment such as a nursing home or senior citizens center

Depression, grief, and loneliness are common among older persons and are often related to the aforementioned developmental tasks. Many individuals experience multiple losses over a short period of time with respect to a previous support network of home, friends, family, and job. These losses, which signify a threat to their own autonomy, independence, and decision making, result in isolation, financial insecurity, diminished coping mechanisms, and a decreased sense of identity, personal value, and societal worth. With aging, individuals begin to question their perception of a "meaningful life"—that is, the potential for further enjoyment, pleasure, and satisfaction.

Separate from biological aging but closely related are the many sociocultural factors that affect how older adults see themselves as competent individuals. The following traits regarding personal goals in life and the values associated with them are significantly related to motivation and learning (Ellison, 1985; Gessner, 1989; Culbert & Kos, 1971):

1. *Independence:* The ability to provide for one's needs is the most important aim of the majority of older persons, regardless of their state of health. Independence gives them a sense of self-respect, pride, and self-functioning so as not to be a burden to others. Health teaching is the tool to help them maintain or regain independence.

2. *Social acceptability:* The approval from others is a common goal of most older adults. It is derived from health, a sense of vigor, and feeling and thinking "young." Despite declining physical attributes, the older adult often has residual fitness and functioning potentials. Health teaching can help to channel these potentials.

3. *Adequacy of personal resources:* Resources, both external and internal, are important considerations when assessing the older adult's current status. Life patterns, which include habits, physical and mental strengths, and economic situation, should

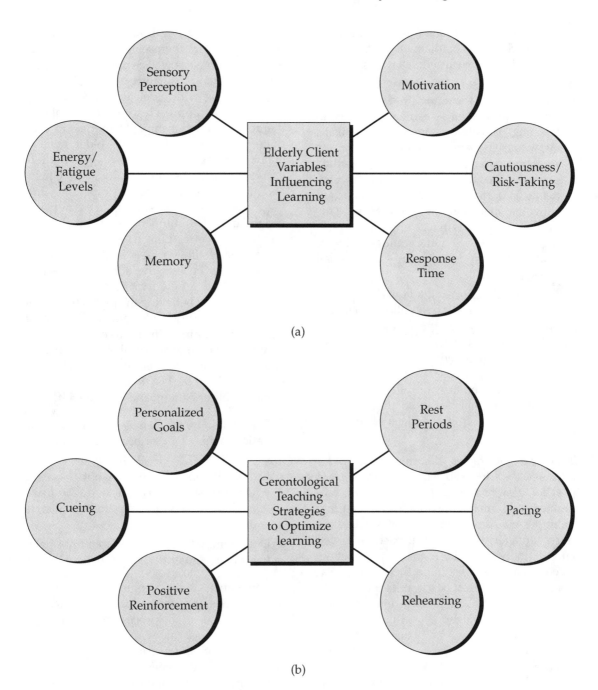

(a)

(b)

FIGURE 5–1    (a) Elderly Client Variables Influencing Learning (b) Gerontological Teaching Strategies
to Optimize Learning.  SOURCE: Reprinted with permission from Rendon, D. C., David, D. K., Gioiella, E.
C., & Tranzillo, M. J. (1986). The right to know, the right to be taught. *Journal of Gerontological Nursing, 12*(12),
34.

be assessed to determine how to incorporate teaching to complement existing regimens with new required behaviors.

4. *Coping mechanisms:* The ability to cope with change during the aging process is indicative of the person's readiness for health teaching. Positive coping mechanisms allow for self-change as older persons draw on life experiences and knowledge gained over the years. Negative coping mechanisms indicate their focus on losses and show that their thinking is immersed in the past. The emphasis in teaching is on exploring alternatives, determining realistic goals, and supporting large and small accomplishments.

5. *Meaning of life:* For well-adapted older persons, having realistic goals allows them the opportunity to enjoy the smaller pleasures in life, whereas less well-adapted individuals may be frustrated and dissatisfied with personal inadequacies. Health teaching must be directed at ways older adults can maintain optimal health so that they can derive pleasure from their leisure years.

**Teaching Strategies** Learning in older adults can be affected by such sociological and psychological factors such as retirement, economics, and mental status. Understanding older persons' developmental tasks will allow nurses to alter how they approach both well and ill individuals in terms of counseling, teaching, and establishing a therapeutic relationship. Nurses must be aware of the fact that older patients will frequently delay medical attention. Social isolation, loneliness, and sensory deprivation may lead to decreased cognitive functioning and perhaps prevent early disease detection and intervention. A decline in psychomotor performance affects their reflex responses and their ability to handle stress. Coping with simple tasks becomes more difficult. The inability of older persons to handle stress has implications with respect to how they care for themselves (food, dress, taking medications) as well as the extent to which they understand the nature of their illnesses.

In working with older adults, reminiscing is a beneficial approach to use to establish a therapeutic relationship. Memories can be quite powerful. Talking with older persons about their experiences—marriage, children, grandchildren, jobs, community involvement, and the like—can be very stimulating. Furthermore, their answers will give the nurse an insight into their humanness, their abilities, and their concerns (Ellison, 1985).

Too many times nurses and other health professionals believe the adage, "You can't teach an old dog new tricks." It is easy to fall into the habit of believing the myths that older people are unteachable and unmotivated (Kick, 1989). Nurses in the role of educators may not even be aware of their stereotypical attitudes toward older adults. To check yourself, think about the last time you gave instruction to an older patient, and ask yourself:

• Did I talk to the family and ignore the patient when I described some aspect of care or discharge planning?

• Did I tell the older person not to worry when he or she asked a question? Did I say, "Just leave everything up to the doctors and nurses"?

• Did I eliminate information that I normally would have given a younger patient?

Remember, older people can learn, but their abilities and needs differ from those of younger persons. The process of teaching and learning is much more rewarding and successful for both the nurse and the patient if it is tailored to fit the older adult's physical, cognitive, motivational, and social differences.

Because changes as a result of aging vary considerably from one individual to another, it is essential to assess each learner's physical, cognitive, and psychosocial functioning level before developing and implementing any teaching plan. It is important to keep in mind that older adults have an overall lower educational level of formal schooling than the population as a whole. Also, they were raised in an era when consumerism and health education were practically nonexistent. As a result, older people may feel uncomfortable in the teaching–learning situation and may be reluctant to ask questions. In the future, as the older population becomes more educated and in tune with consumer activism in the health field, these individuals will likely have an increased desire to participate more in decision making and demand more detailed and sophisticated information. The proliferation of self-help literature and today's expectations for patients and families to take responsibility for self-care result in the present-day need for nurse educators to involve clients more fully in decisions affecting their health (Morra, 1991).

Health education for older persons should be directed at promoting their involvement and changing their attitudes toward learning (Weinrich et al., 1989; Ahroni, 1996). A climate of mutual respect should be cultivated in which they are made to feel important for what they once were as well as for what they are today. Interaction needs to be supportive, not judgmental. Interventions work best when they take place in a casual, informal atmosphere. In the primary care setting, where time is often limited, it may be beneficial to schedule additional time to allow for a more relaxed environment. Individual and situational variables such as motivation, life experiences, educational background, socioeconomic status, health-illness status, and motor, cognitive, and language skills may all influence the ability of the older adult to learn.

Some of the more common aging changes that affect learning and the teaching strategies specific to meeting the needs of the older adult are summarized in Table 5–1. The following are specific tips to abide by when

teaching older persons to create an environment for learning that takes into account major changes in their physical, cognitive, and psychosocial functioning (Picariello, 1986; Hallburg, 1976; Alford, 1982):

Physical Needs

1. To compensate for visual changes, teaching should be done in an environment that is brightly lit but without glare. Visual aids should include large print, well-spaced letters, and the use of primary colors. Bright colors and a visible name tag should be worn by the educator. Because of older persons' difficulty in discriminating certain shades of color, avoid blue, blue-green, and violet hues. Use white or off-white, flat mat paper and black print for posters, diagrams, and other written materials. Keep in mind that tasks that require discrimination of shades of color, such as test strips measuring the presence of sugar in the urine, may present learning difficulties for older patients. Color distortions can have an especially devastating effect on learning regarding medications. Avoid referring to pills by color in guiding patients to take medications as prescribed. Green, blue, and yellow pills may all appear gray to older persons. Additional accommodations should be made to meet physical needs, such as arranging seats so that the learner is reasonably close to the instructor and to any visual aids that may be used. For patients who wear glasses, be sure they are readily accessible, lenses are clean, and frames are properly fitted.

2. To compensate for hearing losses, eliminate extraneous noise, avoid covering the mouth when speaking, directly face the learner, and speak slowly. Female instructors should wear bright lipstick, and male teachers can wear lip gloss. These techniques will assist the learner who may be seeking visual confirmation of what is

being said. Low-pitched voices are heard best, but be careful not to drop your voice at the end of words or phrases. Do not shout, because the decibel level is usually not a problem for hearing-impaired persons. The intensity of sound seems to be less important than the pitch and rate of auditory stimuli. Word speed should not exceed 140 words spoken per minute. Ask for feedback from the learner to determine whether you are speaking too softly, too fast, or not distinctly enough. When addressing a group, microphones are useful aids. Be alert to nonverbal cues from the audience. Participants who are having difficulty with hearing your message may try to compensate by leaning forward, turning the "good" ear to the speaker, or cupping their hands to their ears. Ask older persons to repeat verbal instructions to be sure the entire message was heard and interpreted correctly.

3. To compensate for musculoskeletal problems, decreased efficiency of the cardiovascular system, and reduced kidney function, keep sessions short, schedule frequent breaks to allow for use of bathroom facilities, and allow time for stretching to relieve painful, stiff joints and to stimulate circulation.

4. To compensate for any decline in central nervous system functioning and decreased metabolic rates, set aside more time for the giving and receiving of information and for the practice of psychomotor skills. Also, do not assume that older persons have the psychomotor skills necessary to handle technological equipment for self-paced learning, such as tape recorders, videocassettes, and television. In addition, they may have difficulty with independently applying prostheses or doing dressing changes because of decreased strength and coordination. Be careful not to misinterpret the loss of energy and motor skills as a lack of motivation.

## Cognitive Needs

1. To compensate for a decrease in fluid intelligence, provide older persons with more opportunities to process and react to information and to see relationships between concepts. Research has shown that older adults can learn anything if new information is tied to familiar concepts drawn from relevant past experiences. When teaching, avoid presenting long lists by dividing a series of directions for action into short, discrete, step-by-step messages and then waiting for a response after each one. For instance, if you want to give directions about following different menus depending on exercise levels, instead of saying, "Use menu A if you are not active; use menu B if you are fairly active; use menu C if you are very active," you should say, "You should use menu A if you are not active." Then wait for the learner's response, "That's what I should eat if I'm not very active?" Follow up with the response, "That's right. And if you are fairly active, you should. . . ."

Older persons also tend to confuse previous words and symbols with a new word or symbol being introduced. Again, wait for a response before introducing a new concept or word definition. For decreased short-term memory, coaching and repetition are very useful strategies that assist with recall. Memory can also be enhanced by involving the learner in devising ways to remember how or when to perform a procedure. Because many older adults experience test anxiety, try to explain procedures simply and thoroughly, reassure them, and, if possible, give verbal rather than written tests.

2. Be aware of the effects of medications and energy levels on concentration, alertness, and coordination. Try to schedule teaching sessions before or well after medications are taken and when the person is rested. For example, the patient who has just returned from physical therapy or a diag-

nostic procedure will likely be too fatigued to attend to learning.

3. Be certain to ask what an individual already knows about a healthcare issue or technique before explaining it. Repetition for reinforcement of learning is one thing; repeating information already known may seem patronizing.

4. Convincing older persons of the usefulness of what you are teaching is only half the battle in getting them motivated. You may also have to convince them that the information or technique you are teaching is correct. Anything that is entirely strange or that upsets established habits is likely to be far more difficult for them to learn. As perception slows, the older person's mind has more trouble accommodating to new ways than does the mind of a younger person. Find out about older persons' health habits and beliefs before trying to change their ways or teach something new. For example, many were taught as children that a bowel movement every day is necessary to prevent constipation. You need to identify this belief before trying to teach them to change their dependency on using laxatives.

5. Arrange for brief teaching sessions, because a shortened attention span requires scheduling a series of sessions to provide for sufficient time for learning. In addition, if the material is relevant and focused on the here and now, older persons are more likely to be attentive to the information being presented.

6. Take into account that the process of conceptualizing and the ability to think abstractly become more difficult with aging. Conclude each teaching session with a summary of the information presented and allow for a question and answer period to correct any misconceptions (Figure 5–2).

## Psychosocial Needs

1. Assess family relationships to determine how dependent the older person is on other members for financial and emotional support. In turn, explore the level of involvement by family members in reinforcing the lessons you are teaching and in giving assistance with self-care measures. Do they help the older person to function independently, or do they foster dependency? With permission of the patient, include family members in teaching sessions and enlist their support.

2. Determine availability of resources. A lack of resources can sabotage any teaching plan, especially if your recommendations include expecting older adults to do something they cannot afford to do or lack the means to do, such as buying or renting equipment, having transportation to get to therapy or teaching sessions, purchasing medications, and the like.

3. Encourage active involvement of older adults to improve their self-esteem and to stimulate them both mentally and socially. Teaching must be directed at helping them find meaningful ways to use their talents acquired over a lifetime. Establishing a rapport based on trust can provide them with contact with others as a means to bolster their sense of self-worth.

4. Identify coping mechanisms. No other time in the life cycle carries with it the number of developmental tasks associated with adaptation to loss of roles, social and family contacts, and physical and cognitive capacities. Teaching must include offering constructive methods of coping.

The older person's ability to learn may be affected by the medium chosen for teaching. One-to-one instruction is a method that provides a nonthreatening environment for older adults in which to meet their individual needs and goals by helping them to compensate for their special deficits and promoting their active participation in learning. Group teaching also can be a beneficial approach for fostering social skills and maintaining contact

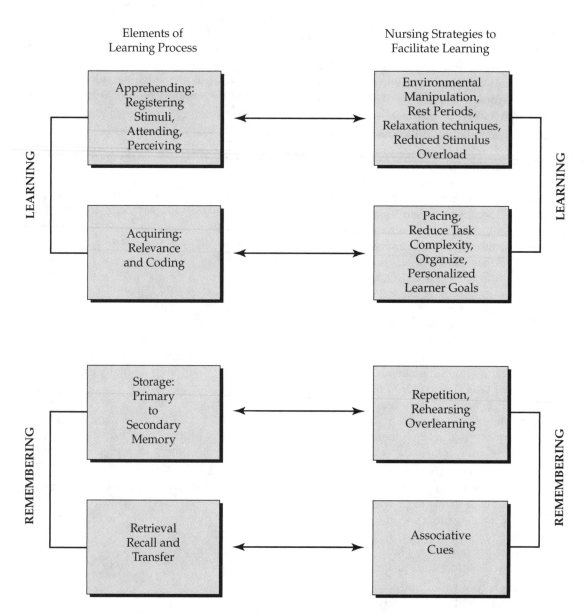

**FIGURE 5–2    A Basic Gerontological Teaching–Learning Model for Nursing** SOURCE: Reprinted with permission from Rendon, D. C., Davis, D. K., Gioiella, E. C., & Tranzillo, M. J. (1986). The right to know, the right to be taught. *Journal of Gerontological Nursing, 12*(12), 36.

with others through shared experiences. Self-paced instructional tools may be very appropriate, but it is important to know the client's previous learning techniques, mental and physical abilities, and comfort levels with certain approaches before assigning any such tools. Many older adults grew up in a time when audiovisual aids did not exist to the extent they do today, and those who have always learned by reading and discussion may not like mediated devices. Introducing new teaching methods and tools, such as use of computer and interactive video formats without adequate instructions on how to operate these technical devices, may inhibit learning by increasing anxiety and frustration levels and may adversely affect self-esteem.

Games, role-playing, demonstration, and return demonstration can be used to rehearse problem-solving and psychomotor skills as long as these methods, and the tools used to complement them, are designed appropriately to accommodate the various developmental characteristics of members of this age group. These teaching methods stimulate learning and can offer opportunities to put knowledge into practice. Written materials, with attention being paid to appropriateness in terms of literacy level and visual impairments in the older adult, are excellent adjuncts to augment, supplement, and reinforce verbal instructions (see Chapters 7, 11, and 12 for specific information on literacy and the design and use of instructional methods and materials).

## THE ROLE OF THE FAMILY IN PATIENT EDUCATION

The role of the family is considered one of the key variables influencing patient care outcomes (Reeber, 1992). The primary motives in patient education for involving family members in the care delivery and decision-making process are to decrease the stress of hospitalization, reduce costs of care, and effectively prepare the client for self-care management outside the healthcare setting. Family caregivers provide critical emotional, physical, and social support to the patient (Gilroth, 1990).

Under the most recent JCAHO accreditation standards, new demands have been placed on healthcare organizations to show evidence that the family is included in patient education efforts. The standards mandate that the instruction of patients and significant others be considered an essential part in the provision of care. Healthcare professionals are responsible for assisting both the patient and his or her family so as to gain the knowledge and skills necessary to meet ongoing healthcare needs (Hartman & Kochar, 1994). Critical (or clinical) pathways have become a popular and effective method to outline specific education needs of the patient and family. These pathways assist in prioritizing and meeting predetermined goals and objectives for learning. Such guidelines provide families with a better understanding of what needs to be learned and when (Barnes, 1995). Interdisciplinary collaboration is a major resource for ensuring continuity of patient and family teaching in and across healthcare settings.

Including the family members in the teaching–learning process helps to ensure a win-win situation for both the client and the nurse educator. Family role enhancement and increased knowledge on the part of the family have positive benefits for the learner as well as the teacher. Clients derive increased satisfaction and greater independence in self-care, and nurses experience increased job satisfaction and personal gratification in helping clients to reach their potentials and achieve successful outcomes (Barnes, 1995).

Orem's (1985) self-care deficit theory, Neuman's (1982) systems theory, Duvall's (1971) family theory, and Erikson's (1963) psychosocial development theory provide the conceptual frameworks for understanding the dynamics of family relationships and the importance of recognizing the developmental stages of the family as influential in achieving teaching–learning outcomes. Although a great deal of attention has been given to the ways in which young and adolescent families function, unfortunately minimal attention has been paid to the dynamics of the complex interactions that characterize the aging family (Phillips, 1989).

In patient education, the nurse may be tempted to teach as many family members as possible. In reality, it is difficult to coordinate the instruction of so many different people. The more individuals involved, the greater the potential for misunderstanding of instruction. The family must make the deliberate decision as to who is the most appropriate person to take the primary responsibility as the caregiver. The nurse educator must determine how the caregiver feels about the role of providing supportive care, how the caregiver feels about learning the necessary information, and what the caregiver's learning style preferences, cognitive abilities, fears and concerns, and current knowledge of the situation are. The caregiver needs information similar to what the patient is given to provide support, feedback, and reinforcement of self-care consistent with prescribed regimens of care. Sometimes the family members need more information than the patient to compensate for any sensory deficits or cognitive limitations the patient may have. Anticipatory teaching with family caregivers can reduce their anxiety, uncertainty, and lack of confidence. What the family is to do is important, but what the family is to expect also is essential information to be shared during the teaching–learning process (Haggard, 1989). The greatest challenge for caregivers is to develop confidence in their ability to do what is right for the patient. Education is the means to help them confront this challenge.

The family can be the educator's greatest ally in preparing the patient for discharge and in helping the patient to become independent in self-care. The patient's family is perhaps the single most significant determinant of the success or failure of the education plan (Haggard, 1989). Rankin and Stallings's (2001) model for patient and family education serves as a foundation for assessing the family profile to determine the family's understanding of the actual or potential health problem(s), the resources available to them, their ways of functioning, and the educational backgrounds, lifestyles, and beliefs of family members.

Education is truly the most powerful tool nurse educators have to ensure safe discharge and the transfer of power to the patient–family dyad. It is imperative that attention be focused on both the assumed and the expected responsibilities of family caregivers. The role of the family has been stressed in each developmental section in this chapter. Table 5–1 outlines the appropriate nursing interventions with the family at different stages in the life cycle.

## SUMMARY

It is important to understand the specific and varied tasks associated with each developmental stage to individualize the approach to education in meeting the needs and desires of learners and their families. Assessment of physical, cognitive, and psychosocial maturation within each developmental period is crucial in determining the strategies to be used to facilitate the teaching–learning process. The younger learner is, in many ways, very different from the adult learner. Issues of dependency, extent of participation, rate of and capacity for learning, and situational and emotional obstacles to learning vary significantly according to phases of development.

Readiness to learn in children is very subject centered and highly influenced by their physical, cognitive, and psychosocial maturation.

Motivation to learn in the adult is very problem centered and more oriented to psychosocial tasks related to roles and expectations of work, family, and community activities. For education to be effective, the nurse in the role of educator must create an environment conducive to learning by presenting information at the learner's level, inviting participation and

feedback, and identifying whether parental and/or peer involvement is appropriate or necessary. Nurses, as the main source of health education, must determine what needs to be taught, when to teach, how to teach, and who should be the focus of teaching in light of the developmental stage of the learner.

## REVIEW QUESTIONS

1. What are the seven (7) stages of development?
2. What is the definition of *pedagogy, andragogy,* and *gerogogy?*
3. Who is the expert in cognitive development? What are the terms or labels used by this expert to identify the key cognitive milestones?
4. Who is the expert in psychosocial development? What are the terms or labels used by this expert to identify the key psychosocial milestones?
5. What are the salient characteristics at each stage of development that influence the ability to learn?
6. What are three (3) main teaching strategies for each stage of development?
7. How do people you know in each stage of development compare with what you have learned about physical, cognitive, and psychosocial characteristics at the various developmental stages?
8. What is the role of the family in the teaching and learning process in each stage of development?
9. How does the role of the nurse vary when teaching individuals at different stages of development?

## REFERENCES

Ahroni, J. H. (1996). Strategies for teaching elders from a human development perspective. *Diabetes Educator, 22*(1), 47–52.

Alford, D. M. (1982). Tips for teaching older adults. *Nursing Life, 2*(5), 60–63.

American Association of Colleges of Nursing. (1994). *AACN Issue Bulletin.* Washington, DC: American Association of Colleges of Nursing.

Babcock, D. E. & Miller, M. A. (1994). *Client Education: Theory & Practice.* St. Louis: Mosby–Year Book.

Banks, E. (1990). Concepts of health and sickness of preschool- and school-aged children. *Children's Health, 19*(1), 43–48.

Barnes, L. P. (1995). Finding the "win/win" in patient/family teaching. *MCN: American Journal of Maternal Child Nursing, 20*(4), 229.

Bille, D. A. (1980). Educational strategies for teaching the elderly patient. *Nursing & Health Care, 1,* 256–263.

Boyd, M. D., Gleit, C. J., Graham, B. A., & Whitman, N. I. (1998). *Health Teaching in Nursing Practice: A Professional Model,* 3rd ed. Norwalk, CT: Appleton & Lange.

Burgireno, J. (1985). Maximizing learning in the adult with SCI. *Rehabilitation Nursing, 10*(5), 20–21.

Burkett, K. W. (1989). Trends in pediatric rehabilitation. *Nursing Clinics of North America, 24*(1), 239–255.

Cauffman, E. & Steinberg, L. (2000). (Im)maturity of judgment in adolescence: Why adolescents may be less culpable than adults. *Behavioral Science Law, 18,* 741–760.

Culbert, P. A. & Kos, B. A. (1971). Aging: Considerations for health teaching. *Nursing Clinics of North America, 6*(4), 605–614.

Day, M. C. (1981). Thinking at Piaget's stage of formal operations. *Educational Leadership, 39,* 44–47.

Duvall, E. M. (1971). *Family Development,* 4th ed. Philadelphia: Lippincott.

Elkind, D. (1984). Teenage thinking: Implications for health care. *Pediatric Nursing, 10*(6), 383–385.

Ellison, S. A. (1985). Geriatric oncology: A developmental approach. *Cancer Nursing,* Supplement 1, 28–32.

Erikson, E. H. (1963). *Childhood and Society,* 2nd ed. New York: Norton.

Erikson, E. H. (1968). *Identity: Youth and Crisis.* New York: Norton.

Falvo, D. R. (1994). *Effective Patient Education: A Guide to Increased Compliance,* 2nd ed. Gaithersburg, MD: Aspen.

Farrand, L. L. & Cox, C. L. (1993). Determinants of positive health behavior in middle childhood. *Nursing Research, 42*(4), 208–213.

Fey, M. S. & Deyes, M. J. (1989). Health and illness self care in adolescents with IDDM: A test of Orem's theory. *Advances in Nursing Science, 12*(1), 67–75.

Gessner, B. A. (1989). Adult education: The cornerstone of patient teaching. *Nursing Clinics of North America, 24*(3), 589–595.

Gilroth, B. E. (1990). Promoting patient involvement: Educational, organizational, and environmental strategies. *Patient Education and Counseling, 15,* 29–38.

Gollop, C. J. (1997). Health information-seeking behavior and older African American women. *Bulletin of the Medical Library Association, 85*(2), 141–146.

Grey, M., Kanner, S., & Lacey, K. O. (1999). Characteristics of the learner: Children and adolescents. *Diabetes Educator, 25*(6), 25–33.

Haggard, A. (1989). *Handbook of Patient Education.* Rockville, MD: Aspen.

Hallburg, J. C. (1976). The teaching of aged adults. *Journal of Gerontological Nursing, 2*(3), 13–19.

Hartman, R. A. & Kochar, M. S. (1994). The provision of patient and family education. *Patient Education and Counseling, 24,* 101–108.

Havighurst, R. (1976). Human characteristics and school learning: Essay review. *Elementary School Journal, 77,* 101–109.

Heiney, S. P. (1991). Helping children through painful procedures. *American Journal of Nursing, 91*(11), 20–24.

Hussey, C. G. & Hirsh, A. M. (1983). Health education for children. *Topics in Clinical Nursing, 5*(1), 22–28.

Jackson, R. H., Davis, T. C., Murphy, P., Bairnsfather, L. E., & George, R. B. (1994). Reading deficiencies in older patients. *American Journal of the Medical Sciences, 308*(2), 79–82.

Johnson-Saylor, M. T. (1980) Seize the moment: Health promotion for the young adult. *Topics in Clinical Nursing, 2*(2), 9–19.

Kennedy, C. M. & Riddle, I. I. (1989). The influence of the timing of preparation on the anxiety of preschool children experiencing surgery. *Maternal-Child Nursing Journal, 18*(2), 117–132.

Kick, E. (1989). Patient teaching for elders. *Nursing Clinics of North America, 24*(3), 681–686.

Knowles, M. (1990). *The Adult Learner: A Neglected Species,* 4th ed. Houston: Gulf.

Knowles, M. S., Holton, E. F., & Swanson, R.A. (1998). *The Adult Learner: The Definitive Classic in Adult Education and Human Resource Development,* 5th ed. Houston: Gulf Publishing.

Kotchabhakdi, P. (1985). School-age children's conceptions of the heart and its function. Monograph 15. *Maternal-Child Nursing Journal, 14*(4), 203–261.

Kray, J. & Lindenberger, U. (2000). Adult age differences in task switching. *Psychology and Aging, 15*(1), 126–147.

Lambert, S. A. (1984). Variables that affect the school-age child's reaction to hospitalization and surgery: A review of the literature. *Maternal-Child Nursing Journal, 13*(1), 1–18.

Levine, M. D. (1983). *Developmental-Behavioral Pediatrics.* Philadelphia: Lippincott.

Matsuda, O. & Saito, M. (1998). Crystallized and fluid intelligence in elderly patients with mild dementia of the Alzheimer type. *International Psychogeriatrics, 10*(2), 147–154.

Milligan, F. (1997). In defense of andragogy. Part 2: An educational process consistent with modern nursing's aims. *Nurse Education Today, 17,* 487–493.

Morra, M. E. (1991). Future trends in patient education. *Seminars in Oncology Nursing, 7*(2), 143–145.

Neuman, B. (1982). *The Neuman System Model.* Norwalk, CT: Appleton-Century-Crofts.

Orem, D. (1985). *Nursing: Concepts of Practice,* 3rd ed. New York: McGraw-Hill.

Palmore, E. (1977). Facts on aging: A short quiz. *Gerontologist, 17*(4), 1–5.

Pearson, M. & Wessman, J. (1996). Gerogogy. *Home Healthcare Nurse, 14*(8), 631–636.

Perrin, E. C., Sayer, A. G., & Willett, J. B. (1991). Sticks and stones may break my bones . . . Reasoning about illness causality and body functioning in children who have a chronic illness. *Pediatrics, 88*(3), 608–619.

Petrillo, M. & Sanger, S. (1980). *Emotional Care of Hospitalized Children,* 2nd ed. Philadelphia: Lippincott.

Phillips, L. R. (1989). Elder-family caregiver relationships: Determining appropriate nursing interventions. *Nursing Clinics of North America, 24*(3), 795–807.

Piaget, J. (1951). *Judgement and Reasoning in the Child*. London: Routlege and Kegan Paul.

Piaget, J. (1952). *The Origins of Intelligence in Children*. New York: International Universities Press.

Piaget, J. (1976). *The Grasp of Consciousness: Action and Concept in the Young Child*. Susan Wedgwood (translator). Cambridge, MA: Harvard University Press.

Picariello, G. (1986). A guide for teaching elders. *Geriatric Nursing, 7*(1), 38–39.

Pidgeon, V. A. (1977). Characteristics of children's thinking and implications for health teaching. *Maternal-Child Nursing Journal, 6*(1), 1–8.

Pidgeon, V. (1985). Children's concepts of illness: Implications for health teaching. *Maternal-Child Nursing Journal, 14*(1), 23–35.

Poster, E. C. (1983). Stress immunization: Techniques to help children cope with hospitalization. *Maternal-Child Nursing Journal, 12*(2), 119–134.

Rankin, S. H. & Stallings, K. D. (2001). *Patient Education: Principles and Practices*, 4th ed. Philadelphia: Lippincott.

Reeber, B. J. (1992). Evaluating the effects of a family education intervention. *Rehabilitation Nursing, 17*(6), 332–336.

Ryberg, J. W. & Merrifield, E. B. (1984). What parents want to know. *Nurse Practitioner, 9*(6), 24–32.

Taylor, K., Marienau, C., & Fiddler, M. (2000). *Developing Adult Learners: Strategies for Teachers and Trainers*. San Francisco: Jossey-Bass.

Theis, S. L. & Merritt, S. L. (1994). A learning model to guide research and practice for teaching of elder clients. *Nursing and Health Care, 15*(9), 464–468.

Vulcan, B. (1984). Major coping behaviors of a hospitalized 3-year-old boy. *Maternal-Child Nursing Journal, 13*(2), 113–123.

Weinrich, S. P. & Boyd, M. (1992). Education in the elderly. *Journal of Gerontological Nursing, 18*(1), 15–20.

Weinrich, S. P., Boyd, M., & Nussbaum, J. (1989). Continuing education: Adapting strategies to teach the elderly. *Journal of Gerontological Nursing, 15*(11), 19–21.

Whitener, L. M., Cox, K. R., & Maglich, S. A. (1998). Use of theory to guide nurses in the design of health messages for children. *Advances in Nursing Science, 20*(3), 21–35.

Woodring, B. C. (2000). If you have taught—have the child and family learned? *Pediatric Nursing, 26*(5), 505–509.

## CHAPTER 6

# Motivation, Compliance, and Health Behaviors of the Learner

*Eleanor Richards*

After completing this chapter, the reader will be able to

1. Define the terms *motivation, compliance,* and *adherence* relevant to behaviors of the learner.

2. Discuss motivation and compliance concepts and theories.

3. Identify incentives and obstacles that affect motivation to learn.

4. Discuss axioms of motivation relevant to learning.

5. Assess levels of learner motivation.

6. Outline strategies that facilitate motivation and improve compliance.

7. Compare and contrast selected health behavior frameworks and their influence on learning.

8. Recognize the unique subroles of the nurse as educator in health promotion.

The nurse as educator needs to understand what drives the learner to learn and what factors promote or hinder the acquisition and application of knowledge. Motivation and compliance, related yet different concepts, are central to the learning situation and are common denominators in many health behavior models.

Although the importance of motivation and compliance as they relate to learning is acknowledged in the literature, there is marginal incorporation of these concepts into educational plans. Educators frequently focus on the learner's level of motivation as an indicator of potential involvement in health education programs. Sands and Holman (1985) noted that compliance often has been used by researchers as a measure of outcomes of these programs. As early as 1974, Becker, Drachman, and Kirscht found motivation to be significantly related to measures of compliance with a medical regimen.

Factors that determine health outcomes are complex. In a review of studies of health behavior, Ross and Rosser (1989) indicated that information alone does not account for changes in health behavior. Knowledge alone does not guarantee that the learner will engage in health-promoting behaviors, nor that the desired outcomes will be achieved. The most well-thought-out educational program or plan of care will not achieve the prescribed goals if the learner is not understood in the context of complex factors associated with motivation and compliance. A thorough understanding of the relationship between the reception of information and the application of information, as well as those factors that impede or promote desired health outcomes, is essential for the nurse as educator.

This chapter discusses the concepts of motivation and compliance as they relate to the learning situation with a focus on health behaviors. The discussion includes factors such as assessment of motivation, obstacles and facilitating factors for motivation and compliance, and motivational axioms. An overview and comparison of selected models of health behaviors is presented with an emphasis on the role of nurse as educator in health promotion.

## MOTIVATION

Motivation, from the Latin *movere*, means to set into motion. *Motivation* has been defined as a psychological force that moves a person toward some kind of action (Haggard, 1989) and as a willingness of the learner to embrace learning, with readiness as evidence of motivation (Redman, 2001). According to Kort (1987), it is the result of both internal and external factors and not the result of external manipulation alone. Implicit in motivation is movement in the direction of meeting a need or toward reaching a goal.

Lewin (1935), an early field theorist, conceptualized motivation in terms of positive or negative movement toward goals. Once an individual's equilibrium is disturbed, such as in the case of illness, forces of approach and avoidance may come into play. He noted that if avoidance endured in an approach–avoidance conflict, there would be negative movement away from a goal. His theory implies the existence of a critical time factor relative to motivation. This time factor, however, is usually not a critical consideration in motivational models of health behavior or motivational research. Ideally, though, the nurse educator's role is to facilitate the learner's approach toward a desired goal and to prevent untimely delays. For example, nursing staff may request an in-service program about clinical pathways. The in-service nurse educator may delay this request to the extent that the staff loses interest in the topic. Although untimely delays may be beyond the control of the educator, every effort should be made to capitalize on the staff's desire and readiness to learn.

Maslow (1943), another well-known early theorist, developed a theory of human motivation that is still widely used in the social sciences. The major premises of Maslow's motivation theory are integrated wholeness of the individual and a hierarchy of goals. Acknowledging the complexity of the concept of motivation, he noted that not all behavior is motivated and that behavior theories are not synonymous with motivation. Many determinants of behavior other than motives exist, and many motives can be involved in one behavior. Using the principles of *hierarchy of needs*—physiological, safety, love/belonging, self-esteem, and self-actualization—Maslow noted the relatedness of needs, which are organized by their level of potency. Some individuals are highly motivated, whereas others are weakly motivated. When a need is fairly well satisfied, then the next potent need emerges. An example of the hierarchy of basic needs is the potent need to satisfy hunger. This need may be met by the nurse who assists the poststroke patient with feeding. The nurse–patient interaction may also satisfy the next most potent needs, those of love/belonging and self-esteem.

There are relationships between motivation and learning; between motivation and behavior; and between motivation, learning, and behavior. Motivation may be viewed in relation to learning in many ways. Redman (2001) categorizes theories of motivation that direct learning as behavioral reinforcers, need satisfaction, reduction of discomforting inconsistencies as a result of cognitive dissonance, allocating causal factors known as attributions, personality in which motivation is acknowledged to be a stable characteristic, expectancy theory encompassing value and perceived chance of success, and humanistic interpretations of motivation that emphasize personal choice. Each theory attempts to address the complex and somewhat elusive quality of motivation.

## Motivational Factors

Factors that influence motivation can serve as incentives or obstacles to achieve desired behaviors. Both creating incentives and decreasing obstacles to motivation pose a challenge for the nurse as educator. The cognitive (thinking processes), affective (emotions and feelings), social, and psychomotor (behavioral) domains of the learner can be influenced by the educator, who can act as a motivational facilitator or blocker.

*Motivational incentives* need to be considered in the context of the individual. What may be a motivational incentive for one learner may be a motivational obstacle to another. For example, a student who is assigned to work with an elderly woman may be motivated when the student holds older persons in high regard. Another student may be motivationally blocked by the same emotional domain because previous experiences with older women, such as a grandmother, were unrewarding.

Facilitating or blocking factors that shape motivation to learn can be classified into three major categories, which are not mutually exclusive:

1. Personal attributes, which consist of physical, developmental, and psychological components of the individual learner

2. Environmental influences, which include the physical and attitudinal climate

3. Learner relationship systems, such as those of significant other, family, community, and teacher–learner interaction.

**Personal Attributes**    Personal attributes of the learner, such as developmental stage, age, gender, emotional readiness, values and beliefs, sensory functioning, cognitive ability, educational level, actual or perceived state of health, and severity or chronicity of illness, can shape an individual's motivation to learn. Functional ability to achieve behavioral outcomes is determined by physical, emotional, and cognitive dimensions. One's perception of disparity between current and expected states of health can be a motivating factor in health behavior and can drive readiness to learn.

The learner's views about the complexity or extent of changes that are needed can shape motivation. Values, beliefs, and natural curiosity can be firmly entrenched and enduring factors that can also shape desire to learn new behaviors. Other factors, such as sensory input and processing of information and short-term and long-term memory, can affect motivation to learn as well. Emerging interest about male–female behavioral and learning differences indicates the need for in-depth research on gender-related characteristics affecting motivation to learn (see Chapter 8).

**Environmental Influences**    Physical characteristics of the learning environment, accessibility and availability of human and material resources, and different types of behavioral rewards influence the motivational level of the individual. The environment can create, promote, or detract from a state of learning receptivity. Pleasant, comfortable, and adaptable individualized surroundings can promote a state of readiness to learn. Conversely, noise, confusion, interruptions, and lack of privacy can interfere with the capacity to concentrate and to learn.

The factors of accessibility and availability of resources include physical and psychological aspects. Can the client physically access a health facility, and once there, will the healthcare personnel be psychologically available to the client? Psychological availability refers to the healthcare system and whether it is flexible and sensitive to patients' needs. It includes factors such as promptness of services, sociocultural competence, emotional support, and communication skills. Attitude influences the client's engagement with the healthcare system.

The manner in which the healthcare system is perceived by the client affects the client's willingness to participate in health-promoting behaviors. Behavioral rewards permeate the foundations of the learner's motivation. Rewards can be extrinsic, such as praise or acknowledgment from the educator or caretaker. Alternatively, they can be intrinsically based, such as feelings of a personal sense of fulfillment, gratification, or self-satisfaction.

**Relationship Systems**    Family or significant others in the support system; cultural identity; work, school, and community roles; and teacher–learner interaction—all influence an individual's motivation. The interactional aspects of motivation are perhaps the most salient because the learner exists in the context of interlocking relationship systems. Individuals are viewed in the context of family/community/cultural systems that have lifelong effects on the choices that individuals make, including healthcare seeking and healthcare decision making. These significant other systems may have even more of an influence on health outcomes than commonly acknowledged, and the health-promoting use of these systems needs to be taken into account by the nurse as educator.

All of these factors interact to address the motivation of the learner. They are not meant to be construed as comprehensive theory constructs, but rather as forces that act on motivation, serving to facilitate or block desire to learn.

## Motivational Axioms

*Axioms* are premises on which an understanding of a phenomenon is based. The nurse as educator needs to understand the premises involved in promoting motivation of the learner. *Motivational axioms* are rules that set the stage for motivation. They include (1) the state of optimum anxiety, (2) learner readiness, (3) realistic goal setting, (4) learner satisfaction/success, and (5) uncertainty-reducing or uncertainty-maintaining dialogue.

**State of Optimum Anxiety**    Learning occurs best when a state of moderate anxiety exists. In this optimum state for learning, one's ability to observe, focus attention, learn, and adapt is operative (Peplau, 1979). Perception, concentration, abstract thinking, and information processing are enhanced. Behavior is directed at a learning or challenging situation. Above this optimum level, at high or severe levels of anxiety, the ability to perceive the environment, concentrate, and learn is reduced. A moderate state of anxiety can be comfortably managed and is known to promote learning. As anxiety escalates, however, attention to external stimuli is reduced, the learner becomes increasingly self-absorbed, and behavior becomes defensively reactionary rather than being cognitively generated.

For example, a patient who has been recently diagnosed with insulin-dependent diabetes and who has a high level of anxiety

will not respond at an optimum level of retention of information when instructed about insulin injections. When the nurse as educator is able to aid the client in reducing anxiety, through techniques such as guided imagery, use of humor, or relaxation tapes, the patient will respond with a higher level of information retention.

**Learner Readiness**    Desire to move toward a goal and *readiness to learn* are factors that influence motivation. Desire cannot be imposed on the learner. It can, however, be critically influenced by external forces and be promoted by the nurse as educator. Incentives are specific to the individual learner. An incentive to one individual can be a deterrent to another. Incentives in the form of reinforcers and rewards can be tangible or intangible, external or internal.

As a facilitator to the learner, the nurse as educator offers positive perspectives and encouragement, which shape the desired behavior toward goal attainment. By ensuring that learning is stimulating, making information relevant and accessible, and creating an environment conducive to learning, educators can facilitate motivation to learn (see Chapter 4 on readiness to learn).

**Realistic Goals**    Goals that are within one's grasp, reasonable, and possible to be achieved are goals toward which an individual will work. Goals that are beyond one's reach are frustrating and counterproductive. Unrealistic goals with loss of valuable time can set the stage for the learner to "give up."

Setting realistic goals is a motivating factor. The belief that one can achieve the task set before him or her facilitates behavior geared toward achieving that goal. Goals should parallel the extent to which behavioral changes are needed. Learning what the learner wants to change is a critical factor in setting realistic goals. Mutual goal setting between learner and educator reduces the negative effects of hidden agendas or the sabotaging of educational plans.

**Learner Satisfaction/Success**    The learner is motivated by success. Success is self-satisfying and feeds one's self-esteem. In a cyclical process, success and self-esteem escalate, moving the learner toward accomplishment of goals. When a learner feels good about step-by-step accomplishments, motivation is enhanced. For example, in the instructor–student relationship, evaluations can be a valuable method of promoting learner success. Clinical evaluations, when focused on demonstration of positive behaviors, can encourage movement toward performance goals. Focusing on successes as a means of positive reinforcement promotes learner satisfaction and instills a sense of accomplishment. On the other hand, focusing on weak clinical performance can reduce students' self-esteem.

**Uncertainty Reduction or Maintenance**    Uncertainty (as well as certainty) can be a motivating factor in the learning situation. Individuals have ongoing internal dialogues that can either reduce or maintain uncertainty. Individuals carry on "self-talk"; they "think things through." When one wants to change a state of health, behaviors will often follow a dialogue that examines uncertainty: "If I stop smoking, then my chances of getting lung cancer will be reduced." On the other hand, when the probable outcome of health behaviors is more uncertain, then behaviors may be uncertainty maintaining: "I am not sure that I need this surgery because the survival rates are no different for those who had this surgery and those who did not." Some learners may maintain current behaviors, given probabilities of treatment outcomes, thus maintaining uncertainty.

Mishel (1990) reconceptualized the concept of uncertainty in illness. She views uncertainty as a necessary and natural rhythm of life, rather than an adverse experience. Uncertainty in sufficient concentration influences

choices and decision making, and it can capitalize on receptivity or readiness for change. Premature uncertainty reduction can be counterproductive to the learner who has not sufficiently explored alternatives. For example, when a staff nurse is uncertain about positions for catheterizing a debilitated female client and is presented with alternatives, then a thinking dialogue is carried out. If the decision to use a particular position is not premature, then uncertainty will promote exploration of alternative positions.

## Assessment of Motivation

How does the nurse know when the learner is motivated? As a generic concept, assessment of motivation to learn has not been adequately addressed in the literature. The lack of adequate, conceptually-based measurement tools could be a factor in this neglect.

Redman (2001) views motivational assessment as a part of general health assessment and states that it includes such areas as level of knowledge, client skills, decision-making capacity of the individual, and screening of target populations for educational programs. Leddy and Pepper (1998) view assessment of motivation in relation to capacity for change. The educator can pose several questions in terms of the learner, such as those focusing on previous attempts, curiosity, goal setting, self-care ability, stress factors, survival issues, and life situations.

Motivational assessment of the learner needs to be comprehensive, systematic, and conceptually based. Cognitive, affective, physiological, experiential, environmental, and learning relationship variables need to be considered. Table 6–1 shows parameters for a comprehensive motivational assessment of the learner.

These multi-theory-based parameters incorporate several perspectives: Bandura's (1986) construction of incentive motivators; Ajzen and Fishbein's (1980) intent and attitude; Becker's (1974) notion of likelihood of engaging in action; Pender's (1996) commitment to a

## TABLE 6–1 Comprehensive parameters for motivational assessment of the learner

**COGNITIVE VARIABLES**

- Capacity to learn
- Readiness to learn
  - Expressed self-determination
  - Constructive attitude
  - Expressed desire and curiosity
  - Willingness to contract for behavioral outcomes
- Facilitating beliefs

**AFFECTIVE VARIABLES**

- Expressions of constructive emotional state
- Moderate level of anxiety

**PHYSIOLOGICAL VARIABLES**

- Capacity to perform required behavior

**EXPERIENTIAL VARIABLES**

- Previous successful experiences

**ENVIRONMENTAL VARIABLES**

- Appropriateness of physical environment
- Social support systems
  - Family
  - Group
  - Work
  - Community resources

**EDUCATOR–LEARNER RELATIONSHIP SYSTEM**

- Prediction of positive relationship

ing–learning is a two-way process. In particular, motivation can be assessed through both subjective and objective means. A subjective means of assessing level of motivation is through dialogue. Through use of communication skills, the nurse can obtain verbal information from the client such as "I really want to maintain my weight" or "I want to have a healthy baby." Both of these statements indicate an energized desire with direction of movement toward an expected health outcome. Nonverbal cues can also indicate motivation, such as browsing through lay literature about healthy pregnancy. Likewise, a staff member or student nurse may express a verbal desire to know more about a specific advanced procedure. A nonverbal motivational cue might be expressed by the staff member or student nurse carefully observing a senior nurse or clinical specialist performing an advanced technique, for example.

Measurement of motivation is another aspect to be considered. Subjective self-reports indicate the level of motivation from the learner's perspective. If desired, self-report measurements could be developed for educational programs. Objective measurement of motivation—an indirect measurement—can be quantified through observation of expected behaviors, the consequence of motivation. These behaviors can be observed in increments as the learner moves toward preset realistic health or practice goals.

plan of action; and Barofsky's (1978) focus on alliance in the learning situation. Additionally, the presence of cognitions in the form of facilitative beliefs proposed by Wright, Watson, and Bell (1996) provide a comprehensive and multidimensional assessment. This proposed multidimensional guide allows for assessment of the level of learner motivation. If responses to dimensions are positive, then the learner is likely to be motivated.

Assessment of learner motivation involves the judgment of the educator, because teach-

## Motivational Strategies

As noted earlier, incentives viewed as appeals or inducements to motivation can be either intrinsically or extrinsically generated. Incentives and motivation are both stimuli to action. Bandura (1986) associates motivation with incentives. He noted, however, that intrinsic motivation, although highly appealing, is elusive. Only rarely does motivation occur without extrinsic influence. Green and Kreuter (1999) note that "strictly speaking we can appeal to people's motives, but we cannot motivate them" (p. 30). Extrinsic incentives are used for motivational strategizing in the educational situation.

Motivational strategies for the nurse as educator are extrinsically generated through the use of specific incentives. The critical question for the nurse as educator to ask is, "What specific behavior, under what circumstances, in what time frame, is desired by this learner?"

Strategizing begins with a systematic assessment of learner motivation, like that outlined in Table 6–1. When an applicable dimension is absent or reduced, then incentive strategizing is likely to move the individual away from the desired outcome. When considering strategies to improve learner motivation, Maslow's (1943) hierarchy of needs can also be taken into consideration. An appeal can be made to the innate need for the learner to succeed, known as achievement motivation (Atkinson, 1964).

In the educational situation, clear communication, including clarification of directions and expectations, is critical. Organization of material in a way that makes information meaningful to the learner, environmental manipulation, positive verbal feedback, and providing opportunities for success are motivational strategies proposed by Haggard (1989). Reducing or eliminating barriers to achieve goals is an important aspect of maintaining motivation.

One particular model developed by Keller (1987), called the Attention, Relevance, Confidence, and Satisfaction (ARCS) Model, focuses on creating and maintaining motivational strategies used for instructional design. This model emphasizes strategies that the educator can use to effect changes in the learner by creating a motivating learning environment.

- **A**ttention introduces opposing positions, case studies, and variable instructional presentations.
- **R**elevance capitalizes on the learners' experiences, usefulness, needs, and personal choices.

- **C**onfidence deals with learning requirements, level of difficulty, expectations, attributions, and sense of accomplishment.
- **S**atisfaction pertains to timely use of a new skill, use of rewards, praise, and self-evaluation.

In motivational strategizing, it would also be beneficial to consider Damrosch's (1991) proposal that client health beliefs, personal vulnerability, efficacy of proposed change, and ability to effect the change are important in patient education efforts. Beliefs are a major construct proposed by Wright, Watson, and Bell (1996) as the heart of healing in families. Facilitating beliefs can promote a desired change, whereas constraining beliefs can restrict options. Challenging constraining beliefs and promoting facilitating beliefs are, therefore, offered as motivational strategies. An understanding of the individual's mental representations or beliefs is also foundational to the Common Sense Model in the representational approach to patient education (Levanthal & Diefenbach, 1991). Beliefs constitute an underacknowledged and understudied phenomenon that needs to be further developed in the education literature in terms of motivational strategizing.

## COMPLIANCE

*Compliance* is a term used to describe submission or yielding to predetermined goals. Defined as such, it has a manipulative or authoritative undertone in which the healthcare provider or educator is viewed as the traditional authority, and the consumer or learner is viewed as submissive. This term has not been well received in nursing, perhaps due to the philosophical perspective that clients have the right to make their own healthcare decisions and to not necessarily follow predetermined courses of action as set by healthcare professionals. Ward-Collins (1998) notes that a diagnosis of noncompliance can be highly subjective. Reflective thought about the relationship between noncompliance and the ethical principle of autonomy is fundamental to education.

Healthcare literature suggests that compliance is the equivalent of the achieved goal to a predetermined regimen. Compliance, as an end unto itself, is different from motivational factors, which are viewed as means to an end.

Compliance to a health regimen is an observable behavior and as such can be directly measured. Motivation, by comparison, is a precursor to action that can be indirectly measured through behavioral consequences or results.

Commitment or attachment to a regimen is known as *adherence*, which may be long-lasting. Both compliance and adherence refer to the ability to maintain health-promoting regimens, which are determined largely by a healthcare provider. A subtle difference separates compliance and adherence. It is possible for an individual to comply with a regimen and not necessarily be committed to it. For example, a patient who is experiencing sleep disturbances may comply with medication as directed for a period of one week. The same patient may not continue to adhere to the regimen for an extended period of time, however, even though the sleep disturbances continue. In this situation, there is no commitment to follow through. Both *compliance* and *adherence* are terms used in the measurement of health outcomes; for the purpose of this chapter, they are used interchangeably.

Healthcare literature has traditionally focused on compliance or adherence to a predetermined regimen. This phenomenon may be the result of an emphasis on cost-effective health care, as seen, for example, in shorter lengths of hospital stays. The successes of educational programs in a fiscally responsible system will ultimately be linked to measurement of patient compliance relative to outcomes.

According to Eraker, Kirscht, and Becker (1984) and Levanthal and Cameron (1987),

patient compliance to health regimens can be viewed from various theoretical perspectives:

1. Biomedical, including patient demographics, severity of disease, and complexity of treatment regimen
2. Behavioral/social learning theory, using the behaviorist approach of rewards, cues, contracts, and social supports
3. Communication feedback loop of sending, receiving, comprehending, retaining, and acceptance
4. Rational belief theory, weighing the benefits of treatment and the risks of disease through the use of cost-benefit logic
5. Self-regulatory systems, in which patients are seen as problem solvers whose regulation of behavior is based on perception of illness, cognitive skills, and past experiences that affect their ability to plan and cope with illness

Compliance is an issue for all healthcare disciplines. The major theories of compliance as described by Eraker et al. (1984) and Levanthal and Cameron (1987) are useful in explaining or describing compliance from a multidisciplinary approach including psychology and education. Fisher (1992) offered a pharmacist's perspective on the measurement of compliance to a medication regimen, with the communication model noted as being the most effective for patient education. It is feasible for the nurse as educator to choose one or a combination of these theoretical perspectives with the goal of compliance to a specific health-promoting regimen.

## COMPLIANCE AND CONTROL

The authoritative aspect of compliance infers that the educator makes an attempt to control, in part, decision making on the part of the learner. Some models of compliance have attempted to balance the issue of control by using terms such as *mutual contracting* (Steckel, 1982) or *consensual regimen* (Fink, 1976).

One way to view the issue of control in the learning situation is through the concept of *locus of control* (Rotter, 1954) and health locus of control (Wallston, Wallston, & DeVellis, 1978). Through objective measurement, individuals can be categorized as "internals," whose health behavior is self-directed, or "externals," whereby others are viewed as more powerful in influencing health outcomes. Externals believe that fate is a powerful external force that determines life's course, whereas internals believe that they control their own destiny. For instance, an external might say, "Osteoporosis runs in my family, and it will 'catch up' with me." An internal might say, "Although there is a history of osteoporosis in my family, I will have necessary screenings, eat an appropriate diet, and do weight-bearing exercise to prevent or control this problem."

Locus of control has been related to compliance with therapeutic regimens. Shillinger (1983) suggests that different teaching strategies are indicated for internals and externals. The literature, however, is inconclusive as to the nature of the relationship between compliance and internals versus externals. Oberle (1991) reviewed a decade of research on locus of control and concluded that the collective results of nursing studies yield little information useful in nursing practice. She noted the existence of problems with nonexperimental designs, issues of reliability and validity, and the multidimensional nature of the construct of locus of control.

Hussey and Guilliland (1989) note that both locus of control and functional literacy level influence compliance. Going beyond poor reading skills, "functional literacy is the idea of being able to function or act on content after reading it" (p. 607). This concept implies that reading skills, although important in assessing a person's level of ability to comprehend written educational material or directions, do not measure one's ability to function or actually carry out regimens following presented content. Functional literacy level in relation to compliance also needs to be assessed by the nurse as educator (see Chapter 7 on literacy).

*Noncompliance* describes resistance of the individual to follow a predetermined regimen. The literature is replete with studies that indicate high levels of patient noncompliance, with estimates of noncompliance ranging from 30% to 50% (Becker & Green, 1975; Sackett & Haynes, 1976). The question of why clients are noncompliant remains largely unanswered.

Research has shown that situational and personality characteristics play a significant role in determining compliance (Luker & Caress, 1989). The educator's self-awareness relative to the learner's personality characteristics and previous history of compliance to health regimens could play an important role in the educational process.

The expectation of total compliance in all spheres of behavior and at all times is unrealistic. At times, noncompliant behavior may be desirable and could be viewed as a necessary defensive response to stressful situations. The learner may use "time-outs" as the intensity of the learning situation is maintained or escalates. This mechanism of temporary withdrawal from the learning situation may actually prove beneficial. Following withdrawal, the learner could reengage, feeling renewed and ready to continue with an educational program or regimen. Viewed in this way, noncompliance is not an obstacle to learning and does not carry a negative connotation.

## HEALTH BEHAVIORS OF THE LEARNER

Motivation and compliance are concepts relevant to health behaviors of the learner. The nurse as educator focuses on health education as well as the expected health behaviors. Health behavior frameworks are blueprints and, as such, serve as tools for the nurse as educator that can be used to maintain desired patient behaviors or promote changes. As a consequence, a familiarity with models and theories that describe, explain, or predict health behaviors will increase the range of health-promoting strategies for the nurse as educator. When these frameworks are understood, the principles inherent in each can be used either to facilitate motivation or to promote compliance to a health regimen. This chapter presents an overview of several models and theories: Health Belief Model, Health Promotion Model, Self-Efficacy Theory, Stages of Change Model, Theory of Reasoned Action, PRECEDE-PROCEED Model, and Therapeutic Alliance Model.

## Health Belief Model

The original *Health Belief Model* was developed in the 1950s from a social psychology perspective to examine why people did not participate in health-screening programs (Rosenstock, 1974). This model was modified by Becker (1974) to address compliance to therapeutic regimens.

The two major premises on which the model is built are the eventual success of disease prevention and curing regimens that involve the clients' willingness to participate and the belief that health is highly valued (Becker, 1990). Both of these premises need to be present for the model to be relevant in explaining health behavior. The model is grounded on the supposition that it is possible to predict health behavior given three major interacting components: individual perceptions, modifying factors, and likelihood of action (Figure 6–1).

Figure 6–1 shows the direction and flow of the interacting components, each of which is

further divided into subcomponents. The individual perceptions component comprises perceived susceptibility or perceived severity of a specific disease. The modifying factors component consists of demographic variables (age, sex, race, ethnicity), socio-psychological variables (personality, locus of control, social class, peer and reference group pressure), and structural variables (knowledge about and prior contact with disease). These variables, in conjunction with cues to action (mass media, advice, reminders, illness, reading material), influence the subcomponent of perceived threat of the specific disease. The third major component, likelihood of action, consists of the subcomponents of perceived benefits of preventive action minus perceived barriers to preventive action. All of the components are directed toward the likelihood of taking recommended preventive health action as the final phase of the model. In sum, individual perceptions and modifying factors interact. An individual appraisal of the preventive action occurs, which is followed by a prediction of the likelihood of action.

The Health Belief Model has been the predominant explanatory model since the 1970s for uncovering differences in preventive health behaviors as well as differences in preventive use of health services (Langlie, 1977). Used to predict preventive health behavior and to explain sick-role behavior, it has been used widely in health behavior research across disciplines such as medicine, psychology, social behavior, and gerontology. The model has also been widely used to study patient behaviors in relation to preventive behaviors and acute and chronic illnesses. Redeker (1988) reviewed the literature on health beliefs and adherence in chronic illness and uncovered studies focused on hypertension, coronary disease, diabetes, renal disease, pulmonary disease, and paraplegia.

Several nursing studies have supported the validity of this model. For instance, Hahn (1993) examined health belief constructs

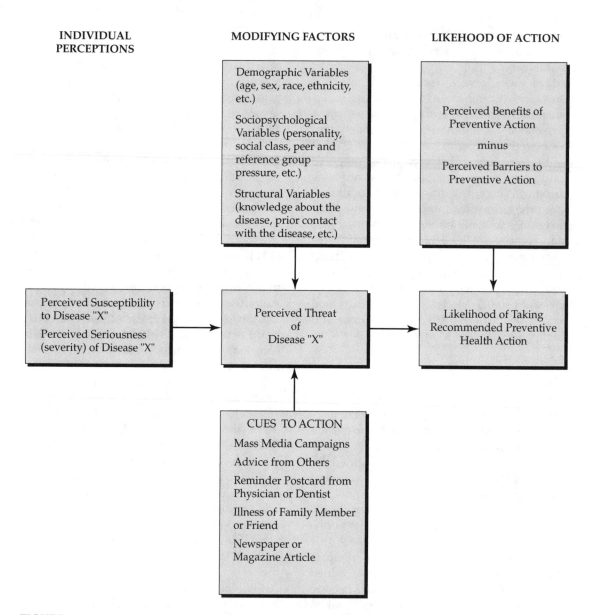

**FIGURE 6–1   The Health Belief Model used as a predictor of preventive health behavior**   Source: From M. Becker, R. Drachman, and J. Kirscht, A new approach to explaining sick-role behavior in low-income populations. (1974). *American Journal of Public Health, 64*(3), 206. Copyright by American Public Health Association. Reprinted with permission.

regarding alcohol and other drug use, including perceived susceptibility, seriousness, barriers, benefits, and parental involvement. In a sample of 200 drug users, study subjects were more likely to perceive their children as susceptible to future alcohol and drug use when compared to nonusers. In their study of adolescent sexuality education, Brock and Beazley (1995) reported a significant correlation between perceived barriers and uninvolved parents of adolescents.

Findings from studies such as these can be operationalized through educational programs specific to high-risk populations. Janz and Becker (1984) reviewed the Health Belief Model literature over a 10-year period and found that the model was robust in predicting health behaviors, with perceived barriers being the most influential factor. In light of this review, the nurse as educator needs to take into consideration the availability of barrier-free educational resources.

## Health Promotion Model (Revised)

The *Health Promotion Model* developed in 1987 and revised by Pender (1996) has been primarily used in the discipline of nursing (Figure 6–2). This model, which describes major components and variables that factor into health-promoting behaviors, has been revised to increase the utility of its predictions and interventions. Its emphasis on actualizing health potential and increasing the level of well-being using approach behaviors rather than avoidance of disease behaviors distinguish this model as a health promotion rather than a disease prevention model.

The sequence of components and variables is clearly outlined. The three major components are as follows: individual characteristics and experiences, behavior-specific cognitions and affect, and behavioral outcome. The revised model includes three new variables: activity-related affect, commitment to a plan of action, and immediate competing demands and preferences. The major component of individual characteristics and experiences consists of two variables: prior related behavior and personal factors. The second major component, behavior-specific cognitions and affect, consists of perceived benefits of action, perceived barriers to action, perceived self-efficacy, activity-related affect, interpersonal influences, and situational influences. The behavioral outcome component consists of commitment to a plan of action, immediate competing demands and preferences, and the health-promoting behavior.

The Health Belief Model and the Health Promotion Model share several schematic similarities, seen in a comparison of Figures 6–1 and 6–2. Both models describe the use of factors or components that impact on perceptions. Sequencing of factors in each of the models, however, shows some schematic dissimilarities. While the Health Belief Model targets the likelihood of engaging in preventive health behaviors, the revised Health Promotion Model targets positive health outcomes.

In a nursing study, Johnson, Ratner, Bottorff, and Hayduk (1993) found partial support for the Health Promotion Model. In their sample of 3000 adults, they discovered that modifying factors had strong direct effects on health-promoting behaviors. As proposed by the model, the modifying factors of age, income, education, and the selected biological characteristic of body mass had indirect effects on health-promoting lifestyles.

Research support for the Health Promotion Model has been shown by Lusk, Kerr, and Ronis (1995), who found significant differences in health-promoting lifestyles in a sample of 638 workers according to job category (blue-collar, skilled trade, and white-collar). Blue-collar workers scored significantly lower on health-promoting lifestyles than did workers in the other two job categories. Significant differences in health-promoting lifestyles were

| Individual Characteristics and Experiences | Behavior-Specific Cognitions and Affect | Behavioral Outcome |

**FIGURE 6–2    Revised Health Promotion Model** Source: From N. Pender, *Health Promotion in Nursing Practice*, 3rd ed., p. 67, 1996. Reprinted by permission of Pearson Education, Inc., Upper Saddle River, NJ.

also found based on gender, exercise, and educational level, but not on marital status or ethnicity. These findings have implications for workplace educational program design.

## Self-Efficacy Theory

Developed from a social-cognitive perspective, the *Self-Efficacy Theory* is based on a per-

son's expectations relative to a specific course of action (Bandura, 1977a, 1977b, 1986). It is a predictive theory in the sense that it deals with the belief that one can accomplish a specific behavior. The belief of competency and capability relative to certain behaviors is a precursor to expected outcomes. Figure 6–3 shows an adaptation of Bandura's efficacy expecta-

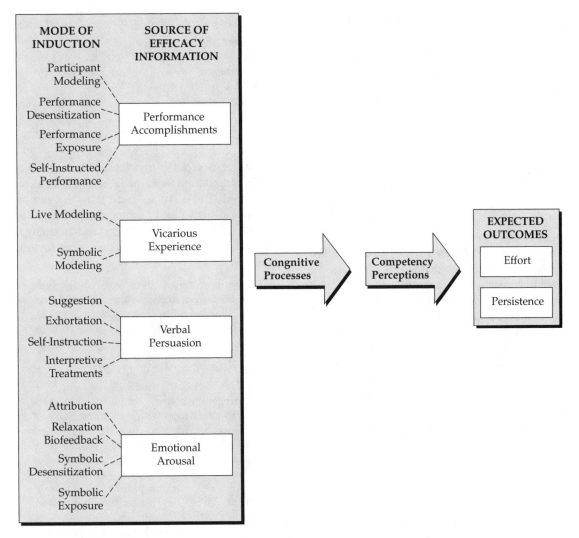

**FIGURE 6–3**    **Determinants of expected outcomes using self-efficacy perceptions** Source: From Albert Bandura, *Social Learning Theory,* © 1977, p. 80. Reprinted by permission of Prentice-Hall, Upper Saddle River, NJ.

tions model extended to include expected outcomes. In this adapted model, self-efficacy is used as an outcome determinant.

According to Bandura (1986), self-efficacy is cognitively appraised and processed through four principal sources of information:

1. Performance accomplishment evidenced in self-mastery of similarly expected behaviors

2. Vicarious experiences such as observing successful expected behavior through the modeling of others

3. Verbal persuasion by others who present realistic beliefs that the individual is capable of the expected behavior

4. Emotional arousal through self-judgment of physiological states of distress

Bandura (1986) notes that the most influential source of efficacy information is that of previous performance accomplishment. Efficacy expectations (expectations relative to a specific course of action) are induced through certain modes. Modes of induction include, but are not limited to, desensitization, self-instruction, exposure, suggestion, and relaxation.

Self-efficacy has proved useful in predicting the course of health behavior. Indeed, nursing literature has addressed linkages between self-efficacy and self-care. Moore (1990) used self-efficacy to teach self-care to older adults. Clark and Dodge (1999) examined self-efficacy as a predictor of disease management in 570 older women with cardiac disease, and found that this precept could be used to constructively manage specific behaviors. Lev (1995) used qualitative methodology to investigate the linkage between self-efficacy–enhancing interventions and self-care in a sample of 73 patients receiving chemotherapy. In this study, interventions—particularly modeling and positive reinforcement—were potentially responsible for positive patient responses.

The self-efficacy model has also been used to investigate the use of preceptors with baccalaureate nursing students. Goldenberg, Iwasiw, and MacMaster (1997) demonstrated significantly increased self-efficacy of these students following a 12-week preceptorship.

The use of the Self-Efficacy Theory for the nurse as educator is particularly relevant in developing educational programs. The behavior-specific predictions of the theory can be used for understanding the likelihood of individuals to participate in existing or projected educational programs. Educational strategies such as modeling, demonstration, and verbal reinforcement, parallel modes of self-efficacy induction.

## Stages of Change Model

Another model that informs the phenomenon of health behaviors of the learner is the *Stages*

| TABLE 6–2   Six stages of change |
| --- |
| • Precontemplation<br>• Contemplation<br>• Preparation<br>• Action<br>• Maintenance<br>• Termination |

*of Change Model* (Prochaska & Di Clemente, 1982). Originating from the field of psychology, this model (see Table 6–2) was developed around addictive and problem behaviors. Prochaska (1996) notes six distinct stages of change: precontemplation, contemplation, preparation, action, maintenance, and termination.

> In the precontemplation stage individuals have no current intention of changing. Strategies involve simple observations, confrontation, or consciousness-raising. In the contemplation stage individuals accept or realize that they have a problem and begin to think seriously about changing it. Strategies involve increased consciousness-raising. In the preparation stage individuals are planning to take action within the time frame of one month. Strategies include a firm and detailed plan for action. In the fourth stage, action, there is overt/visible modification of behavior. This is the busiest stage and strategies include commitment to the change, self-reward, countering (substitute behaviors), creating a friendly environment, and supportive relationships. Maintenance, the fifth stage, is a difficult stage to achieve and may last six months to a lifetime. There are common challenges to this stage, including overconfidence, daily temptation, and relapse self-blame. The strategies in this stage are the same for the action stage. The final stage, termination, occurs when the problem no longer presents any temptation. However, some experts note that termination does not occur, only maintenance becomes less vigilant (p. 5).

The extent to which people are motivated and ready to change is seen as an important construct. It is useful in nursing to stage the client's intentions and behaviors for change as well as strategies that will enable completion of the specific stage. More recent use of the model in nursing research has focused on its value in health promotion and the processes by which people decide to change (or not to change) behaviors. The Stages of Change Model has been used to correlate behaviors with activities such as smoking cessation (Miller, 1999), as well as to examine client decision-making processes for genetic testing (Houlihan, 1999), the latter having implications for staging advanced practice nursing counseling interventions.

## Theory of Reasoned Action

The *Theory of Reasoned Action* emerged from a research program that began in the 1950s and is concerned with prediction and understanding of any form of human behavior within a social context (Ajzen & Fishbein, 1980). It is based on the premise that humans are rational decision makers who make use of whatever information is available to them. Attitudes toward persons are not an integral part of this theory; rather, the focus is on the predicted behavior. This theory is shown as a sequential model in Figure 6–4.

In a two-pronged linear approach, specific behavior is determined by (1) beliefs, attitude toward the behavior, and intention and (2) motivation to comply with influential persons known as referents, subjective norms, and intention. The person's intention to perform can be measured by relative weights of attitude and subjective norms.

In nursing research, Jemmott and Jemmott (1991) found support for the Theory of Reasoned Action in their study on AIDS risk behavior among 103 young, unmarried, sexually active black women. They found that attitude toward condom use was the strongest predictor

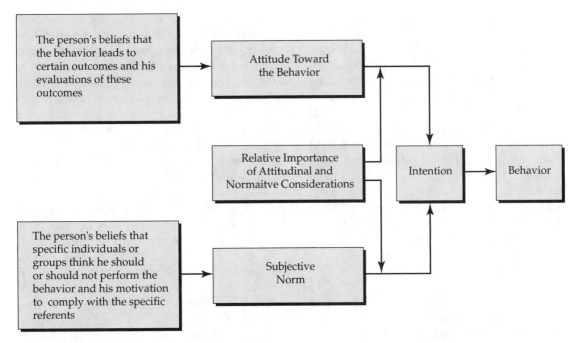

FIGURE 6–4  **Factors determining a person's behavior**  Source: From I. Ajzen and M. Fishbein, *Understanding Attitudes and Predicting Social Behavior*, © 1980, p. 8. Reprinted by permission of Prentice-Hall, Upper Saddle River, NJ.

of behavior, followed by increased support by referents for the intention to use condoms in the following three months. Knowledge of AIDS was not significantly related to attitude toward or actual use of condoms. These researchers' findings indicate that attitudes and the influence of significant others need to be taken into consideration when intervening in risky sexual behavior. Lierman and colleagues (1990) used a restrospective design to test this model while studying breast self-examination. They found significant correlations between intention and actual breast self-examination.

The Theory of Reasoned Action is useful in predicting health behaviors, particularly for educators who want to understand the attitudinal context within which behaviors are likely to change. Nurses as educators need to take beliefs, attitudinal factors, and subjective norms into consideration when designing educational programs relating to intent to change a specific health behavior.

## PRECEDE-PROCEED Model

The *PRECEDE-PROCEED Model* emerged from an epidemiological perspective on health promotion in the hopes of combating leading causes of death (Green & Kreuter, 1999). The model acronym PRECEDE stands for Predisposing, Reinforcing, and Enabling Constructs in Educational Diagnosis and Evaluation, as originally developed by Green, Kreuter, Deeds, and Partridge (1980). Green and Kreuter (1999) further refined the model to include a second component referred to as PROCEED, which means Policy, Regulatory, and Organizational Constructs in Educational and Environmental Development.

Health education, defined as "any combination of learning experiences designed to facilitate voluntary actions conducive to health" (Green & Kreuter, 1999, p. 27), is the core of the model. Green and Kreuter further emphasize that health education is aimed primarily at planning learning experiences that are designed to "predispose, enable, and reinforce voluntary behavior conducive to the health of individuals, groups, or communities" (p. 506). Referring to the centrality of health education, Green and Kreuter (1999) state that "health promotion encompasses health education . . . and is aimed at the complementary social and political actions that will facilitate the necessary organizational, economic, and other environmental supports for the conversion of individual actions into health enhancements and quality-of-life gains" (p. 19). The phases in the PRECEDE component identify priorities and objectives, while the phases in the PROCEED component address criteria for policy, implementation, and evaluation relative to a variety of diagnoses in the PRECEDE phases (Figure 6–5).

The model begins with population self-study/assessment relative to quality of life in phase 1 and ends with outcome evaluation in phase 9. Education—a key and pivotal dimension—is specifically addressed in phases 4 and 5. It is noteworthy that the educational diagnosis phase of this robust model (comprised of predisposing, reinforcing, and enabling factors) synthesizes the Health Belief Model, Self-Efficacy Theory, and Theory of Reasoned Action. The authors note that health behaviors are most heavily influenced by the predisposing factors of knowledge, beliefs, values, attitudes, and confidence.

In several instances, the PRECEDE-PROCEED model has been used in population-based studies. Macrina, Macrina, Horvath, Gallaspy, and Fine (1996) studied hospital-based nurse managers and their nursing staff. They found that formal emergency room policy and formal data collection procedures would enhance educational effectiveness in emergency rooms. In a study of the needs of stroke survivors and their families as perceived by themselves and health professionals, van Veenendaal, Grinspun, and Adriaanse (1996) used the model to identify informational needs. Results included the

PRECEDE

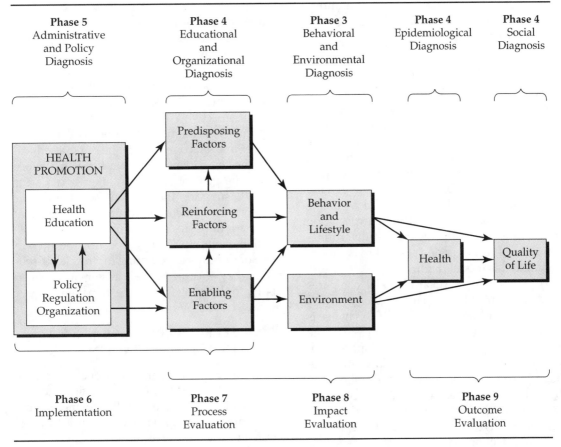

FIGURE 6–5   **The PRECEDE-PROCEED Model for health promotion planning and evaluation** Source: From *Health Promotion Planning: An Educational and Ecological Approach*, 3rd ed., by Lawrence W. Green and Marshall W. Kreuter. Copyright © 1999 by Mayfield Publishing Company. Reprinted by permission of the publisher.

need to address level of education in terms of amount of information given, gaps in information, and sources of information.

Mullen, Hersey, and Iverson (1987) compared the Health Belief Model, Theory of Reasoned Action, and the original PRECEDE Model for usefulness in predicting changes in health behavior in a random sample of 661 adults from ethnically diverse backgrounds. They found that all three models had similar predictive power. The strength of the PRECEDE-PROCEED model, however, lies in its inclusion of interventions from a population needs perspective.

Nurses as educators can use this model when considering implications for social policy change. It has particular relevance for community health nurses, because the model notes that community is "the center of gravity." The design and development of health education programs for specific populations and the use of the perspective of community as client are within the scope of nursing practice and education.

## Therapeutic Alliance Model

Barofsky's (1978) *Therapeutic Alliance Model* addresses a shift in power from the provider to a learning partnership in which collaboration and negotiation with the consumer are key. A therapeutic alliance is formed between the caregiver and receiver in which each participant in this affiliation is viewed as having equal power. The client is viewed as active and responsible, with an outcome expectation of self-care. The shift toward self-determination and control over one's own life is fundamental to this model (Figure 6–6).

The Therapeutic Alliance Model compares the components of compliance, adherence, and alliance. According to Barofsky (1978), change is needed in treatment determinants—change from coercion in compliance, and from conforming in adherence to collaboration in alliance. The power in the relationship between the participants is equalized by alliance. The role of the patient is neither passive nor rebellious, but rather active and responsible. The expected outcomes are not compliant dependence or counterdependence, but responsible self-care.

| COMPLIANCE | ADHERENCE | THERAPEUTIC ALLIANCE |
|---|---|---|
| Dependency | Conforming | Self-Care |

Key: ● Patient Power
○ Provider Power

**FIGURE 6–6   Continuum of the Therapeutic Alliance Model**

Although not originally developed as an educational model, and not well-known in nursing, the usefulness of this model to the nurse as educator is nevertheless acknowledged in the partnership of learning. This interpersonal model is appropriate in the educational process when shifting the focus from the patient as a passive-dependent learner to one of an active learner. It serves as a guide to refocus education efforts on collaboration rather than on compliance. The nurse as educator and the patient as learner form an alliance with the goal of self-care. Luker and Caress (1989) support the notion of therapeutic alliance in patient education, arguing that "nurses have resisted equalizing their role with patients" (p. 715). Advocating the alternative of self-directed learning for the aim of self-care, they encourage the transfer of responsibility for learning from nurse to patient.

## ■ SELECTION OF MODELS FOR HEALTH EDUCATION

Selection of models for educational use can be made with respect to (1) similarities and dissimilarities, (2) nurse as educator agreement with model conceptualizations, and (3) functional utility.

### Similarities and Dissimilarities of Models

Models may be seen as so similar that there would be a negligible difference in choosing one over the other, or they may be seen as so dissimilar that one would be inappropriate for a specific educational purpose. A comparative analysis of the different frameworks reveals that the Health Belief Model and the Health Promotion Model are similar. Each uses comparable salient factors of individual perceptions and competing variables. The differences appear in the models' basic premises and outcomes. The Health Belief Model emphasizes susceptibility to disease and the likelihood of preventive action, whereas the Health Promotion Model emphasizes health potential and health-promoting behaviors.

The Self-Efficacy Theory and the Theory of Reasoned Action are similar in that both focus on the predictions or expectations of specific behaviors. The theories lend themselves more easily to less complex model testing than either the Health Belief Model or Health Promotion Model because the former are more linear in conceptualization. Specificity of behaviors may aid in targeting outcomes of educational programs. The Stages of Change Model is similar to the Self-Efficacy Theory and the Theory of Reasoned Action in the sense that all of these models focus on intent. However, the Stages of Change Model is more simplistic and does not take into account personal characteristics or experiences. It differs from the Self-Efficacy Theory and the Theory of Reasoned Action in that stages and strategies for change in the specific stage are key to interventions.

The Health Belief Model, Health Promotion Model, Self-Efficacy Theory, and Theory of Reasoned Action are similar in that they acknowledge factors such as experiences, perceptions, or beliefs relative to the individual and factors external to the individual that can modify health behaviors. These frameworks also recognize the multidimensional nature, complexity, and probability of health behaviors. The PRECEDE-PROCEED model broadens this perspective to include aggregates and populations.

All of the models acknowledge the importance of the patient in decision making with respect to health behaviors. The differences relate to patient focus, the relative importance of modifying factors, specificity of behavior, and outcomes.

The most dissimilar model is the Therapeutic Alliance Model. Although it is relatively narrow in scope, its simplicity and parsimony are strengths. When applied to the educational arena, the educator–learner relationship is the critical factor. Addressing potentially frustrating patient education situations such as noncompliance, Hochbaum (1980) noted that patient educators, when frustrated, "are unable to understand the apparently irrational and self-destructive action of their patients, and sometimes throw their hands up in despair, bedeviled by the seeming irrationality of the patient's behavior . . . But this behavior may be altogether rational from the patient's perspective" (p. 7). Understanding of the client as learner can be uncovered in the Therapeutic Alliance Model.

## Educator Agreement with Model Conceptualizations

Nurses as educators have belief systems, which may or may not agree with some of the tenets of each of the models presented. Choice of a model, therefore, can be based on the educator's level of agreement with salient factors in each framework.

Likelihood of action is best addressed by the Health Belief Model, while attaining positive health outcomes is the focus of the Health Promotion Model. Attitude and intention are best viewed through the Theory of Reasoned Action. Belief in one's capabilities is best addressed by the Self-Efficacy Theory, and reduction of noncompliance through an educator–learner collaboration by use of the Therapeutic Alliance Model. Staging the individual's readiness for change and developing strategies for interventions are helpful in designing educational programs with the Stages of Change Model. The PRECEDE-PROCEED Model best fits with the beliefs that health education and health promotion are inseparable and that consent for voluntary change of people is necessary before attempting to change social systems.

In scrutinizing each of the models, the attention of the educator may be drawn to other factors as well. Ultimately, the model or models that fit best with the educator's own beliefs are more likely to be chosen.

## Functional Utility of Models

Model selection for educational purposes can also be based on functional utility. Questions to be asked to determine functional utility are as follows:

- Who is the target learner?
- What is the focus of the learning?
- When is the optimal time?
- Where is the process to be carried out?

The question of *who* the learner is deals with whether the target learner is the individual, family, group, or community. The Health Belief Model, Health Promotion Model, Self-Efficacy Theory, Stages of Change Model, and Theory of Reasoned Action are more likely to be used with individuals, families, and groups, with the focus being placed on the individual. It is difficult to talk about collective self-perceptions, collective self-confidence, and collective intention to perform. The models present each of these factors in the context of the individual. The important notion for the nurse as educator to remember is the probability of individual variation. Another consideration in terms of the target learner is categorical groups, such as those considered at high risk and those diagnosed with acute or chronic illnesses.

The functional use of the models can also be determined by the content needed, the timing of the educational experience, and the setting in which the learning is to take place. *What* is needed relates to the focus of the learning and addresses the content to be taught, such as disease processes, specific disease, promotion of wellness, expectations of specific health practices, or focus on self-care. The PRECEDE-PROCEED model is best used as a diagnostic framework for health education programs and health planning (Mullen et al., 1987).

The question of *when* is one of optimal timing and refers to the readiness of the learner, a mutually convenient time, and prevention of untimely delays in moving toward a desired goal. Although considered important in the context of health education, this critical factor has received little specific reference in terms of health promotion models. Except for the Stages of Change Model, timing is an often neglected factor in the models discussed. It is apparent that determining optimal time can be a motivational incentive in terms of meeting health needs of the learner.

Addressing the question of *where* the educational process is to be carried out is another aspect of functional utility. The settings of home, workplace, school, institution, or specific community locations are all options. All of the models discussed in this chapter lend themselves to these diverse settings. The one that is most specific to community locations is the PRECEDE-PROCEED model, which deals with community-based populations (see Chapter 14 on instructional settings).

## ▓ INTEGRATION OF MODELS FOR USE IN EDUCATION

From the previous discussion, it is clear that the integration of various components of health promotion models is advantageous. When salient factors are taken into consideration in light of developmental stages of the learner, an integrated motivational model of learning in health promotion could emerge. Padilla and Bulcavage (1991) advocate a multi-theory approach to promote health behaviors of the learner and note that theories can provide blueprints for interventions. In a more recent approach, Poss (2001) developed a new model synthesizing the Health Belief Model and the Theory of Reasoned Action, noting that a synthesized model is appropriate for the study of persons from varying cultural backgrounds. The development of new models and/or the revision of older models is a necessary step in the evolution of and delivery of health care, and it necessarily affects the educator concerned with motivational behaviors of the learner.

Salient health promotion factors that can be used in a multi-theory approach to health education include, but are not limited to, level of knowledge, attitudes, values, beliefs, perceptions, level of anxiety, self-confidence, skills mastery, past experiences, intention, physiological capacity, sociocultural enablers, environment, educator–learner alliance, resources and reinforcements, mutual and realistic goal setting, hierarchy of needs, quality of life, and voluntary participation in learning.

Developmental stages of the learner incorporate principles of pedagogy (teaching children), andragogy (teaching adults), and gerogogy (teaching the aged) to meet the needs of the learner. A more comprehensive and holistic model for the nurse as educator emerges when learning is viewed along a unidirectional developmental continuum, in combination with salient health promotion factors. (For a discussion on educational approaches with learners at different stages of development, see Chapter 5.)

An example of a multi-theory approach is described by Bille (1980), who considered motivation, readiness to learn, selected concepts from theories of learning, and principles of gerogogy in the development of an educational plan for the older adult. Another multi-theory approach to health instruction is proposed by Wooley (1995), wherein behavior mapping is used as a tool for identifying priorities for health education. This approach incorporates the Health Belief Model, Social Learning Theory, PRECEDE-PROCEED Model, Stages of Change Model, and Theory of Reasoned Action.

## ▄▄▄ THE SUBROLES OF NURSE AS EDUCATOR IN HEALTH PROMOTION

Nurses as educators are in a position to promote healthy lifestyles. Combining content specific to the discipline of nursing, knowledge from educational theories, and health behavior models allows for an integrated approach to shaping health behaviors of the learner. Subroles of the nurse as educator include facilitator of change, contractor, organizer, and evaluator.

### Facilitator of Change

The goal of the nurse as educator is, of course, to promote health. Health education and health promotion are integral to this effort. At the same time, the nurse as educator is an important facilitator of change. When learning is viewed as an intervention, it needs to be considered in the context of other nursing interventions that will effect change. DeTornay and Thompson (1987) proposed that explaining, analyzing, dividing complex skills, demonstrating, practicing, asking questions, and providing closure are effective in facilitating change in the learning situation.

### Contractor

Contracting has been a popular means of facilitating learning. Informal or formal contracts can delineate and promote learning objectives. Similar to the nursing process, *educational contracting* involves stating mutual goals to be accomplished, devising an agreed-upon plan of action, evaluating the plan, and deriving alternatives. (See the discussion of learning contracts in Chapter 10.) The plan of action needs to be as specific as possible and include the *who, what, when, where,* and *how* of the learning process. Responsibilities that are clearly stated aid in evaluating the plan and directing plan revisions.

In light of our changing healthcare system, there needs to be an emphasis on patient–nurse partnerships, because patients are expected to take increasingly more responsibility and control in the decisions that affect their own health. Educational contracting is the key to informed decision making.

When education is viewed in the context of the client, rather than the client in the context of education, learning is individualized. The "fit" between the client as learner and the nurse as educator has the capacity to facilitate learning. Indeed, the "goodness of fit" between these two educational participants can be a motivating factor. Do the client and educator share an understanding of backgrounds or language? Is there a mutual understanding of goal setting? Are health beliefs respected?

A contract involves a trusting relationship. In a mutually satisfying teacher–learner relationship system, trust is a key ingredient. The learner trusts that the nurse as educator possesses a respectable, current body of theoretically-based and clinically-applicable knowledge. The nurse needs to be approachable, trustworthy, and culturally sensitive, because the learner's own health status is often valued as a private matter. In turn, the nurse trusts that when the client enters into an agreement, the learner will demonstrate behaviors that will be health-promoting. Newman and Brown (1986) list the following elements as part of the ideal relationship: both parties have trust and respect; the teacher assumes the student can learn and is sensitive to individual needs; and both feel free to learn and make mistakes.

## Organizer

Organization of the learning situation, including manipulation of materials and space, sequential organization of content from simple to complex, and determining priority of subject matter, is a task taken on by the nurse as educator. Organization of learning material decreases obstacles to learning (Haggard, 1989). Attendance at educational programs or individual sessions can be organized around the target learner as well as significant others to facilitate the learning process and promote motivation to learn.

## Evaluator

Educational programs, like other healthcare projects, need to be accountable to the learner or consumer of the health service. This accountability is ensured by evaluation in the form of outcomes. Of course, self-evaluation, patient evaluation, organization evaluation, and peer evaluation are not new concepts. Evaluative processes are an integral part of all learning.

The nurse as educator is a role that has been challenged. Luker and Caress (1989) make the distinction between patient education and patient teaching, noting that the former is in the province of the clinical specialist. They also note that not all nurses are prepared to be patient educators. The specialist approach to education needs to be investigated in terms of health outcomes as well as impact on professional role.

In the final analysis, application of knowledge that improves the health of individuals, families, groups, or communities is the evaluative measure of learning.

## SUMMARY

Critical components of this chapter have included a discussion of concepts of motivation and compliance, assessment of level of learner motivation, identification of incentives and obstacles that affect motivation and compliance, and discussion of axioms of motivation relevant to learning. In addition, selected health behavior frameworks and their influence on learning have been compared and contrasted, specific strategies that facilitate motivation and compliance have been outlined, and the recognition of the unique role of the nurse as educator in influencing learner motivation and compliance has been addressed.

When information is imparted, accepted, and applied, the foundation is set for change in health behaviors. When people are motivated and know that they can make a difference in their own lives, then a barrier to health has been lifted.

## REVIEW QUESTIONS

1. How are the terms *motivation, compliance,* and *adherence* defined?
2. How do the terms defined in Question 1 relate to one another?
3. What are the three (3) major motivational factors?
4. Which axioms (premises) are involved in promoting motivation of the learner?
5. What are the six (6) parameters for a comprehensive motivational assessment of the learner?
6. What are the six (6) major models or theories used to describe, explain, or predict health behaviors?
7. Which models/theories are used to facilitate motivation and which ones are used to promote compliance to a therapeutic healthcare regimen?
8. What are the basic concepts particular to each model or theory?
9. What are the similarities and differences between the models with respect to who is the target audience, what is the focus of the learning, and where is the education process to be carried out?
10. What are the subroles of the nurse in shaping health behaviors of the learner?

## REFERENCES

Ajzen, I. & Fishbein, M. (1980). *Understanding Attitudes and Predicting Social Behavior.* Englewood Cliffs, NJ: Prentice-Hall.

Atkinson, J. W. (1964). *An Introduction to Motivation.* Princeton, NJ: Van Nostrand.

Bandura, A. (1977a). Self-efficacy: Toward a unifying theory of behavioral change. *Psychological Review, 84*(2), 191–215.

Bandura, A. (1977b). *Social Learning Theory.* Englewood Cliffs, NJ: Prentice-Hall.

Bandura, A. (1986). *Social Foundations of Thought and Action: A Social Cognitive Theory.* Englewood Cliffs, NJ: Prentice-Hall.

Barofsky, I. (1978). Compliance, adherence and the therapeutic alliance: Steps in the development of self-care. *Social Science and Medicine, 12,* 369–376.

Becker, M. (ed.). (1974). *The Health Belief Model and Personal Health Behavior.* Thorofare, NJ: Slack.

Becker, M. (1990). Theoretical models of adherence and strategies for improving adherence. In S. A. Shumaker, E. B. Schron, & J. K. Ockene (eds.), *The Handbook of Human Health Behavior* (pp. 5–43). New York: Springer.

Becker, M. W., Drachman, R. H., & Kirscht, J. P. (1974). A new approach to explaining sick-role behavior in low-income populations. *American Journal of Public Health, 64*(3), 205–216.

Becker, M. H. & Green, L. W. (1975). A family approach to compliance with medical treatment: A selective review of the literature. *International Journal of Health Education, 18,* 173–182.

Bille, D.A. (1980). Educational strategies for teaching the elderly patient. *Nursing and Health Care, 1,* 256–263.

Brock, G. C. & Beazley, R. P. (1995). Using the health belief model to explain parents' participation on adolescents' at-home sexuality education activities. *Journal of School Health, 65*(4), 124–128.

Clark, N. M. & Dodge, J. A. (1999). Exploring self-efficacy as a predictor of disease management. *Health Education and Behavior, 26*(1), 72–89.

Damrosch, S. (1991). General strategies for motivating people to change their behavior. *Nursing Clinics of North America, 26*(4), 833–843.

deTornay, R. & Thompson, M.A. (1987). *Strategies for Teaching Nursing,* 3rd ed. New York: Wiley.

Eraker, S. A., Kirscht, J. P., & Becker, M. H. (1984). Understanding and improving patient compliance. *Annals of Internal Medicine, 100,* 258-268.

Fink, D. L. (1976). Tailoring in the consensual regimen. In D. L. Sackett & R. B. Haynes (eds.), *Compliance with Therapeutic Regimens.* Baltimore: Johns Hopkins University Press.

Fisher, R. C. (1992). Patient education and compliance: A pharmacist's perspective. *Patient Education and Counseling, 19,* 261–271.

Goldenberg, D., Iwasiw, C., & MacMaster, E. (1997). Self-efficacy of senior baccalaureate nursing students and preceptors. *Nurse Education Today, 17*(4), 303–310.

Green, L. W. & Kreuter, M. W. (1999). *Health Promotion Planning: An Educational and Ecological Approach,* 3rd ed. Mountain View, CA: Mayfield.

Green, L. W., Kreuter, M. W., Deeds, S. G., & Partridge, K. B. (1980). *Health Education Planning: A Diagnostic Approach.* Palo Alto, CA: Mayfield.

Haggard, A. (1989). *Handbook of Patient Education.* Rockville, MD: Aspen.

Hahn, E. J. (1993). Parental alcohol and other drug use (AOD) and health beliefs about parent involvement in AOD prevention. *Issues in Mental Health Nursing, 14,* 237–247.

Hochbaum, G. M. (1980). *Patient counseling vs. patient teaching. Education for self-care.* Rockville, MD: Aspen.

Houlihan, G. D. (1999). The evaluation of the "stages of change" model for use in counseling clients undergoing predictive testing for Huntington's disease. *Journal of Advanced Nursing 29*(5), 1137–1143.

Hussey, L. C. & Guilliland, K. (1989). Compliance, low literacy, and locus of control. *Nursing Clinics of North America, 24*(3), 605–610.

Janz, N. K. & Becker, M. H. (1984). The health belief model: A decade later. *Health Education Quarterly, 11*(1), 1–47.

Jemmott, L. S. & Jemmott, J. B. III. (1991). Applying the theory of reasoned action to AIDS risk behavior: Condom use among black women. *Nursing Research, 40*(4), 229–234.

Johnson, J. L., Ratner, P. A., Bottorff, J. L., & Hayduk, L. A. (1993). An exploration of Pender's health promotion model using LISREL. *Nursing Research, 42*(3), 132–138.

Keller, J. M. (1987). Development and use of the ARCS model of instructional design. *Journal of Instructional Development, 10*(3), 2–10.

Kort, M. (1987). Motivation: The challenge for today's health promoter. *Canadian Nurse, 83*(9), 16–18.

Langlie, J. K. (1977). Social networks, health beliefs, and preventive health behavior. *Journal of Health and Social Behavior, 18,* 244–260.

Leddy, S. K. & Pepper, J. M. (1998). *Conceptual Bases of Professional Nursing.* Philadelphia: Lippincott.

Lev, E. (1995). Use of triangulation reveals theoretical linkages and outcomes in a nursing intervention study. *Clinical Nurse Specialist, 9*(6), 300–305.

Levanthal, H. C. & Cameron, L. (1987). Behavior theories and the problem of compliance. *Patient Education Counseling, 10,* 117–138.

Levanthal, H. C. & Diefenbach, M. (1991). The active side of illness cognition. In J. A. Skelton & R. T. Croyle (eds.), *Mental Representation in Health and Illness.* New York: Springer-Verlag, 245–271.

Lewin, K. (1935). *A Dynamic Theory of Personality.* New York: McGraw-Hill.

Lierman, L. M., Young, H. M., Kasprzyk, D., & Benoliel, J. Q. (1990). Predicting breast self examination using the theory of reasoned action. *Nursing Research, 39,* 97–101.

Luker, K. & Caress, A. L. (1989). Rethinking patient education. *Journal of Advanced Nursing, 14,* 711–718.

Lusk, S. L., Kerr, M. J., & Ronis, D. L. (1995). Health promoting lifestyles of blue-collar, skilled trade, and white-collar workers. *Nursing Research, 44*(1), 20–24.

Macrina, D., Macrina, N., Horvath, C., Gallaspy, J., & Fine, P. R. (1996). An educational intervention to increase use of Glasgow Coma Scale by emergency department personnel. *International Journal of Trauma Nursing, 2*(1), 7–12.

Maslow, A. H. (1943). A theory of human motivation. *Psychological Review, 50*(4), 371–396.

Miller, J. (1999). Stages of change theory and the nicotine-dependent client: Direction for decision making in nursing practice. *Clinical Nurse Specialist, 13*(1), 18–22.

Mishel, M. H. (1990). Reconceptualization of the uncertainty in illness theory. *Image: Journal of Nursing Scholarship, 22*(4), 256–262.

Moore, E. J. (1990). Using self-efficacy in teaching self-care to the elderly. *Holistic Nursing Practice, 4*(2), 22–29.

Mullen, P. D., Hersey, J. C., & Iverson, D. C. (1987). Health behavior models compared. *Social Science Medicine, 11,* 973–981.

Newman, F. & Brown, R. (1986). Creating optimal conditions for learning. *Educational Horizons, 64*(4), 188–189.

Oberle, K. (1991). A decade of research in locus of control: What have we learned? *Journal of Advanced Nursing, 16,* 800–806.

Padilla, G. V. & Bulcavage, L. M. (1991). Theories used in patient/health education. *Seminars in Oncology Nursing, 7*(2), 87–96.

Pender, N. (1987). *Health Promotion in Nursing Practice,* 2nd ed. Norwalk, CT: Appleton-Lange.

Pender, N. (1996). *Health Promotion in Nursing Practice,* 3rd ed. Upper Saddle River, NJ: Pearson Education.

Peplau, H. E. (1979). *The Psychotherapy of Hildegard E. Peplau.* Texas: Atwood.

Poss, J. E. (2001). Developing a new model for cross-cultural research: Synthesizing the health belief model and the theory of reasoned action. *Advances in Nursing Science, 23*(4), 1–15.

Prochaska, J. O. (1996). Just do it isn't enough: Change comes in stages. *Tufts University Special Report Diet and Nutrition Letter*. September.

Prochaska, J. O. & Di Clemente, C. C., (1982). Transtheoretical therapy: Towards a more integrative model of change. *Psychotherapy, Theory, and Practice, 19*(3), 276–288.

Redeker, N. (1988). Health beliefs and adherence in chronic illness. *Image: Journal of Nursing Scholarship, 20*(1), 31–35.

Redman, B. K. (2001). *The Practice of Patient Education*, 9th ed. St. Louis: Mosby.

Rosenstock, I. M. (1974). Historical origins of the health belief model. In M. H. Becker (ed.), *The Health Belief Model and Personal Health Behavior*. Thorofare, NJ: Slack.

Ross, M. W. & Rosser, B. R. (1989). Education and AIDS risks: A review. *Health Education Research, 4*(3), 273–284.

Rotter, J. B. (1954). *Social Learning Theory and Clinical Psychology*. Englewood Cliffs, NJ: Prentice-Hall.

Sackett, D. L. & Haynes, R. B. (1976). *Compliance with Therapeutic Regimens*. Baltimore: Johns Hopkins University Press.

Sands, D. S. & Holman, E. H. (1985). Does knowledge enhance patient compliance? *Journal of Gerontological Nursing, 11*(4), 23–29.

Shillinger, F. (1983). Locus of control: Implications for nursing practice. *Image: Journal of Nursing Scholarship, 15*(2), 58–63.

Steckel, S. B. (1982). Predicting, measuring, implementing and following up on patient compliance. *Nursing Clinics of North America, 17*(3), 491–497.

van Veenendaal, H., Grinspun, D. R., & Adriaanse, H. P. (1996). Educational needs of stroke survivors and their family members, as perceived by themselves and by health professionals. *Patient Education and Counseling, 28*(3), 265–276.

Wallston, K. A., Wallston, B. S., & DeVellis, R. (1978). Development of the multidimensional health locus of control (MHLC) scales. *Health Education Monographs*, Spring, 160–170.

Ward-Collins, D. (1998). Noncompliant: Isn't there a better way to say it? *American Journal of Nursing, 98*(5), 17–31.

Wooley, S. F. (1995). Behavior mapping: A tool for identifying priorities for health education curricula and instruction. *Journal of Health Education, 26*(4), 200–206.

Wright, L. M., Watson, W. L., & Bell, J. M. (1996). *Beliefs: The Heart of Healing in Families and Illness*. New York: Basic Books.

## CHAPTER 7

# Literacy in the Adult Patient Population

*Susan B. Bastable*

## CHAPTER HIGHLIGHTS

## KEY TERMS

## OBJECTIVES

After completing this chapter, the reader will be able to

1. Define the terms *literacy, illiteracy, health literacy, low literacy, functional illiteracy, reading, readability, comprehension,* and *numeracy.*

2. Identify the magnitude of the literacy problem in the United States.

3. Differentiate the characteristics of those individuals at risk for having difficulty with reading and comprehension of written and oral language.

4. Discuss common myths and assumptions about the illiterate person.

5. Identify clues that are indicators of reading and writing deficiencies.

6. Assess the impact of illiteracy and low literacy on patient motivation and compliance with healthcare regimens.

7. Recognize the role of the nurse as educator in the assessment of patients' literacy skills.

8. Critically analyze readability and comprehension levels of printed materials using specific formulas and tests.

9. Describe specific guidelines for writing effective education materials.

10. Outline various teaching strategies useful in educating clients with low literacy skills.

11. Recognize the research and policy-making issues that must be addressed to solve the health literacy problem.

Over the past two decades, literacy of the U.S. population has been the subject of increasing interest and concern by educators as well as by government officials, employers, and media experts. Adult illiteracy continues to be a major problem in this country despite public and private efforts at all levels to address the issue through testing of literacy skills and development of literacy training programs. Today, the fact remains that many individuals do not possess the basic literacy abilities to function effectively in our technologically complex society. Many adult citizens have difficulty reading and comprehending information well enough to be able to perform such common tasks as filling out job and insurance applications, interpreting bus schedules and road signs, completing tax forms, or registering to vote.

Ever since the early 1980s, when President Reagan launched the National Adult Literacy Initiative, followed by the United Nations' declaration of 1990 as the International Literacy Year (Belton, 1991; Wallerstein, 1992), illiteracy has become a common topic in the public media nationwide and worldwide. In 1992, the National Adult Literacy Survey (NALS)

conducted by the U.S. Department of Education revealed a shockingly high prevalence of illiteracy in this country (Kirsch et al., 1993). Since then, awareness about illiteracy, thought to be mainly a problem confined to developing countries, has taken on new meaning (Lasater & Mehler, 1998).

Particularly in the past 10 years as a result of the NALS report, nursing and medical literature has focused significant attention on the effects of patient illiteracy on healthcare delivery and health outcomes. Today, the emphasis is on health literacy—that is, the extent to which Americans can read well enough to function successfully in healthcare settings. Although a great deal more research needs to be done on the causes and effects associated with poor health literacy as well as the methods available to screen and teach patients, much has been learned about the magnitude and consequences of the health literacy problem (Ad Hoc Committee, 1999; Fetter, 1999).

With respect to the subject of literacy, the nurse educator's attention specifically focuses on adult patient populations. Rarely do literacy levels become an issue in teaching staff nurses or nursing students because of their level of formal education. It is becoming a concern, however, if the audience for in-service programs includes less educated, more culturally and socioeconomically diverse housekeeping and maintenance staff (Hess, 1998) or if a member of the audience has been diagnosed with a learning disorder such as dyslexia. What must be of particular concern to the healthcare industry are the numbers of consumers who are illiterate, functionally illiterate, or marginally literate. Researchers have discovered that people with poor reading and comprehension skills have disproportionately higher medical costs and more perceived physical and psychosocial problems than do literate persons (Jenks, 1992).

In today's world of managed care, the literacy problem is perceived to have grave consequences. Patients are expected to assume greater responsibility for self-care and health promotion, yet this expanded role depends on increased knowledge and skills. If patients with low literacy abilities cannot fully benefit from the type and amount of information they are typically given, then they cannot be expected to maintain health and manage independently. The result is a significant negative impact on the cost of health care and the quality of life (Brez & Taylor, 1997; Brownson, 1998; Fisher, 1999).

Traditionally, healthcare professionals have relied heavily on printed education materials as a cost-effective and time-efficient means to communicate health messages. For years, nurses and physicians have assumed that the written materials commonly distributed to patients were sufficient to ensure informed consent for tests and procedures, to promote compliance with treatment regimens, and to guarantee adherence to discharge instructions. Only recently have healthcare providers begun to recognize that the scientific and technical terminology inherent in the ubiquitous printed teaching aids is a bewildering set of written instructions little understood by the majority of patients. Unless education materials are written at a level appropriate for their intended audiences, patients cannot be expected to be able or willing to accept responsibility for self-care.

An essential prerequisite to implementing patient education programs is knowing a person's literacy skills. Yet calls for assessment of literacy and recommendations for appropriate interventions for patients with poor literacy skills have largely been ignored. Even though illiteracy and low literacy are quite prevalent in the U.S. population, problems with literacy frequently continue to go undiagnosed (Doak et al., 1996).

This chapter examines the magnitude of the illiteracy problem, the factors that influence readability and comprehension of written health educational materials, the important role nurses play in assessing patients' literacy skills, and the effects of illiteracy on the health and well-being of the public. In addition, the formulas and tests used to evaluate reading skills, readability, and comprehension of printed tools are reviewed, specific guidelines are put forth for writing effective health education materials, and teaching strategies are recommended as a means for breaking down the barriers of illiteracy.

## ▬▬ DEFINITION OF TERMS

*Literacy* is an umbrella term used to describe socially required and expected reading and writing abilities. There is no clear agreement about what it means to be literate in U.S. society. The word *literate* is defined in *Webster's Collegiate Dictionary* (1999) as "an educated person," one who is "able to read and write" (p. 680). More specifically, literacy has been thought of as the relative ability to use printed and written material commonly encountered in daily living. In 1993, the U.S. Department of Education (USDOE) defined literacy as "the ability to use print and written information to function in society, to achieve one's goals, and to develop one's knowledge and potential"(p. 6).

Others have defined literacy based on the number of grade levels of school completed or the equivalent on achievement tests. Many researchers have found, however, that the reported number of years of schooling attended is an inadequate predictor of a person's reading and writing skills (Doak et al., 1996; Jackson et al.,1991; Davis et al., 1990; Winslow, 2001; French & Larrabee, 1999; Kelly, 1999). Many studies have been flawed by the inconsistent and erroneous definitions of literacy, including equating literacy with academic achievement and years of schooling (Adams-Price, 1993). Over time, performance on reading tests has become the conventional method used to measure grade-level achievement. The commonly accepted definition of literacy is the ability to read, understand, and interpret information written at the eighth-grade level or above. On the other end of the spectrum, *illiteracy* is the total inability to read or write, which until now has been relatively rare in our society and which affects less than 5% of all adults in the U.S. population (Doak et al., 1996).

Literacy can be categorized into three general kinds of tasks (Adams-Price, 1993; Fisher, 1999):

- Prose tasks, which measure reading comprehension and the ability to extract themes from newspapers, magazines, poems, and books
- Document tasks, which assess the ability of readers to interpret documents such as insurance reports, consent forms, and transportation schedules
- Quantitative tasks, which assess the ability to work with numerical information embedded in written material such as computing restaurant menu bills, figuring out taxes, interpreting paycheck stubs, or calculating calories on a nutrition checklist.

*Health literacy* refers to how well an individual can read, interpret, and comprehend health information for maintaining an optimal level of wellness. The Ad Hoc Committee on Health Literacy for the Council on Scientific Affairs of the American Medical Association (1999) defined health literacy as "a constellation of skills, including the ability to perform basic reading and numerical tasks required to function in the health care environment" (p. 553). Its 12-member panel, composed of experts in the fields of medicine, nursing, health research, psychology, adult literacy, and health education, identified the scope and consequences of poor health literacy in the United States. They concluded that an individual's functional health literacy is likely to be significantly worse than his or her general literacy skills.

As managed care requires individuals to take more responsibility for self-care and symptom management, health literacy is becoming an important determinant of health status. Poor health literacy may lead to serious negative consequences, such as increased morbidity and mortality, when a person is unable to read and comprehend instructions for medications, follow-up appointments, diet, procedures, and other regimens. Patients cannot be expected to be autonomous and self-directed in navigating the healthcare system if they do not have the ability to follow basic instructions (Fetter, 1999). Health knowledge, health status, and the use of health services are all related to literacy levels.

*Low literacy*, also termed *marginally literate* or *marginally illiterate*, refers to the ability of adults to read, write, and comprehend information between the fifth- and eighth-grade level of difficulty. Low-literate persons have trouble using commonly printed and written information to meet their everyday needs such as reading a TV schedule, taking a telephone message, or filling out a relatively simple application form (Doak et al., 1996).

*Functional illiteracy* means that adults have reading, writing, and comprehension skills below the fifth-grade level; that is, they lack the fundamental education skills needed to function effectively in today's society. Functionally illiterate persons have very limited competency with communication via the written or spoken word; in many cases, they do not understand basic written instructions, audiovisual aids, or even tape recordings. Such individuals are unable to read well enough to understand and interpret what they have read or use the information as it was intended (Doak et al., 1996). For example, functionally illiterate persons may be able to read the words on a label of a can of soup that directs "Pour soup into pan. Add one can water. Heat until hot." However, they cannot comprehend the meaning and sequence of the words to carry through with these directions.

These operational definitions are, at best, approximations. Conventional grade-level definitions of literacy are considered conservative because even an adult with the ability to read at the eighth-grade level will encounter difficulties in functioning in our advanced society. However, although an individual may have poor reading skills, this does not necessarily imply a lack of intelligence. Low literacy or illiteracy cannot be equated with IQ level (Hussey & Guilliland, 1989). A person can be illiterate or low literate, yet intellectually be within at least normal IQ range (Doak et al., 1996).

*Reading, readability,* and *comprehension* are also terms frequently used when determining levels of literacy. Fisher (1999) defines *reading* or *word recognition* as "the process of transforming letters into words and being able to pronounce them correctly" (p. 57). Word recognition scores can be misleading because they are usually three grade levels higher than comprehension scores (Fisher, 1999). Hirsch (2001) addressed the public's confusion between "reading" in the sense of being able to decode words fluently

and "reading" in the sense of being able to comprehend the meaning of words.

*Readability* is defined as the ease with which written or printed information can be read based on a measure of a number of different elements within a given text of printed material that influence with what degree of success a group of readers will be able to read the style of writing of a selected printed passage.

*Comprehension*, on the other hand, is the degree to which individuals understand what they have read (Fisher, 1999). It is the ability to grasp the meaning of a message—to get the gist of it. A healthcare professional can determine whether comprehension of health instruction has occurred by noting whether patients are able to correctly demonstrate or recall in their own words the message that was received. If the elements of logic, language, and experience in health instruction are compatible with and culturally appropriate to the patient's elements, the message will be clear, relevant, and achievable (Barnes, 1992a, 1992b; Doak et al., 1996). A mismatch will likely make the message confusing, incomprehensible, and useless to the patient. Comprehension is affected by the amount, clarity, and complexity of the information presented. The ability to read does not alone guarantee reading comprehension. For example, illness or other disruptive life situations have been found to significantly interfere with comprehension. Patterns of recall—that is, the length of time between information disclosure and the need to remember the information— as well as the nature of the information (how threatening) and the method of presentation also affect understanding (Silva & Sorrell, 1984; Doak et al., 1996; Doak et al., 1998).

Readability and comprehension, therefore, are particularly complex activities involving many variables with respect to both the reader and the actual written material (Owen, Johnson, et al., 1993; Fisher, 1999; Doak et al., 1996). Both are commonly determined by using one

| Table 7–1    Examples of elements that affect readability and comprehension | |
|---|---|
| **Material Variables** | **Reader Variables** |
| Legibility (e.g., print size, spacing) | Health status |
| Organization and flow of content | Perceived threat of illness |
| Concept level | Effects of illness/stress |
| Length of text | Physical and mental energy |
| Sentence structure | Level of motivation |
| Level of vocabulary | Visual and auditory acuity |
| Relevance to the reader | Educational attainment |
| Jargon (medical terminology) | Background knowledge |
| Number of polysyllabic words | Ability to decipher language of message |

or more measurement formulas (see the later discussions of measurement tools in this chapter). Table 7–1 shows examples of elements that affect readability and comprehension.

Another term used when discussing literacy is *numeracy*, which is the ability to read and interpret numbers. Overwhelmingly, those with limited literacy also have limited skills in numeracy (Morgan, 1993; Williams et al., 1995; Fisher, 1999; Doak et al., 1996).

## Literacy Relative to Oral Instruction

To date, very little attention has been paid to the role of oral communication in the assessment of illiteracy. Certainly, inability to comprehend the spoken word or oral instruction above the level of understanding simple words, phrases, and slang words should be considered an important element in the definition or assessment of literacy. Doak et al. (1985) addressed the fact that there is no universally accepted way to test the degree of difficulty with oral language. However, as these authors observed, "it is believed that some of the same characteristics that are critical for written materials will also affect the comprehensibility of spoken language" (p. 40). Much

more research needs to be done on "iloralacy," or the inability to understand simple oral language, as a generic concept of illiteracy (Hirsch, 2001).

## Literacy Relative to Computer Instruction

The literacy issue has always been examined from the standpoint of readability of materials in print. Recently, *computer literacy* has become an increasingly popular topic and a new dimension of the issue of literacy. There is a bright future for the use of computers as educational tools, but this potential is only beginning to be fully realized or appreciated. Those patients who are well educated and career oriented are already likely to be computer literate.

As healthcare organizations and agencies invest more resources in computer technology and software programs, computer literacy of the patient population will become an issue of increasing concern. Computers not only will be used to convey instructional messages, but also will serve as a valuable tool to access additional sources of information (see Chapters 11, 12, and 13). The opportunity to expand patients' knowledge base through telecommunications will require nurse educators to attend to computer literacy levels much in the same way they have begun to recognize the negative effects that illiteracy and low literacy in using print materials have had by restricting the information base of consumers of health care. Evidence suggests that computer software programs can be highly suitable for low-literate patients as long as these individuals have the basic capacity to use computers. The trend toward managed care and home care portends that computers will play an important role in patient teaching. Thus, nurses must begin to advocate for computer literacy in the public they serve (Doak et al., 1996).

## ▬▬ SCOPE AND INCIDENCE OF THE PROBLEM

Literacy has been termed the "silent epidemic," the "silent barrier," and the "silent disability" (Kefalides, 1999; Doak & Doak, 1987). Based on available statistics, it is evident that the United States has significant literacy problems. In 1985, Kozol recognized that with respect to the average level of literacy in our country, the United States ranked only forty-ninth from the top among 159 members of the United Nations.

In 1992, the National Adult Literacy Survey, considered to be the most accurate, detailed, and recent profile on the condition of English language literacy in the United States, revealed surprising statistics (a new NALS survey will be released in 2002). NALS divided a representative sample of 26,000 individuals, aged 16 years and older, into five levels (Level 1 being the lowest and Level 5 being the highest) based on assessment of skills in three areas: prose, document, and quantitative literacy. Twenty-one to twenty-three percent, or approximately 40 to 44 million of the 191 million adults in the country, scored in the lowest levels of the three skill areas and are, therefore, considered to be functionally illiterate. Another 25% to 28%, or approximately 50 million adults, scored in the Level 2 category; that is, they are considered to have low literacy skills. Thus, the total number of illiterate and low-literate adults in the United States conservatively is estimated to be approximately 90 million. This figure represents about one-half of the adult population in this country who have deficiencies in reading, writing, and math skills (Fisher, 1999; Williams et al., 1996). NALS did not specifically test health literacy levels (Ad Hoc Committee, 1999), but the researchers did find those individuals with poor literacy skills to be more often from minority populations, from lower socioeconomic groups, and with poorer health status (TenHave et al., 1997; Fisher, 1999).

In cases of both illiteracy and low literacy, the level of readability is measured in terms of performance, not years of school attendance. Even though the mean reading education level of the U.S. population is at grade 12.6, the mean literacy level is at or below eighth grade; Medicaid enrollees, on average, read at the fifth-grade level (Winslow, 2001). Many

people read two to four grade levels below their reported level of formal education. This deficiency persists because schools have a tendency to promote students for social and age-related reasons rather than for academic achievement alone, patients may report inaccurate histories of years of school attended, and reading skills may be lost over time through lack of practice (Yasenchak & Bridle, 1993; Jackson et al., 1991; Stephens, 1992; Miller & Bodie, 1994; Davidhizar & Brownson, 1999). In addition, although most students taking the Scholastic Aptitude Tests (SATs) graduate from high school, their proficiency in reading and comprehension shows signs of declining (Thomison, 1991).

Thus, at least one out of every four to five Americans lacks the literacy skills and knowledge to cope with the requirements of day-to-day living. For example, one needs to be able to read at the sixth-grade level to understand a driver's license manual, at the eighth-grade level to follow directions on a frozen dinner package, and at the tenth-grade level to read instructions on a bottle of aspirin (Doak et al., 1985). The literacy problem is so widespread that the government, in an effort to reduce traffic accidents, has replaced some conventional printed road signs with road signs using symbols (Loughrey, 1983).

Because of the difficulty inherent in defining and testing literacy, and because few people with limited reading skills admit to having such difficulty, the scope of the literacy problem may be much greater than found in formal studies (Jolly et al., 1993; Brownson, 1998). The above numbers are merely estimates, and the rates have risen steadily over the years. Although many believe the numbers of illiterate persons are greater than the estimates, it is difficult to determine exact numbers because of the ever increasing complexity of the technological and informational demands of our society today. To be literate 100 years ago meant that people could read and write their own name. Today, being literate means that one is able to learn new skills, think critically, problem solve, and apply general knowledge to various situations (Fain, 1994a).

The trend toward an increased proportion of Americans with literacy levels that are inadequate for active participation in our advanced technological society most likely is due to factors such as the following (Baydar et al., 1993; Hayes, 2000; Hirsch, 2001; Weiss et al., 1995):

- A rise in the number of immigrants
- The aging of the population
- The increasing complexity of information
- More people living in poverty
- Changes in policies and funding for public education
- A disparity in the literacy achievements of minority versus nonminority populations

All of these factors correlate significantly with the level of formal schooling attained and the level of literacy ability. Although it was stated previously that research indicates the number of years of schooling is not a good predictor of literacy level, there remains a correlation between someone's educational background and the ability to read. As our society becomes more and more "high tech," with new products and more complicated functions to perform, the basic language requirements needed for survival will continue to rise. A greater number of people are beginning to fall behind, unable to keep up with our increasingly sophisticated world.

Levels of literacy are often seen as indicators of the well-being of individuals, and the literacy problem has greater implications for the social and economic status of the country as a whole. Low levels of literacy have been associated with marginal productivity, high unemployment, minimum earnings, high costs of health care, and high rates of welfare dependency (Baydar et al., 1993; Winslow, 2001; Kelly, 1999; Ziegler, 1998). Illiteracy is considered to be an element contributing to many of the grave social issues confronting the United States today, such as homelessness,

teen pregnancy, unemployment, delinquency, crime, and drug abuse (Fleener & Scholl, 1992). Deficiencies in basic literacy skills compound to create devastating cumulative ignorance for the affected individuals, creating a social burden that is extremely costly for the American people. Reports indicate that poor basic literacy skills are evident in 69% of all those arrested, 85% of unwed mothers, 79% of welfare recipients, 85% of dropouts, and 72% of unemployed people (Johnson & Layng, 1992). Illiteracy and low literacy are not necessarily the reasons for these ills, but the high correlation between literacy levels and social problems is a marker for disconnectedness from society in general (Jenks, 1992).

The decline in reading achievement scores across the United States suggests that the number of people capable of decoding words and comprehending health information written at the high school level and above may actually be dwindling. Those with minimal educational achievement are most likely to be at even greater risk for the conditions that many health education materials attempt to address.

## THOSE AT RISK

Illiteracy has been portrayed "as an invisible handicap that affects all classes, ethnic groups, and ages" (Fleener & Scholl, 1992, p. 740). It is a silent disability. Illiteracy knows no boundaries and exists among persons of every race and ethnic background, socioeconomic class, and age category (Weiss et al., 1995; Duffy & Snyder, 1999). It is true, however, that illiteracy is rare in the higher socioeconomic classes, for example, and that certain segments of the U.S. population are more likely to be affected than others by lack of literacy skills. According to Jackson et al. (1991), Lasater and Mehler (1998), Cole (2000), Winslow (2001), and Hayes (2000), populations that have been identified as having poorer reading and comprehension skills than the average American include the following:

- The economically disadvantaged
- Older adults
- Immigrants (particularly illegal ones)
- Racial minorities
- High school dropouts
- The unemployed
- Prisoners
- Inner-city and rural residents
- Southerners (Louisiana, Texas, and Mississippi report the highest rates of illiteracy in the nation)
- Those with poor health status due to chronic mental and physical problems

With respect to demographics, statistics indicate that 38 million Americans are presently living in poverty and that nearly half (43%) of all adults with low literacy live in poverty (Kelly, 1999). Although the disadvantaged represent many diverse cultural and ethnic groups, including millions of poor white people, one-third of the disadvantaged in this country are minorities, and a larger percentage of minorities fall into the disadvantaged category (see Chapter 8). In the twenty-first century, the major growth in the population will come from the ranks of minority groups. By 2010, one out of every three people in the United States is projected to belong to a racial or ethnic minority (Robinson, 2000); in 53 of the 100 largest cities, minorities will be in the majority. In 1996, the U.S. Census Bureau reported that one in every 10 people living in this country was born in another country. Since 1980, the number of people speaking a language at home other than English has risen by 43% (28.3 million). The birth rate of Latinos, for example, is growing five times faster than the national average, and this population is expected to increase to almost 30 million by the early years of the twenty-first century. By 2010, there is predicted to be 5.5 million more Latino/Hispanic American children, 2.6 million more African American children, and 1.5 million more chil-

dren of other races, but 6.2 million fewer Caucasian children. Nurse educators must recognize how these demographic changes will affect the way in which services need to be rendered, educational materials need to be developed, and information needs to be marketed (Morra, 1991; Robinson, 2000; Denboba et al., 1998).

Many minority and economically disadvantaged people, as well as the prison population—which has the highest concentration of adult illiteracy (Duffy & Snyder, 1999)—are not benefactors of mainstream health education activities, which often fail to reach them. Overall, they are not active seekers of health information because they tend to have weaker communication skills and inadequate foundational knowledge on which to better understand their needs. Many lack enough fluency to make good use of written health education materials (Morra, 1991; Denboba et al., 1998). Areas with the highest percentage of minorities and high rates of poverty and immigration also have the highest percentage of functionally illiterate people. When these people need medical care, they tend to require more resources, have longer hospital stays, and have a greater number of readmissions (Davis et al., 1990; TenHave et al., 1997). The challenge now and in the future will be to find improved ways of communicating with these population groups and to develop innovative strategies in the delivery of medical and nursing care.

Of the Americans older than 65 years of age, two out of five adults (approximately 40%) are considered functionally illiterate (Davidhizar & Brownson, 1999; Brooks, 1998). Individuals older than 85 years of age make up the fastest-growing age group in the country. By the turn of the century, they will account for almost 5 million people. Children born today can expect to live to an average age of 83. Statistics indicate that the U.S. population is growing older as people live longer. By 2020, it is expected that 52 million (or an unprecedented 16.5%) of the U.S. population will be 65 years or older (Gollop, 1997). As time goes on, the older population will be more educated and demand more services. In 1960, only 20% of older people were high school graduates, whereas by the beginning of the twenty-first century, 64% were educated at the high school level. Although these statistical trends indicate there will be a more highly educated group of older adults in the future, the information explosion and rapid technological advances may cause them to fall behind relative to future standards of education.

Today, the illiteracy problem in the aged is due to the facts that not only did these individuals have less education in the past, but also that their reading skills have declined over time because of disuse. If a person does not use a skill, he or she loses the skill. Reading ability can deteriorate over time if not exercised regularly (Brownson, 1998). In addition, cognition and intellectual functioning are affected by aging (Jackson et al., 1994; Weinrich & Boyd, 1992; Pearson & Wessman, 1996; Weiss et al., 1995). The vast majority of older people have some degree of cognitive changes and vision impairments, and about one-fourth have serious hearing loss. Along with these normal physiological changes, many suffer from chronic diseases, and large numbers are taking prescribed medications. All of these conditions can interfere with the ability to learn or negatively affect thought processes, which contributes to the high incidence of illiteracy in this population group.

Beyond the issue of prevalency, illiteracy also presents unique psychosocial problems for the older adult. Because older persons tend to learn material more slowly than do young adults, especially with such tasks that require reading and writing, they may become more easily frustrated in a learning situation (Morra, 1991; Pearson & Wessman, 1996). Furthermore, many older individuals have developed ways to compensate for missing skills through their support network. Lifetime patterns of behavior have been set such that they may lack the motivation to improve their literacy skills (Anscher & Gold, 1991). Today and in the years to come, those

involved with providing health education will be challenged to overcome these obstacles to learning in the aged.

Keeping in mind that illiteracy has been said to run in families from generation to generation, Baydar et al. (1993) conducted an interesting study on childhood and adolescent determinants of literacy in adulthood. These researchers used longitudinal data collected over 20 years from a sample of African American children of teenaged mothers from the Baltimore area, which correlated with nationally representative data. Their aim was to identify early precursors of adulthood literacy levels that could define high-risk groups in each developmental period from early childhood to adolescence. The researchers found that family factors affecting the physical and emotional quality of the home environment (maternal education, family size in early childhood, maternal marital status, and income) as well as early childhood developmental levels (preschool cognitive and behavioral functioning) and educational background of the child (grade repetition or school suspension) were all predictive of literacy in young adulthood.

Cultural diversity, although not considered to be directly related to illiteracy, may also serve as a barrier to effective client education. According to Davidhizar and Brownson (1999), most illiterate adults in this country are white, native-born, English-speaking Americans. However, when examining the proportion of the population that has poor literacy skills, minority ethnic groups are at higher risk. It is estimated that 44% of African Americans and 56% of Hispanic Americans are illiterate or marginally illiterate. According to the NALS report, adults belonging to the four major cultural groups (African American, Hispanic American, Native American, and Asian/Pacific Islander) were more likely than Caucasians to perform at the two lowest literacy levels (Kirsch et al., 1993). Given these demographics, individuals from culturally diverse backgrounds with poor literacy skills are likely to represent a significant proportion of consumers who visit public healthcare facilities (Wilson, 1995). In communicating with clients from cultures different than those of the healthcare providers, it is important to be aware that even though people may speak the English language, the meanings of words and the understanding of facts may vary significantly based on life experiences, family background, and culture of origin, especially if English is the client's second language (Davidhizar & Brownson, 1999).

Hussey and Guilliland (1989) also identified culture as another aspect of literacy. They define *cultural literacy* as "knowing how to communicate without having to explain" (p. 608). In conversation, an individual must be able to understand undertones, voice intonations, and in what context (slang, terminology, or customs) the message is being delivered. Davidhizar and Brownson (1999) stress the importance of assessing other elements of verbal and nonverbal communication, such as emotional tone of speech, gestures, eye contact, touch, voice volume, and stance, between persons of different cultures that may affect the interpretation of behavior and the validating of information received or sent. Educators must be aware of these potential barriers to communication when interacting with clients from other cultures whose literacy skills may be limited (see Chapter 8). Given the increasing diversity of the U.S. population, most currently available written materials are inadequate based on the literacy level of minority groups.

Although most illiterates have had some degree of formal education, the majority have not graduated from high school, are younger than 40 years of age, and live in metropolitan areas; more than 40% are unemployed (Powers, 1988). Thus, individuals with less education, which often includes the groups of low-income persons, older adults, racial minorities, and people with ethnic origins for whom English is a second language, are likely to have more difficulty with reading and comprehending written materials as well as understanding oral instruction (Winslow,

2001). This profile is not intended to stereotype illiterate people but rather to give a broad picture of who most likely lacks literacy skills. It is essential that nurses and other healthcare providers be aware of who might be susceptible to having literacy problems when carrying out assessments on their patient populations.

## MYTHS, STEREOTYPES, AND ASSUMPTIONS

Rarely do people voluntarily admit that they are illiterate. Illiteracy is a stigma that creates feelings of shame, inadequacy, fear, and low self-esteem (Parikh et al., 1996). Most individuals with poor literacy skills have learned that it is dangerous to reveal their illiteracy because of fear that others such as family, strangers, friends, or employers would consider them dumb or incapable of functioning responsibly. In fact, the majority of people with literacy problems have never told their spouse or children of their disability (Quirk, 2000; Parikh et al., 1996; Kelly, 1999; Murphy & Davis, 1997). People also tend to underreport their limited reading abilities because of embarrassment or lack of insight about the extent of their limitation. The NALS report revealed that the majority of adults performing at the two lowest levels of literacy skill describe themselves as proficient in being able to read and/or write English (Kirsch et al., 1993). Because self-reporting is so unreliable and because illiteracy and low literacy are so common, many experts suggest that screening of all patients should be done to identify clients who have reading difficulty to determine the extent of their impairment (Lasater & Mehler, 1998; Wilson, 1995).

The literature contains many examples of illiterates who have managed to keep their secret from others and have successfully held jobs and survived in a world that requires literacy skills (Walker, 1987). Most people with limited literacy abilities are masters at concealment. Typically, they are ashamed by their limitation and attempt to hide the problem in clever ways. Often, they are resourceful and intelligent about trying to conceal their illiteracy and have developed remarkable memories to help them cope with family and career situations (Kanonowicz, 1993; Doak et al., 1996). Many have discovered ways to function quite well in society without being able to read by memorizing signs and instructions, by making intelligent guesses, or by finding employment opportunities that are not heavily dependent on reading and writing skills. As Fain (1994b) points out, illiterate patients "become very good actors, practiced in misdirection and evasion" (p. 16B).

An important thing to remember is that there are many myths about illiteracy. It is very easy for healthcare providers to fall into the trap of wrongly labeling someone as illiterate or, for that matter, assuming that they are literate based on stereotypical images. Walker (1987) addressed some of the most common myths (see also Brooks, 1998; Lasater & Mehler, 1998; Doak et al., 1996; Mayeaux et al., 1996):

Myth #1: Illiterates are stupid and slow learners or incapable of learning at all. (In fact, many illiterates have normal or above-normal intelligence quotients.)

Myth #2: Illiterates can be recognized by their appearance. (In fact, appearance alone is an unreliable basis for judgment because some very articulate, well-dressed people suffer from illiteracy.)

Myth #3: The number of years of schooling completed correlates with literacy skills. (In fact, grade-level achievement does not correspond well to reading ability. The number of years of schooling completed overestimates reading levels by four to five grade levels [Winslow, 2001].)

Myth #4: All illiterates are foreigners, poor, of ethnic or racial minority, and/or from the South. (In fact, illiterate people come from very diverse backgrounds.)

Myth #5: Most illiterates will freely admit that they do not know how to read or do not understand. (In fact, most try to hide their reading deficiencies and will go to great lengths to avoid discovery, even when directly asked about their possible limitations. As Doak says, "People would rather tell you they have a venereal disease than that they can't read" [Jenks, 1992, p. 1069].)

## ASSESSMENT: CLUES TO LOOK FOR

So the question remains: How does one recognize an illiterate person? Identifying illiteracy is not easy because there is no stereotypical pattern. It is an impairment easily overlooked because illiteracy has no particular face, age, socioeconomic status, or nationality (Cole, 2000; Hayes, 2000). Nurses, because of their highly developed assessment skills and frequent contact with patients, are in an ideal position to determine the literacy levels of their clients. Because of the prevalence of illiteracy, nurses should never assume that their patients are literate. Knowing a person's ability to read and comprehend is critical in providing teaching–learning encounters that are beneficial, efficient, and cost-effective.

There are a number of informal clues to watch out for that indicate reading and writing deficiencies. The caveat is not to rely on the obvious but to look for the unexpected. There are so many instances when a patient does not fit the stereotypical image of an illiterate that nurses and physicians have never even considered the possibility. Overlooking the problem has the potential for grave consequences in treatment outcomes and has resulted in frustration for both the patient and the caregiver (Rudolph, 1994; Cole, 2000). Unfortunately, healthcare providers are often hesitant to infer that a patient may have low literacy skills because there is an implication of personal inadequacy associated with the failure to have learned to read (Quirk, 2000; Parikh, 1996).

Because illiterate or semiliterate patients often have had many years of practice at disguising the problem, they will go to elaborate lengths to hide the fact that they do not possess a skill already acquired by most six-year-olds. The observant practitioner should always be on the lookout for possible signs of poor reading ability in a patient. If healthcare providers become aware of a patient's literacy problem, they must convey sensitivity and maintain confidentiality to prevent increased feelings of shame (Quirk, 2000). During assessment, the nurse should take note of the following clues that illiterate patients may demonstrate (Loughrey, 1983; Fain, 1994b; Meade & Thornhill, 1989; Brooks, 1998; Lasater & Mehler, 1998):

- Reacting to complex learning situations by withdrawal, complete avoidance, or being repeatedly noncompliant

- Using the excuse that they were too busy, too tired, too sick, or too sedated with medication to maintain attention span when given a booklet or instruction sheet to read

- Claiming that they just did not feel like reading, that they gave the information to their spouse to take home, or that they lost, forgot, or broke their glasses

- Camouflaging their problem by surrounding themselves with books, magazines, and newspapers to give the impression they are able to read

- Circumventing their inability by insisting on taking the information home to read or having a family member or friend with them when written information is presented

- Asking you to read the information for them under the guise that their eyes are bothersome, they lack interest, or they do not have the energy to devote to the task of learning

- Showing nervousness as a result of feeling stressed by the threat of the possibility of "getting caught" or having to confess to illiteracy

- Acting confused, talking out of context, holding reading materials upside down, or expressing thoughts that may seem totally irrelevant to the topic of conversation

- Showing a great deal of frustration and restlessness when attempting to read, often mouthing words aloud (vocalization) or silently (subvocalization), substituting words they cannot decipher (decode) with meaningless words, pointing to words or phrases on a page, or exhibiting facial signs of bewilderment or defeat

- Standing in a location clearly designated for "authorized personnel only"

- Listening and watching very attentively to observe and memorize how things work

- Demonstrating difficulty with following instructions about relatively simple activities such as breathing exercises or with operating the TV, electric bed, call light, and other simple equipment, even when the operating instructions are clearly printed on them

- Failing to ask any questions about the information they received

- Revealing a discrepancy between what is understood by listening and what is understood by reading

In summary, although it has been clearly pointed out that the level of completed formal education is an inaccurate presumption by which to predict reading level, it is certainly one estimate that nurses should incorporate into their methods of assessment. Negative feedback and clues from the patient in the form of puzzled looks, inappropriate behaviors, excuses, or irrelevant statements may give the nurse the gut feeling that the message being communicated is neither received nor understood. Not only do illiterate patients become confused and frustrated in their attempts to deal with the complex system of health care, which is so dependent on written and verbal information, but also they become stressed in their efforts to cover up their disability.

Nurses, in turn, can feel frustrated when patients with undiagnosed literacy problems seem at face value to be unmotivated and noncompliant in following self-care instructions. Many times nurses wonder why patients make caregiving so difficult for themselves as well as for the provider. It is not unusual for nurses to conclude, "He's too proud to bend," "She's in denial," or "He's just noncompliant—it's a control issue." Nurses must go beyond their own assumptions, look beyond a patient's appearance and behavior, and seek out the less than obvious by conducting a thorough initial assessment of variables to uncover the possibility that a literacy problem exists (Rudolph, 1994). An awareness of this possibility and good skills at observation are key to diagnosing illiteracy or low literacy in the patient population. Early diagnosis will enable nurses to intervene appropriately to avoid disservice to illiterate patients, who do not need condemnation but nurses' support and encouragement.

## ▊▊▊ IMPACT OF ILLITERACY ON MOTIVATION AND COMPLIANCE

In addition to the fact that poor literacy skills affect the ability to read as well as understand and interpret the meaning of written, visual, and verbal instruction, an illiterate or semiliterate person struggles with other significant interrelated limitations with communication that negatively influence healthcare teaching (Barnes, 1992a; Doak et al., 1998; Murphy & Davis, 1997). The person's organization of thought, perception, vocabulary and language/fluency development, and problem-solving skills are adversely affected, too (Brooks, 1998).

Fleener and Scholl (1992) investigated characteristics of self-identified illiterates. For the functionally illiterate, the most common deficiencies found were in phonics, comprehension, and perception. Difficulties in perception were evident in the reversal of letters and words, miscalling letters, and adding and omitting letters. Also, a major problem was comprehension, the calling of words without knowing their meaning. Some individuals needed to read aloud to understand, and others read so slowly that they lost the meaning of a paragraph before they had finished it. Still other subjects perceived difficulty in remembering as a factor in their lack of reading skill.

People with poor reading skills have difficulty analyzing instructions, assimilating and correlating new information, and formulating questions (Barnes, 1992a). They may be reluctant to ask questions because of concerns that their questions will be regarded as incomprehensible or irrelevant. Not only do they probably not know what to ask, but they also do not want anyone to think of them as ignorant or lacking in intelligence.

Hussey and Guilliland (1989) provide a poignant example of a young pregnant girl prescribed antiemetic suppositories to control her nausea. When she had no relief of symptoms, questioning by the nurse revealed that she was swallowing the medication. Obviously, not only did she not understand how to take the medicine, but she also probably had never seen a suppository and was not even able to read the word. She did not ask what it was, probably because she did not know what to ask in the first place, and she may have been reluctant to question the treatment out of fear that she would be regarded as stupid.

If past experiences with learning have been less than positive, illiterates may prefer not knowing the answers to questions and may withdraw altogether to avoid awkward or embarrassing learning situations. They may react to complicated, fast-paced instruction with discouragement, low self-esteem, and refusal to participate because their process of interpretation is so slow. Even when questioned about their understanding, persons with low literacy skills will most likely claim that the information was understood even when it was not (Doak et al., 1996).

Another characteristic of illiterate individuals is that they have difficulty synthesizing information in a way that fits into their behavior patterns. If they are unable to comprehend a required behavior change or cannot understand why it is needed, then any health teaching will be disregarded (Hussey & Guilliland, 1989; Brooks, 1998). For example, cardiac patients who are told via verbal and written instructions to lose weight, increase exercise, decrease dietary fat, and begin taking medications may fail to comply with this regimen because of lack of understanding of the information and how to go about incorporating these changes into their lifestyle.

Persons with poor literacy skills may also think in only concrete, specific, and literal terms. An example of this limitation is the diabetic patient whose glucose levels were out of control even when the patient insisted he was taking his insulin as instructed—injecting the orange and then eating the fruit (Brooks, 1998; Hussey & Guilliland, 1989).

The illiterate or semiliterate person may also experience difficulty handling large amounts of information and classifying it into categories. Patients who need to take several different medications at various times and in different dosages may either become confused with the schedule or ignore the instruction. If asked to change their daily medication routine, a great deal of retraining may be needed to convince them of the benefits of the new regimen.

Another major factor in noncompliance is the lack of adequate and specific instructions about prescribed treatment regimens. Poor literacy skills, which are seldom assessed by healthcare personnel when teaching a patient about medications, tend to limit the patient's ability to understand the array of instructions regarding medication labels, dosage scheduling, adverse reactions, drug interactions, and complications. No wonder those who lack vocabulary, organized thinking, and the ability to formulate questions, coupled with inadequate instruction, become confused and easily frustrated to the point of taking medications incorrectly or refusing to take them at all.

Thus, illiteracy, functional illiteracy, and low literacy significantly affect both motivation and compliance levels (see Chapter 6). What is often mistaken for noncompliance is, instead, the simple inability to comply. Although approximately 21% to 23% of adult patients are functionally illiterate, this statistic is overlooked by many healthcare professionals as a major factor in noncompliance with prescribed regimens, follow-up appointments, and measures to prevent medical complications (Doak et al., 1996). A number of studies have correlated literacy levels with noncompliance (Hussey & Guilliland, 1989; Jolly et al., 1993; Doak et al., 1998; Hussey, 1994). Individuals with poor literacy skills that coincide with inadequate language skills have difficulty following instructions and providing accurate and complete health histories, which are vital to the delivery of good health care. The burden of illiteracy leads patients into noncompliance not because they do not want to comply, but rather because they are unable to do so (Williams et al., 1996; Hayes, 2000).

Numerous research studies indicate that the impact of illiteracy is broader than just the inability to read; it alters the way a person organizes, interprets, analyzes, and summarizes information. Caregivers often overestimate an individual's ability to understand instructions and are quick to label someone as uncooperative. In reality, the underlying problem may be limited cognitive processing that impedes comprehending and following written and oral communication (Lasater & Mehler, 1998).

## ETHICAL AND LEGAL CONCERNS

Sources of printed education materials (PEMs) include healthcare facilities, commercial vendors, government services, voluntary health agencies, nonprofit charitable organizations, pharmaceutical firms, and medical equipment supply companies. These materials are distributed primarily by nurses and physicians and are the major sources of information for patients participating in health programs in many settings. Written health information materials are intended to reinforce learning about health promotion, disease prevention, illness process, diagnostic procedures, drug and treatment modalities, rehabilitative course, and self-care regimens. Unfortunately, many of these sources fail to take into account the educational level, preexisting knowledge base, cultural influences, language barriers, racial or ethnic status, or economic backgrounds of persons with limited literacy skills. Unless patients are competent in reading and comprehending the literature given to them, these tools are useless as adjuncts for health education and are neither a cost-effective nor a time-efficient means for teaching and learning. Materials that are widely distributed, but little or not at all understood, pose not only a health hazard for the patient but also an ethical and legal liability for healthcare providers (French & Larrabee, 1999; Ad Hoc Committee, 1999).

Materials that are too difficult to read or comprehend serve little purpose. Patient education cannot be considered to have taken place if the patient has not gained enough knowledge and requisite skills necessary for self-care. Ultimately, indiscriminate or nonselective use of PEMs can result in complete or partial lack of communication between healthcare providers and consumers (Fisher, 1999; Winslow, 2001).

Initial standards for health education put forth in 1993 by the Joint Commission for Accreditation of Healthcare Organizations (JCAHO) require that "the patient and/or, when appropriate, his/her significant other(s) are provided with education that can enhance their knowledge, skills, and those behaviors necessary to fully benefit from the health care interventions provided by the organization" (JCAHO, 1993, p. 1030). In 1996, JCAHO identified additional standards necessary for client care to meet accreditation mandates. Not only is patient and family (or significant other) instruction required, but education must be provided by all relevant members of the interdisciplinary healthcare team, with special consideration being given to the client's literacy level, educational level, and language. All clients must have an assessment of their readiness to learn and an identification of any obstacles to learning. This new emphasis has prompted healthcare agencies and providers to reexamine their teaching practices, educational materials, and systems of documenting evidence of teaching interventions to better match the reading levels and cultural diversity of the clients being served. The JCAHO standards have specified that education relevant to a person's healthcare needs must be "understandable" and culturally appropriate to the patient and/or significant others. Therefore, PEMs must be written in ways that assist patients in comprehending their health needs and problems to undertake self-care regimens such as medications, diet, exercise therapies, and use of medical equipment (Bernier, 1993; Davidhizar & Brownson, 1999; Fisher, 1999).

Furthermore, the federally mandated Patient's Bill of Rights has established the rights of patients to receive complete and current information regarding their diagnoses, treatments, and prognoses in terms they can understand (Duffy & Snyder, 1999). It is imperative that the reading levels of PEMs match the patients' reading abilities, and vice versa. Compounding the need for appropriately written materials is the fact that research reveals that patients forget within five minutes about one-half of any oral instruction they receive (Boyd, 1988). Failure to retain information combined with inappropriate reading levels of materials used to reinforce or supplement verbal teaching methods may very well decrease compliance, increase morbidity, and encourage misuse of healthcare facilities.

Encouraging self-care through patient education for purposes of health promotion, disease prevention, health maintenance, and rehabilitation is not a new concept to either consumers or providers of health care. However, the constraints of the current healthcare system in the United States have impinged on the professional ability of nurses to provide needed information to ensure self-care that is both safe and effective. Patient education has assumed an even more vital role in assisting patients to independently manage their own healthcare needs given such factors as

- Early discharge
- Decreased reimbursement for direct care
- Increased emphasis on delivery of care in the community and home setting
- Greater demands on nursing personnel time
- Increased technological complexity of treatment
- Assumption by caregivers that printed information is an adequate substitute for direct instruction of patients

These trends do not allow for sufficient opportunities for patients in various healthcare settings to receive the necessary education they need for self-management after discharge. Most outpatient care, such as that given in clinics, doctors' offices, and same-day surgery centers, requires patients and their families to understand both written and oral instruction (Jackson et al., 1991). Consequently, profes-

sional nurses are relying to a greater extent than ever before on PEMs to supplement their teaching (Owen, Porter, et al., 1993). Thus the burden of becoming adequately educated falls on the shoulders of patients, their families, and significant others. Often unprepared because of shortened hospital stays or limited contact with healthcare providers, patients have to assume a greater role in their own recovery and the maximization of their health potential (Stephens, 1992; Zimm, 1998).

The burden also falls on nurses to safeguard the lives of their clients by becoming better, more effective communicators of written health information. Osborne (1999) describes the annual summer institute for healthcare professionals established by the Maine AHEC Health Literacy Center at the University of New England and the NIFL-Health e-mail list sponsored by the National Institute for Literacy as opportunities for healthcare professionals to learn about literacy issues, to share resources with colleagues from around the world, and to acquire skills in writing and critiquing health information documents. Zimm (1998) lists organizations that can provide healthcare professionals with useful information about literacy and health.

It is only recently that research in the area of written health education materials in relation to patients' literacy skills has examined and attempted to answer even the most basic questions, such as the following:

- Do patients read the education literature provided them?
- Are they capable of reading it?
- Can they comprehend what they read?
- Are written materials appropriate and sufficient for the intended target audience?

In our increasingly litigious society, growing attention is being paid by health professionals to informed consent and teaching for self-care via both verbal and written healthcare instruction.

The potential for misinterpretation of instructions not only can adversely affect treatment but also raises serious concerns regarding the legal implications with respect to professional liability when information is written at a level incomprehensible to many patients (French & Larrabee, 1999). A properly informed consumer is not only a legal concern in health care today but an ethical one as well (see Chapter 2).

## READABILITY OF PRINTED EDUCATION MATERIALS

Many studies on literacy have attempted to document the disparity between the reading levels within the patient population and the estimated readability of printed health information. Given that the health of people depends in part on their ability to understand information contained in food labeling, over-the-counter and prescription medication instructions, environmental safety warnings, discharge instructions, health promotion and disease prevention flyers, and the like, the focus of attention on identifying this discrepancy is more than warranted. A substantial body of evidence in the literature indicates that there is a significant gap between patients' reading and comprehension levels and the level of reading difficulty of PEMs (Winslow, 2001).

Healthcare providers are beginning to recognize that the reams of written materials relied on by so many of them to convey health information to consumers are essentially closed to the illiterate patient (Morgan, 1993). For example, look at the lines below:

Laeyo aoiou dxpo quto a uoixyo mnstr.

Mnstr laeyo dxpo guto tzny auoibxgo.

Do they make sense, or are you confused? If they appear unreadable, that is exactly what written teaching instructions look like to someone who cannot read (Loughrey, 1983).

A number of researchers have assessed specific population groups in a variety of healthcare settings based on the ability of patients to meet the literacy demands of written materials related to their care. All of these investigators used commonly accepted readability formulas to test patients' understanding of printed health information. Their findings revealed:

- Patients are better able to understand written materials prepared at grade level five than at grade level nine (Estey et al., 1991).

- Emergency department instructional materials (average tenth-grade readability) are written at a level of difficulty out of the readable range for most patients (Jolly et al., 1993; Williams et al., 1996; Duffy & Snyder, 1999; Lerner et al., 2000).

- A significant mismatch exists between the reading ability of older adults and the readability levels of documents essential to their gaining access to health-related services offered through local, state, and federal government programs (Winslow, 2001).

- A large discrepancy exists between average patient reading comprehension levels and the readability demand of PEMs used in ambulatory care settings (Davis et al., 1990; Lerner, 2000).

- Standard institutional consent forms require college-level reading comprehension (Davis et al., 1990; Doak et al., 1998).

- A variety of education materials available from sources such as the government, health agencies, professional associations, universities, and industries are written beyond the reading ability of the majority of patients (Owen, Porter, et al., 1993; Glanz & Rudd, 1990; Swanson et al., 1990; Williams-Deane & Potter, 1992; Holt et al., 1990).

- An analysis of more than 2000 healthcare publications by Leonard and Cecelia Doak, well-recognized leaders in the field of patient literacy, found that the majority of

PEMs are written in medical school language, which is at a level incomprehensible to the average person (Doak et al., 1996; Jenks, 1992).

• Of the American Cancer Society PEMs commonly used to deliver messages about cancer detection methods, lifestyle risks, and treatment modalities, more than half are written at twelfth-grade level or higher (Meade et al., 1992; Doak et al., 1998; Brownson, 1998).

Thus, numerous investigators have demonstrated that PEMs for patients are written at grade levels that far exceed the reading ability of the majority of patients. Results from these studies reveal that most patient education literature is written above the eighth-grade level, with the average level falling between the tenth and twelfth grade. Many PEMs exceed this upper range, even though the average reading level of adults falls between the fifth- and eighth-grade levels and millions of people in our population read at considerably lower levels (Brownson, 1998; Doak et al., 1998). Furthermore, the education literature indicates that people typically read at least two grade levels below their highest level of schooling and prefer materials that are written below their school level. In fact, contrary to popular belief, sophisticated readers also prefer simplified PEMs when ill and even when well due to the demands of their busy schedules (Lasater & Mehler, 1998; Winslow, 2001).

The conclusion to be drawn is that complex and lengthy PEMs serve no useful teaching purpose if patients are unable to understand them or unwilling to read them. Literacy levels of patients compared with literacy demands of PEMs, whether in hospital or community-based settings, are an important factor in the rehabilitation and recidivism of patients.

The Internet is an excellent resource for nurse educators to locate easy-to-read PEMs.

The Web site *http://www.oshu.edu/bicc-Library/ patiented/links.html#lowlit* is a helpful link to locate low-literacy education materials. The National Cancer Institute also has a Web site at *http://rex.nci.nihgov/NCI-PUB-INDEX/PUBS- EASYREAD.html* for publications with low reading-grade levels (Duffy & Snyder, 1999).

## ▮▮▮ MEASUREMENT TOOLS TO TEST READABILITY OF WRITTEN MATERIALS

Healthcare professionals continually struggle with the task of effectively communicating highly complex and technical information to their consumers, who often lack sufficient background knowledge to understand the sophisticated content of instruction relevant to their care. Whether they author or merely distribute printed education information, nursing and other healthcare practitioners are responsible for ensuring the readability of the materials given to patients. If the readability of education materials matches the patients' literacy levels, consumers may be better able to understand and comply with treatment regimens, thereby reducing the number of readmissions and improving quality of life (Ad Hoc Committee, 1999). Because nurses rely heavily on PEMs to convey necessary information to their clients, the usefulness and efficacy of these materials in terms of readability must be determined.

Readability has been a concern of primary and secondary school educators and educational psychologists for years. In the 1940s, there was a great upswing in attempts by educators and reading specialists to develop systematic procedures by which to objectively evaluate reading materials. Today, more than 40 formulas are available to measure the readability levels of PEMs.

According to George Klare, a noted authority on readability formulas, readers' interest in the subject of instructional material may also influence their comprehension. When interest is high, the formulas may overestimate text difficulty; likewise, when interest is low, they may underestimate difficulty (Pichert & Elam, 1985). Fundamental to the readability of any particular piece of written material is the literacy skills of the reader.

Readability indices have been devised to determine the reading skill required to understand specific written information. Although they can predict a level of reading difficulty of material based on an analysis of sentence structure and word length, they do not take into account the "within" or inherent individual variables that affect the reader or the actual content of the materials (Doak et al., 1996). Even though materials may have similar readability levels as measured by some formula, not all readers will have equal competence in reading them. For example, a patient with a long-standing chronic illness may already be familiar with vocabulary related to the disease and, therefore, may be able to read and understand new materials much more easily than a newly diagnosed patient, even though both patients may have equal reading skill with other types of material (Doak et al., 1985).

As assessment tools, readability formulas are useful but must be employed with caution, because the "match" between reader and material does not necessarily guarantee comprehension. Readability formulas originally were designed as "predictive averages" to rank-order the difficulty of books used in specific grades of school—not to determine exactly which factors contribute to the difficulty of a text. Educators should be careful in assuming that a patient can or cannot read instructional material simply because a formula-based readability score does or does not match the patient's educational level (Pichert & Elam, 1985). Therefore, while readability formulas are easily applied and have proved useful in determining the reading grade-level achievement of a person, when used alone

they are not an adequate index of readability (Doak et al., 1996). Pichert and Elam (1985) make the analogy that "using readability formulas to judge the quality of patient-education materials is like using a urine test to judge diabetes control" (p. 181). While both tests are valid and provide useful information, they can also be misleading, and one must be aware of the practical and theoretical limitations of these formulas for proper use in health education.

Readability formulas are merely one useful step in determining reading comprehension. Many researchers suggest using a multimethod approach to ascertain readability—that is, they suggest applying a number of readability formulas to any given piece of written material as well as taking into consideration the reader and material variables cited previously (Doak et al., 1996; Ley & Florio, 1996). Formula scores are simply rough approximations of text difficulty. Human judgment is always needed in conjunction with formula-based estimates to determine the quality of PEMs.

To objectively evaluate reading materials, two basic methods exist. One method is based on ascertaining the average length of sentences and words (vocabulary difficulty) as exemplified by the various reading formulas. The other method involves measuring patient comprehension and reading skills through the use of a number of standardized tests (see Appendix A). Both methods, although not ideal, are considered to have a sufficient relationship to reading ability to justify their use. The most widely used readability formulas, such as Spache, Flesch, Fog, Fry, and SMOG, rate highly on tests of reliability and predictive validity. They also do not require elaborate training to administer. In addition, the advent of computerized readability analysis has made evaluating reading materials much easier and quicker. All of these methods are most useful to nurse educators for designing and evaluating PEMs.

Readability formulas are mathematical equations, derived from multiple regression analysis, that describe the correlation between an author's style of writing and a reader's skill at decoding words as printed symbols (Doak et al., 1996). In many respects, a readability formula is like a reading test, except that it does not test people but rather written material (Fry, 1977). The first guideline to remember is that readability formulas should not be the only tool used for assessing PEMs. The second rule is to select readability formulas that have been validated on the reader population for whom the PEM is intended. Several formulas are geared to specific types of materials or population groups.

Ley and Florio (1996) conducted an extensive study of the most commonly used formulas and reported on their reliability and validity when used to measure health-related information. As so many readability formulas are available for assessment of reading levels of PEMs, only those that are relatively simple to work with are accepted as reliable and valid and are in widespread use have been chosen for review here.

## Spache Grade-Level Score

What is unique about this formula (Spache, 1953) is that, unlike the other leading formulas that focus largely on the evaluation of materials written for adults, this score is specifically designed to judge materials written for children at grade levels below fourth grade (elementary grades one through three). The Spache Grade-Level Score should not be used to assess adult reading materials (Spache, 1953). The elements used to estimate reading difficulty using the Spache formula are word length; sentence length; the percentage of personal words or personal sentences; the number of syllables, affixes (i.e., prefixes or suffixes), and prepositional phrases; and the number of words outside the Dale "Easy Word List" of 769 words required for formula calcula-

tion. See Appendix A for the method of formula analysis.

## Flesch Formula

This formula was developed as an objective measurement of readability of materials between grade five and college level. Its use has been validated repeatedly over more than 50 years for assessing news reports, adult education materials, and government publications. The Flesch formula is based on a count of two basic language elements: average sentence length in words of selected samples and average word length measured as syllables per 100 words of sample. The reading ease (RE) score is calculated by combining these two variables (Flesch, 1948; Spadero, 1983; Spadero et al., 1980). See Appendix A for the method of formula analysis.

## Fog Index

This formula developed by Gunning (1968) is appropriate for use in determining readability of materials from fourth grade to college level. It is calculated based on average sentence length and the percentage of multisyllabic words in a 100-word passage. The Fog index is considered one of the easier methods because it is based on a short sample of words (100), it does not require counting syllables of all words, and the rules are simple (Spadero, 1983; Spadero et al., 1980). See Appendix A for the method of formula analysis.

## Fry Readability Graph–Extended

The contribution of the Fry formula comes from the simplicity of its use without sacrificing accuracy, as well as its wide and continuous range of testing readability of materials (especially books, pamphlets, and brochures) at the level of grade one through college. A few simple rules can be applied to the Fry Readability Graph to estimate the readability of a wide range of reading materials. This formula plots two language elements—the number of syllables and the number of sentences in three 100-word selections (Fry, 1968; Fry, 1977; Spadero et al., 1980). See Appendix A for directions on how to use the Fry Readability Graph.

## SMOG Formula

This formula by McLaughlin (1969) is recommended not only because it offers relatively easy computation (simple and fast) but also because it is one of the most valid tests of readability (Doak et al., 1996). Whereas other methods base the calculation of grade level on 50% to 75% comprehension, the SMOG method is based on 100% comprehension of material read; that is, if the SMOG formula tests reading material at grade seven, it means all readers able to read at a seventh-grade level should fully comprehend the material. If the same piece of writing were assessed by any of the other formulas, the material would be comprehended by only 50% to 75% of all persons reading at the seventh-grade level. Thus, when using the SMOG formula to calculate the grade level of material, the SMOG results are usually about two grades higher than the grade levels calculated by the other methods (Spadero, 1983). The SMOG formula has been used extensively to judge grade-level readability

of patient education materials. It is the most popular measurement tool because of its reputation for reading-level accuracy, its simple directions, and its speed of use, which is a particularly important factor if computerized resources for analysis of test samples are not available (Meade & Smith, 1991). The SMOG formula measures readability of PEMs from grade four to college level based on the number of polysyllabic words within a set number of sentences to define the grade level needed for complete comprehension. See Appendix A for the method of formula analysis and for an example of how to apply the SMOG formula to a short passage.

In summary, Doak et al. (1996) state that it is critically important to determine the readability of all written materials at the time they are drafted or adopted by using one or more of the many available formulas. They contend that "you cannot afford to fly blind" by using health materials that are untested for readability difficulty. Pretesting PEMs before distribution is the way to be sure they fit the literacy level of the audience for which they are intended. It is imperative that the formulas used to measure grade-level readability of PEMs are appropriate for the type of material being tested in relation to the grade level of the target reader (Table 7–2).

| TABLE 7–2 Appropriate readability formula choice | | | | |
|---|---|---|---|---|
| Formula | Selection Shorter Than 300 Words | Selection Longer Than 300 Words | Entire Piece | Grade Level |
| Spache score | Yes | Yes | Yes | 1–3 |
| Flesch formula | Yes | Yes | Yes | 5 to college |
| Fog formula | Yes (minimum of 100 words) | Yes | Yes | 4 to college |
| Fry Graph | Not recommended | Yes | Yes | 1 to college |
| SMOG formula | Yes | Yes | Yes | 4 to college |

Source: Adapted from Spadero (1980), p. 216.

## Computerized Readability Software Programs

The recent advent of computerized programs has helped tremendously in facilitating the use of readability formulas. Some software programs are capable of applying a number of formulas to analyze one text selection. In addition, some packages are able to identify difficult words in written passages that may not be understood by patients. Dozens of user-friendly, menu-driven commercial software packages can automatically calculate reading levels as well as provide advice on how to simplify text (Mailloux et al., 1995; Doak et al., 1996). Computerized assessment of readability is fast and easy, and it provides a high degree of reliability, especially when several formulas are used. Determining readability by computer programs rather than manually is also more accurate in calculating reading levels because it eliminates human error in scoring and because entire articles, pamphlets, or books can be scanned (Duffy & Snyder, 1999). It is advisable to take an average across several pieces of literature, using several different formulas and software programs, when calculating estimates of readability (Mailloux et al., 1995).

## ■ MEASUREMENT TOOLS TO TEST COMPREHENSION

In addition to the five readability formulas described in the previous section, a number of standardized tests have proved reliable and valid to measure comprehension and reading skills of patients, a relatively new concept in health education (Doak et al., 1996). Usually pre- and post-tests used in institutional settings measure recall of knowledge rather than comprehension and reading skills. However, the determination of patients' reading skills and abilities to comprehend information is essential. Health education materials must serve a useful purpose, both from the stand-point of assisting patients to assume self-care as well as protecting the health professional from legal liability.

The two most popular standardized methods to measure comprehension of written materials are the Cloze test and the listening test. These tests can be used to assess how much a patient understands from reading or listening to a passage of text.

## Cloze Procedure

The Cloze test (derived from the term *closure*) has been specifically recommended for assessing understanding of health education literature. Although it takes more time and resources to compute than do readability formulas, the Cloze procedure has been validated for its adequacy in ranking reading difficulty of medical literature, which typically has a high concept load. This procedure is not a formula that provides a school grade–type level of readability like the formulas already described, but rather takes into consideration the context of a written passage. The Cloze test can be administered to individual patients who demonstrate difficulty comprehending health materials used for instruction. Nevertheless, it is suggested that this test not be administered to every patient in a particular health setting but rather to a representative sample of clients. The Cloze test should be used only with patients whose reading skills are at sixth grade or higher (approximately Level 1 on the NALS scale); otherwise, it is likely that the test will prove too difficult (Doak et al., 1996).

The Cloze test is best used when reviewing the appropriateness of several texts of the same content for a particular audience. The reader may or may not be familiar with the material being tested. This procedure is designed so that every fifth word is systematically deleted from a portion of a text. The reader is asked to fill in the blanks with the exact word replacements. One point is scored for every missing word guessed correctly by the reader. The Cloze score is the total number of blanks filled in correctly by the reader. To be successful, the reader must demonstrate sensitivity to clues related to grammar, syntax, and semantics. If the reader is able to fill in the blanks with appropriate words, this process is an indication of how well the material has been comprehended—that is, how much knowledge was obtained from the set surrounding the blank spaces and how well the information was used to supply the additional information (Doak et al., 1996; Dale & Chall, 1978). The underlying theory is that the more readable a passage is, the better it will be understood even when words are omitted. The resulting score can be converted to a percentage for ease in interpreting and analyzing the data (Pichert & Elam, 1985). A score for the Cloze test is obtained by dividing the number of exact word replacements by the total number of blanks. A score of 60% or better indicates that the passage was sufficiently understood by the patient. A score of 40% to 59% indicates a moderate level of difficulty, where supplemental teaching is required for the patient to understand the message. A score of less than 40% indicates the material is too difficult to be understood and is not suitable to be used for teaching (Doak et al., 1996).

Instead of using packaged Cloze tests available from commercial sources, it is suggested that educators devise their own tests so that the resultant scores will indicate a patient's comprehension of their own instructions. It is not suggested, however, that a Cloze test be administered to every patient, but rather to a representative sample of patients (Doak et al., 1996). Then problem words or sentences within these PEMs can be revised accordingly to make them more understandable. See Appendix A for an outline of the steps for constructing a Cloze test, test scoring methodology, and a sample test.

Because the Cloze procedure is a test of patients' ability to understand what they have read, be sure to be honest about the purpose of the test. You might state that it is important for them to understand what they are to do when on their own after discharge, so you want to be sure they understand the written instructions they will need to follow. Doak et al. (1985) found that most patients are willing to participate in the testing activity. They suggest that the following guidelines should be given to patients before taking the Cloze test:

1. Encourage them to read through the entire test passage before attempting to fill in the blanks.

2. Tell them that only one word should be written in each blank.

3. Let them know that it is all right to guess, but that they should try to fill in every blank.

4. Reassure them that spelling errors are all right just as long as the word they have put in the blank can be recognized.

5. Tell them that this exercise is not a timed test. (If patients struggle to complete the test, tell them not to worry, that it is not necessary for them to fill in all the blanks, and set the test aside to go on to something else less frustrating or less threatening.)

## Listening Test

This test also measures a reader's comprehension skills. Unlike the Cloze test, which may be too difficult for patients who read below the sixth-grade level—that is, those who likely lack fluency and read with hesitancy—the listening test is a good approach to determining what a low-literate patient understands and remembers when listening (Doak et al., 1996).

The procedure for administering the listening test is to select a passage from instructional materials that takes about three minutes to read aloud and is written at approximately the fifth-grade level. Formulate eight to ten questions relevant to the content of the passage by selecting key points of the text. Read the passage to the patient at a normal rate. Ask the listener the questions orally and record the answers. To determine the percentage score, divide the number of questions answered correctly by the total number of questions. The instructional material will be appropriate for the patient's comprehension level if the score is approximately 75% (some additional assistance when teaching the material may be necessary for full comprehension). A score of 90% or higher indicates that the material is too easy for the patient and can be fully comprehended independently. A score of less than 75% means that the material is too difficult and simpler instructional material will need to be used when teaching the patient. Doak et al. (1996) provide examples of a sample passage and questions for a listening comprehension test.

## ■■■■ MEASUREMENT TOOLS TO TEST READING SKILLS

The two most popular standardized methods to measure reading skill are the WRAT and the REALM tests. The TOFHLA is a newer test for the same purpose.

### WRAT (Wide Range Achievement Test)

The WRAT is a word recognition screening test. It is used to assess a patient's ability to recognize and pronounce a list of words out of context as a criterion for measuring reading skills. There are a number of word recognition tests available, but the WRAT requires the least time to administer (approximately 5 minutes as compared with 30 minutes or more for the other tests). Although it is limited to measuring only word recognition and does not test other aspects of reading such as vocabulary and comprehension of text material, this test is nevertheless useful for determining an appropriate level of instruction and for establishing a patient's level of literacy. It is

based on the belief that reading skill is associated with the ability to look at written words and put them into oral language, a necessary first step in comprehension. As designed, it should be used only to test people whose native language is English.

The WRAT tests on two levels: Level I is designed for children 5 to 12 years of age, and Level II is intended for testing persons older than age 12. The WRAT scores are normed on age but can be converted to grade levels (Boyd, 1988). The WRAT consists of a graduated list of 100 words. The patient is asked only to pronounce the words from the list. The individual administering the test listens carefully to the patient's responses and scores those responses on a master score sheet. Next to those words that are mispronounced, a checkmark should be placed. When three words are mispronounced, indicating that the patient has reached his or her limit, the test is stopped. To score the test, the number of words missed or not tried is subtracted from the list of words on the master score sheet to get a raw score. Then a table of raw scores is used to find the equivalent grade rating (GR). For more information on this test, see Doak et al. (1996) and Quirk (2000).

### REALM (Rapid Estimate of Adult Literacy in Medicine)

The REALM test is another reading skills measure that has advantages over the WRAT and other word tests because it measures a patient's ability to read medical and health-related vocabulary, it takes less time to administer, and the scoring is simpler (Duffy & Snyder, 1999; Foltz & Sullivan, 1998). Although it has established validity, this test offers less precision than other word tests (Hayes, 2000). The raw score is converted to a range of grade levels rather than an exact grade level, but this result correlates well with the WRAT reading scores and is quite acceptable to most patients.

The procedure for administering the test is to ask patients to read aloud words from three word lists. Sixty-six medical and health-related words are arranged in three columns, beginning with short, easy words such as *fat, flu, pill,* and *dose,* and ending with more difficult words such as *anemia, obesity, osteoporosis,* and *impetigo.* Patients are asked to begin at the top of the first column and read down, pronouncing all the words that they can from the three lists. The total number of words pronounced correctly is their raw score, which is converted to a grade ranging from third grade and below to ninth grade and higher. For the REALM test, the scoring guide, and validation results summary, see Doak et al. (1996).

## TOFHLA (Test of Functional Health Literacy in Adults)

This test is a relatively new instrument for measuring patients' literacy skills using actual hospital materials, such as prescription labels, appointment slips, and informed consent documents. The test consists of two parts: reading comprehension and numeracy. It has demonstrated reliability and validity, requires approximately 20 minutes to administer, and is available in a Spanish version (TOFHLA-S) as well as English (Parker, et al., 1995; Williams et al., 1995; Quirk, 2000).

Readability formulas and standardized tests for comprehension and reading skills were never designed for the purpose of serving as writing guides. Patient educators may be tempted to write PEMs to fit the formulas and tests, but they should be aware that doing so places emphasis on structure, not content, and that comprehensibility of a written message may be greatly compromised. Pichert and Elam (1985) recommend that readability formulas should be used solely to judge material written without formulas in mind. Formulas are merely methods to check readability, and standardized tests are merely methods to

check comprehension and word recognition. Neither method guarantees good style in the form of direct, conversational writing.

## ▰ INSTRUMENT FOR SUITABILITY ASSESSMENT OF MATERIALS (SAM)

In addition to using formulas and tests to measure readability and comprehension, Doak et al. (1996) have addressed the dilemma of how to rapidly and systematically assess the suitability of instructional materials for a given population of patients. Ideally, instructional tools should be evaluated with a sample of the intended audience, but limited time and resources may preclude such an approach. In response to this dilemma, Doak's group developed the SAM instrument. Not only can SAM be used with print material and illustrations, but it has also been designed to be applied to video- and audiotaped instructions. SAM yields a numerical (percent) score, with materials tested falling into one of three categories: superior, adequate, or not suitable. The application of SAM can identify specific deficiencies in instructional materials that reduce their suitability. SAM includes factors and evaluation criteria to assess the content, literacy demand, graphics, layout and typography, learning stimulation and motivation, and cultural appropriateness of instructional materials being developed or already in use. For directions, a score sheet, and a description of the evaluation criteria, see Chapter 4 of Doak et al. (1996).

## ▰ SIMPLIFYING THE READABILITY OF PRINTED EDUCATION MATERIALS

Readability of written materials depends not only on actual reading skills, which can be measured by standardized tests, but also on those elements within a text such as technical format, concept demand, legibility, literacy level of the material, and accuracy and clarity of the message. It must never be forgotten that knowing the target audience in terms of their level of motivation, reading abilities, experiential factors, and cultural background is also of crucial importance in determining the appropriateness of printed health information as effective communication tools (Meade & Smith, 1991). Even good readers may fail to respond to important health education literature if they lack the motivation to do so or if the material is not appealing to them. Despite the well-documented potential of written materials to increase knowledge, compliance, and satisfaction with care, printed education materials are often too difficult for even motivated patients to read. Clearly, the technical nature of health education literature lends itself to high readability levels, often requiring college-level reading skills to fully comprehend (Winslow, 2001). Even though printed materials are the most commonly used form of media, as currently written, they remain the least effective means for reaching a large proportion of the adult population who have marginal literacy skills (Glanz & Rudd, 1990). What the nurse in the role of patient educator must strive to achieve when designing or selecting health-based literature is a good and proper fit between the material and the reader. Choosing and designing PEMs is a difficult, time-consuming, and challenging task that often becomes the responsibility of the nurse (Winslow, 2001).

Certainly the best solution for improving the overall comprehension and reading skills of patients would be to strengthen their basic general education, but this process will require decades to accomplish (Jackson et al., 1991). What is needed now are ways in which to write or rewrite educational materials commensurate with the current comprehension and reading skills of patients. Nathaniel Hawthorne was once reported to have said, "Easy reading is damned hard writing" (Pichert & Elam, 1985). He was correct in his perception that clear and concise writing is a

task that takes effort and practice. It is possible, though, to reduce the disparity between the literacy demand of written instructional materials and the actual reading level of patients by attending to some basic linguistic, motivational, organizational, and content principles. *Linguistics* refers to the type of language and grammatical style used. *Motivation principles* focus on those elements that stimulate the reader, such as relevance and appeal of the material. *Organizational factors* deal with layout and clarity. *Content principles* relate to load and concept density of information (Bernier, 1993). These elements will be examined as they relate to designing or revising instructional materials for the marginally literate reader.

Prior to writing or rewriting a text for easier reading, however, some preliminary planning steps need to be taken to ensure that the final written material will be geared to the target audience (Doak et al., 1996):

1. Decide what the patient should do or know. In other words, what is the purpose of the instruction? What outcomes do you hope the patient will achieve?

2. Choose information that is relevant and needed by the patient to achieve the behavioral objectives. Limit or cut out altogether extraneous and "nice to know" information such as the history or detailed physiological processes of a disease. Include only survival skills and essential main ideas of who, what, where, and when, with new information related to what the reader already knows. Remember: A person does not have to know how an engine works to drive a car.

3. Select other media to supplement the written information, such as pictures, demonstrations, models, audiotapes, and videotapes. Even poor readers will benefit from written material if it is combined with other forms of delivering a message. Consider the field of advertising, for example. Advertisers get their message across with

words but often in combination with strong, action-packed visuals.

4. Organize topics into chunks that follow a logical sequence. Prioritize to present the most important information first. If topics are of equal importance, proceed from the more general as a basis on which to build to the more specific. Begin with a statement of purpose. In a list of items, place key facts at the top and bottom, because readers best remember information presented first and last in a series.

5. Determine the preferred reading level of the material. If the readers have been tested, preferably write two to four grades below the reading grade-level score. If the audience has not been tested, the group is likely to display a wide range of reading skills. When in doubt, write instructional materials at the fifth-grade level, which is the lowest common denominator, keeping in mind that the average reading level of the population is approximately fifth to eighth grade, that more than 20% read below the fifth-grade level, and that fewer than 50% read above the tenth-grade level. To cover a wide range of reading skills, it is also possible to develop two sets of instructions—one at a higher grade level and one at a lower grade level—and allow patients to select the one they prefer (Table 7–3). Once the reading grade level of a piece of written material is determined, it should be printed on the back of the document in coded form, as the reading level (RL), for easy reference.

The literature contains numerous references related to techniques for writing effective educational materials (Doak et al., 1996; Brooks, 1998; Brownson, 1998; Doak et al., 1998; Duffy & Snyder, 1999; Buxton, 1999; Doak & Doak, 1987; Bernier, 1993; Wong, 1992). Recommendations have been put forth for developing written instructions that can be more easily understood by a wide audience. General guidelines for writing PEMs with

## TABLE 7–3   Example of lowered readability level

### NINTH-GRADE LEVEL

*Smoking contributes to heart disease in the following ways:*

1. When you smoke, you inhale carbon monoxide and nicotine, which causes your blood vessels to narrow, your heart rate to increase, and your blood pressure to go up. All of these factors increase the workload for your heart.

2. Carbon monoxide stimulates your body to produce more red blood cells. The presence of more red cells means that your blood will clot more readily, leading to increased risk of coronary artery disease and stroke.

3. Carbon monoxide and nicotine may also increase your risk of atherosclerotic buildup by causing damage to your artery walls.

4. Smoking raises blood cholesterol level and has been known to cause irregular heartbeats.

### FOURTH-GRADE LEVEL

*Smoking hurts your heart in many ways:*

1. Smoking makes your heart beat faster, raises your blood pressure, and makes your blood vessels smaller. All these things cause your heart to work harder.

2. Smoking makes your blood clot easier. This increases your chance of having a heart attack or a stroke.

3. Smoking makes your cholesterol level go up. It may also damage your blood vessels.

4. Smoking may make your heartbeat less regular.

SOURCE: From Martha Wong, "Self-Care Instructions: Do Patients Understand Educational Materials?" Reprinted with permission of American Association of Critical-Care Nurses from *Focus on Critical Care, 19,*(1), February 1992.

clarity and completeness can be found in Chapter 12.

Although there may be some overlap of information, the strategies described in this section are specific with regard to simplifying written health information for patients with low literacy skills. The key factor in accommodating low-literate patients is to write in plain, familiar language using an easy visual format. The following are some basic linguistic, motivational, organizational, and content principles to adhere to when writing PEMs:

1. Write in a conversational style using the personal pronoun you and the possessive pronoun your. Write in an active voice using the present tense rather than a passive voice using the past or future tense. The message is more personalized, more imperative, more interesting, and easier to understand if instruction is written as "Take your medicine . . ." instead of "Medicine should be taken. . . ." This rule is considered to be the most important technique to reduce the level of reading difficulty and to improve comprehension of what is read. Speaking directly to the reader through personal words and sentences engages the reader. For example:

**LESS EFFECTIVE**

People who sunburn easily and have fair skin with red or blond hair are most prone to develop skin cancer.

The amount of time spent in the sun affects a person's risk of skin cancer.[1]

**MORE EFFECTIVE**

If you sunburn easily and have fair skin with red or blond hair, you are more likely to get skin cancer.

How much time you spend in the sun affects your risk of skin cancer.

2. Use short words with only one or two syllables as much as possible. Rely on sight words, known as high-frequency words, such as there, said, come, stop, house, and go, which are recognized by almost everyone. The key is to choose words that sound familiar and natural and are easy to read and understand, like shot rather than injection and use instead of utilize. Avoid compound words, such as lifesaver, and words with prefixes or suffixes, such as reoccur or emptying, that create multisyllable words. Also, try to avoid technical words and medical terms, and substitute common, nontechnical, lay terms such as stroke instead of cerebral /vascular accident. Be careful to select substitutions carefully, because they may have a different meaning for some people than for others or in one context versus another. For example, if the word medicine is replaced with the word drug, the latter may be interpreted as the illegal variety. Use of modest words is not considered "talking down" to patients; it is considered "talking to" them at a more comfortable level.

3. Spell words out rather than using abbreviations or acronyms. That is should be used instead of i.e. and for example instead of e.g. Abbreviations for the months of the year (e.g., Sept.) or the days of the week (e.g., Wed.) are a real problem for patients with limited vocabulary. Also do not use CVA or NPO, for example, unless these medical abbreviations are clearly defined beforehand in the text.

4. Organize information into "chunks," which improves recall. Use numbers sparingly and only when absolutely necessary. Statistics are usually meaningless and are another source of confusion for the low-literate reader. Limit the number of items in

---

[1] Fry Now, Pay Later. American Cancer Society pamphlet, No. 2611, 1985.

any list to no more than seven. People have a difficult time remembering more than seven consecutive items (Baddeley, 1994).

5. Keep sentences short, preferably not longer than 20 words and less if possible, because they are easier to read and understand for readers with short-term memories. Avoid subordinate (dependent) clauses that make the reading more difficult. The use of commas, colons, or dashes make for long, complex sentences that "turn off" the reader. Titles also should be short and convey the purpose and meaning of the material that follows.

6. Clearly define any technical or unfamiliar words by using apposite phrases or parenthetical expressions—for example, "bacteria (germ)." A glossary of terms is a helpful tool, but defining the terms and spelling out difficult words phonetically immediately following the unfamiliar word within the text are most recommended, for example, "Alzheimer's (pronounced *Altz-hi-merz*)." New vocabulary should be taught in small increments and reviewed frequently (Spees, 1991; Byrne & Edeani, 1984). Standal's (1981) method suggests identifying words whose meanings should be taught to the reader prior to introducing the instructional material to increase comprehensibility and to avoid having to make major revisions to a printed piece.

7. Use words consistently throughout the text. Avoid interchanging of words such as *diet, meal plan, menu, food schedule,* and *dietary prescription,* which merely confuses the reader and can lead to misunderstanding of instruction.

8. Avoid value judgment words such as *excessive* and *regularly.* How much pain or bleeding is excessive? How often is regularly? Use exact terms to describe what you mean by using, for example, a scale of 1–5 or explaining frequency in terms of minutes, hours, or days.

9. Put the most important information first by prioritizing the "need to know."

10. Use advance organizers (topic headings or headers) and subheadings. They clue the reader into what is going to be presented and help focus the reader's attention on the message.

11. Limit the use of connectives such as *however, consequently, even though,* and *in spite of* that lengthen sentences and make them more complex.

12. Make the first sentence of a paragraph the topic sentence, and, if possible, make the first word the topic of the sentence. For example:

**LESS EFFECTIVE**

Even though overexposure to the sun is the leading cause, it isn't necessary to give up the outdoors in order to reduce your chances of developing skin cancer.[1]

**MORE EFFECTIVE**

Enjoying the outdoors is still possible if you take steps to reduce your risk of skin cancer when in the sun.
or
Your chance of skin cancer can be reduced even when enjoying the outdoors.

13. Reduce concept density by limiting each paragraph to a simple message or action and include only one idea per sentence. In the following example, the first paragraph contains at least six concepts. As rewritten, the second paragraph has been reduced to four concepts (and is written using the second person pronoun, which is a much more personalized approach):

A person who has had a stroke may or may not be able to return to his or her former level of functioning, depending on the extent and location of brain damage. Mental attitude, efforts of the rehabilitation team and the understanding of family and friends also affect the patient's progress. Recovery must be gradual, but it should begin the moment the patient is hospitalized. After the patient is tested to determine the extent of brain damage, rehabilitation such as physical, speech, and occupational therapy should begin. Family and friends should be told how to handle special problems the stroke victim may have, such as irrational behavior or difficulty communicating.[2]

Returning to your normal life after a stroke is an important part of your recovery. Each stroke patient is different and your progress depends on where and how much the brain is damaged. Your rehabilitation must be gradual and therapy will begin to meet your needs while you are in the hospital. Your mental attitude, the treatment given by the medical team, and the caring from your family and friends will help you handle special problems.

14. Keep density of words low by not exceeding 30–40 characters (letters) per line.

15. Allow for plenty of white space in margins, and use generous spacing between paragraphs and double spacing between sentences to reduce density. Uncrowded pages seem less overwhelming to the reader with low literacy skills.

16. Keep right margins unjustified because the jagged right margins help distinguish one line from another. In this way, the eye does not have to adjust to different spacing between letters and words as it does with justified type.

17. Design layouts that encourage eye movement from left to right, as in normal reading. In simple drawings and diagrams, using arrows or circles that give direction is helpful, but do not add too many elements to a schematic.

---

2 Adapted from American Heart Association (1983). *An Older Person's Guide to Cardiovascular Health*, National Center, 7320 Greenville Avenue, Dallas, TX: 75321. The information from this booklet is not current and is used for illustrative purposes only.

18. Select a simple type style (serif) and a large font (14 or 18 print size) in the body of the text for ease of reading and to increase motivation to read. A sans serif font (without little hooks at the top and bottom of letters) should be used only for titles to give style to the handout. Avoid *italics, fancy lettering,* or all CAPITAL letters. Low-literate readers are not fluent with the alphabet and need to look at each letter to recognize a word. To facilitate decoding of words in titles, headings, and subheadings, use upper- and lowercase letters, which provide reading cues given by tall and short letters on the type line. Avoid using a large stylized letter to begin a new paragraph.

This looks attractive, but it is confusing to a poor reader who cannot decode the word minus the first letter.

19. Highlight important ideas or terms with bold type or underlining.

20. If using color, employ it consistently throughout the text to emphasize key points or to organize topics. Color, if used appropriately, attracts the reader. Red, yellow, and orange are warm colors that are more eye-catching and easier to read than cold colors such as violet, blue, and green.

21. Create a simple cover page with a title that clearly and succinctly states the topic to be addressed.

22. Limit the entire length of a document—the shorter, the better. It should be long enough just to cover the essential information. Too many pages will "turn off" even the most eager and capable reader.

23. Select paper that is attractive and on which the typeface is easy to read. Black print on white paper is most easily read and most economical. Dull finishes reduce the glare of light, while high-gloss

paper reflects light into the eyes of the reader and is usually too formal and not in harmony with the purpose and informal tone of your message.

24. Use bold line drawings and simple, realistic diagrams. Basic visuals aid the reader to better understand the text information. Use cartoons judiciously, however, because they can trivialize the message and make it less credible. Graphic designs that are strictly decorative should never be used because they are distracting and confusing. Also, never superimpose words on a background design because it makes reading the letters of the words very difficult. Only illustrations that enhance understanding of the text and that relate specifically to the message should be used.

Be careful to use pictures that portray the messages intended. For example, avoid using a picture of a pregnant woman smoking or drinking alcohol because this negative message is dependent on careful reading of the text to correct a faulty impression. The visuals should clearly show only those actions that you want the reader to do and remember.

Use simple subtitles and captions for each picture. Also, be sure drawings are recognizable to the audience. For instance, if you draw a picture of the lungs, be certain they are within the outline of the person's body to accurately depict the location of the organ. The low-literate person may not know what they are looking at if the lungs are not put in context with the body's torso. However, pictures do not necessarily make the text easier to read if the readability level remains high. Be careful that visuals do not communicate cultural bias.

25. Include a summary paragraph to review in a different form what has already been presented. A question-and-answer format using the patient's point of view is an effective way to summarize information

in single units using a conversational style. The following example is adapted from the American Cancer Society pamphlet entitled *Fry Now, Pay Later* (1985):

Q: Am I likely to get skin cancer?

A: If you have spent a lot of time in the sun and if you sunburn easily and have fair skin with red or blond hair, you have a greater chance of getting skin cancer than people with dark skin or people who have stayed out of the strong sunlight.

Q: How can I tell if I have skin cancer?

A: The only way to know for certain if you have a skin cancer is to see your doctor. Your doctor may want to take a sample of skin to test for cancer if you have a problem such as red, scaly patches, a mole that has changed, or an area of the skin that does not heal.

Q: How can I prevent skin cancer?

A: Stay out of direct sunlight between 11 A.M. to 2 P.M. When in the sun, cover up with clothing, wear a wide-brimmed hat, and use sunscreens that block out the sun's harmful rays.

Ask for feedback after patients have read your instructions. Either have patients explain the information in their own words or have them demonstrate the desired behavior. If patients can do so correctly, it is a good indication that the information is understood. Do not ask questions such as "Do you understand?" because you are likely to get a "yes" or "no" answer, not a substantive response.

26. Put the reading level (RL) on the back of a written or revised PEM for future reference—for example, "Skin Cancer" (RL6).

It does not take a great deal of effort, just know-how and common sense, to improve the readability and comprehensibility of instructional materials (see Table 7–4 for a summary of guidelines). The benefits are significant in terms of compliance and quality of care when marginally literate patients are given PEMs that effectively communicate messages they can read and understand.

**TABLE 7–4   Summary of guidelines for designing effective low-literacy printed materials**

**CONTENT**

Clearly define the purpose of the material.

Decide when and how the information will be used.

Use behavioral objectives that cover the main points.

Verify the accuracy of content with experts.

Give "how to" information for the learner to achieve objectives.

Present only the most essential information (three to four main ideas: who, what, where, and when).

Relate new information to what the audience already knows.

Present content relevant to the audience and avoid cultural bias in writing and graphics.

**ORGANIZATION**

Keep titles short, yet use words that clearly convey the meaning of the content.

Provide a table of contents for lengthy material and a summary to review content presented.

Present the most important information first.

Use topic headings (advance organizers).

Make the first sentence of each paragraph the topic sentence.

Include only a few concepts per paragraph.

Use short, simple sentences that convey only one idea at a time; limit the length of the entire text.

Limit lists to no more than seven items.

Present each idea in logical sequence.

**LAYOUT/GRAPHICS**

Select large, easily read print (minimum 12-point type) and use nonglossy paper.

Write headings and subheadings in both lower- and uppercase letters; avoid fancy lettering.

Use bold type or underlining to emphasize important information.

Use lots of white space between segments of information.

Use generous margins and keep right-hand margins unjustified.

Provide a question-and-answer format for patient–nurse interaction.

Select double spacing (between lines of type), type style (serif), and font (print size) for ease of reading.

Design a colorful, eye-catching cover that suggests the message contained in the text.

**LINGUISTICS**

Keep sentences short (8–10 words).

Write in the active voice, using the present tense and the pronouns *you* and *your* to engage the reader.

Use one- to two-syllable words as much as possible; avoid multisyllabic (polysyllabic) words.

Use words familiar and understandable to the target audience.

Avoid complex grammatical structures (i.e., multiple clauses).

Limit the number of concepts.

Focus content on what the audience should do as well as know.

Use positive statements; avoid negative messages.

Use questions throughout the text to encourage active learning.

Provide examples the audience can use to relate to personal experiences/circumstances.

TABLE 7–4    (continued)

**LINGUISTICS**

Avoid using double negatives and value judgment words.

Clearly define terms likely to be unclear to audience.

**VISUALS**

Include simple, culturally sensitive illustrations and pictures.

Use simple drawings, but only if they improve the understanding of essential information.

Choose illustrations and photographs free of clutter and distractions.

Convey a single message or point of information in each visual.

Use visuals that are relevant to the text and meaningful to the audience.

Use drawings recognizable to the audience that reflect familiar images.

Use adult rather than childlike images (use cartoons sparingly).

Use captions to describe illustrations.

Use cues such as arrows, underlines, circles, and color to give direction to ideas and to highlight the most important information.

Use appealing and appropriate colors for the audience (for older adults, use black and white, and avoid pastel shades, especially blue, green, and violet hues).

**READABILITY AND COMPREHENSION**

Perform analysis with readability formulas and comprehension tests to determine reading level of material.

Write materials two to four grade levels below the determined literacy level of the audience.

Pilot-test the material to determine readability, comprehensibility, and appeal before its widespread use.

SOURCE: Adapted from Bernier (1993), p. 42, and from papers from the 16th Annual Conference on Patient Education, Nov. 17–20, 1994, Orlando, FL—sponsored by American Academy of Family Physicians and Society of Teachers of Family Medicine.

Always remember to pilot-test any new materials before printing and distributing them. Not only will this effort save the cost of printing handouts that might not be useful, but patients will have the opportunity to participate in the evaluative process (Brownson, 1998). Readily understandable materials also reduce time and frustration on the part of the nurse educator and avoid the possibility of litigation when better-quality and more appropriate healthcare instructions are used. The important role of printed media to communicate health information should compel all writers of PEMs to use the techniques recommended in this chapter. As Doak and Doak (1987) so aptly summarize, "With so much to be gained, the investments of a little time and thoughtful attention to the materials provided to patients can pay back dividends too important to ignore" (p. 8).

## TEACHING STRATEGIES FOR LOW-LITERATE PATIENTS

Working with illiterate and marginally literate patients requires more than designing simple-to-read instructional literature. It also calls for using alternative and innovative teaching strategies to break down the barriers of illiteracy. Using techniques to improve communication with patients has the potential to greatly enhance their understanding (Mayeaux et al., 1996). Teaching clients with poor reading skills does not have to be viewed as a problem but rather can be seen as a challenge (Dunn et al., 1985). Existing teaching methods and tools can be adapted to meet the logic, language, and experience of the patient who has difficulty with reading and comprehension (Doak et al., 1998). Incidentally, many literate and highly motivated patients also can benefit from some of these same teaching strategies. Many authors (Walker, 1987; Wallerstein, 1992; Fain, 1994b; Meade & Thornhill, 1989; Dunn et al., 1985; Hussey, 1991; Brez & Taylor, 1997; Doak et al., 1998; Winslow, 2001; Mayeaux et al., 1996; Murphy & Davis, 1997; Austin et al., 1995) suggest the following tips as useful strategies for the nurse educator to employ:

1. *Establish a trusting relationship before beginning the teaching–learning process.* Start by getting to know the patients and helping to reduce their anxiety. Because many poor readers have a history of being defensive, the nurse educator must attempt to overcome their defense mechanisms by casting aside barriers such as any preconceived notions, including myths and stereotypes, of illiterates as poor or from racial or ethnic minority groups. Focus on patients' strengths, demonstrate your belief in them as responsible individuals, and be open and honest about what specifically needs to be learned to build up their confidence in their ability to perform self-care activities. Encourage family and friends to help reinforce patients' self-confidence. Remember, you cannot learn for the patient, but you can facilitate learning by providing guidance and support.

2. *Use the smallest amount of information possible to accomplish the predetermined behavioral objectives.* Stick to the essentials, paring down the information you teach to what the patient must learn. Prioritize behavioral objectives, and select only one or two concepts to present and discuss in any one session. Present the context of the message first before giving any new information. Remember, patients with poor reading and comprehension skills are easily overwhelmed.

Information about the history of treatment, general principles, detailed physiology, and extraneous facts of a subject are not necessary for them to know. Keep teaching sessions short, limiting them to no more than 20 to 30 minutes.

3. *Make points of information as vivid and explicit as possible.* Explain information in simple terms, using everyday language and personal examples relevant to the patient's background (Spees, 1991; Byrne & Edeani, 1984; Lerner et al., 2000). Visual aids, such as signs and pictorials, should be large with readable print and contain only one or two messages. For example, a sign reading "NOTHING BY MOUTH" or, worse yet, "NPO" should be changed to "Do Not Eat or Drink Anything" (remember to avoid using all-capital letters and abbreviations). Underlining, highlighting, color coding, arrows, and common international symbols can be used effectively to give directions and draw attention to important information. For example, using different-colored floor tiles that lead to specific areas of the hospital and the use of other visual stimuli and pictorial cues are valuable for increasing independence and safety.

4. *Teach one step at a time.* Teaching in increments and organizing information into chunks help to reduce anxiety and confusion and give enough time for patients to understand each item before proceeding to the next unit of information. Also, a block format gives patients a sense of order, a chance to ask questions, and an opportunity for you to assess their progress and reward them with words of encouragement, praise, and reinforcement every step of the way. In addition, pacing of instruction allows for more adequate time between sessions for learners to assimilate information.

5. *Use multiple teaching methods and tools requiring fewer literacy skills.* Oral instruction contains cues such as tone, gestures, and expressions that are not found in written materials.

However, the spoken word lacks other signals, such as punctuation and capital letters. Therefore, a person with poor reading skills is likely to have some difficulty with comprehending the spoken language as well as with reading. There is no accepted way to test the difficulty level of oral instruction unless a spoken message is first taped, then converted into a written form, and finally a readability formula applied to it. Therefore, exposing patients to repetition and multiple forms of the same message is recommended. Audiotaped instruction, used in combination with other visual resources such as simple lists, pictorials, and videotapes, can help to improve comprehension and reduce learning time. These media forms, as more permanent sources of information, can also be sent home for added reinforcement of health messages. Interactive computer programs allow patients to proceed at their own pace and can be programmed developmentally to match patients' literacy skill levels.

6. *Allow patients the chance to restate information in their own words and to demonstrate any procedures being taught.* Encouraging patients to explain something in their own words may take longer and requires patience on the part of the educator, but feedback in this manner can reveal gaps in knowledge or misconceptions of information. Return demonstration, hands-on practice, role-playing real-life situations, and sharing personal stories in dialogue form are communication modes that provide you with feedback as to the patient's level of functioning. Trying to elicit feedback by asking questions of patients does not always work, because low literates often do not have the right vocabulary or fluency to explain what they do and do not understand. Remember, do not ask questions that will elicit only a "yes" or "no" response because patients will likely respond in the affirmative, even when they have no clue as to what

you are talking about, just so they do not have to admit their ignorance. Furthermore, they are unlikely to ask questions of you for fear of embarrassment at not understanding instructions. Ask open-ended questions, such as "Tell me what you understand about . . . ," to obtain feedback from patients to verify their comprehension. Encouraging patients to repeat instructions in their own words or physically demonstrate an activity is an effective approach to verifying what the patient really understands.

Story typing, a strategy used for low-level readers, is also a helpful technique. While audiotaping, patients listen to your oral instruction, they repeat it in their own words, and then the message (with corrections of any errors in procedural methods) is transcribed into a typed version using the patient's own phrases. In this way, patients can read the message themselves in familiar language as many times as necessary. Story typing is an especially effective technique in teaching functional skills such as administering medications, changing dressings, and the like.

7. *Keep motivation high.* It is important to recognize that illiterate persons may feel like failures when they cannot work through a problem. Reassure patients that it is normal to have trouble with new information and that they are doing well, and encourage them to keep trying. Recognition of progress being made, even in small increments, is motivating to the slow learner. Rewards—not punishments—are excellent motivators. Sticking to the basics and keeping the information relevant and succinct will maintain a patient's interest and willingness to learn.

8. *Build in coordination of procedures.* A way to facilitate learning is to simplify information by using the principles of tailoring and cuing. *Tailoring* refers to coordinating

patients' regimens into their daily schedules rather than forcing them to adjust their lifestyles to regimens imposed on them. Tailoring allows new tasks to be associated with old behaviors. It personalizes the message so that instruction is individualized to meet the patient's learning needs. For example, coordinating a medication schedule to patients' mealtimes does not drastically alter everyday lifestyle and tends to increase motivation and compliance. *Cuing* focuses on the appropriate combination of time and situation using prompts and reminders to get a person to perform a routine task. For example, placing medications where they best can be seen on a frequent basis or keeping a simple chart to check off each time a pill is taken serves as a reminder to comply with taking medications as prescribed. Both of these principles are related to the behavior modification theory and are especially useful techniques to encourage compliance with medications. Because poor readers often cannot decipher schedules, tailoring and cuing can assist them to adhere to time frames.

9. *Use repetition to reinforce information.* Repetition, at appropriate intervals, is a key strategy to use with low-literate clients. Each major point along the way must be reviewed repeatedly, and time must be set aside to remind learners of what has come before and to prepare them for what is to follow. Repetition, in the form of saying the same thing in different ways, is one of the most powerful tools to help patients understand their problems and learn self-care.

All of these teaching strategies are especially well suited to the individual needs of patients with low literacy skills. As noted ear-

lier, nurses must empower consumers by providing health information that is culturally and linguistically appropriate. Creating an open, trusting, and accepting environment that makes it acceptable for the client to say "I don't understand" is the cornerstone of effective communication (Cole, 2000). It is always a challenge to teach patients who, because of illness or a threat to their well-being, may be anxious, frightened, depressed, in denial, or in pain. Patient teaching is even more of a special challenge in today's healthcare environment, when varying degrees of literacy compound the ability of a significant portion of the adult population to understand information vital to their health and welfare.

## RESEARCH AND POLICY-MAKING ISSUES

The Ad Hoc Committee on Health Literacy for the Council on Scientific Affairs of the American Medical Association (1999) acknowledges that, although a great deal has been learned about the magnitude and consequences of the problem of illiteracy and low literacy, further research efforts must focus on four areas:

- Literacy screening
- Methods of health education
- Medical outcomes and economic costs
- Understanding the causal pathway of how health literacy influences health

The Committee also calls for healthcare policies to address the issue of health literacy for the following reasons:

1. Low-literate patients cannot be empowered consumers in a market-driven healthcare system.

2. Patients who cannot understand health-care instructions will not receive quality health care.

3. Healthcare professionals are subject to liability for adverse outcomes by patients who do not understand important health information.

4. Clinical management problems likely result in substantial but avoidable costs for the U.S. healthcare system.

5. Health literacy problems are more prevalent in certain populations (Medicare beneficiaries, Medicaid recipients, and uninsured individuals).

What is needed is a broad policy agenda on health literacy, which is reflected in the objectives of *Healthy People 2010* (U.S. Department of HHS, 2000) and additional research supported by federal and private funding.

## SUMMARY

The ability to learn from health instruction varies for patients, depending on their intellectual skills, educational background, motivational levels, and reading and comprehension skills. The prevalence of functional illiteracy and low literacy is a major problem in the adult population of this country. Nurses, in the role of teachers and interpreters of health information, must always be alert to the potentially limited capacity of patients to grasp the meaning of written and oral instruction. These educators need to know how to identify patients with literacy problems, assess their needs, and choose appropriate interventions that create a supportive environment directed toward helping patients with poor reading and comprehension skills to better and more safely care for themselves. An awareness of the incidence of illiteracy, at-risk populations, and the effects that literacy levels have on motivation and compliance with self-management regimens is key to understanding the barriers to communication between nurses and patients.

The first half of this chapter focused on the magnitude of the illiteracy problem, the myths and stereotypes associated with poor literacy skills, the assessment of variables affecting reading and comprehension of information, and the readability levels of patient education materials. The remainder of the chapter examined in detail the measurement tools available, ways to use them to test for readability and comprehensibility of patient education literature, guidelines for writing effective education materials, and specific teaching strategies to be used to match the logic, language, and experience of the low-literate patient. Data suggest that written materials are an important source of health information to reinforce and complement other methods and tools of instruction. PEMs are the most cost-effective and time-efficient means to communicate health messages, but research suggests that there is a large discrepancy between the average reading skills of patients and the readability level required with written instructional aids. Unless this gap is narrowed, printed sources of information will serve no useful purpose for illiterate and low-literate adult clients.

Removing the barriers to communication between patients and healthcare providers offers an ideal opportunity for nurse educators and other health professionals to work collaboratively to improve the quality of care delivered to consumers. It is our mandated responsibility to teach in understandable terms so that patients can fully benefit from our healthcare interventions.

## REVIEW QUESTIONS

1. What are the definitions of literacy, illiteracy, low literacy, and functional illiteracy?

2. What is the difference between the terms readability and comprehension?

3. Approximately how many million Americans are considered to be illiterate or functionally illiterate? This represents what percentage of the U.S. population?

4. Why are the rates of low literacy and illiteracy on the rise in the United States?

5. Why is the number of years of schooling a poor indicator of someone's literacy level?

6. What segments of the U.S. population are more likely to be at risk for having poor reading and comprehension skills?

7. Why is the low literacy and illiteracy problem greater in older adults than in younger age groups?

8. What are three (3) common myths about persons who are illiterate?

9. What are seven (7) clues that persons who are illiterate may demonstrate as indicators of deficiencies in reading and comprehension?

10. What impact does illiteracy or low literacy have on a person's level of motivation and compliance?

11. How does reliance on printed education materials to supplement teaching pose an ethical or legal liability for nurse educators?

12. Which measurement tools (standardized tests or formulas) are used specifically to test readability, comprehension, and reading skills?

13. What are ten (10) general guidelines to simplify written educational materials for clients with low literacy skills?

14. What five (5) teaching strategies can be used by the nurse educator to make health information more understandable for clients with poor reading and comprehension skills?

## REFERENCES

Adams-Price, C. E. (1993). Age, education, and literacy skills of adult Mississippians. *Gerontologist, 33*(6), 741–746.

Ad Hoc Committee on Health Literacy for the Council on Scientific Affairs, American Medical Association. (1999). Health literacy: Report of the Council on Scientific Affairs. *Journal of the American Medical Association, 281*(6), 552–557.

Anscher, M. S. & Gold, D. T. (1991). Literacy and laryngectomy: How should one treat head and neck cancer in patients who cannot read or write? *Southern Medical Journal, 84*(2), 209–213.

Austin, P. E., Matlock, R., Dunn, K. A., Kesler, C., & Brown, C. K. (1995). Discharge instructions: Do illustrations help our patients understand them? *Annals of Emergency Medicine, 25*(3), 317–320.

Baddeley, A. (1994). The magical number seven: Still magic after all these years? *Psychological Review, 101*(2), 353–356.

Barnes, L. P. (1992a). The illiterate client. *MCN: American Journal of Maternal-Child Nursing, 17*(2), 99.

Barnes, L. P. (1992b). The illiterate client: Strategies in patient teaching. *MCN: American Journal of Maternal-Child Nursing, 13*(3), 127.

Baydar, N., Brooks-Gunn, J., & Furstenberg, F. F. (1993). Early warning signs of functional illiteracy: Predictors in childhood and adolescence. *Child Development, 64*(3), 815–829.

Belton, A. B. (1991). Reading levels of patients in a general hospital. *Beta Release, 15*(1), 21–24.

Bernier, M. J. (1993). Developing and evaluating printed education materials: A prescriptive model for quality. *Orthopedic Nursing, 12*(6), 39–46.

Boyd, M. D. (1988). Patient education literature: A comparison of reading levels and the reading abilities of patients. *Advances in Health Education, 1*, 101–110.

Brez, S. M. & Taylor, M. (1997). Assessing literacy for patient teaching: Perspectives of adults with low literacy skills. *Journal of Advanced Nursing, 25*, 1040–1047.

Brooks, D. A. (1998). Nurse educator: Techniques for teaching ED patients with low literacy skills. *Journal of Emergency Nursing, 24*(6), 601–603.

Brownson, K. (1998). Education handouts: Are we wasting our time? *Journal for Nurses in Staff Development, 14*(4), 176–182.

Buxton, T. (1999). Effective ways to improve health education materials. *Journal of Health Education, 30*(1), 47–50, 61.

Byrne, T. & Edeani, D. (1984). Knowledge of medical terminology among hospital patients. *Nursing Research, 33*(3), 178–181.

Cole, M. R. (2000). The high risk of low literacy. *Nursing Spectrum, 13*(10), 16–17.

Dale, E. & Chall, J. S. (1978). The Cloze procedure: Measuring the readability of selected patient education materials. *Health Education, 9*, 8–10.

Davidhizar, R. E. & Brownson, K. (1999). Literacy, cultural diversity, and client education. *Health Care Manager, 18*(1), 39–47.

Davis, T. C., Crouch, M. A., Wills, G., Miller, S., & Abdehou, D. M. (1990). The gap between patient reading comprehension and the readability of patient education materials. *Journal of Family Practice, 31*(5), 533–538.

Denboba, D. L., Bragdon, J. L., Epstein, L. G., Garthright, K., & Goldman, T. M. (1998). Reducing health disparities through cultural competence. *Journal of Health Education, 29*(5), 47–51.

Doak, C. C., Doak, L. G., Friedell, G. H., & Meade, C. D. (1998). Improving comprehension for cancer patients with low literacy skills: Strategies for clinicians, *CA-A Cancer Journal for Clinicians, 48*(3), 151–162.

Doak, C. C., Doak, L. G., & Root, J. H. (1985). *Teaching Patients with Low Literacy Skills*, 1st ed. Philadelphia: Lippincott.

Doak, C. C., Doak, L. G., & Root, J. H. (1996). *Teaching Patients with Low Literacy Skills*, 2nd ed. Philadelphia: Lippincott.

Doak, L. G. & Doak, C. C. (1987). Lowering the silent barriers to compliance for patients with low literacy skills. *Promoting Health*, July/August, 6–8.

Duffy, M. M. & Snyder, K. (1999). Can ED patients read your patient education materials? *Journal of Emergency Nursing, 25*(4). 294–297.

Dunn, M. M., Buckwalter, K. C., Weinstein, L. B., & Palti, H. (1985). Teaching the illiterate client does not have to be a problem. *Family & Community Health, 8*(3), 76–80.

Estey, A., Musseau, A., & Keehn, L. (1991). Comprehension levels of patients reading health information. *Patient Education and Counseling, 18*, 165–169.

Fain, J. A. (1994a). Assessing nutrition education in clients with weak literacy skills. *Nurse Practitioner Forum, 5*(1), 52–55.

Fain, J. A. (1994b). When your patient can't read. *American Journal of Nursing, 94*(5), 16B, 16D.

Fetter, M. S. (1999). Recognizing and improving health literacy. *MEDSURG Nursing, 8*(4), 226.

Fisher, E. (1999). Low literacy levels in adults: Implications for patient education. *Journal of Continuing Education in Nursing, 30*(2), 56–61.

Fleener, F. T. & Scholl, J. F. (1992). Academic characteristics of self-identified illiterates. *Perceptual and Motor Skills, 74*(3), 739–744.

Flesch, R. (1948). A new readability yardstick. *Journal of Applied Psychology, 32*(3), 221–233.

Foltz, A. & Sullivan, J. (1998). Get real: Clinical testing of patients' reading abilities. *Cancer Nursing, 21*(3), 162–166.

French, K. S. & Larrabee, J. H. (1999). Relationships among educational material readability, client literacy, perceived beneficence, and perceived quality. *Journal of Nursing Care Quality, 13*(6), 68–82.

Fry, E. (1968). A readability formula that saves time. *Journal of Reading, 11*, 513–516, 575–579.

Fry, E. (1977). Fry's Readability Graph: Clarifications, validity, and extension to level 17. *Journal of Reading, 21*, 242–252.

Glanz, K. & Rudd, J. (1990). Readability and content analysis of print cholesterol education materials. *Patient Education and Counseling, 16*, 109–118.

Gollop, C. J. (1997). Health information-seeking behavior and old African American women. *Bulletin of the Medical Library Association, 85*(2), 141–146.

Gunning, R. (1968). The Fog Index after 20 years. *Journal of Business Communications, 6*, 3–13.

Hayes, K. S. (2000). Literacy for health information of adult patients and caregivers in a rural emergency department. *Clinical Excellence for Nurse Practitioners, 4*(1), 35–40.

Hess, V. T. (1998). Literacy and learning for hospital employees. *Journal for Nurses in Staff Development, 14*(3), 143–146.

Hirsch, E.D. (2001). Overcoming the language gap. *American Educator, 4*, 6–7.

Holt, G. A., Hollon, J. D., Hughes, S. E., & Coyle, R. (1990). OTC labels: Can consumers read and understand them? *American Pharmacy, NS30*(11), 51–54.

Hussey, L. C. (1991). Overcoming the clinical barriers of low literacy and medication noncompliance among the elderly. *Journal of Gerontological Nursing, 17*(3), 27–29.

Hussey, L. C. (1994). Minimizing effects of low literacy on medication knowledge and compliance among the elderly. *Clinical Nursing Research, 3*(2), 132–145.

Hussey, L. C. & Guilliland, K. (1989). Compliance, low literacy, and locus of control. *Nursing Clinics of North America, 24*(3), 605–611.

Jackson, R. H., Davis, T. C., Bairnsfather, L. E., George, R. B., Crouch, M. A., & Gault, H. (1991). Patient reading ability: An overlooked problem in health care. *Southern Medical Journal, 84*(10), 1172–1175.

Jackson, R. H., Davis, T. C., Murphy, P., Bairnsfather, L. E., & George, R. B. (1994). Reading deficiencies in older patients. *American Journal of the Medical Sciences, 308*(2), 79–82.

Jenks, S. (1992). Researchers link low literacy to high health care costs. *Journal of the National Cancer Institute, 84*(14), 1068–1069.

Johnson, K. R. & Layng, T. V. J. (1992). Breaking the structuralist barrier: Literacy and numeracy with fluency. *American Psychologist, 47*(11), 1475–1490.

Joint Commission on Accreditation of Healthcare Organizations. (1993). *Accreditation Manuals for Hospitals—1993.* Chicago: JCAHO.

Jolly, T., Scott, J. L., Feied, C. F., & Sandford, S. M. (1993). Functional illiteracy among emergency department patients: A preliminary study. *Annals of Emergency Medicine, 22*(3), 573–578.

Kanonowicz, L. (1993). National project to publicize link between literacy, health. *Canadian Medical Association Journal, 148*(7), 1201–1202.

Kefalides, P. T. (1999). Illiteracy: The silent barrier to health care. *Annals of Internal Medicine, 130*(4), 333–336.

Kelly, C. K. (1999). Helping low-literacy patients: What they don't know can hurt them. *Professional Medical Assistant*, Jan.–Feb., 8–13.

Kirsch, I. S., Jungeblat, A., Jenkins, L., & Kolstad, A. (1993). *Adult Literacy in America: A First Look at Results of the National Adult Literacy Survey.* Washington, D.C.: National Center for Education Statistics, U.S. Department of Education.

Kozol, J. (1985). *Illiterate America.* New York: Doubleday.

Lasater, L. & Mehler, P. S. (1998). The illiterate patient: Screening and management. *Hospital Practice, 33*(4), 163–165, 169–170.

Lerner, E. B., Jehle, D. V. K., Janicke, D. M., & Moscati, R. M. (2000). Medical communication: Do our patients understand? *American Journal of Emergency Medicine, 18*(7), 764–766.

Ley, P. & Florio, T. (1996). The use of readability formulas in health care. *Psychology, Health & Medicine, 1*(1), 7–28.

Loughrey, L. (1983). Dealing with the illiterate patient . . . You can't read him like a book. *Nursing, 13*(1), 65–67.

Mailloux, S. L., Johnson, M. E., Fisher, D. G., & Pettibone, T. J. (1995). How reliable is computerized assessment of readability? *Computers in Nursing, 13*(5), 221–225.

Mayeaux, E. J., Murphy, P. W., Arnold, C., Davis, T. C., Jackson, R. H., & Sentell, T. (1996). Improving patient education for patients with low literacy skills. *American Family Physician, 53*(1), 205–211.

McLaughlin, G. H. (1969). SMOG-grading: A new readability formula. *Journal of Reading, 12*, 639–646.

Meade, C. D., Diekmann J., & Thornhill, D. G. (1992). Readability of American Cancer Society patient education literature. *Oncology Nursing Forum, 19*(1), 51–55.

Meade, C. D. & Smith, C. F. (1991). Readability formulas: Cautions and criteria. *Patient Education and Counseling, 17*, 153–158.

Meade, C. D. & Thornhill, D. G. (1989). Illiteracy in healthcare. *Nursing Management, 20*(10), 14–15.

Miller, B. & Bodie, M. (1994). Determination of reading comprehension level for effective patient health-education materials. *Nursing Research, 43*(2), 118–119.

Morgan, P. P. (1993). Illiteracy can have major impact on patients' understanding of health care information. *Canadian Medical Association Journal, 148*(7), 1196–1197.

Morra, M. E. (1991). Future trends in patient education. *Seminars in Oncology Nursing, 7*(2), 143–145.

Murphy, P. & Davis, T. C. (1997). When low literacy blocks compliance. *RN, 60*(10), 58, 60–63.

Osborne, H. (1999). In other words . . . Getting through . . . Lives can depend on simplifying the written word. *On-Call, 2*(9), 42–43.

Owen, P. M., Johnson, E. M., Frost, C. D., Porter, K. A., & O'Hare, E. (1993). Reading, readability, and patient education materials. *Cardiovascular Nursing, 29*(2), 9–13.

Owen, P. M., Porter, K. A., Frost, C. D., O'Hare, E., & Johnson, E. (1993). Determination of the readability of educational materials for patients with cardiac disease. *Journal of Cardiopulmonary Rehabilitation, 13*(1), 20–24.

Parikh, N. S., Parker, R. M., Nurss, J. M., Baker, D. W., & Williams, M. V. (1996). Shame and health literacy: The unspoken connection. *Patient Education and Counseling, 27*, 33–39.

Parker, R., Baker, D., Williams, M., & Nurss, J. (1995). The test of functional health literacy in adults (TOFHLA): A new instrument for measuring patients' literacy skills. *Journal of General Internal Medicine, 10*, 537–545.

Pearson, M. & Wessman, J. (1996). Gerogogy. *Home Healthcare Nurse, 14*(8), 631–636.

Pichert, J. W. & Elam, P. (1985). Readability formulas may mislead you. *Patient Education and Counseling, 7*, 181–191.

Powers, R. D. (1988). Emergency department patient literacy and the readability of patient-directed materials. *Annals of Emergency Medicine, 17*(2), 124–126.

Quirk, P. A. (2000). Screening for literacy and readability: Implications for the advanced practice nurse. *Clinical Nurse Specialist, 14*(1), 26–32.

Robinson, J. H. (2000). Increasing students' cultural sensitivity: A step towards greater diversity in nursing. *Nurse Educator, 25*(3), 131–135, 144.

Rudolph, R. S. (1994). What Mr. Connor couldn't say. *Nursing, 24*(6), 47–48.

Silva, M. C. & Sorrell, J. M. (1984). Factors influencing comprehension of information for informed consent: Ethical implications for nursing research. *International Journal of Nursing Studies, 21*(4), 233–240.

Spache, G. (1953). A new readability formula for primary-grade reading materials. *Elementary School Journal, 53*(7), 410–413.

Spadero, D. C. (1983). Assessing readability of patient information materials. *Pediatric Nursing, 9*(4), 274–278.

Spadero, D. C., Robinson, L. A., & Smith, L. T. (1980). Assessing readability of patient information materials. *American Journal of Hospital Pharmacy, 37*, 215–221.

Spees, C. M. (1991). Knowledge of medical terminology among clients and families. *Image: Journal of Nursing Scholarship, 23*(4), 225–229.

Standal, T. C. (1981). How to use readability formulas more effectively. *Social Education, 45*, 183–186.

Stephens, S. T. (1992). Patient education materials: Are they readable? *Oncology Nursing Forum, 19*(1), 83–85.

Swanson, J. M., Forrest, K., Ledbetter, C., Hall, S., Holstine, E. J., & Shafer, M. R. (1990). Readability of commercial and generic contraceptive instructions. *Image: Journal of Nursing Scholarship, 22*(2), 96–100.

TenHave, T. R., VanHorn, B., Kumanyika, S., Askov, U., Matthews, Y., & Adams-Campbell, L. L. (1997). Literacy assessment in a cardiovascular nutrition education setting. *Patient Education and Couseling, 31*, 139–150.

Thomison, J. B. (1991). Why Johnny is illiterate. *Southern Medical Journal, 84*(5), 547–548.

United States Department of Education. (1993). *Adult Literacy in America: National Adult Literacy Survey.* Washington, D.C.

United States Department of Health and Human Services. (2000). *Healthy People 2010, vol. II.* Washington, D.C.: U.S. Government Printing Office.

Walker, A. (1987). Teaching the illiterate patient. *Journal of Enterostomal Therapy, 14*(2), 83–86.

Wallerstein, N. (1992). Health and safety education for workers with low-literacy or limited-English skills. *American Journal of Industrial Medicine, 22*(5), 751–765.

*Webster's Collegiate Dictionary*, 10th ed. (1999). Springfield, MA: Merriam Webster.

Weinrich, S. P. & Boyd, M. (1992). Education in the elderly. *Journal of Gerontological Nursing, 18*(1), 15–20.

Weiss, B. D., Reed, R. L., & Kligman, E. W. (1995). Literacy skills and communication methods of low-income older persons. *Patient Education and Counseling, 25*, 109–119.

Williams, D. M., Counselman, F. L., & Caggiano, C. D. (1996). Emergency department discharge instructions and patient literacy: A problem of disparity. *American Journal of Emergency Medicine, 14*(1), 19–22.

Williams, M. V., Parker, R. M., Baker, D. W., Parikh, W. S., Pitkin, K., Coates, W. C., & Nurss, J. R. (1995). Inadequate functional health literacy among patients at two public hospitals. *Journal of the American Medical Association, 274*(21), 1677–1682.

Williams-Deane, M. & Potter, L. S. (1992). Current oral contraceptive use instructions: An analysis of patient package inserts. *Family Planning Perspectives, 24*(3), 111–115.

Wilson, F. L. (1995). Measuring patients' ability to read and comprehend: A first step in patient education. *Nursing Connections, 8*(4), 17–25.

Winslow, E. H. (2001). Patient education materials: Can patients read them, or are they ending up in the trash? *American Journal of Nursing, 101*(10), 33–38.

Wong, M. (1992). Self-care instructions: Do patients understand educational materials? *Focus on Critical Care, 19*(1), 47–49.

Yasenchak, P. A. & Bridle, M. J. (1993). A low-literacy skin care manual for spinal cord injury patients. *Patient Education and Counseling, 22*(1), 1–5.

Ziegler, J. (1998). How literacy drives up health care costs. *Business & Health, 16*(4), 53–54.

Zimm, A. (1998). The need to understand: Addressing issues of low literacy and health. *On-Call, 1*(4), 20–23.

# CHAPTER 8

# Gender, Socioeconomic, and Cultural Attributes of the Learner

*Susan B. Bastable*

## CHAPTER HIGHLIGHTS

## KEY TERMS

gender-related cognitive abilities
socioeconomic status (SES)
poverty circle (cycle)
acculturation
assimilation
cultural assessment
cultural competence
cultural diversity
cultural relativism
culture

culturological assessment
ethnicity
ethnocentrism
ethnomedical
historically underrepresented groups
ideology
minority groups
subcultures
transcultural nursing
stereotyping

## OBJECTIVES

After completing this chapter, the reader will be able to

1. Identify gender-related differences in the learner based on social and hereditary influences on brain functioning, cognitive abilities, and personality characteristics.

2. Recognize the influence of socioeconomics in determining health status and health behaviors.

3. Define the various terms associated with diversity.

4. Identify three approaches within clinical practice, academia, and research to prepare

practitioners to function in a culturally sensitive manner.

5. Examine cultural assessment from the perspective of different models of care.

6. Distinguish between the beliefs and customs of the four major cultural groups in the United States.

7. Suggest teaching strategies specific to the needs of learners belonging to each of the four historically underrepresented groups.

8. Examine ways in which transcultural nursing can serve as a framework for meeting the learning needs of various ethnic populations.

9. Identify the meaning of stereotyping, the risks involved, and ways to avoid stereotypical behavior.

Gender, socioeconomic level, and cultural background have a significant influence on a learner's willingness and ability to respond to and make use of the teaching–learning situation. Two of these factors—gender and socioeconomic status—have been given very little attention to date by nurse educators. The third factor, cultural and ethnic diversity, has been the focus of considerable study in recent years with respect to its effects on learning. Understanding diversity, particularly those variations among learners related to gender, socioeconomics, and culture, is of major importance when designing and implementing education programs to meet the needs of an increasingly unique population of learners.

This chapter explores how individuals respond differently to healthcare interventions through examination of gender-related differences resulting from heredity or social conditioning that affects how the brain functions for learning, the influence of environment on the learner from a socioeconomic viewpoint, and the significant effects cultural norms have on the behaviors of learners from the perspective of the four major subcultures in the United States. In addition, models for cultural assessment and the planning of care are highlighted. This chapter also includes ways to prepare nurses for diversity care and to deal with the issue of stereotyping.

## GENDER DIFFERENCES

Most of the information on gender differences with respect to learning can be found in the educational psychology literature. Nursing literature contains scant information about this subject from a teaching–learning perspective. There are, however, differences between males and females that affect their learning, and this issue needs to be addressed more closely. Two well-established facts exist. First, individual differences within a group are usually greater than differences between groups. Second, studies that compare the sexes seldom are able to separate out genetic differences from environmental influences on behavior (Gage and Berliner, 1998; MacCoby & Jacklin, 1974; Woolfolk, 1998; Ormrod, 1995).

Despite the sophistication of social sciences research, there remains a gap in knowledge of what the sexes would be like if humans were not subject to behavioral conditioning. As no person can survive outside a social matrix, individuals begin to be shaped by their environment right from birth. For example, our U.S. culture exposes girls and boys, respectively, to pink and blue blankets in the nursery, dolls and trucks in preschool, ballet and basketball in the elementary grades, and cheerleading and football in high school. These social influences continue to affect the sexes throughout the life span. However, studies that show gender-related differences in intellectual functioning tend to overestimate their findings. The results of those studies that do not identify gender differences usually fail to get published or little attention is paid to the results (Gage & Berliner, 1998). Thus, the extent to which learning is affected by differences between the sexes remains open to question.

Of course, men and women are different. But the question remains, How are they different when it comes to learning and to what can the differences be attributed? Biological and behavioral scientists have, to date, been unable to quantify the exact impact that genetics and environment have on the brain. Opinions are rampant, and research findings are inconclusive. One fact remains: There are sex differences as to how males and females act, react, and perform in situations affecting every sphere of life. In human relationships, for example, women's intuition tends to pick up subtle tones of voice and facial expressions, whereas men tend to be less sensitive to these communication cues; in navigation, women tend to have difficulty finding their way, while men seem to have a better sense of direction; in cognition, females tend to excel in languages and verbalization, and men demonstrate stronger spatial and mathematical abilities. Scientists are beginning to believe that gender differences have as much to do with the biology of the brain as with the way people are raised (Gorman, 1992).

Some would argue that these examples are representative of stereotyping. Perhaps, but as generalizations these statements seem to hold enough truth that neuroscientists have begun to suspect structural as well as functional differences in the brains of males and females. This suspicion has led to an upsurge in research into the mental lives of men and women.

The field of neuroscience is wide open to exploration as to how the human brain works. Neurobiologists are just at the dawn of understanding exactly which types of sensory input, or experiences, wire the brain and in which ways. Scientists expect that cognitive abilities work much like sensory ones in that they are promoted by those activities to which a person is exposed from birth. Circuits in different regions of the brain are thought to mature at different stages of development. These circuits are critical "windows of opportunity" at different ages for the learning of math, music, language, and emotion and are much more sensitive to life experiences than once believed (Begley, 1996; Hancock, 1996). A baby's brain is like "a work in progress, trillions of neurons waiting to be wired . . . to be woven into the intricate tapestry of the mind" (Begley, 1996, pp. 55-56). Some of the neurons of the brain have been hard-wired by genes, but trillions more are waiting to be connected by the influence of environment. Much like a computer programmer reconfiguring the circuits of a computer, the neurons of the brain have almost infinite potential. "Which keys are typed—which experiences a child has—determines whether a child grows up to be intelligent or dull, fearful or self-assured, articulate or tongue-tied" (Begley, 1996, p. 56). The first three years of life, it is being discovered, are crucial in the development of the mind. The wiring of the brain, a process both of nature and nurture, forms the connections that determine the ability to learn (Nash, 1997).

Thanks to technology, new multimillion-dollar imaging machines are revolutionizing the field of neuroscience. Functional magnetic resonance imaging (FMRI) and the more outdated positron emission tomography (PET) are designed to be able to observe human brains in the very act of cognating, feeling, or remembering (Monastersky, 2001; Speck et al., 2000; Kawamura et al., 2000; Yee et al., 2000). Fifteen years ago, only a few laboratories had access to such advanced technology. Today, 1500 studies are done per year, and the most widely read science journals publish articles that include colorful images of the brain almost weekly. Using the "tools du jour," computer monitors can display "the content of your skull, with all its folds and convolutions that make up your true identity" (Monastersky, 2001, p. A20). Amazing discoveries through brain scanning have been made, such as where the emotion of love resides in the brain. Nevertheless, researchers caution that although machines can measure blood flow in the brain that supports nerve activity, so far no machines can "read" or "interpret" a person's thoughts. The field of brain scanning still has far to go, but its potential is considered by experts to be incredible.

The trend in current studies is to focus on how separate parts of the brain *interact* while performing different tasks rather than focusing on only isolated regions of the brain associated with certain tasks to find out, for example, how the brain processes speech sounds. Cognitive scientists argue that the emphasis in the future needs to be on computational models that can explicitly reveal how cognition works (Monastersky, 2001).

Researchers have already reported that men and women use different clusters of neurons when they read than when their brains are "idling." In a study by Karwamura et al. (2000) focusing on the cerebral localization of the center for reading and writing music of a male patient, the authors concluded that the left side of the brain is involved in this type of task, just as it is in an individual's ability to read and write language. Also, gender differences in brain activity during working memory—an important component for performing many higher functions—have been examined with FMRI. In a study by Speck et al. (2000) of verbal working memory, the amount of brain activity increased with task difficulty. Interestingly, male subjects demonstrated right-sided dominance whereas females showed predominant activity in the left hemisphere, with higher accuracy and slightly slower reaction times than their male counterparts. The results revealed highly significant gender differences in the functional brain organization for working memory, which may be due to gender differences in problem-solving strategies or neurodevelopment of the sexes.

Provocative new studies are revealing that women engage more of their brains when thinking sad thoughts and, possibly, less of their brains when solving math problems. Functional brain data are yielding many new insights supporting the hypothesis that, in general, men and women have brains that work differently. For example, researchers reported that men and women employ different parts of their brains to figure out rhymes. In another study, although men and women were able to perform equally well in math problems, tests indicated that they seemed to use the temporal lobes of the brain differently to figure out problems. In yet another study, when men and women subjects were asked to conjure up sad memories, the front of the limbic system in the brain of women glowed with activity eight times more than in men. These results are just a few examples of some of the tentative, yet tantalizing, findings from research that are beginning to show that male and female identity is a creation of both nature and nurture. Along with genetics, life experiences and the choices men and women make in the course of a lifetime help to mold personal characteristics and determine gender differences in the very way the sexes think, sense, and respond (Begley et al., 1995).

Despite the differences in how men and women feel, act, process information, and perform on cognitive tests, scientists have been able to identify only a few gender differences in the brain structure of humans (Table 8–1). Most gender differences that have been uncovered are quite small, as measured statistically. Even the largest differences in *gender-related cognitive abilities* are not as significant as, for example, the differences found between male and female height. There is a

| TABLE 8–1 Gender differences in brain structure | | |
| --- | --- | --- |
| | Men | Women |
| **TEMPORAL LOBE** | | |
| Regions of the cerebral cortex help to control hearing, memory, and a person's sense of self and time. | In cognitively normal men, a small region of the temporal lobe has about 10% fewer neurons than it does in women. | More neurons are located in the temporal region where language, melodies, and speech tones are understood. |
| **CORPUS CALLOSUM** | | |
| The main bridge between the left and right brain contains a bundle of neurons that carry messages between the two brain hemispheres. | This part of the brain in men takes up less volume than a woman's does, which suggests less communication between the two brain hemispheres. | The back portion of the callosum in women is bigger than in men, which may explain why women use both sides of their brains for language. |
| **ANTERIOR COMMISSURE** | | |
| This collection of nerve cells, smaller than the corpus callosum, also connects the brain's two hemispheres. | The commissure in men is smaller than in women, even though men's brains are, on average, larger in size than women's brains. | The commissure in women is larger than in men, which may be a reason why their cerebral hemispheres seem to work together on tasks from language to emotional responses. |
| **BRAIN HEMISPHERES** | | |
| The left side of the brain controls language, and the right side of the brain is the seat of emotion. | The right hemisphere of men's brains tends to be dominant. | Women tend to use their brains more holistically, calling on both hemispheres simultaneously. |
| **BRAIN SIZE** | | |
| Total brain size is approximately 3 pounds. | Men's brains, on average, are larger than women's. | Women have smaller brains, on average, than men because the anatomical structure of their entire bodies is smaller. However, they have more neurons than men (an overall 11%) crammed into the cerebral cortex. |

SOURCE: Adapted from Begley et al. (March 27,1995), p. 51.

great deal of overlap; otherwise, "women could never read maps and men would always be lefthanded. That flexibility within the sexes reveals just how complex a puzzle gender actually is, requiring pieces from biol-ogy, sociology, and culture" (Gorman, 1992, p. 44).

With respect to brain functioning, there is likely a mix between the factors of heredity and environment that accounts for gender inequities. The following is a list of cognitive abilities and gender-related differences specific to each ability (Gage & Berliner, 1998; MacCoby & Jacklin, 1974; Woolfolk, 1998; Ormrod, 1995):

*General intelligence:* Various studies have not yielded consistent findings on whether males and females differ in general intelligence. When mean differences have occurred, they are small. On IQ tests, during preschool years, girls score higher; in high school, boys score higher on these tests. Differences may be due to greater dropout rates in high school for low-ability boys. Thus, overall no dramatic differences between the sexes have been found on measures of general intelligence.

*Verbal ability:* Girls learn to talk, use sentences, and use a greater variety of words earlier than boys. In addition, girls speak more clearly, read earlier, and do consistently better on tests of spelling and grammar. Originally, researchers believed females performed better than males on measures of verbal fluency, but recent research has questioned this early superiority of females in the verbal domain. On tests of verbal reasoning, verbal comprehension, and vocabulary, the findings are not consistent, and the conclusion is that no significant gender differences in verbal ability exist.

*Mathematical ability:* During the preschool years, there appears to be no gender-related differences in ability to do mathematics. By the end of elementary school, however, boys show signs of excelling in mathematical reasoning, and the differences in math abilities of boys over girls become even greater in high school. Recent studies reveal that any male superiority likely is related to the way math is traditionally taught—as a competitive individual activity rather than as a cooperative group learning endeavor. When the approach to teaching math is taken into consideration, only about a 1% variation in quantitative skills is seen in the general population. In our culture, math achievement differences may result from different role expectations. The findings on math ability and achievement can also be extended to science ability and achievement, as these two subjects are related.

*Spatial ability:* The ability to recognize a figure when it is rotated, to detect a shape embedded in another figure, or to accurately replicate a three-dimensional object is consistently better for males than for females. Of all possible gender-related differences in intellectual activity, the spatial ability of males is consistently higher than that of females and probably has a genetic origin. However, the magnitude of this sex difference accounts for only about 5% of the variation in spatial ability. Interestingly, women surpass men in the ability to discern and later recall the location of objects in a complex, random pattern. Scientists have reasoned that historically men may have developed strong spatial skills so as to be successful hunters, while women may have needed other types of visual skills so as to excel as gatherers and foragers of food (Gorman, 1992). Because differences that exist are declining and can be removed through special training, these factors make it unlikely that any strong gender explanation for the differences exists.

*Problem solving:* The complex concepts of problem solving, creativity, analytical skill, and cognitive styles, when examined, have led to mixed findings regarding gender differences. Men tend to try new approaches in problem solving and are more likely to be "field independent"; that is, they are less influenced by irrelevant cues and more focused on common features in certain learning tasks. Males also show more curiosity and significantly less conservatism than women in risk-taking situations. In the area of human relations, however, women perform better at problem solving than do men.

*School achievement:* Without exception, girls get better grades on average than boys, particularly at the elementary school level. Scholastic performance of girls is more stable and less fluctuating than that of boys.

Although no compelling evidence proves significant gender-linked differences in the areas of cognitive functioning mentioned above, some findings do reveal sex differences when it comes to personality characteristics (Gage & Berliner, 1998; MacCoby & Jacklin, 1974; Woolfolk, 1998; Ormrod, 1995). Most of the observed differences between the sexes in personality and affective behaviors are thought to be largely determined by culture but are, to some extent, a result of mutual interaction between environment and heredity:

*Aggression:* Males of all ages and in most cultures are generally more aggressive than females. The role of the gender-specific hormone testosterone is being investigated as a possible cause of the more aggressive behavior demonstrated by males. However, anthropologists, psychologists, sociologists, and scientists in other fields continue to disagree about whether aggression is biologically based or environmentally influenced. Regardless, male and female roles differ widely in most cultures, with males usually being more dominant, assertive, energetic, active, hostile, and destructive.

*Conformity and dependence:* Females have been found generally to be more conforming and more influenced by suggestion. The gender biases of some studies have

made these findings open to suspicion, however.

*Emotional adjustment:* The emotional stability of the sexes is approximately the same in childhood, but differences do arise in how emotional problems are manifested. Some evidence indicates that adolescent girls and adult females have more neurotic symptoms than males, but this tendency may reflect how society defines mental health in ways that coincide with male roles or the fact that tests to measure mental health usually have been designed by men and, therefore, may be biased.

*Values and life goals:* In the past, men have tended to show greater interest in scientific, mathematical, mechanical, and physically active occupations as well as to express stronger theoretical, economic, and political values. Women have tended to choose literary, social service, and clerical occupations and to express stronger aesthetic, social sense, and religious values. These differences have become smaller over time as women have begun to think differently about themselves, have more freely pursued career and interest pathways, and society has begun to take a more "equal opportunity" viewpoint for both sexes.

*Achievement orientation:* Females are more likely to express achievement motivation in social skills and social relations, whereas men are more likely to try to succeed in intellectual or competitive activities. This difference is thought to be due to sex-role expectations that are strongly communicated at very early ages.

How do the preceding observations on gender differences in intellectual functioning and personality relate to the process of teaching clients whom the nurse as educator encounters? Gender differences need to be investigated further for explanations of how and when females and males learn best. It is very difficult to differentiate between biological and environmental influences simply because these two factors are intertwined and influence each other. The cause, meaning, and outcome of these differences remain speculative at this time (Babcock & Miller, 1994).

The behavioral differences that are well documented include the fact that females have an accelerated biological timetable and, in general, are more prone to have verbal ability. Conversely, males lag behind females in biological development and attention span but tend to excel in visual-spatial ability and mathematical pursuits; during adolescence, they also surpass females in physical strength. With respect to gender differences and aging, men are biologically weaker, as suggested by life-span mortality rates. White females have a life expectancy of approximately 80 years compared to approximately 73 years for white males (U.S. Census Bureau, 2000). However, less is known about women's health because women's health issues have been underrepresented in research efforts, although this trend is changing.

Overall, women are likely to seek health care more often than men do. It is suspected that one of the reasons women have more contact with the healthcare system is that they traditionally have tended to be the primary caretakers of their children, who need pediatric services. In addition, during childbearing years, women seek health services for care surrounding pregnancy and childbirth. Perhaps the reason that men tend not to rely as much as women on care from health providers is because of the sex-role expectation by our society that men should be stronger. They also have a tendency to be risk takers and to think of themselves as more independent. Although men are less likely to pursue routine health care for purposes of health and safety promotion and disease and accident prevention, they typically face a greater number of health hazards, such as a higher incidence of automobile accidents, use of drugs and alcohol, suicide, heart disease, and engaging in dangerous occupations.

## Teaching Strategies

As health educators, nurses must become aware of the extent to which social and heredity-related differences between the genders affect health-seeking behaviors and influence individual health needs. It is imperative for nurses to have an understanding of the intellectual functioning and personality variables that affect how men and women learn, when they learn, what they are most adept at learning, and what they are interested in learning. As stated previously, in some areas males and females display different orientations, learning styles, and levels of success at communicating and learning (see Chapter 4). The differences seem to depend on their interests and past experiences in the biological and social roles of men and women in our society.

Women and men are part of different social cultures, too. They use different symbols, belief systems, and ways to express themselves, much in the same manner that different ethnic groups have distinct cultures (Tear, 1995). In the future, these gender differences may become less pronounced as the sex roles become more blended. For now, one especially must consider society's role in instilling certain characteristic learning behaviors in males and females, however stereotypical they may seem to be. Nurse educators are encouraged to use versatile teaching style strategies so as not to perpetuate stereotypical approaches to teaching and learning with the two genders.

## SOCIOECONOMIC DIFFERENCES

*Socioeconomic status (SES)*, in addition to gender differences, influences the teaching–learning process. SES is considered to be the single most important determinant of health in our society (Pappas et al., 1993; Crimmins & Saito, 2001). SES or socioeconomic class is an aspect of diversity that must be addressed in the context of education and in the process of teaching and learning. Class is the "unmentionable five-letter word" (Rhem, 1998, p. 1). Many people are hesitant to categorize themselves according to class. They also are reluctant to discuss the issue of class differences because of the widespread idea that the United States should be a classless country (Rhem, 1998). It is a myth, though, that America is a society without classes (McGoldrick, 1995). Rhem describes definitions of class as elusive because although class differences are felt everywhere, the question remains as to whether class depends on income level or educational level, on having a rural or an urban background, on the kind of work your parents do, on the inner sense of one's status compared with objective measures, or on a combination of some or all of these factors. If race cannot change and gender (typically) does not change, then understanding what could and should change about class distinctions may prove very useful in helping nurses, as well as other professionals, to reach people of different socioeconomic levels. Class, as universal as race or gender, "hides in the shadows" even though class consciousness is a commonality shared by everyone. Those who are privileged feel embarrassed about their advantages just as much as those who are poor feel embarrassed about their disadvantages (Rhem, 1998).

Social and economic levels of individuals have been found to be significant variables affecting health status and in determining health behaviors (Pappas et al., 1993; Crimmins & Saito, 2001). Approximately 40 million Americans are living in poverty (Morra, 1991). Poverty is defined as an income of less than $13,359 for a family of four living in an urban area. More than one in four American chil-

dren under the age of 18 are classified as impoverished; by 2020, the total number of children living in poverty is expected to reach 20 million (Woolfolk, 1998). Disadvantaged people—those with low incomes, low educational levels, and/or social deprivation—come from many different ethnic groups, including millions of poor white people (Morra, 1991; Woolfolk, 1998). SES takes into account the variables of educational level, family income, and family structure (Woolfolk, 1998; Gage & Berliner, 1998), all of which seem to affect health beliefs, health practices, and readiness to learn.

The relationships among poverty, suboptimal cognitive development, and academic failure have been well established, but the mechanics and processes involved are highly complex and remain poorly understood (Campbell & Ramey, 1994). Heredity and environment usually vary together; that is, people who are genetically related (parents and their children) tend to have similar environments. Evidence suggests that variations in heredity are equally as powerful as variations in environmental conditions in producing individual differences in cognitive ability (Gage & Berliner, 1998). Also, socioeconomic class is correlated with low educational levels. The significant correlation between literacy levels and SES is well documented in Chapter 7.

Although many educators, psychologists, and sociologists have recognized that a cause and effect relationship exists among low SES, low IQ score attainment, and poor quality of life, they are hard-pressed to know what to do about breaking the cycle. So, too, are healthcare providers, who recognize that patients belonging to lower social classes have higher rates of illness, more severe illnesses, and reduced rates of life expectancy. People with low SES, as measured by indicators such as income, education, and occupation, have increased rates of mortality compared to those with higher SES. Pappas et al. (1993) found that an inverse relationship exists between SES and mortality. Individuals who have higher incomes and are better educated live longer and healthier lives than those who are of low income and poorly educated. Thus, one finds a significant disparity between death rates of people of different incomes and educational backgrounds. Crimmins and Saito (2001) also found morbidity rates to be highly related to SES. People with more education and higher incomes have longer life expectancies and experience fewer adverse health events. These disparities in morbidity and mortality rates continue to widen for racial and educational subgroups in the United States (Crimmins & Saito, 2001; Pappas et al., 1993).

These studies demonstrate that the level of socioeconomic well-being is a strong indicator of health outcomes. Such research findings raise serious questions about health differences among our nation's people as a result of unequal access to health care due to SES. These unfortunate health trends are costly to society in general and to the healthcare system in particular. Although adverse health-related behavior and less access to medical care have been found to contribute to higher morbidity and mortality rates, there is newer but still limited research on the effect socioeconomic status has on disability-free or active life expectancy (Guralnik et al., 1993; Crimmins & Saito, 2001).

Social class is measured by one or more of the following types of indices: occupation of parents, income of family, location of residence, and educational level of parents. A number of studies have compared IQ scores of fathers and their sons, with their findings indicating that intelligence levels decrease for both groups as the father's social class goes down. Data clearly show that certain levels of intelligence are typically found in certain occupations and not others. For example, teachers, accountants, and engineers typically score above average in standardized tests of intelligence, whereas lumberjacks, teamsters, and cobblers score below average (Gage & Berliner, 1998). Certain occupations not only require certain levels of academic aptitude, but also attract people of a certain level of measured intelligence.

Whatever the factors that keep particular groups from achieving at higher levels, these groups are likely to remain on the lower end of the occupational structure. This cycle has been coined the *poverty circle* (Gage & Berliner, 1998; Nagoshi et al., 1993) or the *cycle of poverty* (Woolfolk, 1998). Gage and Berliner (1992) describe the poverty circle as follows:

> Parents low in scholastic ability and consequently in educational level create an environment in their homes and neighborhoods that produces children who are also low in scholastic ability and academic attainment. These children grow up and become parents, repeating the cycle. Like them, their children are fit only for occupations at lower levels of pay, prestige, and intellectual demand (p. 61).

Woolfolk (1998) explains that many factors, including poor health care for mothers and children, limited resources, family stress, discrimination, and low-paying jobs, maintain the cycle by which generation after generation are born into poverty.

In addition, Baydar et al. (1993) studied family environmental factors such as maternal education, family size, maternal marital status, and family income as predictors of illiteracy in children and adolescents. They point out that low levels of literacy have been linked to low productivity, high unemployment, low earnings, high rates of welfare dependency, and teenage parenting, all of which are common measures of a society's economic well-being.

Family structure and the home environment are not the only factors affecting proficiency in learning. Hirsch (2001) contends that the alarming verbal and reading gap between rich and poor students "represents the single greatest failure in American public schooling" (p. 5). Many low-income children entering kindergarten have heard only half the words and understand only half the meanings of language than the high-income child has heard and understands. This gap continues to widen along the same trajectory as students progress in each succeeding grade in school. Barriers to equal educational opportunity must be reduced by putting the responsibility on the educational system to become more intensive. That is, we need to develop standards for each grade and make sure each child meets these expectations before being allowed to progress to subsequent grades in school.

The lower socioeconomic classes have been studied more than others probably because the health views of this group deviate the most from those viewpoints espoused by health professionals who care for this group of individuals. People from the lower social stratum have been characterized as being indifferent to the symptoms of illness until poor health interferes with their lifestyle and independence. Their view of life is one of a sense of powerlessness, meaninglessness, and isolation from middle-class knowledge of health and the need for preventive measures, such as vaccination for their children (Lipman et al., 1994; Winkleby et al., 1992).

The high cost of health care may well be a major factor affecting health practices of people in the lower socioeconomic classes. Individuals with adequate financial and emotional resources are able to purchase services and usually have support systems on which to rely to sustain them during recovery or augment their remaining functions after the course of an acute illness. Conversely, individuals deprived of monetary and psychosocial resources are at a much greater risk for failing to reach an optimal level of health and well-being.

Just as socioeconomic status can have a negative effect on illness, so too can illness have devastating implications for a person's socioeconomic well-being. A catastrophic or chronic illness can lead to unemployment, loss of health insurance coverage or ineligibility for health insurance benefits, enforced social isolation, and a strain on social support

systems. Without the socioeconomic means to counteract these threats to their well-being, impoverished individuals may be powerless to improve their situation. These multiple losses tax the individual, their families, and the healthcare system.

Low-income groups are especially affected by changes in federal and state assistance in the form of Medicare and Medicaid. The spiraling costs associated with illness and consequent overuse of the healthcare system have resulted in increased interest on the part of the public and healthcare providers to control costs. Today, more emphasis is being given to health promotion, health maintenance, and disease prevention. The push for healthcare reform in this country has resulted in widespread efforts targeted toward the concept of managed care. Although such reform has not yet been realized at the national level, local and state legislators, hospital administrators, healthcare providers, health insurers, and others are consolidating their attempts to make healthcare reform a reality. For some, managed care means the reallocation of healthcare dollars to selected groups who will share the monies as well as the risks of keeping people healthy. It also means the opportunity to contain costs and eliminate duplication or misuse of tertiary healthcare services (Kinsey, 1995).

The current trends in health care, as a result of these economic concerns, are directed toward teaching individuals how to attain and maintain health. The nurse plays a key role in educating the consumer about avoiding health risks, reducing illness episodes, establishing healthful environmental conditions, and accessing healthcare services. The primary targets for these initial efforts at using public dollars to support managed care comprise the populations currently receiving medical assistance, such as low-income families in urban and rural areas. Kinsey (1995) believes that if planning is careful and collaborative between all parties concerned, including the consumer, managed care could yield positive outcomes.

If health resources could become more accessible and appropriate for socioeconomically deprived individuals, allowing them to stabilize and improve their health indices and maximize their family life, then society could realize true savings. However, achievement of these goals is contingent on many factors, such as collective public interest and deemphasis on profit motives, to find ways to ensure individual and family well-being and to improve the society's health overall. This author warns, however, that managed care, if not properly designed and carried out, could pose a threat to the health of low-income groups if their needs are neglected.

## Teaching Strategies

Educational interventions by nurses for those who are socially and economically deprived have the potential for yielding short-term benefits in meeting these individuals' immediate healthcare needs. However, more research must be done to determine whether teaching can ensure the long-term benefits of helping deprived people develop the skills needed to reach and sustain independence in self-care management. Nurse educators must be aware of the probable effects of low SES on an individual's ability to learn as a result of suboptimal cognitive functioning, poor academic achievement, low literacy, high susceptibility to illness, and disintegration of social support systems. Low-income people are at greater risk for these factors that can interfere with learning, but one cannot assume that everyone at the poverty or near-poverty level is equally influenced by these threats to their well-being. To avoid stereotyping, it is essential that each individual or family be assessed to determine their particular strengths and weaknesses for learning. In this way, teaching strategies unique to particular circumstances can be designed to assist socioeconomically deprived individuals in meeting their needs for health care.

Nevertheless, it is well documented that individuals with literacy problems, poor educational backgrounds, and low academic achievement are likely to have low self-esteem, feelings of helplessness and hopelessness, and low expectations. They also tend to think in concrete terms, are more focused on satisfying immediate needs, have a more external locus of control, and have decreased attention spans. They have difficulty in problem solving and in analyzing and synthesizing large amounts of information (Woolfolk, 1998; Gage & Berliner, 1998). With these individuals, the nurse educator will most likely have to rely on specific teaching methods and tools similar to those identified as appropriate for intervening with clients who have low literacy abilities (see Chapter 7).

## ▓▓ CULTURAL DIFFERENCES

At the beginning of the twenty-first century, more than one-quarter (28.6%) of the U.S. population is estimated to consist of people from culturally diverse groups (U.S. Census Bureau, 2000). People of minority have been predicted to be the majority in 53 of the 100 largest cities at that time (Morra, 1991). Also, future projections are for a continued increase in the number of legal and illegal immigrants and refugees coming into this country (Andrews, 1992). Therefore, in the immediate years to come, the major growth in the U.S. population and in the workplace will come from the ranks of historically underrepresented racial and ethnic groups. By 2080, people belonging to cultural subgroups will account for more than half (51%) of the U.S. total population. If predictions prove true, it will be the first time in U.S. history that minority subgroups will become the majority of the total population. If the present demographic trends continue, when this historical milestone is reached, the racial and ethnic composition of this country will be 23.4% Hispanics, 14.7% blacks, and

12% Asian and others (Morra, 1991). As of the year 2000, according to the U.S. Census Bureau, the current composition of the U.S. population was 71.3% whites, 12.2% blacks, 11.2% Hispanics, 3.8% Asian/Pacific Islanders, and 0.7% American Indians.

To keep pace with a society that is increasingly more culturally diverse, nurses will need to have sound knowledge of the cultural values and beliefs of specific ethnic groups as well as be aware of individual practices and preferences (Price & Cordell, 1994; Spicer et al., 1994; Rooda & Gay, 1993; Price & Cortis, 2000). In the past, healthcare providers have experienced difficulties in caring for clients whose cultural beliefs differ from their own, because beliefs about health and illness vary considerably among cultural groups. Lack of cultural sensitivity by healthcare professionals has resulted in millions of dollars wasted annually through misuse of healthcare services, the alienation of large numbers of people, and the misdiagnosis of health problems with often tragic and dangerous consequences. In addition, certain underrepresented groups are beginning to demand culturally relevant health care that respects their cultural rights and incorporates their specific beliefs and practices into the delivery of care. This expectation is in direct conflict with the unicultural, Western, biomedical paradigm taught in many nursing and other healthcare provider programs across the country. Andrews (1992) suggested that a serious conceptual problem exists within the nursing profession because nurses are presumed to understand and be able to meet the healthcare needs of a culturally diverse population, even though they do not have the formal educational preparation to do so.

## Definition of Terms

Before examining the major cultural subgroups within the United States, it is imperative to define the following terms commonly used in dealing with the subject of culture.

*Acculturation:* A willingness to modify one's own culture as a result of contact with another culture (Purnell & Paulanka, 1998). This term describes an individual's adaptation to the customs, values, beliefs, and behaviors of a new country. The degree of acculturation depends on many factors, such as time and willingness to assimilate to the traditions, values, and beliefs of another culture (Falvo, 1994). For example, some individuals may live in an adopted country for their entire lives but continue to cherish and practice the traditions, values, and beliefs of their original culture.

*Assimilation:* The willingness of a person emigrating to a new culture to gradually adopt and incorporate characteristics of the prevailing culture (Purnell & Paulanka, 1998).

*Cultural assessment:* "A systematic appraisal of beliefs, values, and practices conducted in order to determine the context of client needs and to tailor nursing interventions" (Tripp-Reimer & Afifi, 1989, pp. 613–614).

*Cultural competence:* A conscious process of demonstrating knowledge and understanding of a client's culture so as to recognize, accept, and respect cultural differences and to be able to incorporate these cultural beliefs and practices about wellness and illness into the delivery of care by adapting interventions to be congruent with the client's culture (Purnell & Paulanka, 1998; Denboba et al., 1998).

*Cultural diversity:* A term meaning "representing a variety of different cultures" (Purnell & Paulanka, 1998, p. 481). People are engaged in cultural diversity when they interact with others from a culture different from their own.

*Cultural relativism:* Implies that "the values every human group assigns to its conventions arise out of its own historical background and can be understood only in the light of that background" (Tripp-Reimer, 1982, p. 181). As Tripp-Reimer explains, the definitions of *ethnocentrism* and *cultural relativism* are two sides of the same coin, the first denoting the perspective of the health professional's culture and the second denoting the client's perspective.

*Culture:* A complex concept that is an integral part of each person's life and includes knowledge, beliefs, values, morals, customs, traditions, and habits acquired by each person as a member of a society. Purnell and Paulanka (1998) define culture as "the totality of socially transmitted behavioral patterns, arts, beliefs, values, customs, lifeways, and all other products of human work and thought characteristic of a population of people that guide their worldview and decision making" (p. 2).

*Culturological assessment:* Defined by Leininger (1978) as a "systematic appraisal or examination of individuals, groups, and communities as to their cultural beliefs, values, and practices to determine explicit needs and intervention practices within the cultural context of the people being evaluated" (pp. 85–86).

*Ethnicity:* A dynamic and complex concept referring to "how members of a group perceive themselves and how, in turn, they are perceived by others. . . . When ethnic identity is strong, individuals maintain ethnic group values, beliefs, behaviors, perspectives, language, culture, and ways of thinking" (Price & Cordell, 1994, p. 163). Ethnicity specifies a population subgroup that shares a common heritage of customs, characteristics, language, and history (Rempusheski, 1989). Incorporated in culture is ethnicity—the biological and racial background of an individual that may be linked to culture or separate from it. For example, someone's ethnic background may be French, but because he or she emigrated to another country several generations ago, the person may identify with the culture of the adopted country (Falvo, 1994).

*Ethnocentrism:* A concept describing "the universal tendency of human beings to think that their ways of thinking, acting, and believing are the only right, proper, and natural ways . . . Ethnocentrism perpetuates an attitude that beliefs that differ greatly from one's own are strange, bizarre, or unenlightened, and therefore wrong" (Purnell & Paulanka, 1998, p. 3).

*Ethnomedical:* A concept of illness incorporating the relationship of humans with the universe, bridging culture with a sensitivity toward the traditional practices of specific ethnic groups (Mail et al., 1989).

*Historically underrepresented groups:* A more politically sensitive and correct term used as a substitute for the word *minority*.

*Ideology:* Consists of the thoughts, attitudes, and beliefs that reflect the social needs and desires of an individual or ethnocultural group (Purnell & Paulanka, 1998).

*Minority groups:* The U.S. Census Bureau (2000) defines minority groups in this country as follows: Blacks (African, Haitian, and Dominican Republic descents), Hispanics (Mexican, Cuban, Puerto Rican, and other Latino descents), Asian/Pacific Islanders (Japanese, Chinese, Filipino, Korean, Vietnamese, Hawaiian, Guamian, Samoan, and Asian Indian descents), and American Indians (Eskimos and hundreds of tribes of Native Americans).

*Subcultures:* Ethnocultural groups of people "who have experiences different from those of the dominant culture by virtue of status, ethnic background, residence, religion, education, or other factors that functionally unify the group and act collectively on each member with a conscious awareness of these differences . . . subcultures differ from the dominant ethnic group and share beliefs according to the primary and secondary characteristics of diversity" (Purnell & Paulanka, 1998, p. 3).

*Transcultural nursing:* Defined by Leininger (1978) as "a formal area of study and practice focused on a comparative analysis of different cultures and subcultures in the world with respect to cultural care, health and illness beliefs, values and practices with the goal of using this knowledge to provide culture-specific and culture-universal care to people" (p. 493). Transcultural nursing, sometimes also referred to as *cross-cultural* or *intercultural nursing,* is a crossing over, spanning, or interacting with a culture other than one's own. It provides a framework for meeting the healthcare needs of culturally diverse groups.

## Approaches to Delivering Culturally Sensitive Care

Given our rapidly changing world and the significant increased geographical mobility of people around the globe, the reality is that our healthcare system and our educational institutions must respond by shifting from a dominant monocultural, ethnocentric focus to a more multicultural, transcultural focus. Tripp-Reimer and Afifi (1989) describe the interpretation of American cultural ideal from a historical perspective:

In the United States, the myth of the melting pot emerged largely from a combination of a cultural ideal of equality and a European ethnocentric perspective. This myth promoted the notion that all Americans are alike—that is, like white, middle-class persons. For many years, the notion that ethnicity should be dis-

counted or ignored was prominent in the delivery of health care, including health teaching programs. . . . the majority of health education programs have been one of two types: those developed by whites for use with white patients, or preexisting white programs adapted to an ethnic group by layering a thin veneer of cultural information over the white-based format. Recently, however, ethnicity has emerged as an important consideration for the effective delivery of health education programs (p. 613).

The question posed by Leininger (1994) remains, "How can nurses competently respond to and effectively care for people from diverse cultures who act, speak, and behave in ways different than their own?" Studies indicate that health professionals are often unaware of the complex factors influencing clients' responses to health care. In conducting a nursing assessment, six cultural phenomena need to be taken into account: communication, personal space, social organization, time, environmental control, and biological variations (Figure 8–1).

According to Anderson (1990), the cultural meanings that shape clients' experiences are not being taken into account when care is planned by practitioners. Strategies must be implemented to enhance the profession's ability to deliver care to culturally diverse populations in the United States as well as abroad (Hahn, 1995). Price and Cordell (1994) outlined a four-step approach to help nurses provide culturally sensitive patient teaching (Figure 8–2).

Hegyvary (1992) encourages the nursing profession to carefully consider the full meaning of diversity, not only as the reality of the future but as an exciting present-day challenge and opportunity for enrichment.

Andrews (1992) suggested three approaches for the nursing profession to undertake to prepare its practitioners for the future:

1. Within clinical practice settings, nursing staff from culturally diverse backgrounds

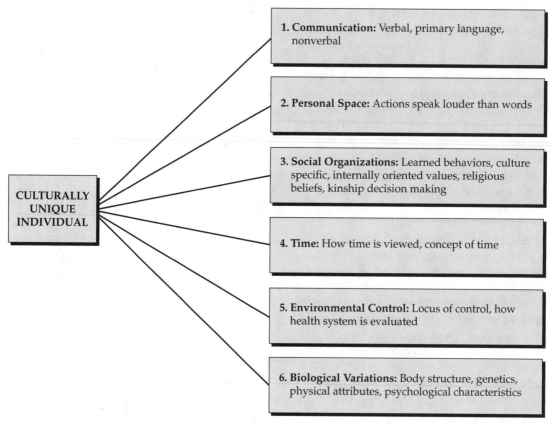

**FIGURE 8–1   Six Cultural Phenomena**  SOURCE: Adapted from Giger, J. N. & Davidhizar, R. E. (1995), *Transcultural Nursing: Assessment and Intervention*, 2nd ed., p. 9. St. Louis: Mosby–Year Book.

should be hired and promoted in increasing numbers. By design or by default, the nursing profession has a very homogeneous membership. It is imperative that minority issues be explored and recommendations from the profession be widely disseminated. There is a need for continuing education programs to raise the awareness of staff nurses about their own culturally based values, beliefs, and practices and to increase their knowledge base about culture-specific health-related beliefs and practices of others whom they are likely to encounter within their specialty areas of practice.

2. Within academic settings, undergraduate and graduate nursing programs have made steady progress in integrating cultural concepts into the nursing curricula. Nevertheless, more concentrated effort is needed from nurse educators who have formal, in-depth preparation in transcultural, cross-cultural nursing with perspectives from the related disciplines of anthropology and sociology. Teaching must focus on culturological assessment, biocultural variations in health and illness, and cultural differences in communication, religious beliefs, nutrition, aspects of aging, and the like. Teaching–learning strategies to integrate cultural

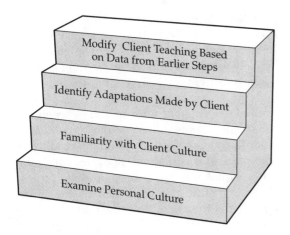

**FIGURE 8–2    Four-Step Approach to Providing Culturally Sensitive Care** SOURCE: Reprinted with permission from Price, J. L. & Cordell, B. (1994). Cultural diversity and patient teaching. *Journal of Continuing Education in Nursing, 25*(4), 164.

concepts into the curriculum include simulated games, values clarification exercises, consciousness-raising encounter groups, and field experiences.

3. Within the field of research, cross-cultural studies in both basic and applied research domains are needed. Funding agencies and private foundations must be encouraged to support cross-cultural studies, most of which place heavy emphasis on qualitative research methods. The debate over quantitative versus qualitative research methodology should cease, because a combination of methods provides useful data and allows researchers to achieve optimal results.

## Cultural Assessment

The *Nurse–Client Negotiations Model* has been developed for the purpose of cultural assessment and planning for care of culturally diverse people. However, the concepts advanced in this model are relevant for any nurse–client interaction, regardless of the client's background and situation (Anderson, 1987, 1990). The Negotiations Model recognizes discrepancies that exist between notions of the nurse and client about health, illness, and treatments. It attempts to bridge the gap between the scientific perspectives of the nurse and the popular perspectives of the client.

Fundamental to understanding this model, one must recognize that most social systems include three structural arenas of health care within which sickness is reacted to and experienced (Figure 8–3). The concept of popular, professional, and folk arenas (sectors) is used to compare medical systems as cultural systems. Each arena or domain possesses its own model for explaining health and illness (Kleinman, 1978; Anderson, 1987):

- The *popular arena* (sector) comprises the family context of sickness and care, including the social network and community perspective. In both Western and non-Western societies, approximately 70% to 90% of sickness is managed solely within this domain.

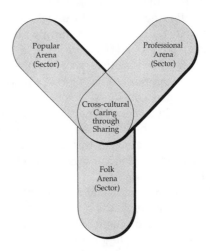

**FIGURE 8–3    Cultural Systems in the Context of Health and Illness Care** SOURCE: Adapted from Anderson, J. M. (1987). The cultural context of caring. *Canadian Critical Care Nursing Journal*, December, 8

- The *professional arena* (sector) consists of scientific medicine (Western and cosmopolitan) and professionalized healthy traditions as practiced by nursing, medical, and other health professionals.
- The *folk arena* (sector) consists of nonprofessional healing specialists, often referred to as "healers."

The Nurse–Client Negotiations Model serves as a framework to attend to the "culture of the nurse" as well as the "culture of the client." In addition to the professional culture, each nurse has his or her own personal beliefs and values, which may operate without the nurse being fully aware of them. These beliefs and values may influence nurses' interactions with patients and families. Each arena (sector) in the model can be viewed as a sociocultural system with its own values, norms of behavior, beliefs, and ways of explaining health and illness. Explanations of the same phenomena may yield different interpretations based on the cultural perspective of the layperson or the professional. Anderson (1987) provided examples of different perspectives of the same intervention: Putting lightweight bedclothes on a patient may be interpreted by family members as placing their loved one at risk for "getting a chill," whereas the nurse will use this technique to prevent or reduce a fever; a Jehovah's Witness family considers a blood transfusion for their child as contamination of the child's body, whereas the nurse and other healthcare team members believe a transfusion is a lifesaving treatment. The important aspect of this model is that it can open lines of communication between the nurse and the patient/family so that each understands how the other interprets or values a problem or practice such that they respect one another's goals.

According to the Negotiations Model, the nurse should not begin negotiation with the premise that predefined problems exist for which there is an acceptable list of solutions. Instead, the nurse should find out clients' understanding of their situation, their interpretations of illness and symptoms, the symbolic meanings they attach to an event, and their notions about treatment. The goal is to actively involve clients in the learning process so as to acquire healthy coping mechanisms and styles of living. *Negotiation* implies a mutual exchange of information between the nurse and clients, whereby the nurse learns from the clients about their understanding of the particular situation, and, in turn, the nurse explains to the clients about the professional scientific model. Together, the nurse and clients then need to engage in a transaction to work out how the popular and scientific perspectives can be reconstructed to achieve goals related to the individual client's interests.

General areas to assess when first meeting the client include the following: the client's perceptions of health and illness; his or her use of traditional remedies and folk practitioners; the client's perceptions of nurses, hospitals, and the care delivery system; his or her beliefs about the role of family and family member relationships; and his or her perceptions of and need for emotional support (Anderson, 1987). According to Anderson (1990), the following questions, although not exhaustive, can be used as a means for understanding the client's perspectives or viewpoints and can serve as the basis for negotiation:

- What do you think caused your problem?
- Why do you think the problem started when it did?
- What does your sickness do to you? How does it work?
- How severe is your illness? Will it have a short- or long-term course?
- What kinds of treatments do you think you should receive?
- What are the most important results you hope to obtain from your treatments?
- What major problems does your illness cause you?
- What do you fear most about your illness?

The processes involved are known as *cultural negotiation* and *cultural brokerage*—acts of translation in which messages, instructions, and belief systems are linked or manipulated between the professional and layperson with respect to determining the health problem and the treatment preferred (Tripp-Reimer & Afifi, 1989; Jezewski, 1993). Crucial to the processes is to elicit and acknowledge the client's point of view regarding the illness experience. The integration of concepts from the social sciences is essential if nurses are to practice competently in a culturally sensitive manner.

The *Culturally Competent Model of Care* proposed by Campinha-Bacote (1995) is another model for conducting a thorough and sensitive cultural assessment. *Cultural competence* is defined as a set of congruent behaviors, attitudes, and policies that enable a system, agency, or professional to work effectively in a cross-cultural situation. Through this model, cultural competence is seen as a continuous process involving four

components: cultural awareness, cultural knowledge, cultural skill, and cultural encounter. *Cultural awareness* is the process of becoming sensitive to interactions with other cultural groups; it requires nurses to examine their biases and prejudices toward others of another culture or ethnic background. *Cultural knowledge* is the process in which nurses acquire an educational foundation with respect to various cultural world views. *Cultural skill* involves the process of learning how to conduct an accurate cultural assessment. *Cultural encounter* encourages nurses to expose themselves in practice to cross-cultural interactions with clients of diverse cultural backgrounds. All four components are essential if one is to deliver culturally competent nursing care (Figure 8–4).

Nurse educators who are competent in cultural assessment and negotiation likely will be the most successful at designing and implementing teaching programs. They also will be

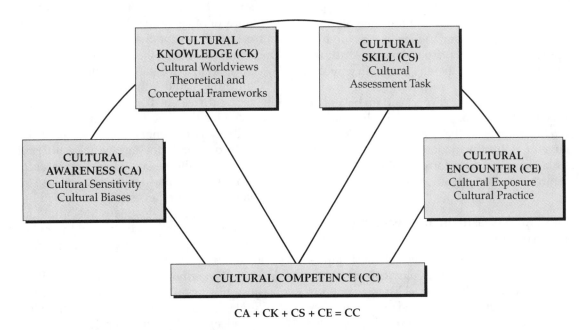

FIGURE 8–4  **Culturally Competent Model of Care**  SOURCE: Reprinted with permission from Campinha-Bacote, J. (1995). The quest for cultural competence in nursing care. *Nursing Forum, 30*(4), 20.

able to assist their colleagues in working with clients who may be considered "uncooperative," "noncompliant," or "difficult;" help with identifying potential areas of cultural conflict; and devise teaching interventions that minimize conflict. Nurses must understand how the reactions of practitioners influence labeling of clients' behaviors and, therefore, eventually influence nurse–client interactions (Anderson, 1987, 1990). There is one very important caveat to remember:

> Although it is crucial to understand cultural context in developing and carrying out effective health education programs, nurses must be especially careful not to over-generalize or stereotype clients on the basis of their cultural heritage. Just because someone belongs to a particular ethnic group does not necessarily mean they adhere to all the beliefs, values, customs, and practices of that ethnic group. As a note of caution, nurses should never assume a client's learning needs or preferred treatment programs simply based on the individual's ethnicity.

As Andrews and Boyle (1995) so aptly explained, "Sometimes cultural stereotyping may be perpetuated when a recipe-like approach to clients from specific cultural groups is used: i.e., there is a tendency by the nurse to view all members of a group homogenously and to expect certain beliefs or practices because of presumptions that may or may not apply to the client" (p. 50). Knowledge of cultural variations should serve only as background cues for obtaining additional information through assessment.

## General Assessment and Teaching Interventions

The nurse in the role of educator must implement successful teaching interventions using the universal skills of establishing rapport, assessing readiness to learn, and using active listening to assess and understand problems. Tripp-Reimer and Afifi (1989) point out the need

for nurses to assess the established customs that influence the behavior one is attempting to change. The implications of cultural heritage are sometimes difficult to detect in our pluralistic society. As a component of the teaching process, assessment should attempt to determine health beliefs, values, and practices, keeping in mind that belonging to an ethnic group does not always mean a person follows or "buys into" all of the traditions or customs of the group to which they have affiliation. Given that culture affects the way someone perceives a health problem and understands its course and possible treatment options, it is essential to carry out a thorough assessment prior to establishing a plan of action for long-term behavioral change.

Different cultural backgrounds not only create different attitudes and reactions to illness, but can also influence how people express themselves, both verbally and nonverbally, which may prove difficult to interpret. For example, eliciting a patient's explanation for the etiology of a problem will help to reveal whether the cause is attributed by the patient to a spiritual intervention, a hex, an imbalance in nature, or other culturally based beliefs. The nurse should accept the client's explanation (most likely reflecting the beliefs of the support system as well) in a nonjudgmental manner.

Culture also guides the way an ill person is defined and treated. For example, some cultures believe that once the symptoms disappear, illness is no longer present. This belief can be problematic for individuals suffering from an acute illness such as a streptococcal infection, when a one- or two-day course of antibiotic therapy relieves the soreness in the throat. It is also problematic for the individual afflicted with a chronic disease that is manifested by periods of remission or exacerbation.

Readiness to learn must also be assessed from the standpoint of a person's culture because this factor is a key element in cross-cultural education. Patients and their families, for instance, may believe that behavior change is context specific, such that they will adhere to a recommended medical regimen while in the hospital setting but fail to follow through with the guidelines once they return to the home setting. In addition, the nurse and other healthcare providers must be cautious not to assume that the values espoused by professionals are equally important or cherished by the patient and significant others. Consideration must also be given to barriers that might exist, such as time, financial, and environmental variables, which may hinder readiness to learn (see Chapter 4). Finally, the client needs to believe that new behaviors are not only possible but also beneficial if behavioral change is to be maintained over the long term.

The following specific guidelines for assessment should be used regardless of the particular cultural orientation of the client (Anderson, 1987):

1. *Observe the interactions between patient and family members and among family members.* Determine who makes the decisions, how decisions are made, who is the primary caregiver, what type of care is given, and what foods and other objects are important to the patient and family.

2. *Listen to the patient.* Find out what the patient wants, how the patient's wants differ from what the family wants and they differ from what you think is appropriate.

3. *Consider communication abilities and patterns.* Be aware of nonverbal behaviors and etiquettes of interaction that may be acceptable or unacceptable to the patient and family, the patient's primary language, which may be different from your own, and manners of speaking (rate of speech, expressions used) that can enhance or hinder understanding.

4. *Explore customs or taboos.* Observe behaviors and ask to clarify beliefs and practices that may restrict care or treatment.

5. *Determine the notion of time.* Become oriented to the patient's and family's sense of time and importance of time frames.

6. *Be aware of cues for interaction.* Determine which approaches are appropriate for patients and families with respect to how to comfortably address the person(s) with whom you are interacting and the symbolic objects or the activities that provide comfort and security.

These guidelines will assist in the exchange of information between the nurse and patient/family. The patient–nurse role is a mutual one in which the nurse is both learner and teacher and the client is also both learner and teacher. The goal of negotiation is to arrive at a way of working together in a collaborative fashion so as to solve a problem or to determine a course of action. To care for someone, the nurse must know who he or she is, know who the other party is, and be able to bridge the gap between each other (Anderson, 1987).

## Use of Translators

If the client speaks a foreign language, whenever possible the client's primary language should be used. When the nurse does not fluently speak the same language, it is necessary to secure the assistance of a translator. Translators may be family members, neighbors and friends, other healthcare staff, or professional interpreters.

For many reasons, the use of family or friends for translation of communication is not as desirable as using professionally trained interpreters. First, family members and friends may not be sufficiently fluent to assume the role. Second, they may choose to omit portions of the content they believe to be unnecessary or unacceptable. Third, their presence may inhibit peer communication and violate the patient's right to privacy and confidentiality (Baker et al., 1996; Poss & Rangel, 1995). Thus it is optimal if professionally trained interpreters can be used. They can translate instructional messages verbatim, and they work under an established code of ethics and confidentiality. If there is no bilingual person available to facilitate communication, the AT&T Language Line provides 24-hour access to translators who are fluent in 144 languages (Duffy & Snyder, 1999).

In teaching clients who are only partially fluent in English, the following strategies, adapted from Tripp-Reimer and Afifi (1989) and Poss & Rangel (1995), are recommended to help the nurse alter the style of interaction when no translator is used:

- Speak slowly and distinctly, allowing for twice as much time as a typical teaching session would take.

- Use simple sentence structures, relying on a direct subject-verb pattern and an active rather than passive voice.

- Avoid technical terms (e.g., use *heart* rather than *cardiac*, or *stomach* rather than *gastric*), medical jargon (e.g., use *blood pressure* rather than *BP*), and American idioms (e.g., *red tape* or *I heard it straight from the horse's mouth*).

- Organize instructional material in the sequence in which the plan of action should be carried out.

- Make no assumptions that the information given has been understood. Ask for clients to explain in their own words the protocol, and, if appropriate, request a return demonstration of a skill that has been taught.

## THE FOUR MAJOR CULTURE GROUPS

Given the fact that there exist hundreds of ethnic minority subgroups in the United States, and many more worldwide, it is impossible to address the cultural characteristics of each one of them. The following is a review of the beliefs and health practices of the four major cultural groups in this country identified by the U.S. Census Bureau—Hispanics, Blacks, Asian/Pacific Islanders, and American Indi-

ans, who are the historically underrepresented groups accounting for more than one-quarter (28.6%) of the U.S. population. These groups are recognized by the U.S. government as disadvantaged due to low income, low education, and/or sociocultural deprivation.

It must be remembered that one of the most important roles of the nurse as educator is to serve as an advocate for clients—as a representative of their interests. If nurses are to assume this role, then their efforts should be directed at making the healthcare setting as similar to the client's natural environment as possible. To do so, they must be aware of clients' customs, beliefs, and lifestyles and be willing to take the responsibility for making adaptations in the institutional environment.

The following references have been used for information on the four cultural groups to be discussed and are recommended as sources of additional information on particular tribes or subgroups not identified: Purnell and Paulanka (1998), Kelly and Fitzsimmons (2000), Spector (1991), Chideya (1999), Caudle (1993), Chachkes and Christ (1996), Cantore (2001), Lowe and Struthers (2001), Gollop (1997), Parker and Kiatoukaysy (1999), Jackson (1993), Westberg (1989), Cohen (1991), Kniep-Hardy and Burkhardt (1977), Shomaker (1981), Perry (1982), Galanti (1991), Horton and Freire (1990), and Smolan et al. (1990).

## Hispanic American Culture

According to the U.S. Census Bureau (2000), Hispanics are the fastest-growing minority group in the United States. They now represent 11.9% of the total population of the United States. It is projected that in another 100 years Hispanics will make up approximately 25% of the population. There has been a tremendous increase in the numbers of Hispanics since 1970 as a result of a higher birth rate in this group than the rest of the population, a significant increase in immigration, as well as improved census procedures.

Hispanic Americans derive from diverse origins. Although sometimes referred to as *Latinos*, the term *Hispanic* is used by the U.S. Census Bureau to label this heterogeneous group of Americans with varied backgrounds in culture and heritage who are of Latin American or Spanish decent or who use the Spanish language in their homes (Caudle, 1993). The largest group comprises Mexicans (60% of the population), followed by Puerto Ricans, Central and South Americans, and Cubans. They are found in every state but are concentrated in just 10 states. California and Texas together have one-half of the Hispanic population, but other large concentrations are found in New York, New Jersey, Massachusetts, Florida, Illinois, Arizona, New Mexico, and Colorado. Nurse educators who practice in the Southwestern states are most likely to encounter Mexicans, those practicing in the Northeast states will most likely be caregivers for Puerto Ricans, and nurses in Florida will be delivering care to a large number of Cubans. Also, Hispanics are more likely to live in metropolitan areas than are non-Hispanics (Torres, 1994; Purnell & Paulanka, 1998; Caudle, 1993; Spector, 1991). While Hispanic Americans have many common characteristics, each subgroup has unique characteristics.

Hispanics have particular healthcare needs that must be addressed. They are disproportionately affected by certain cancers, alcoholism, drug abuse, obesity, hypertension, diabetes, adolescent pregnancy, dental disease, and HIV/AIDS. Unlike in non-Hispanic whites, homicide, AIDS, and perinatal conditions rank in the top ten as causes of mortality. Hispanics are more prone to certain diseases, are less likely to receive preventive care, often lack health insurance, and have less access to health care than whites living in the United States.

Unfortunately, both the curricula in nursing schools nationwide and the literature in nursing with respect to patient education efforts geared toward Hispanic Americans have paid little attention to the healthcare needs of this minority group. Although Hispanics are a culturally diverse group of people with varying health needs, avenues for including Hispanic healthcare issues in nursing curricula have been minimal and especially need to be developed in schools located in areas with high concentrations of this population group. Fluency in Spanish as a foreign language is a necessity, or at least highly recommended, when practitioners are responsible for delivering care to this growing, underserved, culturally diverse group. Spanish-speaking people represent 54% of all non–English-speaking persons in the United States.

In proportion to the U.S. population, Hispanics are underrepresented in nursing education. Only 3% of all graduates of basic nursing programs are of Hispanic descent. Far too few graduates are available to satisfy the increasing need for Hispanic healthcare professionals. The lack of representation of this minority group in the health professions is not thought to result from low aspirations on their part. Indeed, many Hispanic high school students rank health/medical services, along with business and engineering, as one of their top ten career choices. Unfortunately, the often poor academic achievement of Hispanics in high schools and colleges is associated with a number of factors related to socioeconomic and educational disadvantages.

Access to health care by Hispanics is limited both by choice and by unavailability of health services. Only one-fifth of Puerto Ricans, one-fourth of Cubans, and one-third of Mexicans see a physician during the course of a year. Even when Hispanics have access to the healthcare system, they may not receive the care they need. Difficulty in obtaining services, dissatisfaction with the care provided, and inability to afford the rising costs of medical care are major factors that discourage them from using the healthcare system.

Approximately 23% of Hispanic families live below the poverty line; members of this group are 2 1/2 times more likely to be below the poverty level than members of other groups in the United States. Economic disadvantage leaves little disposable income for paying out-of-pocket expenses for health care. When they do seek a regular source of care, many Hispanics rely on public health facilities, hospital outpatient clinics, and emergency rooms (Westberg, 1989; Andersen et al., 1986; Caudle, 1993).

The health beliefs of Hispanics also affect their decisions to seek traditional care. Many studies dating back to the 1940s on Hispanic health beliefs and practices stressed exotic folklore practices, such as their use of herbs, teas, home remedies, and over-the-counter drugs for treating symptoms of acute and chronic illnesses. In addition, Hispanics place a high degree of reliance on health healers, known as *curenderos* or *esperitistas*, for health advice and treatment.

Other studies also have reported that illnesses of Mexican Americans could be organized into the following categories (Markides & Coreil, 1986; Caudle, 1993; Spector, 1991):

1. Diseases of "hot" and "cold," believed to be due to an imbalanced intake of foods or ingestion of foods at extreme opposites in temperature. In addition, cold air was thought to lead to joint pain, and a "cold womb" resulted in barrenness in women. Heating or chilling was the cure for parts of the body afflicted by disease.

2. Diseases of dislocation of internal organs, cured by massage or physical manipulation of body parts.

3. Diseases of magical origin, caused by *mal Ojo* or "evil eye," a disorder of infants and children as a result of a woman's looking admiringly at someone else's child without touching the child, resulting in crying, fitful sleep, diarrhea, vomiting, and fever.

4. Diseases of emotional origin, attributed to sudden or prolonged terror called *Susto*.

5. Folk-defined diseases, such as *latido*.

6. "Standard scientific" diseases.

Additional studies in the 1950s and 1960s focused primarily on mental health issues. These studies suggested the existence of an "epidemiological paradox." Unlike other socioeconomically disadvantaged minority groups, Mexican Americans in particular were found to have low rates of psychiatric problems, probably explained by strong family ties that protected them against stress. More recent research concludes that Southwestern Hispanics' health status is determined by key health indicators on infant mortality, life expectancy, and mortality from cardiovascular disease, cancer, and measures of functional health. This research reveals that the health of Hispanics is much closer to that of whites than to blacks, with whom Hispanics share similar socioeconomic conditions. Concerning the incidence of diabetes and infectious and parasitic diseases, however, Hispanics are clearly at a disadvantage in relation to whites.

Possible explanations for the relative advantages and disadvantages in health status of Hispanics involve such factors as cultural practices favoring reproductive success, early and high fertility contributing to low breast cancer but high cervical cancer rates, dietary habits linked to low cancer rates but high prevalence of obesity and diabetes, genetic heritage, extended family support reducing the need for psychiatric services, and low socioeconomic status that contributes to increased infectious and parasitic diseases. Alcoholism also represents a crucial health problem for many Hispanic Americans. As the Hispanic population becomes more acculturated, certain risk factors conducive to cardiovascular disease and certain cancers are expected to play larger roles in this group (Markides & Coreil, 1986; Purnell & Paulanka, 1998).

Today, the literature disagrees about the extent and frequency to which Hispanics use home remedies and folk practices. In the Southwestern United States, 21% of the Hispanic population has been found to use herbs and other home remedies to treat illness episodes—twice the proportion reported in the total U.S. population. Other studies claim that the use of folk practitioners has declined and practically disappeared in some Hispanic subgroups. Knowing where people get their health information can provide clues to practitioners as to how to reach particular population groups. One study indicated that Mexican Americans receive almost as much information from mass media sources (TV, magazines, and newspapers) as they do from physicians and nurses. As a consequence, mass media could play an important role in disseminating information to a large portion of the Mexican American population.

Because of the centrality of the family in Hispanic peoples' lives, the extended family serves as the single most important source of social support to its members. This culture is characterized by a pattern of respect and obedience to elders as well as a pattern of male dominance. Caregivers' focus, therefore, needs to be on the family rather than on the individual. It is likely, for example, that a woman would be reluctant to make a decision about her or her child's health care without consulting her husband first. Changes are occurring, however, as Hispanic women are taking jobs outside the home. Also, children are picking up the English language more quickly than their parents and are ending up in the powerful position of acting as interpreters for their parents. The heavy reliance on family has been linked to Hispanics' low utilization of healthcare services. In addition, levels of education correlate highly with access to health care—that is, the less education possessed by the head of the household, the poorer the family's health status and access to health care (Westberg, 1989; Spector, 1991; Purnell & Paulanka, 1998). Hispanics are more likely than the general U.S. population

to read English below the fourth-grade level and to have lower educational attainment than non-Hispanic whites (Massett, 1996).

**Teaching Strategies**   Only about 40% of Hispanics have completed four years of high school or more, and only 10% have completed college, as compared with approximately 80% and 20%, respectively, of the rest of the non-Hispanic population (Purnell & Paulanka, 1998). Both the educational level and the primary language of Hispanic clients need to be taken into consideration when selecting instructional materials (Massett, 1996). Sophisticated teaching methods and tools would be inappropriate for those who have minimal levels of education. The age of the population can also affect health and patient education efforts. Because the Hispanic population is young as a total group (30% are younger than 20 years of age), the school system is an important setting for educating members of the Hispanic community. Morbidity, mortality, and risk factor data also provide clues to the areas in which patient education efforts should be directed. As mentioned earlier, Hispanics have higher rates of diabetes, AIDS, obesity, alcohol-related illnesses, and mortality from homicide than the general population. All of these topics should be targeted for educational efforts at disease prevention and health promotion (Caudle, 1993).

Until recently, little data existed regarding patient education for Hispanic Americans. Purnell and Paulanka (1998), Spector (1991), and Caudle (1993) have contributed significantly to our understanding of the traditions and practices surrounding health and illness in the various Hispanic subgroups. A few earlier studies reviewed by Westberg (1989) are congruent with the findings of these authorities and have implications for patient education. In a study focusing on the educational and emotional needs of Hispanic women who were hospitalized for prenatal care, the women revealed that they were so nervous in talking to physicians that they would forget to ask questions and, when they did, would forget the doctor's answers; they found it difficult to talk with health professionals about their "private parts"; and they found it easiest to talk with those practitioners with whom they had met on prior visits.

Other studies indicate that education programs in the school system for Hispanic students on alcohol and drug abuse and on cardiovascular disease risk reduction proved successful if

- Cultural beliefs were observed.

- The educator was first introduced by an individual accepted and respected by the learners.

- Family members were included.

- The community was encouraged to take responsibility for resolving the health problems discussed.

Another study investigated mass media's ability to increase health knowledge and awareness as well as stimulate responses in the Hispanic population to the problems communicated through these instructional tools. Researchers concluded that regular radio and TV broadcasts delivering public service announcements in Spanish can be an effective health education strategy. Moreover, print materials, the most heavily relied-on medium by healthcare practitioners to inform the Spanish-speaking population, must be carefully assessed for linguistic appropriateness and cultural sensitivity (Massett, 1996).

The following general suggestions are useful when designing and implementing education programs for Hispanic Americans (Westberg, 1989; Caudle, 1993; Spector, 1991; Purnell & Paulanka, 1998):

1. Encourage Hispanics to be involved in planning education programs.

2. Identify those Hispanics in the community who are not currently recipients of health education services.

3. Consider developing outreach programs, such as mass media segments, to reach the unmet needs of underserved Hispanics.

4. Identify the Hispanic American subgroups (e.g., Mexicans, Cubans, and Puerto Ricans) in the community whose needs differ in terms of health beliefs, language, and general health status so that education programs can be targeted to meet their distinct ethnic needs.

5. Be aware of individual differences within subgroups as to age, years of education, income levels, job status, and degree of acculturation.

6. Take into account the special health needs of Hispanic Americans with respect to incidences of diseases and risk factors to which they are vulnerable—diabetes, AIDS, obesity, alcohol-related illnesses, homicide, and accidental injuries.

7. Be aware of the importance of the family so as to direct education efforts to include all interested family members. Remember that Hispanic families are usually willing to provide support to each other and decision making usually rests with the male and elder authority figures in the family.

8. Provide adequate space for teaching to accommodate family members who typically accompany patients seeking health care.

9. Be cognizant of the importance of the Roman Catholic religion in the lives of Hispanics when dealing with such issues as contraception, abortion, and family planning.

10. Demonstrate cultural sensitivity to health beliefs by respecting ethnic values and taking time to learn about Hispanic beliefs.

11. Consider other sources of care that Hispanics might be using, such as home remedies, before they enter or while they are within the healthcare system.

12. Be aware of the modesty felt by some Hispanics, especially women and girls, who may be particularly uncomfortable in talking about sexual issues in mixed company.

13. Display warmth, friendliness, and tactfulness when developing a relationship with Hispanics, because they expect healthcare providers to be informal and interested in their lives.

14. Determine whether Spanish is the most comfortable language for the client in which to converse and read. Many Hispanics prefer to speak Spanish but are not proficient in reading this language.

15. Speak slowly and distinctly, avoiding the use of slang and idioms if the client has limited proficiency in English.

16. Do not assume that a nod of the head or a smile indicates understanding of what has been said. For Hispanics who are not familiar with English and because they respect authority, it is not uncommon for them to display nonverbal cues that may be misleading or misinterpreted by the receiver. Ask clients to repeat in their own words what they have been told to determine their level of understanding.

17. If interpreters are used, be sure they speak the dialect used by the learner. Be certain that the interpreter "interprets" rather than just "translates" so that the real meaning of instructions gets across. Also, be sure to talk to the client, not to the interpreter.

18. Provide written and audiovisual materials in Spanish that reflect cultural appropriateness. An increasing number of patient education materials are available strictly in Spanish or have been prepared for a bilingual audience.

19. Locate the hotline telephone number in the community that provides a direct link to Spanish-speaking interpreters who can assist healthcare providers in communicating with non–English-speaking patients.

A review of the literature indicates that much more must be learned about the Hispanic American population with respect to their cultural beliefs and their health and education needs. Given the limited knowledge available, it is evident that many members of this cultural group are not receiving the kind and amount of health services they desire and deserve. Nurse educators—and particularly in those regions of the country densely populated with these ethnic subgroups—need to extend themselves to Hispanics in a culturally sensitive manner to effectively and efficiently address the needs of this rapidly growing segment of the U.S. population.

## Black American Culture

At the present time, members of the Black American culture make up the largest historically underrepresented group in the United States, but this situation is expected to change in the near future due to the rapid growth of the Hispanic population. Currently, Black Americans constitute 12.2% of the U.S. population as compared with 11.9% for Hispanics (U.S. Census Bureau, 2000).

The cultural origins and heritage of Black Americans are quite diverse. Their roots are mainly from Africa and the Caribbean Islands. They speak a variety of languages, including French, Spanish, African dialects, and various forms of English. The one distinguishing factor of this group is the length of time many of these people have had to acculturate to the American "way of life," adapting to a number of the beliefs and practices of Western medicine. Quite a few black families have ancestors who settled in America many generations ago. Although the cultural heritage of the black subgroups varies, it is possible to make some generalizations about their cultural beliefs and traditions, particularly those customs and beliefs of the more recent immigrants or those that were carried through the generations from colonial times, when blacks were held as slaves. It must be pointed out that there are few recent studies conducted specifically investigating the Black American culture. Perhaps this omission has arisen because their cultural heritage has been blended into the social fabric of America over time as blacks were exposed to whites with whom they lived and served (Spector, 1991; Purnell & Paulanka, 1998).

Unfortunately, a disproportionate number of people from the Black American culture are disadvantaged as a result of poverty and low educational attainment. Many black families are exposed to numerous risk factors simultaneously as a result of the poor environmental conditions in which they live. Black children born to teenaged mothers, for example, were found to be approximately four times as likely to have low scores on achievement tests. Poor learning outcomes in these children have been linked to their exposure to poverty, low maternal educational level, absence of a father or father figure in the home, and the like. Another potential risk factor with respect to learning is urban residence. In a comparison of urban and rural communities, individuals living in urban areas were twice as likely to have behavioral and reading problems than members of families living in rural settings. This prevalence is believed to largely result from the many stressors (e.g., crowded and noisy living conditions) found in the urban setting. In addition, the urban school systems were found to provide less than optimal settings for the acquisition of skills and information (Luster & McAdoo, 1994).

Black Americans constitute a large segment of blue-collar workers and are not well represented in managerial and professional positions of employment. Discrimination in employment and job advancement is thought to be a major variable contributing to problems with career mobility. The government has taken major steps in the past 30 years to reverse discrimination in social and employment settings so as to give Black Americans more equal opportunities, but the majority of working-class blacks still do not typically advance to higher-level occupations.

Increased exposure to hazardous working conditions has also resulted in a greater incidence of occupation-related diseases and illnesses among this population. Black American males, for example, are at increased risk for developing cancer and stress-related diseases such as hypertension and other cardiovascular illnesses associated with low-paying, insecure, dead-end jobs.

Obesity is another major problem among Black Americans. Food to them is a symbol of health and wealth, and a higher than ideal body weight is viewed as positive by this ethnic group.

Poverty and low educational attainment have also had major consequences for the Black American community in terms of social and medical issues. Although black families value education highly, there continues to be a greater than average high school dropout rate among blacks, and many individuals remain poorly educated with concomitant literacy problems. Low educational levels and socioeconomic deprivation are strongly correlated with higher incidences of disease, poor nutrition, lower survival rates, and a decreased quality of life in general. In addition, the majority of blacks reside in inner-city areas where exposure to violence and pollution puts them at greater risk for disease, disability, and death. The average life span of Black Americans is 6.5 years shorter than that of white Americans due to high death rates from cancer, cardiovascular disease, cirrhosis, diabetes, accidents, homicides, and infant mortality. Also, blacks are at higher risk for drug addiction, teenaged pregnancy, and sexually transmitted diseases. Thirty percent of reported cases of AIDS are found in the black population, even though Black Americans represent less than 13% of the U.S. population.

Purnell & Paulanka (1998) reported findings that the Black American belief system emphasizes three major themes:

1. The world is a hostile and dangerous place to live.

2. The individual is vulnerable to attack from external forces.

3. The individual is considered helpless with few internal resources to combat adversity.

Furthermore, many Black Americans are pessimistic about human relationships and tend to be suspicious of healthcare professionals, seeking the assistance of physicians and nurses only when absolutely necessary. Folk practitioners are held in higher esteem than the Western biomedical healthcare team.

Black Americans of African descent have been found by sociologists and anthropologists to have similarities with respect to the importance of extended family. Common to the black culture is the concept of extended family, consisting of several households, with the older adults often taking the leadership role within the family constellation. Respect for elders and ancestors is valued. They are held in high esteem because living a long life indicates that the individual had more opportunities to acquire much experience and knowledge. Decision making regarding healthcare issues is, therefore, often left to the elders. Family ties are especially strong between grandchildren and grandparents. It is not unusual for grandmothers to want to stay at the hospital bedside when their grandchildren are ill. This extended family network provides emotional, physical, and financial support to members during times of illness

and other crises (Spector, 1991; Purnell & Paulanka, 1998).

Beliefs, consisting of knowledge, opinions, and faith that dispose persons to demonstrate certain kinds of behavior, are not necessarily dependent on the degree to which they correspond to reality. The strength of a belief also does not depend on its congruence with other beliefs held by the individual. In a study of black teenaged women in a prenatal clinic, their beliefs were shown to contribute to noncompliance relating to prevention of pregnancy. Although these women believed contraception was appropriate, birth control pills and IUDs were considered unacceptable because they were felt to alter menstrual cycles and thus cause illness (Horn, 1983). The understanding of young black women of how contraceptives work, what they do, and how pregnancy occurs is handed down through a rich description of events by their mothers and other female relatives. Becoming a mother at a young age, although not highly desirable or condoned by black women, does have a fairly high level of acceptance in this cultural group (Purnell & Paulanka, 1998). In fact, black women do not perceive negative sanctions within their culture if they do not meet the ideal norm of getting an education or job prior to marriage and children. Families are supportive of their members if they need help.

Black people often have strong religious values, and these religious beliefs may extend to their feelings about illness and health. A majority of Black Americans find inner strength from their trust in God. Some believe that whatever happens is God's will. This belief has led to the perception that Black Americans have a fatalistic view of life (Purnell & Paulanka, 1998) and are governed by a relatively strong external locus of control.

A common folk practice, known as voodoo, consists of beliefs about spirits inhabiting the world: All animate and inanimate objects have good or evil spirits. A religious priest, witch doctor, or medicine man has the power to appease or release hostile spirits. Illness, or disharmony, is thought to be caused by evil spirits because a person failed to follow religious rules or the dictates of ancestors. Curative measures involve finding the cause of an illness—a hex or a spell placed on a person by another or the breaking of a taboo—and then finding someone with magical healing powers or witchcraft to rid the afflicted individual of the evil spirit(s). Some black American families also continue to practice home remedies such as the use of mustard plasters, taking of herbal medicines and teas, and wearing of amulets to cure or ward off a variety of illnesses and afflictions (Spector, 1991; Purnell & Paulanka, 1998).

**Teaching Strategies**   In teaching Black Americans preventive and promotion measures, as well as caring for them during acute and chronic illnesses, the nurse must explore the client's value systems. Generally, any folk practices or traditional beliefs should be respected and allowed (if not harmful) and incorporated into the recommended treatment or healthcare interventions used by Western medicine. The following discussion offers more specific recommendations for rendering culturally appropriate care for Black Americans.

Black Americans tend to be very verbal and express feelings openly to family and friends. However, they are much more private about family matters when in the company of strangers. The volume of their voices tends to be louder than in other cultures and they express their thoughts in a more dynamic manner, but these types of behaviors should not be perceived as necessarily reflecting anger or frustration. Black Americans feel comfortable with less personal space than do some other ethnic groups. However, direct eye contact by others outside of their culture can be misinterpreted by blacks as aggressive behavior. They are also more present- than past- or future-oriented. Thus, they tend to be

more relaxed about specific time frames, evincing a more circular rather than linear sense of time. Health providers must be careful not to misinterpret nonverbal and verbal behaviors when delivering care and must be flexible in the timing of appointments, as blacks will usually keep their appointments but may not always be on schedule.

Even though Black Americans are very informal when they interact among themselves, they prefer to be greeted in a more formal manner with the use of their surnames, which demonstrates the respect and pride they have in their family heritage. Traditionally, the family structure has been matriarchal; this pattern persists to the present day due to a high percentage of households run by a female single parent. It is imperative that healthcare providers acknowledge the dominant role that black women play in decision making and the importance of sharing health information directly with them. Grandmothers continue to play a central role in the Black American family and are often involved in providing economic support and child care for their grandchildren.

With respect to prevalent diseases and health issues within this population group, hypertension continues to be the most serious health problem. Approximately 25% of Black Americans are hypertensive, and the group as a whole suffers higher morbidity and mortality rates from this disease than do other Americans. Also, blacks are more than three times more likely to develop kidney failure associated with hypertension and, as stated previously, they are at higher risk for being victims of violence, accidents, disabilities, obesity, and cancer. Nurse educators must concentrate on disease prevention measures, institute early screening for high blood pressure as well as for signs and symptoms of other diseases common in this population, and provide culturally congruent health education to improve the overall health status of Black Americans. Strong family ties encourage individuals to be treated by the family before seeking care from health professionals. This cultural practice may be a factor contributing to the delay or failure of blacks to seek treatment of diseases at the early stages of illness. An effective approach to providing care can be to institute health screening programs in conjunction with community and church activities where the entire family is present.

Due to economic factors, Black Americans are likely to have less ready access to healthcare services. Lack of culturally relevant care, perceptions of racial discrimination, and a general distrust of both healthcare professionals and the healthcare system are also identified barriers to Black Americans seeking the health care they need. Establishing a trusting relationship, therefore, is an essential first step if blacks are to receive and accept the health services they require and deserve. Recognizing their unique responses to health and illness based on their spiritual and religious foundations, their strong family ties, and other traditional beliefs is essential if therapeutic interventions developed by the healthcare team are to be successful. Efforts to recruit more blacks into the nursing profession would help most assuredly to reduce some of the barriers to caring for this population of Americans.

## Asian/Pacific Islander Culture

People from Asian countries and the Pacific Islands constitute this cultural group. Mainly as a result of World War II, the Korean War in the 1950s, the fall of the South Vietnam government in 1975, and the successive disintegrations of the governments of Laos and Cambodia, the West Coast region of the United States, in particular, has been occupied by Southeast Asian refugees. More than 45,000 Vietnamese, Cambodians, and Laotians settled in the San Francisco Bay area alone, and 29,000 officially resettled in Washington state (Schultz, 1982; Kubota & Matsuda,

1982). The states of New York, New Jersey, and Texas also have experienced a large influx of Asian peoples, particularly from China, the Philippines, and Japan. In the decades following political and social upheavals in Southeast Asia, almost three-quarters of a million people of Asian/Pacific Islander origin immigrated into the United States. Presently, more than 10 million Asian/Pacific Islanders (3.8% of the total U.S. population) live in the country (U.S. Census Bureau, 2000).

The medical system of the Asian/Pacific Islander countries and the culture and religion of these peoples need to be understood to successfully deal with their health issues. The language barrier has proved to be the biggest problem in providing healthcare services to these populations. Many misconceptions can occur because the Southeast Asian languages are not as technical as English. Although Asian/Pacific Islander people have been classified as a single ethnic group by many researchers and census takers, and although many presume that the culture of all these people is the same, in fact a wide variety of cultural, religious, and language backgrounds are represented by this designation. Some similarities exist among members of the Asian/Pacific Islander group, but there are also many differences (Purnell & Paulanka, 1998). By understanding the basic philosophical tenets of the Southeast Asian clients, whether they are refugees or immigrants, or first-, second-, or third-generation Americans, nurses and other healthcare practitioners can be better prepared to understand, if not accept, their cultural differences and varied behavior patterns (Kubota & Matsuda, 1982).

According to Kubota and Matsuda (1982), the major philosophical orientation of the Asian/Pacific Islander people is a blend of four philosophies—Buddhism, Confucianism, Taoism, and Phi. Four common values are strongly reflected in all of these philosophies:

1. Male authority and dominance

2. "Saving face" (conduct as a result of a sense of pride)

3. Strong family ties

4. Respect for parents, elders, teachers, and other authority figures

Based on data from Kubota and Matsuda (1982), Schultz (1982), Purnell and Paulanka (1998), and Spector (1991), the following is a brief review of the beliefs and healthcare practices of the Asian/Pacific Islander people.

**Buddhism** The fundamental belief of Buddhism is that all existence is suffering. The continuation of life, and therefore suffering, arises from desires and passions, and the ultimate solution lies in the cessation of personal desire. According to the Buddhist philosophy, no humans are limited to a single existence terminating in death. Instead, everyone is reincarnated. "Ultimate salvation lies in the elimination of the self, which is to be gained by an understanding of the causality of things—a condition known as enlightenment, or nirvana, a state that cannot be described" (Kubota & Matsuda, 1982, p. 21). Cambodians, who are particularly strongly influenced by the Buddhist philosophy, strive to accumulate religious merits or good deeds to ensure a better life to come. They adhere to a deep belief in karma, whereby things done in this existence will help or hinder their ascension on the ladder to nirvana. Good deeds, sharing, donating, and being generous and kind are all ways to accumulate merits.

**Confucianism** The moral values and beliefs of Southeast Asians are heavily influenced by the Confucianism philosophy. In this concept, the moral personality is the focus. Two predominant moral qualities, developed through cultivation of the personality, include humaneness (the attitude shown toward others) and a sense of moral duty and obligation (attitudes persons display toward themselves). The principles that guide the social

behavior of people who adhere to Confucianism are described next.

*Patterns of authority* Five relationships run from inferior to superior to form a pattern of obligation and authority in the family as well as in social and political realms:

1. Son (child) to father

2. Wife to husband

3. Younger brother to older brother

4. Friend to friend

5. Subject to ruler

These patterns of authority and obligation influence decision making and social interactions. For example, a friend is to regard a friend as a younger or older brother. Women's subservience to men is reflected in a woman's behavior to always seek the advice of her husband when making decisions. This authority needs to be respected by nursing staff when, for instance, a woman refuses to choose a contraceptive method until she asks for her husband's advice and permission.

*Man in harmony with the universe* In the Confucian system, people are seen as being between heaven and earth, and life has to be in harmony with the universe. An example of this principle in action is when an Asian responds passively to new information, quietly accepting it rather than actively seeking to understand and clarify it. Given this typical behavior, it is important for the nurse when instructing the client to ask for an explanation of the information to ascertain if it was understood.

*Ancestor worship* Concern for the moral order of relationships is reflected in a deep reverence for tradition and prescribed rites. Great emphasis is placed on funerals, etiquette for mourning, and the sharing of a communal meal with the dead.

The Asian/Pacific Islander culture values harmony in life and a balance of nature. Shame is something to be avoided, families are the center of life, elders are respected, and ancestors are worshiped and remembered. Children are highly valued because they carry on the family name and are expected to care for aging parents. The woman's role is one of subservience throughout her entire life—follow the advice of parents while unmarried, the husband's advice while married, and the children's advice when widowed. This subservient role is in direct conflict with U.S. social and family values, which expect women to take a more independent, assertive, and self-determined role.

**Taoism**  The Tao philosophy has its roots in the belief of two opposing magical forces in nature, the negative (*yin*) and the positive (*yang*), which affect the course of all material and spiritual life. The basic concepts of Chinese philosophy, the beliefs in *tao* (the way of nature) and *yin* and *yang* (the principle of balance), stress that human achievement in harmony with nature should be accomplished through "nonaction." Common also is the idea that good health depends on the balance between hot and cold. Equilibrium of hot and cold elements produces good health. Drugs, natural elements, and foods are classified as either hot or cold. It is believed that sickness can be caused by eating too much hot or cold food. If a child has a stomachache, for example, the mother considers the diet. Hot foods include meats, sweets, and spices. Cold foods include rice and vegetables.

The Chinese believe in strong family ties, respect for elders, and the authority of men as the head of the household. As a consequence, sons are highly valued. Illness is believed to result from an imbalance in the forces of nature. Ill health is believed to be a curse from heaven, with mental illness being the worst possible curse, because the individual was irresponsible in not obtaining the right amount of rest, food, and work.

**Phi**  *Phi* worship is a belief in the spirits of dead relatives or the spirits of animals and nature. *Phi* range from bad to good. If a place has a strong *phi*, the individual must make an offering before doing anything in that place, such as building a house or tilling the land. If someone violates a rule of order, an atmosphere of bad *phi* can result in illness or death. Redemption can be sought from a *phi* priest as a hope of getting relief from suffering. Offerings are made and special rites are performed to rid the person of a bad *phi*.

Worshipers of this philosophy respect elders and avoid conflict by doing things in a pleasant manner. Those who adhere to the *phi* philosophy are hospitable and generous, show respect to others in the way a person is addressed, and tend to prize hard work and ambition.

For people of the Asian/Pacific Islander ethnic group, marked cultural differences confront them when they live in the United States with respect to ways of life, ways of thinking, values orientation, social structure, and family interactions (Chao, 1994). Children may adapt quickly to acculturation, but the older generations tend to have difficulty. Their medical practices, like their other unique cultural practices, differ significantly from Western ways. The health-seeking behaviors of immigrants are crisis oriented, following the pattern in their homelands where medical care was not readily available. They tend to seek health care only when seriously ill. Reinforcement is needed to encourage them to come for follow-up visits after an initial encounter with the healthcare system. Sometimes they are viewed by practitioners as noncompliant when they do not do exactly what is expected of them, when they withdraw from follow-up treatments, or when they do not keep prearranged appointments.

Asians make great use of herbal remedies to treat fevers, diarrhea, and coughs. Dermabrasion, often misunderstood by U.S. practitioners, is a home remedy to treat a wide variety of problems such as headaches, cold symptoms, and fever and chills. In their traditional healthcare system, Asian individuals rely on folk medicines from healers, sorcerers, and monks. Western medicine is thought to be "shots that cure," and Asian patients expect to get medicine (injections or pills) whenever they seek medical help in the United States. If no medication is prescribed, the person, if not given an explanation, may feel that care is inadequate and fail to return for future care. Common to many Southeast Asians is the idea that illnesses, just like foods, are classified as hot and cold, which coincide with the *yin* and *yang* philosophy of the principles of balance. If a disease is considered hot in origin, then giving cold foods is thought of as the proper treatment.

Conflict and fear are the most likely responses to laboratory tests and having blood drawn because of the belief that removing blood makes the body weak and that blood is not replenished. Fear of surgery may result from the belief that souls inhabit the body and may be released. Loss of privacy leading to extreme embarrassment and humiliation is another major fear.

**Teaching Strategies** Respect is automatically endowed on most healthcare providers and teachers because they are seen as knowledgeable. Asians are sensitive and formal people, so making a friendly and non-threatening approach to them is necessary before giving care. They must be given permission to ask a question but are not offended by questions from others.

Language barriers are usually the first and biggest obstacle to overcome in dealing with people of Asian/Pacific Islander descent. Translators can be used to facilitate interactions. The learning style of Asians is essentially passive—no personal opinions, no confrontations, no challenges, and no outward disagreements—and learning is done by repetition and rote memorization of information. It must be remembered that decision making is a family affair. Consequently, family members need to be included, especially the male authority figure, in the process of deciding the best solution for a situation.

Nurses and other healthcare practitioners should be aware that in the Asians' wish to "save face" for themselves and others, they avoid being disruptive and will agree to what is said so as not to be offensive. They are easily shamed, so patients must be reassured and told what is considered acceptable behavior by Western moral and legal standards. Nods of the head do not necessarily mean agreement or understanding. Questions directed to them need to be asked in several ways to confirm that they understand any instructional messages given.

## Native American Culture

The U.S. Census Bureau (2000) has identified more than 2 million people (0.7% of the U.S. population) who are of Native American (American Indian or Native Alaskan) descent living in the United States. Of these people, approximately 1 million are eligible for health services provided by the federal government. Medical care to American Indian people has a long history. As far back as 1832, the War Department undertook a smallpox vaccination campaign for tribes of American Indian people, largely to protect military troops from infection. In 1849, healthcare responsibility was transferred to the newly created Bureau of Indian Affairs. In 1954, the Department of Health, Education, and Welfare of the U.S. Public Health Service (USPHS) took over jurisdiction. Today, the Indian Health Service (IHS) of the USPHS maintains responsibility for providing health care to more than 500 distinct tribes of American Indians and Native Alaskans, including Eskimo and Aleut tribes (Mail et al., 1989; Lowe & Struthers, 2001).

The largest of the Native American tribes are the Navajo. Other tribes of significant size are the Cherokee, Sioux, Chippewa, and Pueblo. These tribes reside primarily in the northwestern, central, and southwestern regions of the United States. The term *Native American* will be used throughout this section of the chapter to include both the American Indian and Native Alaskan people.

The current challenge to healthcare practitioners is to integrate Western medicine with traditional non-Western tribal folk medicine to provide cross-cultural health education to Native Americans in reservation-based communities across the nation. To do so, nurses must understand contemporary Native American cultural patterns, including theories of disease causality and associated therapies. It is also essential for nursing professionals to become focused on a more "ethnomedical" orientation of delineating the nature and consequences of illness problems and disease interventions, rather than adhering to the biomedical orientation of defining diseases and illness interventions. In the ethnomedical context, the concept of illness incorporates the relationship of humans with their universe—a concept that bridges culture with a sensitivity toward the daily practices inherent within specific ethnic groups. The challenge for the nurse educator is to understand the world perspective of contemporary American Indian and Native Alaskan people that sets them apart from non–Native Americans (Mail et al.,1989; Lowe & Struthers, 2001; Cantore, 2001).

As outlined by Primeaux (1977), Purnell and Paulanka (1998), Spector (1991), Lowe and Struthers (2001), and Cantore (2001), Native American culture has the following major characteristics:

1. A spiritual attachment to the land and harmony with nature

2. An intimacy of religion and medicine

3. Emphasis on strong ties to an extended family network, including immediate family, other relatives, and the entire tribe

4. The view that children are an asset, not a liability

5. A belief that supernatural powers exist in animate as well as in inanimate objects

6. A desire to remain Native American and avoid acculturation, thereby retaining one's own culture and language

7. A lack of materialism, time consciousness, and a desire to share with others

Unless the awareness of non–Native American healthcare workers is raised, these common characteristics can easily be overlooked by them when care is being provided to the Native American client. Although Anglo-American culture and Western healthcare practices have been integrated to some extent into the Native American way of life, the preceding characteristics still predominate today to set American Indians and Native Alaskans apart as a unique cultural group.

Native Americans see a close connection between religion and health. When a family member becomes ill, witchcraft is still perceived by some tribes as the real cause of illness. In traditional societies, witchcraft functions to supply answers to perplexing or disturbing questions. It also explains personal insecurities, intragroup tensions, fears, and anxieties. Witches, with their supernatural powers, have served as convenient scapegoats on which to blame the misfortunes in life and provided tribes with a mechanism for social control. It is hypothesized that as the cultural practices of witchcraft were increasingly denigrated by missionaries and bureaucrats, substitutions such as compulsive drinking and frequent use of narcotics (peyote) emerged as culturally sanctioned outlets for aggressive impulses and frustrations. These behaviors were seen as less disruptive than demonstrating overt hostilities. This hypothesis has been proposed as an explanation of the high prevalence of substance abuse by Native Americans. Some Native American tribes still practice witchcraft but tend to deny it as a reality because of the negative stereotype and stigma attached to it by outsiders. Nevertheless, the intimacy between religion and medicine persists and is exhibited in the form of "sing" prayers and ceremonial cure practices. However, few nurses would think of providing space and privacy for several relatives to be able to conduct a ceremony for a hospitalized family member.

Some Native American tribal beliefs also require incorporating the medicine man (*shaman*) into the system of care given to patients. It is important to realize that the central and formal aspects of Native American medicine are ceremonial, embracing the notion of a supernatural power. Although the ceremonies vary from tribe to tribe, the ideas of causation and cure are common to all Native Americans. The ritual performed is determined by the signs and symptoms of an illness. Sometimes rituals are conducted by family members. Cornmeal, from the sacred food of corn, is one item that is frequently used in a variety of curative ceremonies. The nurse must demonstrate legitimate respect for such ritualistic symbols and ceremonial activities (Primeaux, 1977).

To be considered really poor in the Native American world is to be devoid of relatives. The family and tribe are of utmost importance, a belief that children learn from infancy (Primeaux, 1977). It is not unusual for many family members—sometimes large groups of 10 to 15 people—to arrive at the hospital and camp out on the hospital grounds to be with their sick relative. Talking is unnecessary, but simply being there is highly important for everyone concerned. Hospital personnel have often labeled this behavior as useless and disruptive and deem the patient and family to be uncooperative. Grandmothers, in particular, have great importance to a sick child, and they frequently must give permission for a child to be hospitalized and treated. The Native American kinship system, in fact, allows for a child to have several sets of grandparents, aunts, uncles, cousins, brothers, and sisters. Sometimes a number of women substitute as a mother figure for a child, which may cause role confusion for the non–Native American healthcare provider.

Children are given a great deal of freedom and independence to learn by their decisions and live by the consequences of their actions. Their entire childhood years consist of experiential learning to develop skills and self-confidence to function as adults. They may appear "spoiled," but in fact they are taught self-care and respect for others at a very early age. Outside of their private domain, Native American children tend not to be very competitive or assertive. This behavior can be seen in children in the public school system. To call attention to oneself is interpreted by Native Americans as "showy" and inappropriate. Children are doted on by family members, and, in turn, they have high regard for their elders. In fact, the older adults in Native American communities are highly respected and looked to for advice and counsel.

Another characteristic of Native Americans is that they generally are not very future oriented; they take one day at a time and do not feel they have control over their own destiny. This attitude or way of thinking has proved to be a significant obstacle when health educators have attempted to provide preventive care. Time is seen as being on a continuum with no beginning and no end. Native Americans tend not to live by clocks and schedules. In fact, many of their homes do not have clocks, and family members eat meals and do other activities when they please. They are more casual in their approach to life than many non–Native American people. This lack of time consciousness and pressure is a crucial factor to be remembered by healthcare providers when a prescribed regimen calls for the patient to follow a medication, exercise, or dietary schedule. Inattention to time also can interfere with their keeping scheduled appointments, although lack of funds rather than time seems to be the main cause of missed appointments.

Another aspect of time is reflected in their belief that death is just a part of the life cycle—a much healthier and more accepting attitude toward dying than that held by most Anglo-Americans. Their grief process is culturally very different. Funerals are accompanied by large feasts and the sharing of gifts with relatives of the deceased. There is no belief in a life hereafter as a reward for a lifetime of good deeds while on earth. Life after death is, instead, viewed as an opportunity to join the world of long-ago ancestors. Their view of death is closely related to their opinion about the appropriate disposal of amputated limbs. Because diabetes is so prevalent in the Native American population, it is important to know that they usually want to reclaim an amputated body part for proper burial.

Sharing is another core value of Native Americans. The concept of "being" is fundamental, and there is little stress on achievement or the worth of material wealth. Individuals are valued much more highly than material goods. Overall, Native Americans are a proud, sensitive, cooperative, passive people, devoted to tribe and family, and willing to share possessions and self with others. They are very vulnerable when it comes to their pride and dignity. They can be easily offended by nonsensitive caregivers. In terms of human relationships, it is important to note that Native Americans believe that to look someone in the eye is considered disrespectful. Some tribes feel that looking into the eyes of another person reveals and may even steal someone's soul. As a friendly handshake and eye contact are acceptable and even expected in the Anglo-American culture, it must be acknowledged that these gestures do not have the same meaning for the Native American. In fact, eye contact by Anglo-American definition is interpreted to mean that someone is paying attention, is interested, or understands. Non–Native American healthcare workers, therefore, may consider lack of eye

contact to mean that these patients are shiftless, shifty, uninterested in learning, or inattentive, when in fact all along they were taking in the message of instruction being given. If asked, they can often repeat verbatim what someone just said to them. As Primeaux (1977) so aptly comments, "Perhaps the notion of being spoken to rather than with has importance here" (p. 94).

The health problems faced by Native Americans are undergoing significant change. In the first half of the twentieth century, acute and infectious diseases were prevalent and were the principal cause of death. Today, as a result of increased life expectancy, Native Americans are succumbing to many lifestyle diseases and chronic conditions. Chief among the causes of morbidity and mortality are heart disease, cancer, diabetes, and drug and alcohol abuse—all of which to some extent are amenable to educational intervention.

**Teaching Strategies**  Patient educators need to focus on giving information about these diseases and risk factors, emphasize the teaching of skills related to changes in diet and exercise, and help clients to build positive coping mechanisms to deal with emotional problems (Hosey & Stracqualursi, 1990). For the most part, acute and infectious diseases, with the exception of a recurrence in tuberculosis, are no longer a major cause of illness and death among Native Americans thanks to greater availability of drug therapy, early case findings, improved sanitary conditions, and better provision of health education. Another positive influence has been the greater availability of community health representatives (CHRs), indigenous community outreach workers who have played a significant role in case finding, early diagnosis, and reinforcement of patient and other health education recommendations. As Mail et al. (1989) stated: "Involving the CHR in patient education is an important cross-cultural consideration, because this is the individual who will reinforce behavior changes with the community and home" (p. 97).

Although all Native Americans share some of the core beliefs and practices of their culture, each tribe is unique in its customs and language. Finding the ways and means to integrate Western medicine with the traditional Native American folk medicine in caring for the varied needs of this population group presents a challenge to the nurse educator as well as a learning opportunity for the recipient of health education services.

## PREPARING NURSES FOR DIVERSITY CARE

America is no longer the homogeneous society it once was. Today, myriad cultures are present in the United States, and we face an increasing trend toward global migration of people and globalization of nursing practice. The delivery of appropriate health care now and in the future will depend on use of a culturally informed approach that goes beyond simple language translation and an understanding of the characteristics of different cultures. As caregivers, we must learn how to relate to people (both patients and fellow healthcare practitioners) from a variety of cultural backgrounds and discover the cultural meaning of various health events (Dreher, 1996). The nursing profession must be prepared to establish a new paradigm for creating and managing diversity within our workforce as well as within a new healthcare marketplace consisting of consumers and staff from multicultural backgrounds. Diversity has the potential to positively affect our profession by increasing organizational effectiveness, creating greater access to care, lifting morale of patients and staff, and enhancing productivity in the workforce (Thomas & Ely, 1996; Marquand, 2001).

As a result of former President Clinton's national leadership to eliminate cultural disparities in health by the year 2010, the U.S. Department of Health and Human Services (HHS) established the Initiative to Eliminate Racial and Ethnic Disparities in Health. This "2010 Initiative" is cause for the nursing profession to eradicate discrepancies in health outcomes among minority populations. The profession needs to do so in both the academic and the practice settings and through clinical research (Carol, 2001).

One important step to assure culturally competent nursing care in this new century is to increase minority representation in nursing. We need to recruit and retain more minority students and faculty to expand diversity within our ranks. Unfortunately, the nursing workforce comprises less than 10% of people from minority groups, whereas more than 28% of the total U.S. population belongs to a variety of cultural subgroups (Robinson, 2000).

Another initiative to break down cultural barriers to health care is to strengthen multicultural perspectives in the curriculum of nursing education programs (Kelley & Fitzsimmons, 2000). Innovative nursing education means incorporating social values that recognize diverse lifestyles and acknowledge multicultural and multiracial perspectives (Sims & Baldwin, 1995). As Dreher (1996) points out, nurses must not only better understand the cultural characteristics and traits of patients and families from different ethnic backgrounds, but also improve the relationship between nurses and clients from different cultural backgrounds. Nurses must be able to create an environment in which people are encouraged to express themselves and freely describe their needs. As Dreher (1996) so aptly states, "Transcending cultural differences is more than an appreciation of cultural diversity. It is transcending one's own investment in the social and economic system as one knows it and lives it" (p. 4). Nurse educators must concentrate on the cultural strategies that are needed to help individuals and groups negotiate the healthcare system.

### ■■■ STEREOTYPING: IDENTIFYING THE MEANING, THE RISKS, AND THE SOLUTIONS

In addressing the diversity issues of gender, socioeconomics, and culture, one must acknowledge the risks of stereotyping inherent in discussing these three attributes of the learner. Throughout this chapter, it has been explicitly recognized that differences exist in learning based on gender, socioeconomics, and culture and often require alternative approaches to teaching. It is important to realize that differences should not be equated with judgments as to what is good or bad, right or wrong; rather, one should not ignore the need to attend to these differences in a sensitive, open, and fair manner. Nurse educators must relate to each person as an individual with an awareness that although a person can be considered as a member, or may identify with members, of a certain group or subgroup, the individual has his or her own abilities, experiences, preferences, and practices when it comes to learning needs, learning styles, and readiness to learn— all factors that influence lifestyle behaviors.

Nevertheless, given that we all have been socialized in subtle and not so subtle ways according to our own diversity attributes, socioeconomic and political backgrounds, and other life exposures, it is imperative to acknowledge the prejudices, biases, and stereotypical tendencies that can come into play when dealing with others like or unlike ourselves. We must consciously attempt to recognize these possible attitudes and the effect they may have on others in our care.

To address the dangers of stereotyping on more than just a superficial level, this section examines examples of what constitutes unacceptable forms of stereotyping, what common pitfalls can arise in dealing with diversity, and what can be done to avoid stereotypical behaviors in ourselves and others. *Stereotyping* is defined by Purnell and Paulanka (1998) as "an oversimplified conception, opinion, or belief about some aspect of an individual or group" (p. 490). Such a generalization is made about the motives thought to underlie the behaviors of any person or people. Woolfolk (1998) describes stereotyping as a schema that organizes knowledge or perceptions about a person or group.

Actually, stereotyping can be positive or negative, depending on how, where, when, why, and with whom the term is used. Under Woolfolk's definition, for example, stereotyping can be a useful and legitimate process employed as an organizing or classifying system if based on logical reasoning and accumulated facts. A system of organization and classification helps people to identify and understand information—for example, "he's Jewish," "she's Italian," or "they're Democrats." Conversely, stereotyping can be negative if it is used to place people in a mold or an artificial, unfair position based on oversimplification without true substantiation by facts. Negative stereotyping leads to disrespect, dehumanization, and denigration of others and serves as a barrier to equality and fairness toward others. Stereotyping deserves a bad name when associated with bias or clichés. There is a huge emotional component to stereotyping. The language that we use, the attitudes that we project, the conclusions that we draw, and the context in which we employ stereotyping all determine its positive or negative quality.

Unfortunately, classification by association is often perfunctory and, therefore, laden with bias. Stereotyping in this sense is used to label someone. For example, we, as Americans, think of ourselves as the freedom fighters and liberty lovers of the world; in the same breath, we may describe members of other groups or nationalities as violators of human rights or terrorists. Simple appearance, such as a beard, attire, or form of speech, can be the basis of broad and deep prejudices. We particularly tend to use an excuse to classify individuals when we do not like or respect people whose backgrounds, attitudes, abilities, values, or beliefs are different from or opposed to our own or are misunderstood or misinterpreted. Stereotyping, conscious or subconscious, results in intolerance toward others and engenders the belief that our way is the only or the right way. Corley and Goren (1998) discuss the ways in which labeling, stereotyping, and stigmatizing responses by nurses tend to marginalize patients.

Tear (1995) discussed gender stereotypes in the workplace. She states that these alleged "masculine" and "feminine" attitudes have, unfortunately, "so permeated our culture that fair-minded members of both sexes are likely to reach mistaken conclusions about each other" (p. A14). Intergender tensions exist, she points out, due to misunderstandings caused by differences in communication patterns of the sexes. Popular culture encourages society to view certain forms of communication as expressions of stereotypical attitudes rather than as language habits. For example, many gender theories label women as attentive listeners and men as poor listeners when, in fact, listening behavior is not a measure of attentiveness but a matter of behavioral style. Men, when listening, move around and make sporadic eye contact, whereas women are likely to remain still and maintain steady eye contact with occasional nodding or smiling. As a result, the listening style of men is often misinterpreted as inattentive or rude, and the style of females is often mistaken for encouragement or agreement with what is being said. Interruption is another example of communication differences between the sexes. Men frequently speak in a steady flow and interrupt each other to take turns, whereas women tend to speak with frequent pauses to allow others to have their say. Pause-free male speech is often misinterpreted as a device to discourage females from participating and as an attempt to be pushy. The tendency for females to pause in speaking is seen as being timid or courteous. These misinterpretations, according to Tear (1995), reinforce stereotypes of men as dominating, insensitive and controlling and women as unassertive, passive, and oversensitive.

Educational psychologists have long addressed gender stereotyping in school settings. It used to be that an extensive list of personality differences between the sexes would be included in psychology textbooks; most recent research, however, reveals that these sex-role lists are gender biased. Today, it is recognized that few personality characteristics associated with gender are consistent across cultures, except for aggression. Males across cultures have been found to be more aggressive (dominant, assertive, hostile, destructive) than females, which can substantially affect the teaching and learning process (Gage & Berliner, 1998). Research in the past 20 years has documented that teachers interact more actively with boys by asking them more questions, giving them more feedback (praise and positive encouragement), and providing them with more specific and valuable comments and guidance. In these subtle ways, these stereotypical expectations are reinforced (Woolfolk, 1998).

Attitudes toward sex-role competencies have been perhaps the greatest and most prevalent kind of stereotyping. Gender bias has produced a true dichotomy in equality in education, employment, and other social spheres. It was only in the twentieth century that women began to attain equal opportunities, both culturally and economically. Stereotypical attitudes persist, however. Although much more attention is being paid to this issue, we have a long way to go to rid our society of gender bias.

Nurse educators must concentrate on treating the sexes equally when providing access to health education, delivering health and illness care, and designing health education materials that contain bias-free language. For example, avoid gender-specific terms and choose words that minimize ambiguity in gender identity, unless critical to the content. Avoid using the pronouns *he* or *she* and instead use the plural pronoun *they*. Avoid beginning or ending words with *man* or *men*, such as "man-made," "mankind," or "chairmen." Do not specify marital status unless necessary by using *Ms.* instead of *Mrs.* Guidelines for nonsexist language can be found in *McGraw-Hill Guidelines for Bias-Free Publishing* or *The Bias-Free Word Finder*.

With respect to socioeconomics, age, ethnicity and race, religion, or disabilities, stereotyping most definitely exists. Throughout this chapter, there are many cautions against stereotyping of individuals and groups. For example, just because someone belongs to a specific cultural group does not necessarily mean that the individual adheres to all of the beliefs and practices of that particular culture. Thorough and accurate assessment of the learner is the key to determining the particular abilities, preferences, and needs of each individual. As with issues of gender, you should choose words that are accurate, clear, and free from bias whenever speaking or writing about various individuals or groups. Refer to someone's ethnicity, race, religion, age, and socioeconomic status only when it is essential to the content being addressed. The term *member of a historically underrepresented group* rather than the term *minority* is the preferred terminology. *Older adult* or *older people/persons* is more politically and socially correct than the term *elderly*. Do not label a member of a special population as a *disabled person* but rather as a *person with a disability*. It is more appropriate and more acceptable to refer to a *person with diabetes*

rather than a *diabetic* or to a *person with AIDS* rather than an *AIDS victim*. To avoid negative stereotyping, you are reminded of the many references used in this chapter, particularly Purnell and Paulanka (1998) and Chideya (1999), and in Chapters 7 and 9 of this text that focus on maintaining sensitivity to the concepts and language of various groups with whom the nurse interacts. The descriptions presented here of differences in group characteristics and attributes are general; although the findings of one or more studies do not represent universal truth, there are plenty of scientific data from anthropology, sociology, psychology, education and social psychology, nursing, and medicine to support these descriptions.

As a nurse educator, ask yourself the following questions:

- Do I use neutral language when teaching clients and families?

- Do I confront bias when evidenced by other healthcare professionals?

- Do I request information equally from clients regardless of gender, socioeconomic status, age, or culture?

- Are my instructional materials free of stereotypical terminology and expressions?

- Am I an effective role model of equality for my colleagues?

- Do I treat all clients with fairness, respect, and dignity?

- Does someone's appearance influence (raise or lower) my expectations of that person's abilities or affect the quality of care I deliver?

- Do I routinely assess the educational backgrounds, experiential backgrounds, personal attributes, and economic resources of clients to ensure appropriate health teaching?

- Am I knowledgeable enough of the cultural traditions of various groups to provide sensitive care in our pluralistic society?

It is easy to stereotype someone, not of out of malice, but out of ignorance. Nurse educators have a responsibility to keep informed of the most current information about various gender attributes, socioeconomic influences, and cultural traditions that affect teaching and learning. Every day, research in nursing, social science, psychology, and medicine is yielding information that will assist in planning and revising appropriate nursing interventions to meet the needs of our diverse client populations.

## SUMMARY

This chapter explored the influence of gender, socioeconomic status, and cultural beliefs on both the ability and willingness of clients to learn healthcare measures. The in-depth examination of these three factors serves as an explanatory model for certain behaviors observed or potentially encountered in a teaching–learning situation. Even though the emphasis of this chapter was on patients or members of the general public from various ethnic groups with whom nurse educators interact, an understanding of gender differences, socioeconomic influences, and cultural characteristics can also be a useful source of information when teaching nursing students or staff who may come from a variety of backgrounds and orientations.

The most important message to remember from this chapter is the care one must take not to stereotype or generalize common characteristics of a group to all members associated with that particular group. If the nurse does not know much about a culture, that lack of knowledge is acceptable. The more important point is to ask clients about their beliefs, rather than just assuming they abide by the tenets of a certain cultural group. In that way, nurses can avoid offending the learner. The educator must be cautious to treat each learner as an individual and to ascertain the extent to which they ascribe to, exhibit beliefs in, or adhere to ways of doing things that might affect learning. Both men and women live in a double environment—an outer layer of natural resources and climate and an inner layer of culture and innate strengths and weaknesses—which influences how they perceive and respond to their world (Griffith, 1982). Nurses as professionals should constantly strive to improve the delivery of care to all people regardless of their gender orientation, ethnic origin, creed, nationality, or socioeconomic background (Holtz & Bairan, 1990). There is much more for nurses to know about how these three factors of gender, socioeconomics, and culture affect the teaching–learning process before we can competently, confidently, and sensitively deliver care to satisfy the needs of our socially, intellectually, and culturally diverse clientele.

## REVIEW QUESTIONS

1. What are five (5) gender-related differences in cognitive functioning and personality characteristics that affect learning?
2. What does the latest research indicate about the affect environment versus heredity has on learning?
3. In what ways does socioeconomic status negatively affect a person's health and, conversely, how does illness impact an individual's socioeconomic well-being?
4. How does socioeconomic status of individuals influence the teaching-learning process?

5. What is meant by the term *poverty circle*?
6. What is a more politically acceptable term for the word *minority*?
7. What is the definition of each of the following terms: *culture, ethnicity, ethnocentrism, acculturation,* and *ethnomedical*?
8. How can the concept of transcultural nursing be applied to the assessment and teaching of clients from culturally diverse backgrounds?
9. What are the six (6) cultural phenomena that should be taken into account when conducting a nursing assessment?
10. Which four (4) components are included in the Culturally Competent Model of Care?
11. What can the nurse do to avoid cultural stereotyping?
12. What are the four (4) major cultural groups in the United States?
13. What are the salient characteristics of each of the four (4) major cultural groups?
14. Which teaching strategies are most appropriate to meet the needs of individuals from each of the four (4) major cultural groups?

## REFERENCES

Andersen, R. M., Giachello, A. L., & Aday, L. A. (1986). Access of Hispanics to health care and cuts in services: A state-of-the-art overview. *Public Health Reports, 101*(3), 238–252.

Anderson, J. M. (1987). The cultural context of caring. *Canadian Critical Care Nursing Journal,* December, 7–13.

Anderson, J. M. (1990). Health care across cultures. *Nursing Outlook, 38*(3), 136–139.

Andrews, M. M. (1992). Cultural perspectives on nursing in the 21st century. *Journal of Professional Nursing, 8*(1), 7–15.

Andrews, M. M. & Boyle, J. S. (1995). Transcultural nursing care. In *Transcultural Concepts in Nursing Care,* 2nd ed. Philadelphia: Lippincott.

Babcock, D. E. & Miller, M. A. (1994). *Client Education: Theory and Practice.* St. Louis: Mosby–Year Book.

Baker, D. W., Parker, R. M., Williams, M. V., Coates, W. C., & Pitkin, K. (1996). Use and effectiveness of interpreters in an emergency department. *Journal of the American Medical Association,* 275(10), 783–788.

Baydar, N., Brooks-Gunn, J., & Furstenberg, F. F. (1993). Early warning signs of functional illiteracy: Predictors in childhood and adolescence. *Child Development, 64,* 815–829.

Begley, S. (February 19, 1996). Your child's brain. *Newsweek,* 55–62.

Begley, S., Murr, A., & Rogers, A. (March 27, 1995). Gray matters. *Newsweek,* 48–54.

Campbell, F. A. & Ramey, C. T. (1994). Effects of early intervention on intellectual and academic achievement: A follow-up study of children from low-income families. *Child Development, 65,* 684–698.

Campinha-Bacote, J. (1995). The quest for cultural competence in nursing care. *Nursing Forum, 30*(4), 19–25.

Cantore, J. A. (2001). Earth, wind, fire and water. *Minority Nurse,* Winter, 24–29.

Carol, R. (2001). Taking the initiative. *Minority Nurse,* Fall, 24–27.

Caudle, P. (1993). Providing culturally sensitive health care to Hispanic clients. *Nurse Practitioner, 18*(12), 40, 43–44, 46, 50–51.

Chachkes, E. & Christ, G. (1996). Cross cultural issues in patient education. *Patient Education & Counseling, 27,* 13–21.

Chao, R. K. (1994). Beyond parental control and authoritarian parenting style: Understanding Chinese parenting through the cultural notion of training. *Child Development, 65,* 1111–1119.

Chideya, F. (1999). *The Color of our Future.* New York: William Morrow.

Cohen, D. (ed.). (1991). *The Circle of Life: Rituals from the Human Family Album.* New York: Harper-Collins.

Corley, M. C. & Goren, S. (1998). The dark side of nursing: Impact of stigmatizing responses on patients. *Scholarly Inquiry for Nursing Practice: An International Journal, 12*(2), 99–118.

Crimmins, E. M. & Saito, Y. (2001). Trends in healthy life expectancy in the United States, 1970–1990: Gender, race, and educational differences. *Social Science & Medicine, 52,* 1629–1641.

Denboba, D. L., Bragdon, J. L., Epstein, L. G. Garthright, K., & Goldman, T. M. (1998). Reducing health disparities through cultural competence. *Journal of Health Education, 29*(5), 47–53.

Dreher, M. C. (1996). Nursing: A cultural phenomenon. *Reflections*, 4th Quarter, 4.

Duffy, M. M. & Snyder, K. (1999). Can ED patients read your education materials? *Journal of Emergency Nursing, 25*(4), 294–297.

Falvo, D. R. (1994). *Effective Patient Education: A Guide to Increased Compliance*, 2nd ed. Gaithersburg, MD: Aspen.

Gage, N. L. & Berliner, D. C. (1992). *Educational Psychology*, 5th ed. Boston: Houghton Mifflin.

Gage , N. L. & Berliner, D. C. (1998). *Educational Psychology*, 6th ed. Boston: Houghton Mifflin.

Galanti, G. A. (1991). *Caring for Patients from Different Cultures*. Philadelphia: University of Pennsylvania Press.

Giger, J. N. & Davidhizar, R. E. (1995). *Transcultural Nursing: Assessment and Intervention*, 2nd ed., St. Louis: Mosby–Year Book.

Gollop, C. J. (1997). Health information-seeking behavior and older African American women. *Bulletin of the Medical Library Association, 85*(2), 141–146.

Gorman, C. (January 20, 1992). Sizing up the sexes. *Time*, 42–51.

Griffith, S. (1982). Childbearing and the concept of culture. *Journal of Obstetrics, Gynecological, and Neonatal Nursing, 11*(3), 181–184.

Guralnik, J. M., Land, K. C., Blazer, D., Fillenbaum, G. G., & Branch, L. C. (1993). Educational status and active life expectancy among older blacks and whites. *New England Journal of Medicine, 329*(2), 110–116.

Hahn, M. (1995). Providing health care in a culturally complex world. *Advance for Nurse Practitioners*, November 43–45.

Hancock, L. (February 19, 1996). Why do schools flunk biology? *Newsweek*, 59.

Hegyvary, S. T. (1992). From diversity to enrichment. *Journal of Professional Nursing, 8*(5), 261.

Hirsch, E. D. (2001). Overcoming the language gap. *American Educator*, Summer, 5–7.

Holtz, C. & Bairan, A. (1990). Personal contact: A method of teaching cultural empathy. *Nurse Educator, 15*(3), 13, 23, 28.

Horn, B. (1983). Cultural beliefs and teenage pregnancy. *Nurse Practitioner*, September, 38–39.

Horton, M. & Freire, P. (1990). *We Make the Road by Walking*. Philadelphia: Temple University Press.

Hosey, G. M. & Stracqualurski, F. (1990). Designing and evaluating diabetes education material for American Indians. *Diabetes Educator, 16*(5), 407–414.

Jackson, L. E. (1993). Understanding, eliciting, and negotiating clients' multicultural health beliefs. *Nurse Practitioner, 18*(4), 30–43.

Jezewski, M. A. (1993). Culture brokering as a model for advocacy. *Nursing & Health Care, 14*(2), 78–85.

Kawamura, M., Midorikawa, A., & Kezuka, M. (2000). Cerebral localization of the center for reading and writing music. *NeuroReport, 11*(14), 3299–3303.

Kelley, M. L. & Fitzsimmons, V. M. (2000). *Understanding Cultural Diversity: Culture, Curriculum, and Community in Nursing*. Boston: Jones and Bartlett Publishers.

Kinsey, K. K. (1995). Risky business: Managing the health care of urban low-income families. *Holistic Nursing Practice, 9*(4), 41–53.

Kleinman, A. (1978). Concepts and a model for the comparison of medical systems as cultural systems. *Social Science & Medicine, 12*, 85–93.

Kniep-Hardy, M. & Burkhardt, M. A. (1977). Nursing the Navajo. *American Journal of Nursing, 77*(1), 95–96.

Kubota, J. & Matsuda, K. J. (1982). Family planning services for southeast Asian refugees. *Family & Community Health, 5*(1), 19–25.

Leininger, M. (1978). *Transcultural Nursing: Concepts, Theories and Practices*. New York: Wiley.

Leininger, M. (1994). Transcultural nursing education: A worldwide imperative. *Nursing & Health Care, 15*(5), 254–257.

Lipman, E. L., Offord, D. R., & Boyle, M. H. (1994). Relation between economic disadvantage and psychosocial morbidity in children. *Canadian Medical Association Journal, 151*(4), 431–437.

Lowe, J. & Struthers, R. (2001). A conceptual framework of nursing in Native American culture. *Journal of Nursing Scholarship*, 3rd Quarter, 279–283.

Luster, T. & McAdoo, H. P. (1994). Factors related to the achievement and adjustment of young African American children. *Child Development, 65*, 1080–1094.

MacCoby, E. E. & Jacklin, C. N. (1974). *The Psychology of Sex Differences.* Stanford, CA: Stanford University Press.

Mail, P. D., McKay, R. B., & Katz, M. (1989). Expanding practice horizons: Learning from American Indian patients. *Patient Education & Counseling, 13,* 91–102.

Markides, K. S. & Coreil, J. (1986). The health of Hispanics in southwestern U.S.: An epidemiological paradox. *Public Health Reports, 101*(3), 253–265.

Marquand, B. (2001). On the front lines of diversity. *Minority Nurse,* Fall, 46–49.

Massett, H. A. (1996). Appropriateness of Hispanic print materials: A content analysis. *Health Education Research, 11*(2), 231–242.

McGoldrick, M. (1995). *You Can Go Home Again.* New York: W. W. Norton.

Monastersky, R. (November 2, 2001). Land mines in the world of mental maps. *Chronicle of Higher Education,* A20–A21.

Morra, M. E. (1991). Future trends in patient education. *Seminars in Oncology Nursing, 7*(2), 143–145.

Nagoshi, C. T., Johnson, R. C., & Honbo, K. A. (1993). Family background, cognitive abilities, and personality as predictors of education and occupational attainment across two generations. *Journal of Biosocial Science, 25*(2), 259–276.

Nash, J. M. (1997). Fertile minds. *Time, 149*(5), 48–56.

Ormrod, J. E. (1995). *Educational Psychology: Principles and Applications.* Englewood Cliffs, NJ: Prentice-Hall.

Pappas, G., Queen, S., Hadden, W., & Fisher, G. (1993). The increasing disparity in mortality between socioeconomic groups in the United States, 1960 and 1986. *New England Journal of Medicine, 329*(2), 103–109.

Parker, M. & Kiatoukaysy, L. N. (1999). Culturally responsive health care: The example of the Hmong in America. *Journal of the American Academy of Nurse Practitioners, 11*(12), 511–518.

Perry, D. S. (1982). The umbilical cord: Transcultural care and customs. *Journal of Nurse-Midwifery, 27*(4), 25–30.

Poss, J. E. & Rangel, R. (1995). Working effectively with interpreters in the primary care setting. *Nurse Practitioner, 20*(12), 43–44, 46–47.

Price, J. L. & Cordell, B. (1994). Cultural diversity and patient teaching. *Journal of Continuing Education in Nursing, 25*(4), 163–166.

Price, K. M. & Cortis, J. D. (2000). The way forward for transcultural nursing. *Nurse Education Today, 20,* 233–243.

Primeaux, M. (1977). Caring for the American Indian patient. *American Journal of Nursing, 77*(1), 91–94.

Purnell, L. D. & Paulanka, B. J. (1998). *Transcultural Health Care: A Culturally Competent Approach.* Philadelphia: F. A. Davis.

Rempusheski, V. F. (1989). The role of ethnicity in elder care. *Nursing Clinics of North America, 24*(3), 717–724.

Rhem, J. (1998). Social class and student learning. *National Teaching & Learning Forum, 7*(5), 1–4.

Robinson, J. H. (2000). Increasing students' cultural sensitivity. *Nurse Educator, 25*(3), 131–135.

Rooda, L. & Gay, G. (1993). Staff development for culturally sensitive nursing care. *Journal of Nursing Staff Development, 9*(6), 262–265.

Schultz, S. L. (1982). How Southeast-Asian refugees in California adapt to unfamiliar health care practices. *Health & Social Work, 7*(2), 148–156.

Shomaker, D. M. (1981). Navajo nursing homes: Conflict of philosophies. *Journal of Gerontological Nursing, 7*(9), 531–536.

Sims, G. P. & Baldwin, D. (1995). Race, class, and gender considerations in nursing education. *Nursing & Health Care, 16*(6), 316–321.

Smolan, R., Moffitt, P., & Naythons, M. (1990). *The Power to Heal: Ancient Arts and Modern Medicine.* New York: Prentice Hall Press.

Speck, O., Ernst, T., Braun, J., Koch, C., Miller, E., & Chang, L. (2000). Gender differences in the functional organization of the brain for working memory. *NeuroReport, 11*(11), 2581–2585.

Spector, R. E. (1991). *Cultural Diversity in Health and Illness,* 3rd ed. Norwalk, CT: Appleton & Lange.

Spicer, J. G., Ripple, H. B., Louie, E., Baj, P., & Keating, S. (1994). Supporting ethnic and cultural diversity in nursing staff. *Nursing Management, 25*(1), 38–40.

Tear, J. (November 20, 1995). They just don't understand gender dynamics. *Wall Street Journal,* A14.

Thomas, D. A. & Ely, R. J. (1996). Making differences matter: A new paradigm for managing diversity. *Harvard Business Review, 74*(5), 79–90.

Torres, S. (1994). A challenge to nursing education: Meeting the health care needs of the Hispanic community. *Deans Notes: A Communication Service to Nursing School Deans, Administrators, and Faculty, 15*(5).

Tripp-Reimer, T. (1982). Barriers to health care: Variations in interpretation of Appalachian client behaviors by Appalachian and non-Appalachian health professionals. *Western Journal of Nursing Research, 4*(2), 179–191.

Tripp-Reimer, T. & Afifi, L. A. (1989). Cross-cultural perspectives on patient teaching. *Nursing Clinics of North America, 24*(3), 613–619.

U.S. Census Bureau. (2000). *Population estimates program.* Washington, DC: U.S. Census Bureau.

Westberg, J. (1989). Patient education for Hispanic Americans. *Patient Education & Counseling, 13,* 143–160.

Winkleby, M. A., Jatulis, D. E., Frank, E., & Fortmann, S. P. (1992). Socioeconomic status and health: How education, income, and occupation contribute to risk factors for cardiovascular disease. *American Journal of Public Health, 82*(6), 816–820.

Woolfolk, A. E. (1998). *Educational Psychology,* 7th ed. Boston: Allyn and Bacon.

Yee, S-H., Liu, H-L., Hou, J., Pu, Y., Fox, P. T., & Gao, J-H. (2000). Detection of the brain response during a cognitive task using perfusion-based event-related functional MRI. *NeuroReport, 11*(11), 2533–2536.

## CHAPTER 9

# Special Populations

*Kay Viggiani*

## CHAPTER HIGHLIGHTS

## KEY TERMS

habilitation
rehabilitation
disability
sensory deficits
hearing impairment
visual impairment
learning disability
input and output disabilities
attention deficit disorder

developmental disability
mental illness
spinal cord injury
brain injury
expressive and receptive aphasia
dysarthria
chronic illness
adaptive computing

## OBJECTIVES

After completing this chapter, the reader will be able to

1. Describe how visual and hearing deficits require adaptive intervention.

2. Identify the various teaching strategies that are effective with learning disabilities.

3. Describe the different physical and mental disabilities for appropriate adaptation of the teaching–learning plan.

4. Enhance the teaching–learning process for someone with a communication disability.

5. Discuss the effects of a chronic illness on people and their families as well as on the teaching–learning process.

6. Describe adaptive computing and its application for people with disabilities.

Teaching others to be independent in self-management of their lives is a critical and challenging role for the nurse in any setting and with any population of individuals. However, the teaching–learning process is especially challenging when dealing with patients—and, in some instances, even nursing staff, nursing students, or hospital personnel—who have altered functional status due to a disabling condition affecting their physical, cognitive, or sensory capacities. The educational component of the practice of nursing becomes paramount in importance as the nurse's efforts are directed toward assisting the disabled and their significant others to maintain already established patterns of living or to develop new ones to accommodate changes in functional ability.

The terms *habilitation* and *rehabilitation* are frequently used to differentiate approaches for both managing developmental and acquired types of disabilities. "Habilitation includes all the activities and interactions that enable an individual with a disability to develop new abilities to achieve his or her maximum potential, whereas rehabilitation is the relearning of previous skills, which often requires an adjustment to altered functional abilities and altered lifestyle" (Burkett, 1989, p. 239). Thus, habilitation and rehabilitation are futuristic processes that focus on helping the disabled learn to live with their disability in their own environment through identification and use of tools that allow them to cope with the ramifications of their altered functional status.

Unfortunately, an increasing number of individuals are faced with having to deal with a disability caused by an injury, a disease, or a birth defect that is permanent and has long-term consequences on their mode of living. Nurses and other healthcare providers need to be prepared to provide those services that will meet the demands of a broad range of clients whose problems and situations are the result of a developmental or acquired disability. With respect to patient populations, the

teaching–learning process is an integral element in the habilitation and rehabilitation of disabled clients who need assistance in making the transition from being a recipient of care to assuming a self-care role. Certainly the disabled patient's family members and significant others are also major players in the habilitation and rehabilitation experience. Education of the client and the client's family is the key factor in preparing them for self-care as they make the transition from the hospital or extended-care facility to the home setting. Weeks (1995) supports the idea that family caregivers need and want information on how to best assist their newly disabled adult family member. An appropriate educational program can foster independence in the client and family by helping them to acquire new information, develop new skills, make changes required to achieve competencies in functional activities, assume behaviors that will aid in recovery and the prevention of future disability, and adapt to future situations (Diehl, 1989).

If we stopped for a moment to conjure up a mental picture of the disabled, what would we envision? The people in this special population group may look like the average person, but then again, they may not. Some will have overt physical disabilities, whereas others may have a cognitive or mental impairment that on the surface may make them indistinguishable from anyone else. The one thing that they will have in common is a problem that makes learning more difficult for them. For the purpose of this chapter, the term *disability* is defined as "the inability to perform some key life functions and is often used interchangeably with functional limitations" (Dittmar, 1989, p. 7).

On July 26, 1990, President George H. W. Bush signed into law the Americans with Disabilities Act (ADA). The definition of disability under the ADA is "a physical or mental impairment which substantially limits one or more of the major life activities of the individual." A "major life activity" includes functions such as caring for oneself, standing, lifting, reaching, seeing, hearing, speaking, breathing, learning, and walking. This significant legislation extends civil rights protection to an estimated 43 million Americans with disabilities. The first part of the law, effective January 1992, mandated accessibility to public accommodations. In July 1992, the second part of the law went into effect, requiring employers to make "reasonable accommodations" in hiring people with disabilities (Merrow & Corbett, 1994). Thus, the ADA legislation makes it illegal to discriminate on the basis of a disability in the areas of employment, public service, public accommodations, transportation, and telecommunications. This statute provides the foundation on which all facets of society will be free of discrimination, including the healthcare system. Therefore, we can expect to find people with disabilities in every setting in which nurses practice, such as schools, clinics, hospitals, nursing homes, and occupational and home-care settings. Persons with special needs caused by a disability will expect nurses and other healthcare professionals to provide appropriate instruction adapted to their needs.

The role of the nurse in teaching the disabled client continues to evolve, as more than ever before clients expect and are expected to assume greater responsibility as self-care agents. Here, the focus is on wellness and strengths—not limitations—of the individual. The family is increasingly becoming involved in their disabled member's rehabilitation efforts, and individuals with disabilities are expecting and demanding to be a part of community life. Because of the complex needs of the disabled as a special population group, the nurse's role, out of necessity, must be an integral part of an interdisciplinary team effort. It is imperative that nurses, physicians, social workers, physical therapists, psychologists, occupational and speech therapists, and other healthcare workers be involved in planning for the care of disabled persons and their fam-

ilies, in dealing with educational issues, and in designing and promoting an environment conducive to learning (Diehl, 1989). We must become aware of the tangible barriers that exist as well as the interventions and technologies that are available to help special populations overcome those barriers (Cunningham, 2001).

This chapter on special populations is a unique aspect of this book on the role of the nurse as educator. Few other publications address the subject or suggest nursing interventions involving teaching self-care measures to individuals with a wide range of disabilities. Although the information presented here focuses specifically on patient populations, the same principles of teaching and learning can be extrapolated to apply to other categories of learners. For example, the nurse educator may be responsible in the position of in-service educator, faculty member, or staff development coordinator for teaching hospital personnel or nursing students who may have a physical or learning disability. This chapter provides an overview of some of the more common disabilities. It addresses the learning problems inherent in population groups with various types of deficits and highlights the role of the nurse as educator in designing and implementing specific teaching strategies that can be used to overcome communication difficulties. It also suggests ways in which nurse educators can incorporate appropriate adaptations into their teaching plans to accommodate the needs of disabled patients and their families. A resource list is provided in Appendix B as a further reference to the reader who seeks additional information about a specific disability.

## THE NURSE AS EDUCATOR'S ROLE IN ASSESSMENT

Application of the teaching–learning process is intended to promote changes in clients that support their optimal recovery and a return to life within the community. Learning must take place in the cognitive, psychomotor, and affective domains to assist disabled individuals to make the necessary adaptations.

Prior to teaching, assessment is always the first step in determining the needs of clients with respect to the nature of their problems, the short- and long-term consequences of their disability, the effectiveness of the coping mechanisms they employ, and the type and extent of sensorimotor, cognitive, perceptual, and communication deficits they experience. The nurse must determine the extent of clients' knowledge with respect to their disability, the amount and type of new information needed to effect a change in behavior, and clients' readiness to learn. At this initial stage, it is imperative that the nurse educator not only obtain feedback from the clients, but also use assessment skills of observation, testing, and interviewing of family members and significant others as well as taking into account the findings of the team of healthcare professionals.

Diehl (1989) outlines the following questions to be asked when determining the disabled person's readiness to learn:

1. Do the individual and family members demonstrate an interest in learning by requesting information or posing questions in an effort at problem solving or determining their needs?

2. Are there barriers to learning such as low literacy or vision or hearing impairments? If so, is the client willing and able to use supportive devices?

3. What learning style best suits the client in processing information and applying it to self-care activities?

4. Is there congruence between the goals of the client and family?

5. Is the environment conducive to learning?

6. Does the client value the learning of new information and skills as a means to achieve functional improvement? Does the client correlate learning with the opportunity to regain an optimal level of functioning?

The prerequisite to the role of the nurse as teacher and provider of care is to serve as a mentor to patients and family in coordinating and facilitating the multidisciplinary services required to assist disabled persons in attaining optimal functioning. The family and significant others, as the disabled person's support system in the community, must be invited right from the beginning to take an active part in learning information as it applies to assisting with self-care activities for their loved ones.

## TYPES OF DISABILITIES

The disabilities affecting millions of Americans can be categorized into two major types: mental and physical. These disabilities may have a neurological, physiological, or cognitive basis, can affect thinking processes, and may involve sensorimotor/neuromuscular functioning. These disabilities may result from injury, disease, heredity, or congenital defect. For purposes of simplification so as to review the more common disabilities encountered by the nurse in practice, the following seven categories have been chosen for discussion: sensory deficits, learning disabilities, developmental disabilities, mental illness, physical disabilities, communication disorders, and chronic illness. Included within the section discussing each category are the specific teaching strategies that should be used to meet the needs of the learner who has a particular disability.

## SENSORY DEFICITS

### Hearing Impairments

People with impaired hearing—both the deaf and the hard of hearing—have a complete loss or a reduction in their sensitivity to sounds.

Strong (1996) explains that "[the word] 'deaf' with a lowercase 'd' is used to refer to the physical condition of hearing loss, whereas 'Deaf', with an uppercase 'D' is used to refer to special collectives and attitudes arising out of interaction among people with hearing losses. The distinction was first made by Woodward (1972) and is standard in most of the literature on sociocultural aspects of deafness" (p. xi). *Hearing impairment* is a term used to describe any type of hearing loss, the etiology of which may be related to either conductive or sensorineural problems resulting from congenital defect, trauma, or disease.

Currently about 10% of Americans (approximately 26 million people) have some degree of hearing loss, ranging from mild to profound (McCafferty, 2002), and a recent national health survey estimates that hearing loss among 18–44 year olds increased by 17% between 1971 and 1990 (Stock, 2002). Approximately 1.8 million people in this country are deaf. For those who are deaf, "being a recipient of health care services is similar to being in a foreign country without fluency in the native language" (Harrison, 1990, p. 113). Regardless of the degree of hearing loss, any person with a hearing impairment faces communication barriers that interfere with efforts at patient teaching. Hearing loss poses a very real communication problem because deaf and hearing-impaired individuals may also be unable to speak or have limited verbal abilities and often have poor vocabularies. This is especially true for adults who are prelingually deaf—that is, who have been deaf since early childhood. They and speakers of other languages share many of the same problems in learning English.

In many families with deaf children, American Sign Language (ASL) is used in the home and is the children's first language. For other children who are raised in an environment where Deaf culture predominates, ASL is the medium of social communication among peers, which reinforces English as a second language. Most, if not all, of these children have difficulty achieving native-like fluency in English, a fact related in the oft-quoted statistics that the average deaf student leaves high school with the ability to read at the fourth- or fifth-grade level (Trybus & Karchner, 1977).

It is clear that individuals who are deaf will have different skills and needs depending on the type of deafness and how long they have been without a sense of hearing. For those persons who have been deaf since birth, they will not have had the benefit of language acquisition. As a result, they may not possess understandable speech and may have limited reading and vocabulary skills as well. Most likely, their primary modes of communication will be sign language and lipreading. If deafness has occurred after language has been acquired, they may speak quite understandably and have facility with reading and writing, and some lipreading abilities. If deafness has occurred in later life, often caused by the process of aging, affected individuals will probably have poor lipreading ability, but their reading and writing skills should be within average range, depending on their educational and experiential background. If aging is the cause of hearing loss, *visual impairments* may also be a compounding factor. Because vision and hearing are two common sensory losses in the older adult, these deficits pose major communication problems when teaching older clients.

Deaf and hearing-impaired persons, like other individuals, will require health care and health education information at various periods during their life. Although you as the nurse educator will encounter many differences among people who are deaf, there is one common denominator—they will always rely on their other senses for information input, especially their sense of sight. For patient education to be effective, then, communication must be visible.

Because there are several different ways to communicate with a person who is deaf, one of the first things you need to do is ask your client to identify communication preferences. Sign language, written information, lipreading, and visual aids are some of the common choices. It is true that one of the simplest ways to transfer information is through visible communication signals such as hand gestures and facial expressions; however, this method will not be adequate for any lengthy teaching sessions. The following modes of communication are suggested as ways to decrease the barriers of communication and facilitate teaching and learning for hearing-impaired patients in any setting in which you may practice.

**Sign Language**   For most deaf people whose native language is ASL, sign language is often the preferred mode of communication. If you do not know ASL, you need to obtain the services of a professional interpreter. Sometimes a family member or friend of the patient skilled in signing is willing and available to act as a translator during teaching sessions. However, prior to enlisting the assistance of an interpreter, always be certain to obtain the patient's permission because information communicated regarding health issues may be considered personal and private. If the information to be taught is confidential, it is advised that family or friends should not be enlisted as an interpreter. Hiring a certified language interpreter is often the best strategy.

When considering the services of an interpreter, be certain that the deaf individual is the one who has made the choice. If a professional interpreter is requested by a deaf patient in a health facility receiving federal funds, it is required by federal law that one be secured (Section 504 of the Rehabilitation Act of 1973, PL 93-112). If the patient cannot provide the names of interpreters, contact the Registry of Interpreters of the Deaf (RID) in your state. This registry can provide an up-to-date list of qualified sign language interpreters.

When working with an interpreter, be sure to stand or sit next to the interpreter. Talk at a normal pace, and look and talk directly to the deaf person when speaking.

**Lipreading**   One common misconception among hearing persons is that all people who are deaf can read lips. This assumption is potentially dangerous (DiPietro, 1979). Only about 40% of English sounds are visible on the lips. Therefore, only a skilled lip-reader will obtain any real benefit from this form of communication.

If the individual can lip-read, it is not necessary to exaggerate your lip movements, because this action will distort the movements of the lips and interfere with interpretation of your words. If lipreading is preferred, you must be sure to provide sufficient lighting on your face and remove all barriers from around your face such as gum, pencils, hands, and surgical masks. Beards, mustaches, and protruding teeth also present a challenge to the lip-reader. Because less than half of the English language is visible on the lips, supplement this form of communication with signing or written materials.

**Written Materials**   Written information is probably the most reliable way to communicate, especially when understanding is critical. In fact, always write down the important information as a supplement to the spoken word even when the person is versed in lipreading. Written communication is the safest approach, even though it is time-consuming and sometimes stressful.

Keeping in mind that the average reading comprehension of deaf adults is at the fourth-grade level (Trybus & Karchner, 1977), be certain to provide printed patient education materials that match the readability level of your audience. When putting information in writing for your client who is deaf, keep the message as simple as possible. For instance, instead of writing, "When running a fever, take two aspirin," revise your message to read, "For a fever of 100.5°F or more, take two aspirin." Remember that a person with low reading skills often interprets words literally; therefore, the word *running* could be confusing because it is often used in the context of someone who is "running to the store," for example (see the guidelines for writing or revising educational materials for low-literacy patients in Chapter 7). Visual aids such as simple pictures, drawings, diagrams, models, and the like are also very useful media as a supplement to increase understanding of written materials.

**Verbalization by the Client**   Sometimes clients who are deaf will choose to communicate through speaking, especially if you have established a rapport and a trusting relationship with them. Often the tone and inflection of the patient's voice will be different than normal speech, so you must give yourself time for listening carefully. Listen without interruptions until you become accustomed to the person's particular voice intonations and speech rhythms. If you still have trouble understanding what a client is saying, try writing down what you hear, which may help you to get the gist of the message.

**Sound Augmentation**   For those patients who have a hearing loss but are not completely deaf, hearing aids are often a useful device. Clients who have already been fitted for a hearing aid should be encouraged to use it, and you should be sure it is readily accessible, fitted properly, turned on, and with the batteries in working order. If the client does not have a hearing aid, with permission of the patient and family you should make a referral to an auditory specialist, who can determine whether such a device is appropriate for your patient. Another means by which sounds can be augmented is by cupping your hands around the client's ear or using a stethoscope in reverse; that is, the patient puts the

stethoscope in his or her ears, and you talk into the bell of the instrument (Babcock & Miller, 1994).

If the patient can hear better out of one ear than the other, always stand or sit nearest to the side of the "good" ear. Be sure to slow your speech, provide adequate time for the patient to process your message and to respond, and avoid shouting.

**Telecommunications**   Telecommunication devices for the deaf (TDD) are an important resource for patient education. Television decoders for closed-caption programs are an important tool for further enhancing communication. Caption films for patient education are also available free of charge through Modern Talking Pictures and Services. Under federal law, these devices are considered to be "reasonable accommodations" for deaf and hearing-impaired persons.

In summary, the following guidelines suggested by Navarro and Lacour (1980, p. 26) should be applied when using any of the aforementioned modes of communication:

- Be natural:

  - Don't be rigid and stiff or attempt to over articulate your speech.

  - Use simple sentences.

  - Be sure to get the person's attention by a light touch on the arm before you start to talk.

  - Face the patient and stand no more than six feet from the patient when trying to communicate.

- Be considerate and refrain from

  - Talking and walking at the same time.

  - Bobbing your head excessively.

  - Talking with your mouth full, while chewing gum, and so forth.

  - Turning your face away from the deaf person while communicating.

–Standing directly in front of a bright light, which may cast a shadow across your face, or glare directly into the patient's eyes.

–Placing an IV in the hand the patient will need for sign language.

No matter what methods of communication for teaching you and your client choose, it is important you confirm that your health messages have been received and understood. It is essential that patient comprehension is validated in a nonthreatening manner. In attempts to avoid embarrassing or offending one another, patients as well as healthcare providers will often acknowledge with a smile or a nod in response to what either one is trying to communicate when, in fact, the message is not understood at all. To ensure that the health education requirements of deaf or hearing-impaired patients are being met, the nurse educator must find effective strategies to communicate the intended message clearly and precisely while at the same time demonstrating acceptance of individuals by making accommodations to suit their needs (Harrison, 1990). Patients who have lived with a hearing impairment for a while usually can tell you what modes of communication work best for them.

## Visual Impairments

In the United States, a person is determined to be legally blind if vision is 20/200 or less in the better eye with correction or if visual field limits in both eyes are within 20 degrees diameter. People lose their vision and may be rendered legally blind for a variety of reasons: infections, accidents, poisoning, or congenital degeneration such as retinitis pigmentosa. Most recently, blindness in AIDS patients as a result of infection has been associated with the end stages of this disease.

Visual impairment is especially common among older persons. According to the 2000 census, more than 2.5 million individuals older than age 65 are severely visually impaired (U.S. Census Bureau, 2000). The four leading eye diseases associated with the aging process are macular degeneration, cataracts, glaucoma, and diabetic retinopathy (Figure 9–1). Severe visual impairment after correction with glasses is defined as the inability to read newspaper print. Using this standard, studies of nursing home residents indicate that about 30% to 50% are considered to be significantly visually impaired (Nelson, 1991).

If you suspect that patients are legally blind but have not been evaluated by a low-vision specialist, you should put them in contact with the local Blind Association. Patients may require assistance in negotiating the complex system of obtaining services from the local Commission for the Blind and Visually Handicapped. Fortunately, many devices are available to help legally blind persons maximize their remaining vision. Patients who are without sight most likely have had services and are familiar with which adaptations work best for them. However, depending on patients' situations and the circumstances under which you are teaching, you may want to further investigate their background to assure yourself that you are using the most appropriate format and tools for communicating with visually impaired clients.

The following are some tips you might find helpful in caring for a blind or visually impaired patient:

• Secure the services of a low-vision specialist, who can prescribe optical devices such as a magnifying lens (with or without a light), a telescope, a closed-circuit TV, or a pair of sun shields, any of which will enable you to adapt your teaching material to meet the needs of your particular client.

• Persons who have long-standing blindness have learned to develop a heightened acuity of their other senses of hearing, taste, touch, and smell. Usually their listening skills are particularly acute, so avoid the tendency to shout. Just because

Major diseases causing serious vision impairment that cannot be corrected with conventional spectacles or lenses are cataract, macular degeneration, glaucoma, and diabetic retinopathy. People who have advanced stages of these diseases have difficulty performing ordinary visual tasks, like reading.

**MACULAR DEGENERATION**—The deterioration of the macula, the central area of the retina, results in an area of decreased central vision. Peripheral, or side, vision remains unaffected. This is the most prevalent eye disease.

**CATARACT**—An opacity of the lens results in diminished acuity but does not affect the field of vision. There are no blind spots, but the person's vision is hazy overall, particularly in glaring light.

**GLAUCOMA**—Chronic elevated eye pressure in susceptible individuals may cause atrophy of the optic nerve and loss of peripheral vision. Early detection and close medical monitoring can help reduce complications.

**DIABETIC RETINOPATHY**—Leaking of retinal blood vessels in advanced or long-term diabetes can affect the macula or the entire retina and vitreous, producing blinding areas.

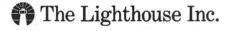

The Lighthouse Inc.

FIGURE 9–1  **Photo Essay on Partial Sight (Low Vision)**  SOURCE: Reprinted courtesy of The Lighthouse Inc., New York, New York.

they have impaired vision does not mean they cannot hear you well. Unlike a sighted person, the blind cannot attend to nonverbal cues such as hand gestures, facial expressions, and other body language. Before approaching a visually impaired person, always announce your presence, identify yourself, and explain clearly why you are there and what you are doing. Because their memory and recall also are better than the abilities of most sighted persons, you can use this talent to maximize learning (Babcock & Miller, 1994). When conveying messages, rely on their auditory and tactile senses as a means to help them assimilate information from their environment.

- When explaining procedures, be as descriptive as possible. Expound on what you are doing, and explain any noises associated with treatments or the use of equipment. Allow the patient to touch, handle, and manipulate equipment. Use the patient's sense of touch when you are in the process of teaching psychomotor skills as well as when the client is learning to return demonstrate.

- Because blind persons are unable to see shapes, sizes, and the placement of objects, tactile learning is an important technique to use when teaching. For example, such patients can identify their medications by feeling the shape, size, and texture of tablets and capsules. Gluing pills to the tops of bottle caps and putting medications in different-sized or -shaped containers will aid in blind persons' ability to identify various medications (Boyd et al., 1998). In this way, they will be able to be more self-sufficient in following their prescribed regimens. Keeping items in the same place at all times will help them independently locate their belongings. Arranging things in front of them in a regular clockwise fashion will facilitate learning to perform a task that must be accomplished in an orderly, step-by-step manner (McConnel, 1996).

- When using printed or handwritten materials, enlarging the print (font size) or handwriting is typically an important first step for those who have diminished sight.

- Color is a key factor in whether a visually impaired person can distinguish objects. Be sure to assess on which medium your client sees better—black ink on white paper or white ink on black paper. Colors and varying hues of color, other than black and white, are more difficult to discriminate by the older person with vision problems.

- Proper lighting is of utmost importance in assisting the legally blind person to read the printed word. Regardless of the print size and the color of the type and paper used, if the light is insufficient, the visually impaired person will have a great deal of difficulty reading print or working with objects.

- Providing contrast is a very helpful technique. For example, using a dark placemat with white dishes or serving black coffee in a white cup will allow persons with visual problems to better see items in front of them.

- Providing a template (writing guide) for signing their name or writing checks and addressing envelopes is a way to encourage independence.

- Large-print watches and clocks with either black or white backgrounds are available through the local chapter of the Blind Association.

- Audiotapes and cassette recorders are very useful tools. Today, many health education texts as well as other printed health information materials are available as "talking books" and can be obtained through the Library of Congress in Washington, D.C., or through your state library for the blind and visually handicapped. It is important to remember that these services are also available for people with other disabilities as well. Oral instruction can be audiotaped so that blind patients can listen to the information as often as they wish at another time and place. Repetition allows the opportunity for memorization to reinforce learning.

- The computer is a popular and useful tool for this population of learners. Although they are costly, some computers have synthetic speech as well as Braille keyboards.

- Most blind associations either have a Braille library or can direct you to appropriate resources for information written in Braille. If your client can read Braille and you have a large amount of printed material for patient education, local blind associations may Braille the materials so they can be used by the visually impaired learner.

- If you are assisting the person who is blind to ambulate, always use the "sighted guide" technique; that is, allow the person to grasp your forearm while you walk about one-half step ahead of them. Another resource person to help with ambulation is an orientation and mobility instructor. These specialists are available in most school districts and the local Association for the Blind.

Diabetes education consumes a great deal of a nurse educator's teaching time because of the high incidence of this disease in the American population. Diabetic retinopathy is a major cause of blindness, so it is likely that you will be teaching at least some visually impaired patients who are also in need of diabetes education. This situation presents a unique challenge to the nurse. Persons who have lost their sight due to diabetic retinopathy probably have already mastered some of the necessary skills to care for themselves; however, it is also possible for visually impaired persons to be diagnosed at a later time with diabetes. In either case, at some point in the course of their lives, these persons will need to learn how to use appropriate adaptive equipment.

In 1993, a task force consisting of representatives from groups of diabetes educators and rehabilitation teachers for the blind developed a document entitled *Adaptive Diabetes Education for Visually Impaired Persons* (ADEVIP). ADEVIP provides consistent practice guidelines for the care of diabetics who are visually handicapped. Fortunately, there also has been continuous improvement in the equipment used for self-monitoring of blood glucose levels. Available now are easy-to-use monitors with large display screens or voice instructions. Just as several devices for monitoring blood glucose levels have been developed, several nonvisual adaptive devices for measuring insulin are also available. It is evident that the teamwork between diabetes educators and rehabilitation specialists has led to the development of a variety of useful mechanisms that allow blind diabetic patients the opportunity to care for themselves and achieve both a successful medical outcome and a good rehabilitation outcome (Baker, 1993).

## LEARNING DISABILITIES

What exactly constitutes a *learning disability* has been the subject of a great deal of controversy over the years. Educators and psychologists alike have debated this very issue (Dykman et al., 1983; Kirk & Kirk, 1983; Knowles & Knowles, 1983; McLoughlin & Natick, 1983; Ysseldyke & Allgozzine, 1983). In 1981, the National Joint Committee on Learning Disabilities defined learning disabilities as "a generic term that refers to a heterogeneous group of disorders manifested by significant difficulties in acquisition and use of listening, speaking, reading, writing, reasoning or mathematical abilities" (Hammill et al., 1981, p. 336). These disorders are intrinsic to the individual and presumed to be due to central nervous dysfunction (Kirk & Kirk, 1983). Today, this definition still stands as the accepted working definition for purposes of assessment, diagnosis, and categorization of an array of perceptual processing deficits. Other general terms for a learning disability are *minimal brain dysfunction, attention deficit disorder (ADD), dyslexia,* and *hyperactivity.*

An estimated 10% to 15% of the overall U.S. population is considered to be learning disabled; approximately 6% to 10% of school-aged children are diagnosed with a learning disability, and an additional 20% have some degree of learning disability (Greenberg, 1991). In the past, a learning disability was thought to be a problem involving only children. Now, however, evidence supports the belief that most individuals do not "outgrow" the problem. Indeed, the rate of learning disabilities in adults is probably similar to the rate in children. A national study recently conducted by the American Council on Education found that the proportion of full-time college students with learning disabilities has more than tripled in the last two decades—from less than 3% in 1978 to 9% in 1998 (Zirkel, 2000). The majority of people with learning disabilities have language and/or memory deficits. If you compound their problem with the stresses and anxieties caused by illness and subsequent hospitalization or the pressures of having to perform in an academic setting, you can be assured that they find themselves in a situation that is not at all conducive to learning.

Individuals with learning disabilities appear normal and have been found to have at least average, if not superior (gifted), intelligence. Some very famous and successful people in world history are thought to have had some type of learning disability—Leonardo daVinci, Woodrow Wilson, George Patton, Winston Churchill, Nelson Rockefeller, and Albert Einstein. Even though there is a large discrepancy between a learning disabled person's intellectual abilities and his or her performance levels, no cause-and-effect relationship exists: Those who exhibit this discrepancy are not necessarily learning disabled. Table 9–1 lists common myths and corresponding facts about learning disabilities. Learning disabilities are not caused by retardation, emotional disturbances, physical impairments (blindness or deafness), or environmental dep-

| TABLE 9–1   Myths and facts |
|---|
| *Myth:*  Children are labeled "learning disabled" because they can't learn. |
| *Fact:*  They can learn, but their preferred learning modality must be identified. |
| *Myth:*  Children who have a learning disability must be spoken to more slowly. |
| *Fact:*  Those who learn auditorily may become impatient with slower speech and stop listening; those who learn visually would benefit more from seeing the information. |
| *Myth:*  Children who are learning disabled just have to try harder. |
| *Fact:*  Telling these children to try harder is a turnoff. They already do try hard. |
| *Myth:*  Children outgrow their disabilities. |
| *Fact:*  Children do not outgrow their disabilities. They develop strategies to compensate for and minimize their disabilities. |
| *Myth:*  Children with learning disabilities should be treated like everyone else. |
| *Fact:*  That treatment would be unfair; they would not get what they need. |
| *Myth:*  Nearly all children with a learning disability are boys. |
| *Fact:*  Boys are more often referred for proper identification of learning disabilities because they are more overt in acting out their frustrations. |

SOURCE: Copyright 1991, The American Journal of Nursing Company. Reprinted from *MCN: American Journal of Maternal Child Nursing*, Sept/Oct, 1991, vol. 16, no. 5. Used with permission.

rivation such as lack of educational opportunity or cultural diversity (Greenberg, 1991).

The factors that may affect learning in a learning disabled person are memory, language, motor, and integrative processing disabilities. These factors fall under two general headings: "input" and "output" disabilities. *Input disabilities*, which refer to the process of receiving and recording information in the brain, include visual perceptual, auditory perceptual, integrative processing, and memory disorders. *Output disabilities*, which refer to the process of orally responding and performing physical tasks, include language and motor disorders. Although these problems and their associated characteristics are frequently identified in reference to disabled children in particular, many of the characteristics of these problems can apply equally well to an older person who has not been diagnosed as learning disabled until later in adulthood. It is important to remember that a learning disabled individual can experience one type of learning disability or a combination thereof. Greenberg (1991) outlines the characteristics of these learning disability problems and the teaching strategies useful in assisting the learning disabled to acquire behaviors required for autonomy in self-care.

## Input Disabilities

**Visual Perceptual Disorders**  This type of disability results in an inability to read or difficulty with reading (dyslexia). Letters of the alphabet may be seen in reverse or rotated order—for example, *d* is *b* and *p* is *q* or *g*. Letters also may be confused with one another such as *was* being perceived as *saw*. In addition, the individual may have trouble focusing on a particular word or group of words. There may be a "figure ground" problem, such that the person is unable to attend to a specific object within a group of objects, such as finding a cup of juice on a food tray. Furthermore, judging distances or positions in space or dealing with special relationships may prove difficult, resulting in the person's bumping into things, being confused about left hand–right hand or up and down, or being unable to throw a ball or do a puzzle.

People with visual perceptual deficits tend to be auditory learners. With these individuals, visual stimulation should be kept to a minimum. Visual materials such as pamphlets or books are ineffective unless the content is explained orally or the information is read aloud. If visual items are used, only one item should be given at any one time with a sufficient period in between times to allow for the information to be focused on and mastered. Because persons with visual perceptual deficits usually learn best through hearing, using CDs and audiotapes (with or without earphones) and verbal instruction are keys in helping them learn. Recall and retention of information can be assessed by oral questioning, allowing learners to express back to you in oral form what they understand and remember about the content that has been presented.

**Auditory Perceptual Disorders**  This type of disability is characterized by the inability to distinguish subtle differences in sounds—for example, "blue" and "blow" or "ball" and "bell." There also may be a problem with auditory "figure ground," such that the sound of someone speaking cannot be identified clearly when others are speaking in the same room. Auditory "lags" may occur, whereby sound input cannot be processed at a normal rate. Parts of conversations may be missed unless one speaks at a speed that allows the disabled person enough time to process the information. During instruction, it is important to limit the noise level and eliminate distractions in the background. Using as few words as possible and repeating them when necessary (using the same words to avoid confusion) are useful strategies. Direct eye contact helps keep the learner focused on the task at hand.

Visual teaching methods such as demonstration–return demonstration, gaming (e.g., puppetry), modeling, and role-playing, as well as provision of visual instructional tools such as written materials, pictures, charts, films, books, puzzles, printed handouts, and the computer are the best ways to communicate information. Using hand signs for key words when giving verbal instructions and allowing the learner to have hands-on experiences and opportunities for observation are useful techniques. Directions for learning via these methods and tools should be in written form. The visual learner may intently watch your face for the formation of words, expressions, eye movements, and hand gestures. Awareness to these details may have developed as a compensatory strategy to aid comprehension. If the learner does not understand something being taught, he or she may exhibit frustration in the form of irritability and inattentiveness.

Individuals with either visual or auditory perceptual problems often rely on tactile learning as well. They enjoy doing things with their hands, want to touch everything, prefer writing and drawing, engage in physical exploration, and enjoy physical movement through sports activities.

**Integrative Processing Disorders**   Recording information in the brain requires that the information be organized and processed if it is to be used correctly. An inability to sequence or abstract visual, auditory, or tactile stimuli is characteristic of this type of disability. A child who has difficulty sequencing information may read and understand the word *dog* as *god* because the letters *d*, *o*, and *g* are processed in the incorrect order. Thought sequencing also may progress from the middle to the end rather than normally (i.e., starting at the beginning). Abstraction is the inability to infer meaning from words or phrases; that is, the specific intended meaning of words or thoughts is misunderstood. For example, a person who has difficulty with abstractions may interpret "window shopping" or "blowing smoke" in the literal rather than the figurative sense.

Those with an integrative processing disability need specific explanations. You should avoid using confusing phrases, puns, or sarcasm with such patients. Frequently ask the person to repeat or demonstrate what was learned to immediately clear up any misconceptions.

**Short-Term or Long-Term Memory Disorders**   Once information is recorded and integrated in the brain, it must be stored and made ready for retrieval. Normally, most people can retrieve information fairly quickly and without much effort from either their short-term or long-term memories. *Short-term memory* refers to information that is remembered as long as one is attending to it—for example, being able to remember what you have been told recently or taking a telephone order and then being able to write it down completely soon after you have hung up the phone. *Long-term memory* consists of information that has been repeated and stored and becomes available whenever you think about it, such as being able to remember someone's telephone number (or your own, for that matter) over a long period of time. Individuals with short-term memory deficits may be unable to recall what they learned an hour before, but they may be able to recall the information at a later point in time. People with both short- and long-term memory disabilities need brief, frequent, repetitive teaching sessions for constant reinforcement of information.

## Output Disabilities

**Language Disorders**   There are two types of oral language—spontaneous (initiating a conversation) and demand (asking a question). With spontaneous language, persons select a topic, organize their thoughts, and choose the correct words to express themselves orally. Demand language occurs when someone else starts a conversation and poses questions for another person to answer. In response to demand language, the language disabled person may panic and answer, "Huh?" or "What?" or "I don't know." If you detect this response pattern, allowing sufficient time either to process the information received or to formulate a response will reduce barriers to communication as a result of anxiety and frustration. For persons with either type of language disability, the greatest gift you can give them is time—time to process internal thoughts, to find words, and then to speak for the purpose of initiating a conversation or responding with answers to questions.

Although there is no one way to ensure results, the following are some adaptive techniques:

- Provide information on tape, or give a learner the option of responding to questions orally with a tape recorder.
- Use hand signs for key words when giving verbal directions.
- Use hands-on experience or observation.
- Highlight important information.
- Use a computer.
- Capitalize on teachable moments.
- Use puzzles.
- Appeal to all senses—auditory, visual, and tactile.
- Use mnemonics (Table 9–2).
- Use a cognitive map (Figure 9–2).
- Use an active reading strategy such as SQ3R (skim, question, read, rehearse, revise).

**Motor Disorders** Learning psychomotor tasks will be difficult if the individual has problems with performing gross and fine motor tasks. Often people with this type of disability will avoid such tasks because of

| TABLE 9–2    Mnemonics |
| --- |
| **P** artner |
| **R** esponsible |
| **E** nthusiastic |
| **C** oach |
| **E** valuation |
| **P** atience |
| **T** eacher |
| **O** pen-minded |
| **R** ole model |

inadequate motor skills. For example, they will shy away from using writing as a form of communication because it requires fine motor coordination to accomplish. Instead of forcing them to handwrite, providing a tape recorder to allow them to demonstrate their knowledge of information is a good substitute. Depending on the disabled person's auditory and visual strengths, computers, typewriters, and preprinted materials may prove helpful tools for teaching and learning. Safety also is always a concern for those with gross motor difficulties because they are prone to clumsiness, stumbling, or falling. The environment should be kept as uncluttered as possible to avoid injury and embarrassment.

## Attention Deficit Disorder

The ability to pay attention is an important prerequisite to success in school and work. Any difficulty with attending skills can have an adverse effect on learning. The American Psychiatric Association holds that *attention deficit disorder* is an appropriate term to use in such cases because in these persons difficulties are prominent and almost always present. Three major subtypes of ADD are attention deficit disorder with hyperactivity (ADDH), attention deficit disorder without hyperactivity (ADDNOH), and attention deficit disorder, residual type.

The onset of ADD is before the age of seven years. Estimates of the prevalence of ADD range from 1.2 to 2.0 percent of all school-aged children. The exact cause of ADD is unknown, but its primary characteristics are signs of inattention and impulsivity that are developmentally inappropriate. The child often fails to finish projects, seems not to listen, is easily distracted, and has difficulty concentrating. Other thoughts, sights, or sounds keep getting in their way, especially when the task is difficult or uninteresting. The child acts before thinking, switches from activity to activity, requires much supervision, and has difficulty

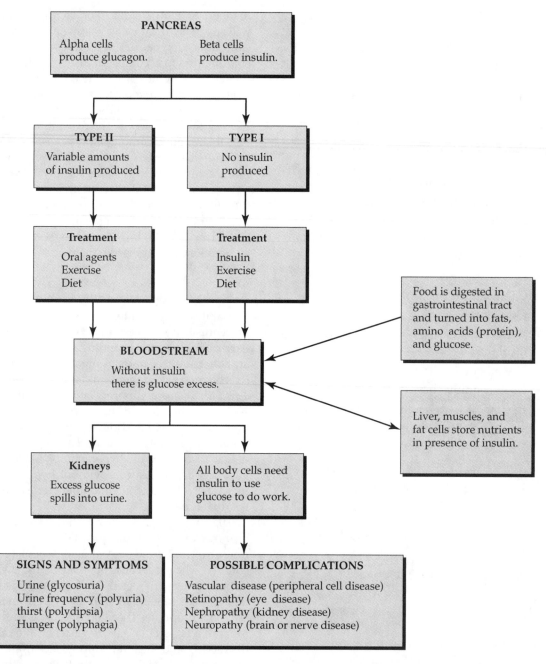

FIGURE 9–2    Diabetes Mellitus Cognitive Map

with organization of time, work, and belongings. Hyperactivity (ADDH) often accompanies the inattentiveness and impulsivity. The older child and adolescent may be extremely restless and fidgety. His or her behavior tends to be haphazard, poorly organized, and not goal directed. ADD, residual type, is sometimes used to identify older adolescents who were previously identified as ADDH at a younger age but who no longer exhibit hyperactivity.

ADD affects children with average ability as well as those who are gifted. This problem and other learning disabilities frequently occur together. Often, medication therapy is the treatment of choice for children with ADD. Before embarking on any educational intervention with these children, have an open discussion with the child and the parents to determine what works best for them. Most older children have been involved in special programs at school that, among other things, help the child use specific learning strategies consistently, which is of primary importance.

Provide new information to such patients in a quiet environment, which may necessitate using another place for the teaching session than the child's hospital room. When giving instructions or assigning a task, give directions one at a time, and divide the work into small parts. Reward achievement, and ignore inappropriate behavior. Eliminate as much distraction as possible. Encourage the older child to keep a notebook and to write the instructions down.

In summary, it is important to stress that learning disabled people are not mentally retarded; they just learn differently. They may have one or more disabilities, ranging from mild to severe. The challenge is to determine how the client learns best and then to adapt your teaching strategies to meet their preferred style of learning—auditory, visual, or tactile. The most reliable way to determine what accommodations need to be made in your teaching approach is to ask learning disabled individuals about problems they encounter in processing information and what they find to be the most appropriate instructional methods and tools to help them with learning. In the case of children, questions should be directed to both the child and the parents. Individuals' strengths and weaknesses with respect to learning can be identified through direct, individualized assessment. A teaching plan can then be developed to promote learning through use of strategies that compensate for or minimize the effect of their disability (Greenberg, 1991).

## DEVELOPMENTAL DISABILITIES

Parental response to the birth of a child with a disability is similar to the grieving process experienced by families after the death of a loved one. A typical reaction is, "Why me?" (Fraley, 1992). Shock or disbelief prevails, and when the reality settles in, the family attempts to integrate the child into the family structure. Enormous amounts of time and physical and psychological energy are expended during this difficult period. A large proportion of these children are born with a developmental disability.

The Developmental Disabilities Act of 1978 defined a *developmental disability* as a severe chronic state that is present before 22 years of age and is likely to continue indefinitely. It may be caused by either a mental or a physical impairment or by a combination of the two. The individual who is developmentally disabled has substantial limitations in at least three of the following major life activities: self-care, receptive and expressive language learning, mobility, self-direction, capacity for independent living, and economic self-sufficiency. In 1975, Public Law (PL) 94-142, the Education of All Handicapped Children's Act, mandated state grant money be made available to provide all children with disabilities with a free and appropriate public education. In 1986, PL

99-457 amended the earlier law to provide special funding for educating all eligible preschool children with disabilities, ages three through five, to help states develop early intervention programs for infants and toddlers (birth through age two), and to require states to use qualified providers of special education and related services. In 1990, PL 101-476 made additional changes to the law, including a name change to Individuals with Disabilities Education Act (IDEA). Under Part B of IDEA, all eligible preschool and school-aged children with disabilities are entitled to receive a free and appropriate education, including special education and related services. According to the *Fifteenth Annual Report to Congress* (U.S. Department of Education, 1993), nearly 5 million children have received services under IDEA.

The manner in which the mentally retarded are provided services has gone through a major transformation in much the same way that the care of the mentally ill has changed. Mandated early intervention and inclusion have increased the presence of such children and young adults in all facets of society, including hospitals and outpatient clinics. Many nurses are limited in their ability to provide holistic care for this population. Indeed, most nursing staff lack prior experience and often feel uncomfortable caring for these children. This problem becomes acute when the nurse is faced with trying to help the child understand particular treatments or tasks. Especially because the real experts in caring and working with these children are their parents, it is a wise nurse who invites the parents to participate and assist the nursing staff during their child's hospitalization. However, caution should prevail, as the hospitalization may be the parents' only respite from an arduous care schedule.

Managing the treatment of persons with developmental disabilities is accounting for an increasing portion of healthcare practice today. Because developmental disabilities usually are diagnosed during infancy and are

likely to last a lifetime, nurses must acquire sensitivity to family issues and learn to be flexible in their approaches to meet the intellectual, emotional, and medical concerns of clients with special needs. Webb et al. (2000) describe an innovative, collaborative project to help nursing students understand how best to care for those with a developmental disability.

When planning a teaching intervention, keep in mind the client's developmental stage, not his or her chronological age. If the child does not communicate verbally, the nurse should note whether certain nonverbal cues, such as gestures, signing, or other symbols, are used for communication purposes. Most mentally retarded children are incapable of abstract thinking. Although the majority can comprehend simple explanations, concrete examples must be given. For example, instead of saying, "Lunch will be here in a few minutes," show a clock and point to the time. For children scheduled to have surgery, giving them a surgical mask to play with will help dispel fears they may have when entering the operating room.

Always remember that facial expression and voice tone are more important than words spoken. Be sure the family explains any nonverbal cues for a "yes" or "no" response, and then try to ask questions in a manner requiring a "yes" or "no" answer. Lavish any positive behavior with great praise. Keep the information simple, concrete, and repetitive. Be consistent, but firm, setting appropriate limits. Be careful not to dominate any teaching session, but let the child actively participate and have a sense of accomplishment. Assign simple tasks with simple directions. Show what is to be done, rather than relying on verbal commands. Give only one direction at a time. A reward system often works very well with such patients. Stickers with familiar childhood characters placed on their bed or pajamas can remind the child of a job well done. "Children with developmental deviations have the potential for greater variability in their responses to hospitalization than their unaffected peers" (Vessey, 1988, p. 54).

## MENTAL ILLNESS

Approximately one-third of the adult population in the United States at some point in time meets the diagnostic criteria for a mental disorder (National Institute of Mental Health, 1991) and at least 12% of children younger than 18 years of age suffer one or more mental disorders (National Advisory Mental Health Council, 1990). These statistics reveal the relative prevalence of *mental illness* in our society and indicate that nurses will often care for patients with a psychiatric problem as a primary or secondary diagnosis.

Until about 1886, the mentally ill were restrained in iron manacles. With the advent of pharmacotherapy in the 1950s, the life of a person with a mental illness began to change. The discovery of the various neuroleptic and antidepressant drugs was a major contribution to the improved quality of life for the mentally ill. Previously dependent clients were now able to live outside of an institution. For the last 25 years, the care of the mentally ill has been moving into community health centers, and clients are spending less time confined to a mental health facility and more time in the community, at work, at home, and at play.

The 1990s have been referred to as the "Decade of the Brain," with new discoveries linking biochemistry with human behavior and conditions of mental health and illness (Haber et al., 1997). The quality of treatments and, therefore, the quality of life for those with mental illness can only improve. It is incumbent upon nurses to examine their own feelings about mental illness so they can enter into a viable teaching–learning relationship.

Although teaching clients with mental disorders requires the same basic principles of patient teaching, there are some specific teaching strategies to consider. In nonpsychiatric settings, the client is usually better able to describe what it is that he or she needs to learn. This capability assumes that the client is ready and motivated to learn. For example, the emotional threat that a person perceives as a result of a psychiatric disorder may result in an increased anxiety level and subsequently begin a chain of physiological reactions that then decrease his or her readiness to learn (Haber et al., 1997).

As with any other nursing intervention, the first step is to begin with a comprehensive assessment. In this case, it is wise to determine whether the consumer has any cognitive impairment or inappropriate behavior as well as to assess the patient's level of anxiety. High anxiety can make learning nearly impossible. Despite the nurse's best efforts, clients with a mental disorder may not be able to identify their need to learn and may not be sufficiently ready to learn. However, the nurse may not be able to wait for "readiness" to happen. Therein lies the challenge. In fact, persons with mental disorders *are* able to learn given the right circumstances and strategies. For instance, it is extremely important that the family or significant other participate in the health education of the client. Therefore, when planning your teaching session, prepare to include the family or significant other. Also keep in mind when planning your teaching strategies that people with mental illness may experience difficulty in processing information and verbally communicating information. In addition, they may experience decreased concentration and are easily distracted, which does limit their ability to stay on task.

The following is a summary of three essential strategies that have proved successful when teaching people with mental illness (Haber et al., 1997):

1. Teach by using small and brief words, repeating information over and over—use

mnemonics, write down important information by placing it on index cards, and use simple drawings or symbols. Be creative.

2. Keep sessions short and frequent. For instance, instead of a one-hour session, break the learning period into four 15-minute sessions.

3. Involve all possible resources, including the client and his or her family. Actively involve them to help determine the client's learning styles as well as the best way to reinforce content. Consider using computer-assisted instruction, videotapes, and role-modeling with clients.

As with any teaching program, it is important to set goals and determine outcomes with the client. The specific goals depend on individual learning outcomes as well as overall learning outcomes. These would include changing clients' health-related behavior and empowering clients to take as much control over their health as possible.

In spite of all the great strides made in the treatment of mental illness, the mentally ill person still faces the problems of being stigmatized. Nurse educators may need to explore teaching strategies that have been successful in the field of mental health. Education programs for the mentally ill are few and far between. Their needs for learning are great, but they are often not given the same opportunities for educational programs as those persons with physical disabilities.

Motivating the patient with a chronic mental illness can be challenging. A certificate of recognition may be given to each patient when he or she completes a program, which can be a powerful motivator. To have a positive effect on the quality of life of the chronically mentally ill, provide useful information. Independence and self-management remain goals for this special population, as with all other populations. Therefore, the nurse as educator will need to consider the strategies available from all specialties to meet the challenge of teaching the person with a mental illness.

## PHYSICAL DISABILITIES

### Spinal Cord Injury

One of the major physical disabilities afflicting the U.S. population is *spinal cord injury*. Approximately 10,000 new spinal cord injuries occur each year in the United States (National Center for Injury Prevention and Control, 1999), which translates into about 40 people per million annually in the population (National Spinal Cord Injury Statistical Center, 1999).

The spinal cord–injured population has benefited directly from the introduction of advanced technologies. Not only are people surviving, but they are also living a greatly improved quality of life. Before 1945, the survival prognosis for people with paraplegia or quadriplegia was very poor (Zejdlik, 1992). By the 1970s, several regional spinal cord injury centers had been established across the country. With more sophisticated techniques and equipment came improved mobility, less complications, and better restoration of musculoskeletal functions (Norris et al., 1982).

Residual impairment from spinal cord injury affects all areas of life—physical, social, psychological, vocational, and spiritual. Typically, spinal cord–injured persons are males between the ages of 16 and 30 years old. Fifty-six percent of new spinal cord injuries occur within this age range, and 82% of them involve men (National Spinal Cord Injury Statistical Center, 1999).

Spinal cord injury is sudden and devastating, both to the person and to the family. The adjustment is difficult and continuous. During the rehabilitation phase of the hospitalization, all interventions are driven by the goal of independent living. As mentioned, spinal cord injuries occur most frequently in young adult males. Normally, this is a difficult stage of development, and families are already struggling with the young adult's need for independence. Very often when the person is ready for discharge, the home environment is unstable, as the family is also attempting to readjust to the disability. It is quite possible the family may be at a different phase of adjustment than the client. At the same time, both the disabled person and the family are faced with the task of redefining roles. Fink (1967), a psychologist, described four sequential phases of recovery: shock, defensive retreat, acknowledgment, and adaptation. With the shortened lengths of stay for both the critical and rehabilitation phases of hospitalization, the newly injured person and the family have less time to reach the adaptation phase. Many families will agree that the adjustment is ongoing, with new challenges greeting them every day.

Initially, most spinal cord injury centers provide comprehensive rehabilitation. However, the skills required to maintain physical equilibrium are many. Often the quantity of information is overwhelming, and the spinal cord–injured persons find themselves plagued with frequent hospital readmissions. The most common problems are urinary tract infections and skin breakdown. Very often the knowledge to prevent such complications is there, but it is just a matter of individualizing the approach to make it fit the person's lifestyle.

Much of the rehabilitation as it relates to patients' functional living is actually done by trial and error. It is wise to remember that most teenagers' concerns center on their friends, especially a boyfriend or girlfriend. Due to the importance of peer relationships during adolescence and a preoccupation with body image, even if teenagers are taught something, it is possible they will be unable to focus on the extensive information being offered.

Before developing strategies that allow learners to bypass the disability, the nurse must consider some common obstacles. These issues might be within or related to the learner's ability to participate in the learning process. In this circumstance, learner readiness is important. *Readiness* is the learner's ability in terms of physical and mental development. Readiness in both respects is necessary for effective teaching (Lubkin, 2002; Haggard, 1989). As most nurses know, presenting important health-related information is only half the challenge. The other half is patients' ability to accept and use the information to change or improve their health status. Denial is the most frequent obstacle to learning readiness in the young spinal cord–injured patient. Although the object of this denial is often the bowel program, denial frequently reappears whenever a task seems overwhelming. Although denial may be an effective coping mechanism, it can also interfere with learning readiness.

Another obstacle to learning readiness is the lack of physical endurance. This weakness may be especially apparent in the older client. In this situation, it may be prudent to involve a friend or family member to ensure that a relief person will be able to take over when the client's energy level is inadequate.

In her work with rehabilitation patients, Vance (1992) cited secondary gains of retained behaviors or attitudes as an obstacle to learning readiness. Seen frequently when the learning leads to role changes related to dependence or independence, in this situation either clients or caregivers may view new information as a threat to their role as patient or caregiver. For example, it is now possible for a person with quadriplegia to drive. If the client has been transported by a good friend for several years, the friend may view this new independence as a serious threat to his or her role as caregiver. It would be imperative for the nurse to deal with this issue from the beginning and, if warranted, refer both parties for counseling.

Lack of readiness will occur when any physical or emotional limitations are present. A nursing diagnosis of noncompliance would be inappropriate when the underlying etiology is learner readiness. Before the teaching plan is implemented, every attempt should be made to determine the client's readiness to learn.

All too often the need for sharing is overlooked. Patients and their families need to have a positive vision of the future, and feelings of isolation can quickly overwhelm them. One way to remedy this problem is by using the group approach to teaching, whereby recovered spinal cord–injured persons are included in some of the teaching sessions. In this way, newly injured persons can benefit from the "trials and errors" of those who have gone before them. It is critical to understand that significant others and children need support throughout this experience, too. Everyone has to work through the injury at their own pace.

It is imperative that at whatever juncture the nurse encounters a person with a spinal cord injury, a careful assessment of the patient's learning readiness be carried out first. Next, the family and, most important, the immediate caregiver, who may or may not be a family member, must be involved. With the appropriate support and knowledge, the client and family will be successful in learning and maintaining independence.

## Brain Injury

A fall, car accident, gunshot wound, or blow to the head are just a few potential causes of traumatic *brain injury*. More than 2 million traumatic brain injuries (TBI) occur each year in the United States, of which 1 million are treated in hospitals and 500,000 are serious enough to require hospital admission (National Center for Injury Prevention and Control, 1999). *Closed head injury* refers to nonpenetrating injury. *Open head injury* refers to penetrating injury resulting in brain tissue exposure and disruption of normal protective barriers.

Most members of this special population, ages 15 to 24 years, were previously healthy and active young people. Often, these persons suffer from behavior and personality changes, as well as an impairment in cognitive ability, following their TBI. "Disturbances in learning and memory, rate of information processing, and adaptive or executive functions are common cognitive sequelae" (Tate et al., 1991, p. 117). There is also a growing number of older individuals surviving a closed head injury. The same or similar cognitive deficits also afflict this population.

The amount of deficits usually depends on the severity and location of the injury. Cognitive impairments may include poor attention span, slowness in thinking, confusion, difficulty with short-term and long-term memory, distractibility, impulsive and socially inappropriate behaviors, poor judgment, and mental fatigue, as well as difficulty with organization and problem solving. Difficulty in the area of reading and writing may also be present. In addition, the person may have acquired a hearing loss. As might be expected, communication will more than likely be an issue.

The treatment of people with severe brain injury is most often divided into three stages:

1. Acute care (in an intensive care unit)

2. Acute rehabilitation (in an inpatient brain-injured rehabilitation unit)

3. Long-term rehabilitation after discharge (at home or in a long-term care facility)

At every stage, there are many hurdles to conquer. Once the person's life is assured and the physical condition improves, the patient is discharged from the acute care unit. It is at this point that someone not familiar with traumatic brain injuries might wonder why a person who looks healthy and independent still needs rehabilitation. For this reason, families need to be kept up-to-date on their loved one's prognosis from the very beginning. Throughout the rehabilitation process, family

**TABLE 9–3   Guidelines for effective teaching of the brain-injured patient**

| DO | DON'T |
|---|---|
| Use simple rather than complex statements. | Stop talking or trying to communicate. |
| Use gestures to complement what you are saying. | Speak too fast. |
| Give step-by-step directions. | Talk down to the person. |
| Allow time for responses. | Talk in the person's presence as though he or she is not there. |
| Recognize and praise all efforts to communicate. | |
| Ensure the use of listening devices. | Give up (instead, seek the assistance of a speech-language pathologist). |
| Keep written instructions simple, with a small amount of information on each page. | |

teaching must be consistent and thoughtful, as most of the residual impairments are not visible, with the exception of the sensorimotor deficits. The communication, cognitive-perceptual, and behavioral changes may be dramatic. "The combined effects of these multiple deficits following a TBI create tremendous psychosocial consequences for patients and their families. Especially in the early stages of the injury, patients are not able to handle normal routine social situations" (Grinspun, 1987, p. 63). However, the most difficult problem for the family is the recognition that their relative will probably never be the same person again. In fact, personality changes present the biggest burden for the family. Studies have shown that the level of the family stress is directly related to personality changes and the relative's own perception of the symptoms arising from the head injury (Grinspun, 1987).

Although most of the literature deals with the importance of family inclusion during the rehabilitation period, it is clear that brain-injured persons will always need the involvement of their family. Again, the benefits of participation in family groups are immeasurable in this area. Considerable strength is gained from group participation, and learning is accomplished through a friendly, informal approach. Of particular importance for brain-injured persons and

their friends and family is the need for unconditional acceptance.

Learning needs for this population center on the issues of client safety and family coping. Safety issues are related to cognitive and behavioral capabilities. Families are faced with a life-changing event and will require ongoing support and encouragement to take care of themselves. Recovery may take several years, and most often the person is left with some form of impairment. Tate et al. (1991) reported a frequency of 70% for each of the symptoms of personality change, slowness, and poor memory in the head-injured population.

Table 9–3 lists some "dos" and "don'ts" for effective teaching of the person with a brain injury.

## COMMUNICATION DISORDERS

"Communication is a universal process by which human beings exchange ideas, impart feelings and express needs" (Adkins, 1991, p. 74). Communication occurs in a variety of ways, including drama, music, literature, and art. It is verbal and nonverbal, and there are both sending and receiving components. Stroke, or cerebrovascular accident, is the most common cause of impaired communication. As is true with the other disabilities discussed in this chapter, a stroke is a major crisis for both the person and the family. Many of the strategies discussed for teaching spinal cord injury patients are also applicable to an educational program for the person with a stroke. This discussion will cover some useful strategies appropriate for working with a person with impaired communication such as aphasia.

Each year, 150 to 200 per 100,000 Americans suffer a stroke (Edwards, 2000). Stroke is a more common occurrence in older adult men and in the African American population. Perceptual deficits such as neglect and denial as well as spatial disturbances may also affect a person's ability to communicate (Olson, 1991). One of the most common residual deficits of a stroke is a problem with language. Language involves not only speaking but also conveying and comprehending thoughts and ideas, as well as understanding and using symbols sequentially and grammatically (Boss, 1986).

Aphasia is a communication problem, either with speaking, writing, or understanding. It may be defined as a multiple-modality loss of language ability, usually caused by damage to the dominant hemisphere (Adkins, 1991). When you prepare to work with someone with aphasia, it is necessary to determine which type of aphasia—expressive or receptive—is present. If your involvement with the client occurs during the early stage of rehabilitation, the speech therapist would be a good teammate.

The function of language primarily resides in the left hemisphere of the brain. Most often when an injury affects the dominant cerebral hemisphere (usually the left), the result is *expressive aphasia*. About three-quarters of the overall population has a dominant left hemisphere. Expressive aphasia occurs when an injury damages the inferior frontal gyrus, just anterior to the facial and lingual areas of the motor cortex, known as Broca's area (Table 9–4). Because Broca's area is so near the left motor area, the stroke often

leaves the person with right-sided paralysis as well.

Wernicke's area of the brain (Table 9–4) is located in the temporal lobe and is needed for auditory and reading comprehension. When this area is affected, persons are left with *receptive aphasia*. Although their hearing is unimpaired, they are nevertheless unable to understand the significance of the spoken word.

It is important to remember that although persons with both types of aphasia are unable to communicate verbally or have difficulty doing so, it does not mean they are intellectually impaired. The inability to communicate verbally is one of the most frustrating experiences. Speech therapy should be one of the earliest interventions, and the nurse will need to incorporate those strategies into the teaching–learning plan. Every effort must be made to establish communication at some level. Remember, regardless of how severe the communication deficit, it is almost always possible to have stroke patients communicate within their own environment in some manner and to some extent.

## Expressive Aphasia

In the event structured speech therapy is not available, the nursing staff will need to develop their own plan of care. When working with expressive aphasia, you might try having the person recall word images, first by naming commonly used objects (e.g., spoons, knives, forks) and then those objects in the immediate environment (e.g., bed, table). Another strategy is having the person repeat words spoken by the nurse. It is wise to begin with simple terms and work progressively to the more complex.

These exercises may be carried out frequently during the day, keeping the sessions short. Most people tire when sessions are longer than 30 minutes. Often their speech will become slurred, and they will experience men-

**Table 9-4  Clinical features of aphasia**

| Type | Involved Anatomy | Expression | Auditory Comprehension | Written Comprehension | Naming | Word/Phrase Repetition | Ability to Write |
|---|---|---|---|---|---|---|---|
| Broca's (motor, expressive) | Precentral gyrus, Broca's area | Nonfluent, telegraphic, may be mute | Subtle deficits | Subtle deficits | Impaired | Impaired | Impaired |
| Wernicke's (receptive, sensory) | Superior temporal gyrus | Fluent but content inappropriate | Impaired | Impaired | Severely impaired | Impaired | Impaired |
| Global (mixed) | Frontal-temporal area | Nonfluent | Severely impaired | Impaired | Severely impaired | Impaired | Severely impaired |
| Conductive (central) | Arcuate fasciculus | Fluent | Intact | Intact | Impaired | Severely impaired | Impaired |
| Anomic (amnesic) | Angular gyrus | Fluent | Intact | Intact | Severely impaired | Intact | Subtle deficits |
| Transcortical sensory (TCSA) | Periphery of Broca's and Wernicke's areas (watershed zone) | Fluent | Impaired | Impaired | Impaired | Intact | Severely impaired |
| Transcortical motor (TCMA) | Anterior, superior, or lateral to Broca's area | Nonfluent, speech initiation difficult | Intact | Subtle deficits | Impaired | Intact | Impaired |

SOURCE: Reprinted by permission from Schofield Bronstein, Judith M. Popvich, and Christina Stewart-Amidei, *Promoting Stroke Recovery: A Research-Based Approach for Nursing*. Table 11–1. St. Louis: Mosby-Year Book, 1991.

tal fatigue. In a following section of this chapter, you will find some helpful information regarding adaptive computing. People with expressive aphasia will find computers a wonderful tool to assist in their efforts to communicate.

## Receptive Aphasia

When working with someone with receptive aphasia, you need to establish a means for nonverbal communication. Usually the tone of voice, facial expressions, gestures, and even pantomime will be effective in conveying a message. Most often, these persons are unaware of their impairment and will speak in what sounds like a correct statement, but on examination the words do not make sense. Speak more slowly and slightly louder to the person with receptive aphasia, as auditory stimulation seems to be effective. When comprehension and memory span increase, the person will begin to respond appropriately.

Aphasic persons also have trouble with retention and recall. It seems old personal memories return first and recent events take longer to reappear.

"It is a lonely, isolated world for those who cannot communicate with other human beings" (Jennings, 1981, p. 39). As we attempt to work with and engage in a teaching–learning intervention, we must be aware of our own attitudes. The effort to communicate with someone without our usual speech and language is one of the more frustrating experiences. Be sure to take time out and reflect on the rewards of assisting the client and family in overcoming this barrier.

Encouragement and explanation when teaching persons with aphasia will go a long way in ensuring client participation and recovery. Keep your teaching sessions filled with praise, and always acknowledge the client's frustration. Keep distractions to a minimum. Be sure the radio and television are turned off so you have the full attention of the client. Always have one person speak at a time. Speak slowly, and be sure to stand where the client is able to

see your face (Norman & Baratz, 1979). In teaching people with aphasia, it is easy to overestimate their understanding of speech. Often they will smile and agree when they are actually understanding only half of the message. Providing enough time and constantly checking to be sure the message is fully understood without chastising the client is the challenge.

Blanco (1982, p. 34) suggests the following general guidelines:

- Don't use baby talk.
- Speak in normal tones.
- Speak in short, slow, simple sentences.
- Allow the person time to answer.

Be patient, slow the person's response down, and involve the family. While working with a person with this type of language deficit, the nurse should also be aware that it may extend into the reading modality. Little is known about this aspect of the disability or how many stroke patients suffer from the inability to read. In a study carried out by Loughrey (1992), a small group of patients with aphasia were able to improve their reading ability. Two methods of reteaching reading were used: a multisensory technique and a visual-verbal technique. Both were successful in improving the subjects' ability to recognize and use their newly acquired words. Although teaching reading is not a usual nursing responsibility, the nurse educator may choose to encourage the family to try and help their loved one relearn reading by using these promising techniques.

## Dysarthria

Many people with degenerative disorders, such as Parkinson's disease, multiple sclerosis, and myasthenia gravis, also have dysarthria. *Dysarthria* is a problem with the voluntary muscle control of speech. It occurs as a consequence of damage to the central or peripheral nervous system and affects the same muscles used in eating and speaking. The result is unintelligible speech. "The degree of unintelligibility will be directly related to the severity of the dysarthria" (Dreher, 1981, p. 347).

Several types of dysarthria exist: flaccid, spastic, ataxic, hypokinetic, or mixed. The difference in symptoms for each type depends not on the underlying disease but on the site in the nervous system that the disease strikes (Dreher, 1981). Although the incidence of the various types is unknown, this category of communication problems will certainly increase as the medical treatments for the various brain diseases improve and people live longer. Those who do survive will need help in overcoming all the residual social and communication problems.

Currently, Parkinson's disease is managed very well with medication, and there is ongoing research in the medical management of multiple sclerosis and myasthenia gravis. The intervention of a physical therapist may help improve the function of various muscles used for speech. There are also some helpful mechanical devices, such as a prosthetic palate, which is used to control hypernasality. Another useful tool is sign language, which may be used if the person's arm and hand muscles are unaffected. The nurse should work with the speech therapist to determine whether any of the other nonverbal aids would be appropriate, such as communication boards or a portable electronic voice synthesizer. With the advent of the adaptive computer, the possibilities are limitless.

To improve communication with the dysarthric person, Dreher (1981) makes the following suggestions:

- Be sure the environment is quiet, because you are listening to a person whose speech muscles are weak and uncoordinated. A careful listener may discern a consistent pattern in the sound errors.
- Ask the speaker to repeat unclear parts of the message. Concentration and intention will aid clarity.

- Do not simplify your message. Dysarthria does not affect comprehension.
- Ask questions that need only short answers, to prevent exhausting the dysarthric patient with the great effort to shape sounds.
- Encourage the person to use more oral movement to produce each syllable, to slow the overall rate of speaking, and to speak more loudly.
- Ask the patient who is extremely unintelligible to gesture, write, or point to messages on a communication board.

### Laryngectomy

The American Cancer Society reports that 30,000 laryngectomies are performed in the United States each year. Most of these people return to society as useful citizens. Cancer of the larynx is five times more common in men than in women, and it occurs most often in persons older than 60 years of age.

Until recently, *esophageal speech* was the primary method for speaking after a laryngectomy. Esophageal speech involves taking air into the upper part of the esophagus and adapting its normal sphincters to vibrate like vocal cords. With practice, the new voice sounds quite natural. Motivation and persistent effort are essential in learning this new kind of speech. Encouragement and support of the family as well as the clients are also critical for success. About 75% of all clients who have their larynx removed acquire some sort of speech, and most people return to work in one to two months.

*Tracheoesophageal speech* is a more rapid restoration of speech. The speech is closer to normal in rate and phrasing, and it is more pleasing than that created with an electrolarynx. On the other hand, it means the person must rely on a prosthesis, and the tracheoesophageal fistula may undergo stenosis. The tracheoesophageal puncture (TEP) was first successfully performed in 1980. In this procedure, a tracheoesophageal puncture is made

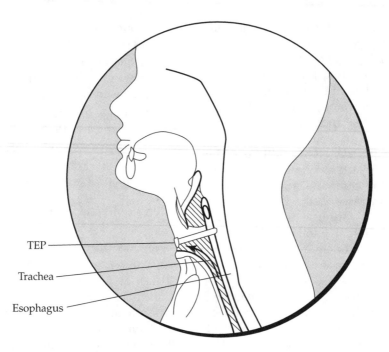

TEP

Trachea

Esophagus

FIGURE 9–3    **Tracheoesophageal Puncture**

to create a tracheoesophageal fistula large enough to permit the insertion of a valve prosthesis (Figure 9–3). The prosthesis is a hollow silicone tube that is open at the tracheal end and closed with a horizontal slit at the laryngopharyngeal end. When the person talks, air pressure opens the closed end, permitting air to enter the laryngopharynx. When the person stops talking, the laryngopharyngeal end closes, preventing saliva from draining into the trachea. Because air is diverted from the trachea into the esophagus, this form of speech is referred to as tracheoesophageal speech (Phipps et al., 1995). During such speech, the stoma needs to be occluded. Education of the person and family includes what to do if the prosthesis comes out.

If an individual is unable to learn esophageal speech in 60 to 90 days after surgery, a speech aid such as a vibrator or an electronic artificial larynx is recommended. This battery-powered, handheld device has a vibrating diaphragm that a person with a laryngectomy presses against the soft tissues of the neck. The newer models permit a more natural type of speech.

As previously noted, many of the people with laryngectomies are older and often have a difficult time adjusting to their new condition. If they are unable to use any of the aforementioned interventions, the nurse needs to be vigilant about preventing "silent suffering" and social isolation. It is essential that contact with other people remain intact. If none of the assistive speech devices work, then other means of nonverbal communication need to be adopted.

Measures to improve communications with a person with a laryngectomy are listed by speech pathologist, Barbara Dreher (1981):

• Seek a quiet environment, because esophageal speech is quieter and less intelligible than normal speech.

- Watch the speaker's lips, because articulation is the same as before and mouth movements give clues.

- Do not alter your message. The laryngectomee's comprehension should be the same as before surgery.

- If you don't understand the speaker, repeat what you think the person said, and ask for more information.

- Encourage the laryngectomee who has not yet learned esophageal speech, or can't learn it, to write or gesture to communicate.

Losing the ability to communicate can be an isolating, depressing experience. It is of particular concern in this day and age of increased technology, when it is easy to lose sight of the human touch as the universal means of communication.

## ▅▅▅ CHRONIC ILLNESS

Lubkin (2002) states that *chronic illness* constitutes the United States' number one medical malady. It is impossible within the confines of this chapter to cover specific teaching strategies for each chronic illness. Unlike acute illnesses, which usually have a clearly defined beginning and end, chronic illness is permanent. It is never completely cured. It requires the full involvement of its victims. Every aspect of life is affected—physical, psychological, social, economical, and spiritual. Because successful management of a chronic illness is a lifelong process, the development of good learning skills is a matter of survival.

The learning process for individuals with a chronic illness begins with rehabilitation at the moment of the disability. From the onset of the problem, patients and their families need to acquire knowledge about the disease and arrive at an early understanding of its effects on their lives. Families need information and education to deal with the limitations and changes in their loved one's lifestyle. There is often a conflict between feelings of dependence and the need to be independent. Sometimes the energy and focus of maintaining independence are overwhelming, both physically and emotionally. Often, living with a chronic illness includes a loss and or change in roles. When people suffer from role loss (e.g., a father who is no longer able to keep his job), their self-esteem may also be affected. If there are lingering issues surrounding the individual's role loss and self-esteem, it is best to hold off teaching until they are resolved.

Controlling symptoms is a major time-consuming activity of those with a chronic illness such as myasthenia gravis or multiple sclerosis. In a study of people with myasthenia gravis focusing on regimens and regimen-associated problems in adults, Hood (1990) discovered that persons with this disorder follow regimens to maximize their physical strength. When they encountered adverse effects with their regimens, they figured out methods to lessen regimen-associated problems. This information supports the work of Strauss et al. (1984, p. 16), who identified the following eight key problem areas experienced by chronically ill patients:

1. Prevention of medical crisis and the management of problems once they occur

2. Control of symptoms

3. Carrying out of prescribed regimens and the management of problems attendant on carrying out the regimens

4. Prevention of, or living with, social isolation that causes lessened control with others

5. Adjustment to changes in the course of the disease, whether it moves downward or enters remission

6. Attempts at normalizing both interactions with others and lifestyle

7. Funding (finding the necessary money to pay for treatments or to survive despite partial or complete loss of employment)

**8.** Confronting attendant psychological, marital, and family problems

When working with a person with a chronic illness who must manage a sometimes complex therapeutic regimen (as in a diabetic regimen), it is easy to see how the label of noncompliance might enter the assessment. The truth is, the person with a chronic illness requires more than just teaching—that is, the acquiring of information. Acquisition of knowledge does not necessarily help people gain the new skills needed to deal with the problems of everyday life. Integration of the new knowledge into solutions that will provide clients with normalization will make the learning meaningful and, most important, useful. Nurses need to remember to encourage people to work with their particular regimen and individualize it as necessary.

## The Family and Chronic Illness or Disability

Families' reaction and perception of the chronic illness or disability rather than the illness or disability itself influence all aspects of adjustment. Families are usually the care providers and the support system for the disabled person, and they need to be included in all the teaching–learning interactions. The literature has documented that family participation does have a profound influence on the success of a client's rehabilitation program. Rehabilitation nurses have learned to assess clients' and families' learning needs and then develop a teaching plan. When the client and family are assessed, it is important to note what the family considers a high-priority learning need. Most often it will be related to the family member's perceived lifestyle change (Will I be able to garden? Go for lunch with friends?). It is important that the nurse assist the client and family to identify problems and develop mutually agreed-upon goals. Adaptation is key. Communication between and among family members is cru-

cial. If a family has open communication, the nurse is in a good position to help the family mobilize so as to obtain needed emotional and educational support.

The client and family educational process also needs to take into consideration where the family is at in coping with their relative's disability. "Having a disabled individual within the family unit requires that all other members adapt to a new family structure" (Fraley, 1992, p. 108). A chronic illness or disability can either destroy or strengthen family unity. Siblings and children of the disabled person may be at a different stage of acceptance. Denial may be present during the initial diagnosis of a disability. Later, as the client and his or her family realize the permanency and the consequence of the illness or disability, the nurse may witness periods of anger, guilt, depression, fear, and hostility. As these feelings dissipate, readjust the teaching lessons to fit the new circumstances; flexibility is vital to a successful outcome. Be sure to treat each family member as unique, and recognize that some family members may never adjust. Table 9–5 lists some of the most common sources of tension in client and family education as adapted from LaRocca (1994).

Nurses need to value their teaching role when they work with the family having a disabled member. Unlike families dealing with an acutely ill member, families with permanently disabled members will have intermittent contact with the healthcare system throughout their lives. Therefore, whenever teaching sessions are required, the families' availability should be a primary consideration. Given adequate support and resources, families with a chronically ill family member can adapt, make adjustments, and live healthy, happy, full lives.

## ▬▬▬ ADAPTIVE COMPUTING

The growth of modern technology has invaded all areas of our lives. Without a doubt, the personal computer has become the tech-

| TABLE 9–5   Relieving external tensions in client and family education | |
|---|---|
| Problem | Response |
| **FAMILY DYNAMICS** | |
| Client or family member feels overwhelmed | Goal setting: Help family refocus on tasks at hand. Review goals that have been attained to boost morale. |
| Anxiety and fear of performing complex procedures | Establish an atmosphere of acceptance. Don't be in a hurry. Offer opportunities for talk and questions. Reassure client and family that they have made the right treatment choice. |
| Emotions associated with chronic or terminal conditions | Provide opportunities to express feelings. Offer referrals to community resources. |
| Caregiver burnout and illness | Simplify client management where possible (e.g., scheduling drug doses to reduce nighttime treatment). Remain accessible. Remember: When caregiver needs are not being met, resentments increase. Provide information on respite care. |
| Client fatigue, especially with chronic illness | Help the client identify individual tolerance for tiredness in planning for as much active participation in the family life as possible. |
| Young clients are frequently overwhelmed by complex emotions about their illness and therapy | Encourage both children and adolescents to use artwork to express their feelings. Suggest support groups. Offer support to parents and siblings who must alter their family lifestyle. |
| **GERIATRIC CONSIDERATIONS** | |
| An increase in the number of drugs taken daily (on average four or more per day) increases the potential for adverse reactions | Use only one pharmacy so that one source keeps track of medications. Continually evaluate all drugs taken for need, safety, compatibility, potential adverse reactions, and expiration dates. |
| Decreased visual acuity | Use teaching materials with large, bold type. Encourage the use of a magnifying glass. |

SOURCE: Adapted by permission from *Mosby's Home Health Nursing Pocket Consultant*. St. Louis: Mosby-Year Book, 1995.

nology that has had the greatest impact. As Max Cleland states, "The real disabled people of the future are going to be those who don't have a computer to use" (Green & Brightman, 1990). Until recently, however, computers have been inaccessible to individuals with a disability. Yet, when adaptive computing has been made available, disabled individuals have experienced dramatic changes in their lives. Computers with the appropriate adaptations have liberated people from social isolation and feelings of helplessness and instilled feelings of self-worth and independence. *Adaptive computing* is relatively new; it refers to the professional services and the technology (both hardware and software) that make computing technology accessible for persons with disabilities (Merrow & Corbett, 1994).

Since the enactment of the ADA in 1990, the diversity of our client population has grown to include more individuals with disabilities in every practice setting, including community health, schools, occupational health, and, of course, rehabilitation nursing. As nurses' understanding of adaptive computing is enhanced, so will their ability to advocate, recommend, and assist persons to attain the appropriate equipment and training. Adaptive computing not only enables independence, but also is a useful tool for health promotion activities. Just about every type of disability mentioned in this chapter could benefit from the use of adaptive computers. Merrow and Corbett (1994) discovered that the healthcare literature includes a number of research studies describing the use of computers with various populations, such as the older adult, the physically disabled in long-term rehabilitation, the blind and visually impaired, and people with quadriplegia.

Internetworking now provides access to education about adaptive computing for persons with disabilities and their families, for health service providers and educators, and for anyone interested and involved in computer resources for the disabled. Burgstahler (1997) describes a three-credit college course entitled Adaptive Computer Technology, which she offers worldwide over the Internet through the University of Washington. This distance-learning course surveys the field of adaptive technology and includes topics such as interface devices, computer applications, compensatory tools, information technology access, implementation strategies, and legal issues. It demonstrates how technology has the potential to improve the lives of people with disabilities by giving them the tools to become more independent, more productive, and better able to participate in a wide range of life experiences related to employment, education, and recreation.

## Assessment of Potential Barriers to Access

Although the personal computer has been proven to change the life of a person with even the most severe disability, the fact remains that it is a very individualized process. Personalized computer solutions are those that respond to a particular person, not to the particular disability (Green & Brightman, 1990). Merrow and Corbett (1994) identified six barriers to computer access:

1. The environment, which includes the room, the table or desk on which the computer sits, and the actual hardware (computer). For example, can the person in a wheelchair fit the wheelchair under the desk?

2. Input, which are the devices responsible for getting information into the computer (the keyboard or the mouse). People with no useful movement in their arms may benefit from a head pointer or a mouth stick.

3. Output devices, or the part of the computer responsible for sending the information back to the user, such as the monitor and printer. Aside from the obvious problem posed for the person with a visual impairment, the person with a learning disability or an acquired brain injury may have a problem interpreting output. The solution may be as simple as using slotted paper that permits the reading of one line at a time, reducing the glare, or decreasing the rate of text scrolling.

4. Documentation, the "written" text that describes how to operate the hardware or software. The problem is that this information is often written in "computerese." Some cognitive or physical disabilities present a barrier to accessing the instructions. For example, a person may not be able to physically handle a computer manual, but a manual in a spiral-bound book would be accessible. A person with a learning disability may do well with instructions if they are auditory or pictorial.

5. Support, which comes in two forms: cognitive and human support. For example, one of the participants in the Links and Frydenberg study (1989) was unwilling to attempt a word processing course, so she was assigned a simpler software program first; once it was mastered, she completed the entire computer program. Human support consists of someone who sets up the equipment and is also around to help answer questions and troubleshoot. Several agencies and organizations provide this kind of service as well as training.

6. Training, which needs to be supplied regarding the use of the hardware, software, and adaptations. Merrow and Corbett (1994) stated that training is probably the second greatest obstacle in adaptive technology. The greatest obstacle is finding out which devices are available and which ones best fit an individual's need.

## Types of Adaptations

Whether the area of impairment is mobility, hearing, seeing, communicating, or a learning disability will determine the type of adaptation. If the problem lies in the area of input, then the person needs to investigate and find the best keyboard or mouse adaptation. Head pointers and mouth sticks have already been mentioned, but many others exist, including voice recognition systems. Joysticks and trackballs are often used to simulate mouse movements. They are ideal alternatives to the mouse because they can be positioned in unique places and activated with different parts of the body, such as the chin or even the mouth. A trackball looks like a mouse turned upside down. It is very useful for people who do not have a wide range of movement in their arms or hands.

People with communication problems, especially those who are unable to speak or whose speech is difficult to understand, can nevertheless use the computer to add a whole new dimension to their lives. Within the last 10 years, the technology for impaired speech has made great strides. Several software packages are available for patients with such problems (see Appendix B). Visual feedback systems are devices that enable the computer to display graphic representation of spoken sounds. Using them, a person can work to match the correct displayed speech pattern. Computer-based electronic augmentative communication aids help people to use a synthetic voice to speak out loud (Green & Brightman, 1990).

Hearing-impaired and deaf persons can benefit from adaptive computing as well. The greatest challenge to this population, however, usually is not the computer, but training on the computer.

The visually impaired and those who are blind can benefit from adaptive computing, too. As previously noted, there is a wide range of visual impairment, ranging from a person with low vision to a person who is blind. It is obvious that the problem with this population relates to output—in other words, the monitor and the printer. There are many types of adaptive devices that can enable individuals with vision impairment to use a personal computer—everything from large-size monitors to large-print software. For people who are unable to see the screen at all, a solution may be to have the computer "speak" the screen contents. Another solution for computer users who are blind, and especially for individuals who are deaf, is tactile output. The images on the screen are converted into Braille or output on a device known as Opt-a-con, which gives the person an exact tactile representation of the letters and lines.

Learning disability problems can often be solved with a creative software package. For example, "Outliners," a type of thought processor, are programs that help people organize their ideas. They are very helpful in writing papers or reports. Sometimes the Outliners' software can be used in place of a word processor. Some experts feel the software may be the best place to start almost any kind of writing.

Every computer-based solution is the result of a carefully planned, individually determined process. Individuals with a disability are the experts on what works best for them. However, some guidelines should be considered when selecting the best adaptive computer. The best computer solution for individuals with disabilities will allow for independent and effective use. Other criteria include affordability, portability, flexibility, and simplicity of learning. If these criteria are met, then the adaptive computer is probably in compliance with the ADA's "reasonable accommodations."

O'Leary et al. (1991) reviewed the literature and determined that there were certain characteristics of the older adult that would probably ensure successful computer usage. They determined that the client must

- Be oriented.
- Have an attention span and short-term memory exceeding five minutes.
- Not be agitated or combative.

Adaptive computing is here to stay. While computer technology will probably be forever changing, the process for ensuring individualized computer solutions will remain much the same. When that process is pursued, the benefits will prove to be enormous. It is exciting to reflect on the positive, possibly life-changing effect the personal computer can have on the lives of individuals with a disability. It has the potential of changing what it means to be disabled. Within the role of nurse as teacher is the client advocate component. As client advocate, the nurse can work with the multidisciplinary team, including the computer specialist, to enable special populations to participate in all of life's experiences. Thanks to what adaptive personal computers will be able to do, people with disabilities will be more among us. Just think of all the opportunities for client teaching, health promotion, and counseling when a person using a modem is able to gain access to telecommunication.

## SUMMARY

The shock of any disability, whether it occurs at the beginning of life or toward the end, has a tremendous impact on individuals and their families. At the onset and all through the habilitation or rehabilitation process, the patient and family are met with new information to be learned, as successful habilitation or rehabilitation means acquiring knowledge and applying it to their situation. Inner strength and courage are attributes needed to face each new day, as the effort to live a "normal" life never ends. The physical, social, emotional, and vocational implications of living with a disability necessitate the nurse as educator to be well prepared to meet any member of this special population right where they are in their struggle to live independently.

## REVIEW QUESTIONS

1. How do the terms *habilitation* and *rehabilitation* differ from one another?

2. What are the major causes of disabilities?

3. Which six (6) questions should be asked by the nurse educator when assessing a disabled person's readiness to learn?

4. What are the two (2) major types of disabilities?

5. What are the seven (7) categories of disabilities?

6. When should the nurse educator enlist the help of a professional interpreter rather than a member of the family when teaching a hearing impaired person?

7. What are ten (10) tips you might find helpful in teaching a blind or visually impaired person?
8. What are the four (4) types of input disabilities and the two (2) types of output disabilities?
9. What are the three (3) subtypes of Attention Deficit Disorder (ADD), what are the characteristic behaviors of persons with ADD, and what are the educational interventions that should be used when teaching people with ADD?
10. How does the Developmental Disabilities Act of 1978 define *developmental disability* and what

subsequent laws have been enacted to protect children with mental and/or physical impairments?
11. What is the most common obstacle to learning readiness in the young spinal cord-injured male?
12. Which of the four (4) communication disorders is caused by a problem with the voluntary muscle control of speech?
13. What are six (6) barriers to computer access for persons with disabilities?

## REFERENCES

Adkins, E. R. H. (1991). Nursing care of the client with impaired communication. *Rehabilitation Nursing, 16*(2), 74–76.

Babcock, D. E. & Miller, M. A. (1994). *Client Education: Theory and Practice.* St. Louis: Mosby.

Baker, S. S. (1993). Teamwork between the health care community and the blind rehabilitation system. *Journal of Visual Impairment and Blindness, 87*(9), 349–352.

Blanco, K. M. (1982). The aphasic patient. *Journal of Neurosurgical Nursing, 14*, 34–37.

Boss, B. J. (1986). The neuroanatomical and neurophysiological basis for learning. *Journal of Neuroscience Nursing, 18*(5), 256–264.

Boyd, M. D., Gleit, C. J., Graham, B. A., & Whitman, N. I. (1998). *Health Teaching in Nursing Practice,* 3rd ed. Stamford, CT: Appleton & Lange.

Bronstein, K. S., Popovoch, J., & Stewart-Amidei, C. (1991). *Promoting Stroke Recovery: A Research-based Approach for Nurses.* St. Louis: Mosby–Year Book.

Burgstahler, S. (April 1997). Teaching on the Net: What's the difference? *T.H.E. Journal*, 61–64.

Burkett, K. W. (1989). Trends in pediatric rehabilitation. *Nursing Clinics of North America, 24*(1), 239–255.

Cunningham, C. (2001). Breaking the barriers to math and science for students with disabilities. *Syllabus*, February, 41–42.

Diehl, L. N. (1989). Client and family learning in the rehabilitation setting. *Nursing Clinics of North America, 24*(1), 257–264.

DiPietro, L. (1979). *Deaf Patients, Special Needs, Special Responses.* Washington, DC: National Academy of Gallaudet College.

Dittmar, S. (1989). *Rehabilitation Nursing.* St. Louis: Mosby–Year Book.

Dreher, B. (1981). Overcoming speech and language disorders. *Geriatric Nursing, 2*, 345–349.

Dykman, R. A., Ackerman, P. T., Holcomb, P. J., & Boudreau, A. Y. (1983). Physiological manifestations of learning disability. *Journal of Learning Disabilities, 16*(1), 46–53.

Edwards, P. A. (2000). *The Specialty Practice of Rehabilitation: A Core Curriculum,* 4th ed. Glenville, IL: Association Rehabilitation Nurses.

Fink, S. L. (1967). Crisis and motivation: A theoretical model. *Archives of Physical Rehabilitation, 48*, 492–597.

Fraley, A. M. (1992). *Nursing and the Disabled: Across the Life Span.* Boston: Jones and Bartlett.

Green, P. & Brightman, A. J. (1990). *Independence Day: Designing Computer Solutions for Individuals with Disability.* Allen, TX: DLM.

Greenberg, L. A. (1991). Teaching children who are learning disabled about illness and hospitalization. *MCN: American Journal of Maternal Child Nursing, 16*(5), 260–263.

Grinspun, D. (1987). Teaching families of traumatic brain-injured adults. *Critical Care Nursing Quarterly, 10*(3), 61–72.

Haber, J., Krainovich-Miller, B., McMahon A. L., & Price-Hoskins, P. (1997). *Comprehensive Psychiatric Nursing.* St. Louis: Mosby.

Haggard, A. (1989). *Handbook of Patient Education.* Rockville, MD: Aspen.

Hammill, D. D., Leigh, J. E., McNutt, G., & Larsen, S. C. (1981). A new definition of learning disabilities. *Learning Disability Quarterly, 4*, 336–342.

Harrison, L. L. (1990). Minimizing barriers when teaching hearing-impaired clients. *MCN: American Journal of Maternal Child Nursing, 15*(2), 113.

Hood, L. J. (1990). Myasthenia gravis: Regimens and regimen-associated problems in adults. *Journal of Neuroscience Nursing, 22*(16), 358–364.

Jennings, S. (1981). Communicating with your aphasic patients. *Journal of Practical Nursing, 31,* 22–23.

Kirk, S. A. & Kirk, W. D. (1983). On defining disabilities. *Journal of Learning Disabilities, 16*(1), 20–21.

Knowles, B. S. & Knowles, P. S. (1983). A model for identifying learning disabilities in college-bound students. *Journal of Learning Disabilities, 16*(1), 39–42.

LaRocca, J. C. (1994). *Handbook of Home Care IV Therapy.* St. Louis: Mosby–Year Book.

Links, C. & Frydenberg, H. (1989). Microcomputer skills training program for the physically disabled in long term rehabilitation. *Physical & Occupational Therapy in Geriatrics, 6*(3/4), 133–140.

Loughrey, L. (1992). The effects of two teaching techniques on recognition and use of function words by aphasic stroke patients. *Rehabilitation Nursing, 17*(3), 134–137.

Lubkin, I. M. (2002). *Chronic Illness: Impact and Interventions,* 5th edition. Boston: Jones and Bartlett.

McCafferty, L. A. E. (January 21, 2002). Sounds of understanding: Nurses can help spot and treat hearing loss. *Advance for Nurses,* 5.

McConnel, E. A. (1996). Clinical do's & don'ts: Caring for a patient with a vision impairment. *Nursing, 26*(5), 28.

McLoughlin, J. A. & Natick, A. (1983). Defining learning disabilities: A new and cooperative direction. *Journal of Learning Disabilities, 16*(1), 21–23.

Merrow, S. L. & Corbett, C. (1994). Adaptive computing for people with disabilities. *Computers in Nursing, 12*(4), 201–209.

National Advisory Mental Health Council. (1990). *National Plan for Research on Child and Adolescent Mental Disorders* (DHHS pub. #90-1683). Rockville, MD: National Institute of Mental Health.

National Center for Injury Prevention and Control. (April 15, 1999). Division of Acute Care Rehabilitation Research and Disability Prevention. *http://www.CDC.gov/NCIPC/dacrrdp/dacrrdp.htm.*

National Institute of Mental Health. (1991). *Caring for People with Severe Mental Disorders: A National Plan of Research to Improve Services* (DHHS pub. #91-1762). Washington, DC: U.S. Government Printing Office.

National Spinal Cord Injury Statistical Center. (1999). *Spinal Cord Injury: The Facts and Figures.* Birmingham, AL: University of Alabama at Birmingham.

Navarro, M. R. & Lacour, G. (1980). Helping hints for use with deaf patients. *Journal of Emergency Nursing, 6*(6), 26–28.

Nelson, K. (1991). *Projected Increase in the Prevalence of Severe Visual Impairment among Elderly Americans.* New York: American Foundation for the Blind.

Norman, S. & Baratz, R. (1979). The brain-damaged patient: Approaches to assessment, care, and rehabilitation. Understanding aphasia, pt. 4. *American Journal of Nursing, 79,* 2135–2138.

Norris, W. C., Wharton, G., Noble, C., & Strickland, S. (1982). The spinal injury learning series: An experimental test. *Archives of Physical Medicine, Rehabilitation, 63*(6), 243–248.

O'Leary, S., Mann, C., & Perkash, I. (1991). Access to computers for the older adults: Problems and solutions. *American Journal of Occupational Therapy, 45*(7), 636–642.

Olson, E. (1991). Perceptual deficits affecting the stroke patient. *Rehabilitation Nursing, 16*(14), 212–213.

Phipps, W. J., Cassmeyer, V. L., Sands, J. K., & Lehman, M. K. (1995). *Medical Surgical Nursing,* 5th ed. St. Louis: Mosby.

Stock, S. (January 21, 2002). When silence isn't golden. *Advance for Nurses,* 28–29.

Strauss, A. L., Corbin, J., Fagerhaugh, S., et al. (1984). *Chronic Illness and Quality of Life,* 2nd ed. St. Louis: Mosby.

Strong, M. (1996). *Language Learning and Deafness.* New York: Cambridge University Press.

Tate, R. L., Fenelon, B., Manning, M. L., & Hunter, M. (1991). Patterns of neuropsychological impairment after severe blunt injury. *Journal of Nervous and Mental Disease, 179*(3), 117–126.

Trybus, P. & Karchner, M. (1977) School achievement scores of hearing impaired children: National data on achievement status and growth patterns. *American Annuals of the Deaf Directory of Programs and Services, 122,* 62–69.

U.S. Census Bureau. (2000). *Population Estimates Program.* Washington, D.C.: U.S. Census Bureau.

Vance, J. L. (1992). Learning readiness in rehabilitation patients. *Rehabilitation Nursing, 17*(3), 148–149.

Vessey, J. (1988). Care of the hospitalized child with a cognitive developmental delay. *Holistic Nursing Practice, 2*(2), 48–54.

Webb, M., Tittle, M., & VanCott, M. L. (2000). Increasing students' sensitivity to families of children with disabilities. *Nurse Educator, 25*(1), 43–47.

Weeks, S. K. (1995). What are the educational needs of the prospective family caregiver of newly disabled adults? *Rehabilitation Nursing, 20*(5), 256–260.

Ysseldyke, J. & Allgozzine, B. (1983). LD or not LD: That's not the question! *Journal of Learning Disabilities, 16*(1), 29–31.

Zejdlik, C. P. (1992). *Management of Spinal Cord Injury,* 2nd ed. Boston: Jones and Bartlett.

Zirkel, P. A. (2000). Sorting out which students have learning disabilities. *The Chronicle of Higher Education, 47*(15), B15–B16.

# PART III

# Techniques and Strategies for Teaching and Learning

## CHAPTER 10

# Behavioral Objectives

*Susan B. Bastable*

With appreciation to Cynthia Sculco, Ed.D., R.N. for her contribution to the first edition of this chapter.

## CHAPTER HIGHLIGHTS

## KEY TERMS

behavioral (learning) objectives
goal
taxonomy
cognitive domain
affective domain
psychomotor domain

transfer of learning
selective attention
intrinsic and augmented feedback
teaching plans
learning contracts
learning curve

## OBJECTIVES

After completing this chapter, the reader will be able to

1. Identify the difference between goals and objectives.

2. Recognize opposing viewpoints regarding the use of behavioral objectives in education.

3. Demonstrate the ability to write behavioral objectives accurately and concisely using the three components of condition, performance, and criterion.

4. Cite the most frequent errors made in writing objectives.

5. Distinguish between the three domains of learning.

6. Explain the instructional methods appropriate for teaching in the cognitive, affective, and psychomotor domains.

7. Develop teaching plans that reflect internal consistency between elements.

8. Describe the importance of learning contracts as an alternative approach to structuring a learning experience.

9. Recognize the role of the nurse educator in formulating objectives for the planning, implementation, and evaluation of teaching and learning.

In previous chapters, the characteristics and attributes of the learner with respect to learning needs, readiness to learn, and learning styles have been addressed. Clearly, assessment of the learner is an essential first step in the teaching–learning process. Assessment determines what the learner needs to know, when and under what conditions the learner is most receptive to learning, and how the learner actually learns best. Before a decision can be made about selecting the content to be taught or choosing the instructional methods and materials to be used to change learner behavior, the educator must first decide what the learner is expected to accomplish. Client needs are determined by identifying the gaps in the learner's knowledge, attitudes, or skills. Identification of needs is a prerequisite to formulating behavioral objectives that serve to guide subsequent planning, implementation, and evaluation of teaching and learning.

Historically, noted educators and education psychologists of this century have developed approaches to writing and classifying behavioral objectives that offer teachers assistance in organizing instructional content for learners functioning at various levels of ability. Mager (1997) has been the primary educator credited with developing a system for writing behavioral objectives that serves to help teachers make appropriate instructional decisions as well as to assist learners in understanding what they need and are expected to know. The underlying principle has been, if one does not know where he or she is going, how will the person know when he or she has arrived? In addition, the taxonomic system devised by Bloom and associates (1956) for categorizing learning objectives according to a hierarchy of behaviors has been the cornerstone of teaching for almost a half-century.

The two dimensions to the preparation of behavioral objectives include the technique of writing objectives and the ordering of these behaviors according to their type and complex-

ity. Both the formulation of objectives and the concept of taxonomy pertain to the nature of the knowledge to be learned, the behaviors most relevant and attainable for a particular learner or group of learners, and the sequencing of knowledge and experiences for learning.

The skill in preparing and classifying behavioral objectives is a necessary function of the educator's role, whether teaching patients and their families in healthcare settings, teaching staff nurses in in-service and continuing education programs, or teaching nursing students in academic institutions. The importance of understanding the systems of writing and categorizing behavioral objectives for the purpose of specifying learner outcomes is imperative if data yielded from educational efforts are to be consistent and measurable. Additionally, the knowledge and utilization of these techniques are becoming essential because of the need to quantify and justify the costs of teaching others in an environment characterized by ever-increasing cost-containment pressures.

This chapter examines the role of behavioral objectives for effective teaching; describes how to write clear and precise behavioral objectives; explores the levels of achievement in the taxonomic hierarchy of cognitive, affective, and psychomotor domains; and outlines the development of teaching plans and learning contracts. All of these elements provide a framework for the successful instruction of the learner.

## CHARACTERISTICS OF GOALS AND OBJECTIVES

As a basis for discussion and prior to differentiating between what is a goal and what is an objective, it is important to clarify the meaning of the terms *educational or instructional objectives* and *behavioral or learning objectives*. Although often used synonymously, these sets of terms can be distinguished from one another. Educational or instructional objectives are used to identify the intended outcomes of the education process, whether in reference to an aspect of a program or a total program of study. Behavioral or learning objectives, on the other hand, make use of the modifier behavioral or learning to denote that they are action-oriented rather than content-oriented and learner-centered rather than teacher-centered. Behavioral objectives describe what the learner will be able to do following a learning situation.

The terms *goal* and *objective* are often used interchangeably—albeit incorrectly, because there does exist a real difference between the two terms. This distinction must be clearly understood by nurse educators. Time span and specificity are the two factors that differentiate goals from objectives, and vice versa (Haggard, 1989).

A *goal* is the final outcome of what is achieved at the end of the teaching–learning process. Goals are global and broad in nature; they serve as long-term targets for both the learner and the teacher. Goals are the desired outcomes of learning that are realistically achievable in weeks or months. They are considered multidimensional in that a number of objectives are subsumed under or incorporated into an overall goal.

An *objective*, in contrast, is a specific, single, unidimensional behavior. Objectives are short-term in nature and should be achievable at the conclusion of one teaching session or within a matter of a few days following a series of teaching sessions. According to Mager (1997), an objective describes a performance that learners should be able to exhibit before they are considered competent. A behavioral objective is the intended result of instruction, not the process or means of instruction itself. Objectives are statements of specific or short-term behaviors that lead step-by-step to the more general, overall long-term goal. Subobjectives reflect aspects of a main objective and are also written as specific state-

ments of short-term behaviors that lead to the achievement of the primary objective. Objectives and subobjectives specify what the learner will be able to do as a result of being exposed to one or more learning experiences. Objectives must be achieved before the goal can be reached. They must be observable and measurable to be able to determine whether they have been met by the learner. Objectives can be thought of as advance organizers, statements that inform the learner of what is expected from a cognitive, affective, or psychomotor perspective to meet the intended outcome (Babcock & Miller, 1994). Objectives are derived from a goal and must be consistent with and related to that goal. As an analogy, a goal can be thought of as an entire pie and the objectives as individual pieces of the pie that make up the goal.

Together, objectives and goals form a map that provides directions (objectives) as to how to arrive at a particular destination (goal). For example, a goal might be that a diabetic patient will learn to manage diabetes. To accomplish this goal, which has been agreed on by both the nurse and the patient, specific objectives must be outlined to address changes in behavior such as the need to learn diet therapy, insulin administration, exercise regimens, stress management, and glucose monitoring. The objectives to accomplish the goal become the blueprint for attaining the desired outcomes of learning. The successful achievement of predetermined objectives is, in part, the result of appropriate instruction. Certainly, many other factors, such as learner motivation and ability to perform, are also key to the successful demonstration of specific behaviors before overall competence by the learner can be declared.

If the teaching–learning process is to be successful, the setting of goals and objectives must be a mutual decision on the part of both the teacher and the learner. Both parties must participate in the decision-making process and "buy into" the immediate objectives and ultimate goals. Involving the learner right from the start in creating goals and objectives is absolutely crucial. Otherwise, time and effort on the part of the educator and the learner may be wasted, because the learner may choose to reject the content if it is deemed from his or her perspective to be unimportant, irrelevant, impractical, or something already known. Goal and objective setting for any educational experience should be as much a responsibility of the learner as of the teacher. Blending what the learner wants to learn with what the teacher has determined that the learner needs to know into a common set of objectives and goals provides for an educational experience that is mutually accountable, respectful, developmental, and fulfilling (Reilly & Oermann, 1990).

Objectives and goals must also be clearly written, realistic, and learner-centered. If they do not precisely state what the learner is expected to do in the short and long term, respectively, then there are no clear guideposts to follow or an obvious end result for which to strive in the learning process. If goals and objectives are too difficult to achieve, the learner will become easily discouraged, which dampens motivation and interferes with the ability to comply. For instance, a goal that a patient will maintain a *salt-free* diet is likely to be impossible to accomplish or adhere to over an extended period of time. Establishing a goal of maintaining a *low-salt* diet, with the objectives of learning to avoid eating and preparing high-sodium foods, is a much more realistic and achievable expectation of the learner.

Goals and objectives must be directed to what the learner is expected to be able to do, not what the teacher is expected to teach. Educators must be sure not only that their teaching remains objectives-oriented but also that the objectives are learner-centered to keep both them and the learners targeted on results, not on the act of teaching.

## THE DEBATE ABOUT USING BEHAVIORAL OBJECTIVES

Educators have made strong arguments for and against the use of behavioral objectives for teaching and learning. Certainly behavioral objectives are not a panacea for all the problems encountered in the planning, implementation, and evaluation of education (Reilly & Oermann, 1990). The following list, outlined by Arends (1994), Reilly and Oermann (1990), Haggard (1989), and Durbach, Goodall, and Wilkinson (1987), present some common arguments by educators against using behavioral objectives:

- The understanding by experienced educators of learners' needs is so sophisticated that the exercise of writing behavioral objectives is superfluous.

- The practice of writing specific behavioral objectives leads to reductionism, a format that reduces behavioral processes into equivalents that do not reflect the sum total of the parts.

- Objectives writing is a time-consuming task, requiring more effort for development than is warranted by their effect on an instructional program, such that the cost benefit does not justify the amount of time required to formulate them.

- The preparation of objectives is merely a pedagogic exercise often expressing the teacher's expectations of the outcome of teaching and precluding the opportunity for learners to seek their own objectives.

- Predetermined objectives, with their emphasis on precise and observable learner behaviors, force teachers and learners to attend only to specific areas, which stifle creativity and interfere with the freedom to learn and to teach.

- The writing of specific objectives is incompatible with the complex field of study such as nursing because an infinite number of objectives are possible for almost any subject or topic.

- Behavioral objectives are unable to capture the more intricate cognitive processes that are not readily observable and measurable.

The rationale for using behavioral objectives, however, far outweighs the arguments against their use. The following considerations justify the need for writing behavioral objectives (Ferguson, 1998). Careful construction of objectives

- Helps to keep educators' thinking on target and learner-centered.
- Communicates to others, both learners and healthcare team members alike, what is planned for teaching and learning.
- Helps learners understand what is expected of them so they can keep track of their progress.
- Forces the educator to organize educational materials so as not to get lost in content and forget the learner's role in the process.
- Encourages educators to question their own motives—to think deliberately about why they are doing things and analyze what positive results will be attained from accomplishing specific objectives.
- Tailors teaching to the learner's particular circumstances and needs.
- Creates guideposts for teacher evaluation and documentation of success or failure.
- Focuses attention not on what is taught but on what the learner will come away with once the teaching–learning process is completed.
- Orients both teacher and learner to the specific end result of instruction.
- Makes it easier for the learner to visualize performing the required actions.

Robert Mager (1997), a recognized authority on preparing behavioral objectives, points out three other major advantages to writing explicit objective statements:

1. They provide a sound basis for the selection or design of instructional content, methods, and materials.
2. They provide learners with the means to organize their efforts and activities toward accomplishing the intent of instruction.
3. They allow for a determination as to whether an objective has, in fact, been accomplished.

As Mager (1997) states, "If you don't know where you're going, how will you know which road to take to get there?" (p. 14). That is, before the educator prepares instruction, before materials and teaching methods are selected, before the means to evaluate learning is chosen, it is important to clearly and concisely state just what the intended results of instruction are to be. To paraphrase Mager's thinking, mechanics do not select repair tools until they know what has to be fixed, surgeons do not choose instruments until they know what operation is to be performed, and builders do not buy construction materials before drafting a blueprint.

Haggard (1989) summarized the following questions that arise if objectives are not always written:

- How will anyone else know what objectives have been set?
- How will the educator evaluate and document success or failure?
- How will learners keep track of their progress?

The writing of objectives is not merely a mechanical task but a synthesizing process. The process of developing behavioral objectives not only helps educators explore their own knowledge, values, and beliefs about the entire spectrum of teaching and learning, but also encourages them to examine the experiences, values, motivations, and knowledge of the learner. The time and effort expended in writing objectives represent a thoughtful deliberation about the knowledge, attitude, and skill requirements needed by the learner in meeting the desired level of competency. The educator and learner work together to compose objectives and goals that focus on what is to be accomplished in the short and long run. This process provides direction that helps the educator identify the time that will be needed for teaching, the clues as to how the learner best acquires information, the teaching methods that will work most effectively, and the best ways to evaluate the learner's progress. In addition, the process of stating well-written objectives encourages the educator to seriously contemplate what is worth teaching and what is worth spending time to accomplish. Also, the process can serve to highlight the value of an existing instructional program and provide the basis for improving a current teaching plan. Thus, the setting of objectives and goals is considered by many educators to be the initial, most important consideration in the education process (Haggard, 1989; Mager, 1997).

## WRITING BEHAVIORAL OBJECTIVES

Well-written behavioral objectives give learners very clear statements about what is expected of them and assist teachers in being able to measure learner progress toward achieving outcomes of learning. Over the past three decades, Robert Mager's (1997) approach to writing behavioral objectives has been widely accepted among educators. His message to educators is that for objectives to be meaningful, they must precisely, clearly, and very specifically communicate the teacher's instructional intent (Arends, 1994).

According to Mager (1997), the format for writing concise and useful behavioral objectives includes the following three important characteristics:

1. *Performance:* Describes what the learner is expected to be able to do or perform to demonstrate the kinds of behaviors the teacher will accept as evidence that objectives have been achieved. Activities performed by the learner may be visible, such as "writing" or "listing," or invisible, such as "identifying" or "recalling."

2. *Condition:* Describes the testing situation or constraints under which the behavior will be observed or the performance is expected to occur.

3. *Criterion:* Describes how well or with what accuracy the learner must be able to perform for the behavior to be considered acceptable; the standard, quality level, or amount of performance defined as satisfactorily demonstrating mastery. It is the level of competence that a learner must achieve.

The preceding characteristics translate into the following questions: (1) What should the learner be able to do? (2) Under what conditions should the learner be able to do it? (3) How well must the learner be able to do it?

A fourth component must also be included that describes the "who" to ensure that the behavioral objective is learner-centered. For education in health care, the learner may be the patient, family members or significant others of the patient, staff nurses, or student nurses. Thus, behavioral objectives are statements that communicate *who* will *do what* under *what conditions* and *how well* (Cummings, 1994). The more complete the statements of objectives, the better the objectives will serve to communicate exactly what is expected of the learner and what is the intent of instruction. To link the behavioral objectives together, the following three steps are recommended:

1. Identify the testing situation (condition).

| TABLE 10–1   The three-part method of objective writing | | |
|---|---|---|
| Condition (Testing Situation) | Performance (Learner Behavior) | Criterion (Quality of Accuracy) |
| | The learner will be able to: | |
| Without using a calculator | solve | 5 out of 6 problems |
| Using a model | demonstrate | the correct procedure |
| Following group discussion | list | at least two reasons |
| After watching a video | select | with 100% accuracy |

2. State the learner and the learner's behavior (performance).

3. State the performance level (criterion).

For example: "Following a 20-minute teaching session on hypoglycemia (*condition*), Mrs. Smith will be able to identify (*performance*) three out of four major symptoms of low blood sugar (*criterion*)."

Table 10–1 outlines the three-part method of objective writing. Table 10–2 gives samples of well-written and poorly written objectives.

It is important to note, however, that there are really two accepted approaches to writing behavioral objectives, depending on the audience of learners. Reilly and Oermann (1990) distinguish between what are known as specific behavioral objectives versus general behavioral objectives. With both types of objectives, the learners and the behaviors to be learned must be clearly stated. The difference between the two types of objectives lies in the desirability of including the conditions of learning and the criteria for the level of performance expected.

*Specific behavioral objectives* are close-ended statements that incorporate the condition and criterion for learning, which make them more prescriptive and predictive for the measurement of outcomes. This relatively linear format for writing specific behavioral objectives is an asset to help focus the learning process on a step-by-step basis, especially when a low-level skill is the intended outcome. For example, when teaching a patient to test blood glucose levels or teaching a nurse a new procedural protocol for a dressing change, the writing of

| TABLE 10–2   Samples of written objectives |
|---|

**WELL-WRITTEN OBJECTIVES**

After watching a demonstration on suctioning, the staff member will be able to correctly suction a tracheostomy tube using aseptic technique.

Following a class on hypertension, the patient will be able to state three out of four causes of high blood pressure.

On completing the reading materials provided on the care of a newborn, the mother will be able to express any concerns she has about caring for her baby after discharge.

**POORLY WRITTEN OBJECTIVES**

The patient will be able to prepare a menu using low-salt foods (*condition and criterion missing*).

Given a list of exercises to relieve low back pain, the patient will understand how to control low back pain (*performance not stated in measurable terms, criterion missing*).

To demonstrate crutch walking postoperatively to the patient (*teacher-centered*).

specific behavioral objectives is preferred. *General behavioral objectives,* which do not include the condition or criterion for learning, are open-ended statements that lend themselves to be used in evaluating higher cognitive skills. This format is more appropriate for stating outcomes of an academic program, when knowledge of the learner is not expected to be just an accumulation of designated parts, but rather an integration and synthesis of broader concepts and theories over time. As such, the writing of general behavioral objectives is more compatible when teaching nurses in a staff development program or nursing students in a course within a professional program of study. It allows teachers to be more creative in teaching and accomodates acceptable variations in the learner that foster the creative expression of ideas and knowledge.

It is important to recognize the existence of and distinction between these two types of behavioral objectives. In this chapter, however, the focus will be on writing specific behavioral objectives appropriate for the learning of particular skill sets by patients and staff.

## Performance Words with Many or Few Interpretations

When writing behavioral objectives using the format suggested by Mager (1997), the recommendation is to use precise action words (verbs as labels, known as verbals) that are open to few interpretations when describing learner performance.

An objective is considered useful only when it clearly states what a learner must demonstrate for mastery in a knowledge, attitude, or skill area. A performance verb describes what the learner is expected to *do.* A performance may be overt, visible, or audible—for example, the learner is able to *list,* to *write,* to *state,* or to *walk.* These performances are directly observable. A performance also may be invisible—for example, the learner is able to *identify,* to *solve,* to *recall,* or to

*recognize.* Any performance, visible/audible or invisible, described by a "doing" word is measurable.

If a word is used to describe something a learner can *be,* then it is not a "doing" word but rather a "being" word. Examples of being words, known also as abstractions, are to *understand,* to *know,* to *enjoy,* or to *appreciate* (Mager, 1997). Understanding, knowing, enjoying, and appreciating are considered abstract states of being and cannot be directly measured but merely inferred from performances. Therefore, verbs that signify an internal state of thinking, feeling, or believing should be avoided because they are difficult to measure or observe.

It is impossible to identify all behavioral terms that may be used in objective writing. The important thing to remember in selecting verbs to describe performance is that they are specific, can be observed or measured, and are action-oriented. The lists in Table 10–3 give examples of verbals that, on the one hand, are too broad, ambiguous, and imprecise to evaluate and, on the other hand, are specific and relatively easy to measure (Gronlund, 1985).

## ▪▪▪ COMMON MISTAKES WHEN WRITING OBJECTIVES

In formulating behavioral objectives, there are a number of common pitfalls that can easily be made by the novice as well as by the seasoned educator. The most frequent errors in writing objectives are

- To describe what the instructor rather than the learner is expected to do.

- To include more than one expected behavior in a single objective (avoid using the compound word *and* to connect two verbs—e.g., the learner will select *and* prepare).

- To forget to include all three components of condition, performance, and criterion.

| TABLE 10–3    Verbals with many or few interpretations | | |
|---|---|---|
| **Terms with Many Interpretations**<br>**(Not Recommended)** | **Terms with Few Interpretations**<br>**(Recommended)** | |
| to know | to apply | to explain |
| to understand | to choose | to identify |
| to appreciate | to classify | to list |
| to realize | to compare | to order |
| to be familiar with | to contrast | to predict |
| to enjoy | to construct | to recall |
| to value | to define | to recognize |
| to be interested in | to describe | to select |
| to feel | to demonstrate | to state |
| to think | to differentiate | to verbalize |
| to learn | to distinguish | to write |

SOURCE: Adapted from Gronlund, N. E. (1985). *Stating Objectives for Classroom Instruction*, 3rd ed. New York: Macmillan.

- To use terms for performance that are subject to many interpretations, not action-oriented, and difficult to measure.

- To write an objective that is unattainable given the ability level of the learner.

- To write objectives that do not relate to the stated goal.

- To clutter an objective by including unnecessary pieces of information.

- To be too general so as not to clearly specify the expected outcome.

## TAXONOMY OF OBJECTIVES ACCORDING TO LEARNING DOMAINS

A *taxonomy* is a mechanism used to categorize things according to their relationships to one another. In science, for example, taxonomies are devices used to classify plants and animals in a systematic and logical fashion (Arends, 1994). In the late 1940s, psychologists and educators became concerned about the need to develop a system for defining and ordering

levels of behavior according to their type and complexity (Reilly & Oermann, 1990). Bloom et al. (1956) and Knathwohl and associates (1964) developed a very useful taxonomy, known as the *Taxonomy of Educational Objectives*, as a tool for systematically classifying behavioral objectives. This taxonomy, which became widely accepted as a standard aid for planning as well as evaluating learning, is divided into three broad categories or domains: cognitive, affective, and psychomotor. Inherent in the concept of taxonomy is the notion that although the three domains of learning are described as existing as separate entities, they are, in fact, interdependent and can be experienced simultaneously. Humans do not possess thoughts, feelings, and actions in isolation of one another and typically do not compartmentalize learning. The affective domain influences the cognitive domain, and vice versa; the processes of thinking and feeling influence psychomotor performance, and vice versa (Menix, 1996).

In the *Taxonomy of Educational Objectives*, the objectives in each domain are ordered in a taxonomic form of hierarchy. Behavioral objectives are classified into low, medium, and high levels with simple behaviors listed first (designated by numbers 1.0 or 2.0) and the more complex behaviors listed last (designated by numbers 5.0 or 6.0). Subobjectives are listed under the main objective and are designated by numbers that range between whole numbers (e.g., 2.1, 3.9, 5.6, or 6.8). Inherent in the concept of hierarchy is the idea that learners must successfully achieve behaviors at the lower levels of the domains before they are able to adequately learn behaviors at the higher levels of the domains.

## The Cognitive Domain

The *cognitive domain* is known as the "thinking" domain. Learning in this domain involves the acquisition of information and refers to the learner's intellectual abilities, mental capacities, and thinking processes. Objectives in this domain are divided into six levels, each specifying cognitive processes ranging from the simple (knowledge) to the more complex (evaluation), as listed and described in the following section (Bloom et al., 1956).

### Levels of Cognitive Behavior

*Knowledge* (1.00–1.99): ability of the learner to memorize, recall, define, recognize, or identify specific information, such as facts, rules, principles, conditions, and terms, presented during instruction.

*Comprehension* (2.00–2.99): ability of the learner to demonstrate an understanding or appreciation of what is being communicated by translating it into a different form or recognizing it in a translated form, such as grasping an idea by defining it or summarizing it in his or her own words (knowledge is a prerequisite behavior).

*Application* (3.00–3.99): ability of the learner to use ideas, principles, abstractions, or theories in particular and concrete

situations, such as figuring, writing, reading, or handling equipment (knowledge and comprehension are prerequisite behaviors).

*Analysis* (4.00–4.99): ability of the learner to recognize and structure information by breaking it down into its constituent parts and specifying the relationship between parts (knowledge, comprehension, and application are prerequisite behaviors).

*Synthesis* (5.00–5.99): ability of the learner to put together parts and elements into a unified whole by creating a unique product that is written, oral, pictorial, and so on (knowledge, comprehension, application, and analysis are prerequisite behaviors).

*Evaluation* (6.00–6.99): ability of the learner to judge the value of something, such as an essay, design, or action, by applying appropriate standards or criteria (knowledge, comprehension, application, analysis, and synthesis are prerequisite behaviors).

Table 10–4 lists verbs commonly used in writing cognitive-level behavioral objectives.

### Examples of Behavioral Objectives in the Cognitive Domain

*Analysis level:* "After reading handouts provided by the nurse educator, the family member will calculate the correct number of total grams of protein included on average per day in the family diet."

*Synthesis level:* "Given a sample list of foods, the patient will devise a menu to include foods from the four food groups (dairy, meat, vegetables and fruits, and grains) in the recommended amounts for daily intake."

**Teaching in the Cognitive Domain**  A variety of teaching methods and tools exist for the primary purpose of developing cognitive abilities. The methods most often used to stimu-

| TABLE 10–4    Commonly used verbs according to domain classification |
|---|

**COGNITIVE DOMAIN**

*Knowledge:* choose, circle, define, identify, label, list, match, name, outline, recall, report, select, state

*Comprehension.* describe, discuss, distinguish, estimate, explain, generalize, give example, locate, recognize, summarize

*Application:* apply, demonstrate, illustrate, implement, interpret, modify, order, revise, solve, use

*Analysis:* analyze, arrange, calculate, classify, compare, conclude, contrast, determine, differentiate, discriminate

*Synthesis:* categorize, combine, compile, correlate, design, devise, generate, integrate, reorganize, revise, summarize

*Evaluation:* appraise, assess, conclude, criticize, debate, defend, judge, justify

**AFFECTIVE DOMAIN**

*Receiving:* accept, admit, ask, attend, focus, listen, observe, pay attention

*Responding:* agree, answer, conform, discuss, express, participate, recall, relate, report, state willingness, try, verbalize

*Valuing:* assert, assist, attempt, choose, complete, disagree, follow, help, initiate, join, propose, volunteer

*Organization:* adhere, alter, arrange, combine, defend, explain, express, generalize, integrate, resolve

*Characterization:* assert, commit, discriminate, display, influence, propose, qualify, solve, verify

**PSYCHOMOTOR DOMAIN**

*Perception:* attend, choose, describe, detect, differentiate, distinguish, identify, isolate, perceive, relate, select, separate

*Set:* attempt, begin, develop, display, position, prepare, proceed, reach, respond, show, start, try

*Guided response mechanism and complex overt response:* align, arrange, assemble, attach, build, change, choose, clean, compile, complete, construct, demonstrate, discriminate, dismantle, dissect, examine, find, grasp, hold, insert, lift, locate, maintain, manipulate, measure, mix, open, operate, organize, perform, pour, practice, reassemble, remove, repair, replace, separate, shake, suction, turn, transfer, walk, wash, wipe

*Adaptation:* adapt, alter, change, convert, correct, rearrange, reorganize, replace, revise, shift, substitute, switch

*Origination:* arrange, combine, compose, construct, create, design, exchange, reformulate

SOURCE: Adapted from Gronlund, N.E. *(1985). Stating Objectives for Classroom Instruction,* 3rd ed. New York: Macmillan.

late learning in the cognitive domain include lecture, one-to-one instruction, and computer-assisted instruction (see Chapter 11). Verbal, written, and visual tools are all particularly successful in supplementing the teaching methods to help learners master cognitive content. For example, Napholz and McCanse (1994) report the effectiveness of using interactive video as an instructional tool to increase efficiency in cognitive learning by nursing students.

Content knowledge can be gained by exposure to all types of educational experiences, including the process methods used primarily for affective and psychomotor learning. Cognitive knowledge, however, is an essential prerequisite for the learner to engage in other educational activities such as group discussion or role-playing. Otherwise, what results is "pooled ignorance." For example, clients cannot adequately learn through group discussion if they do not possess an accurate and at least basic knowledge level of the subject at hand to draw on for purposes of discourse. Participating in a group discussion experience is not the same thing as engaging in a brainstorming session. Brainstorming does not necessarily require prior knowledge of information about issues or problems to be explored.

Cognitive domain learning is the traditional focus of most teaching. In education of patients, nursing staff, and students, emphasis remains on the sharing of facts, theories, concepts, and the like. Cognitive processing—that is, the means through which knowledge is acquired—has taken precedence over psychomotor skill development and the learning of affective behaviors (Ellis, 1993). Perhaps this emphasis has occurred because educators typically feel more confident and more skilled in being the "giver of information" rather than being the facilitator and coordinator of learning. Lecture and one-to-one instruction are the most often used, albeit abused, teaching methods. Both of these instructional approaches, when taught in a typical fashion, are directed almost exclusively at the cognitive domain.

## The Affective Domain

The *affective domain* is known as the "feeling" domain. Learning in this domain involves an increasing internalization or commitment to feelings expressed as emotions, interests, attitudes, values, and appreciations. Whereas the cognitive domain is ordered in terms of complexity of behaviors, the affective domain is divided into categories that specify the degree of a person's depth of emotional responses to tasks. It represents the degree to which feelings or attitudes toward complex phenomena are incorporated into one's personality or value system (Reilly & Oerman, 1990; Arends, 1994).

Although nurse educators recognize the need for individuals to learn in the affective domain, constructs such as attitudes, beliefs, and values cannot be directly observed but can only be inferred from words and actions (Maier-Lorentz, 1999). Educators tend to be less confident and more challenged in writing behavioral objectives for the affective domain

because it is difficult to develop easily measurable objectives and evaluation of learning outcomes is based on inferences of someone's observed behavior.

Competencies in the affective domain relate to the development of a value system. Behavior is guided by notions held by an individual and society as to what is considered good and right. Thus affective competencies involve moral reasoning and ethical decision making. For staff nurses, competency in the affective domain is required to intervene with clients in a humanistic and caring manner. Reilly and Oermann (1990) differentiate between the terms *beliefs*, *attitudes*, and *values*. *Beliefs* are what an individual perceives as reality; *attitudes* represent feelings about an object, person, or event; and *values* are operational beliefs that guide actions and ways of living. Maier-Lorentz (1999), acknowledging the difficulty in writing and measuring specific objectives in the affective domain, presents a rating scale to evaluate learning outcomes for a gerontological nursing in-service program that measures beliefs, attitudes, and values of staff using a Likert scale.

Objectives in the affective domain are divided into five categories, each specifying the associated level of affective responses as listed and described in the following section (Bloom et al., 1956; Krathwohl et al., 1964).

### Levels of Affective Behavior

*Receiving* (1.00–1.99): ability of the learner to show awareness of an idea or fact or a consciousness of a situation or event in the environment. This level represents a willingness to selectively attend to or focus on data or to receive a stimulus.

*Responding* (2.00–2.99): ability of the learner to respond to an experience, at first obediently and later willingly and with satisfaction. This level indicates a movement beyond denial and toward voluntary acceptance, which can lead to feelings of pleasure or enjoyment as a result of some new experience (receiving is a prerequisite behavior).

*Valuing* (3.00–3.99): ability of the learner to regard or accept the worth of a theory, idea, or event, demonstrating sufficient commitment or preference to be identified with some experience seen as having value. At this level, there is a definite willingness and desire to act to further that value (receiving and responding are prerequisite behaviors).

*Organization* (4.00–4.99): ability of the learner to organize, classify, and prioritize values by integrating a new value into a general set of values, to determine interrelationships of values, and to harmoniously establish some values as dominant and pervasive (receiving, responding, and valuing are prerequisite behaviors).

*Characterization* (5.00–5.99): ability of the learner to integrate values into a total philosophy or world view, showing firm commitment and consistency of responses to the values by generalizing certain experiences into a value system or attitude cluster (receiving, responding, valuing, and organization are prerequisite behaviors).

Table 10–4 lists verbs commonly used in writing affective-level behavioral objectives.

## Examples of Behavioral Objectives in the Affective Domain

*Receiving level:* "During a group discussion session, the patient will admit to any fears he may have about needing to undergo a repeat angioplasty."

*Responding level:* "At the end of one-to-one instruction, the child will verbalize feelings of confidence in managing her asthma using the Peak Flow Tracking Chart."

*Characterization level:* "Following a series of in-service education sessions, the staff

nurse will display consistent interest in maintaining strict hand-washing technique to control the spread of nosocomial infections to patients in the hospital."

**Teaching in the Affective Domain** A variety of teaching methods have been found to be reliable in helping the learner acquire elements of the affective domain. Questioning, case study, role-playing, simulation gaming, and group discussion sessions are examples of instructional methods that can be used to prepare nursing staff and students as well as patients and their families to incorporate values and to explore attitudes, interests, and feelings in the process of developing affective behaviors. Another powerful tool for affective teaching is role-modeling of desired behaviors by the educator.

Nurse educators have been encouraged to attend to the needs of the whole person by recognizing that learning is subjective and values-driven (Schoenly, 1994). For practicing nurses, affective learning is especially important because they are constantly faced with ethical issues and value conflicts. In addition, our increasingly pluralistic society requires nurses to respect the racial and ethnic diversity in the population groups served by healthcare providers (Reilly & Oermann, 1990). Advancing technology also places nurses in advocacy positions when patients, families, and other healthcare professionals are constantly grappling with treatment decisions. In turn, patients and family members are faced with making moral and ethical choices as well as learning to internalize the value of complying with prescribed treatment regimens and incorporating health promotion and disease prevention practices into their daily lives.

The environment in which teaching and learning take place is important to the successful achievement of affective behavioral outcomes. A trusting relationship and an open, empathetic, accepting attitude by the educator toward clients are necessary to secure client interest and involvement in learning. Staff nurses' beliefs, attitudes, and values significantly influence their affective behavior and, thus, the quality of nursing care they deliver. A nurse's personal value system must coincide with the values of the nursing profession. Three American Nurses Association documents, *Code of Ethics for Nurses with Interpretive Statements* (2001), *Standards of Clinical Nursing Practice* (1998), and *Nursing's Social Policy Statement* (1995), provide educators with sources of professional values for teaching staff nurses in the affective domain (Maier-Lorentz, 1999).

Unfortunately, adequate weight is not usually given to teaching in the affective domain. The educator's focus more often emphasizes cognitive processing and psychomotor functioning with little time set aside for exploration and clarification of learner feelings, emotions, and attitudes (Ellis, 1993; Rinne, 1987).

Schoenly (1994) examined affective teaching strategies that can be used to assist learners in acquiring affective domain behaviors. Once appropriate objectives and an accepting climate have been established, the following educational interventions can be selected and implemented:

*Questioning:* Although the lecture method is usually identified with helping the learner gain cognitive skills, the technique of careful questioning during the lecture process can assist in meeting objectives in the affective domain. Affective questioning increases interest and motivation to learn about feelings, values, beliefs, and attitudes regarding a topic under study. Low-level affective questions are directed at stimulating learner awareness and responsiveness to a topic, midlevel affective questioning assists in determining the strength of a belief or the internalization of a value, and high-level affective questioning probes

for information about the depth of integration of a value.

*Case study:* This method can assist the learner in developing problem solving and critical thinking skills through exploration of participant attitudes, beliefs, and values. Using learning groups with the reader assuming the role of a key player in the situation (nurse, family member, patient) rather than as a neutral observer will help in eliciting affective behavioral responses.

*Role-playing:* This method provides an excellent opportunity to practice new behaviors and explore feelings, attitudes, and values; to problem solve; and to resolve personal problems associated with human circumstances. Role-playing allows the learner to "walk in someone else's shoes," but without the actual risk, thereby gaining empathy for the reality of another's situation. Being an observer during role-playing can sensitize the learner to the phenomenon, while active participation in role-playing energizes the learner to attend and respond to the phenomenon under consideration.

*Simulation gaming:* Process games, controlled by the participants and with flexible rules, are more appropriate for accomplishing affective behavioral objectives than content games, which are characterized by structured roles and specific rules and are better for cognitive learning. Simulation gaming promotes active involvement of the learner in goal-directed, although not necessarily competitive, activities. Debriefing following gaming is an important aspect of the technique; it provides an opportunity for guidance in the application and assimilation of the experience.

*Group discussion:* This method provides an opportunity for clarifying personal values as well as exploring social values and moral issues. Value clarification involves identifying and sharing personal values for the purpose of increasing self-awareness and self-discovery. Values inquiry involves investigating the value systems of various ethnic groups. Both approaches provide the chance for in-depth learning of affective behaviors.

The affective domain encompasses three levels that govern attitudes and feelings:

* The intrapersonal level includes personal perceptions of one's own self, such as self-concept, self-awareness, and self-acceptance.

* The interpersonal level includes the perspective of self in relation to other individuals.

* The extrapersonal level involves the perception of others as established groups.

All three levels are important in affective skill development and can be taught through a variety of methods specifically geared to affective-domain learning (Richards & Vicary, 1985).

Affective learning is a part of every type of educational experience, even though the primary focus for learning may be on either the cognitive or the psychomotor domain. Learner feelings or emotions cannot help but be aroused to some extent when exposed to all types of new educational experiences (Bucher, 1991). Without a doubt, learning is a multidimensional process that can occur formally or informally in structured or unstructured settings (Andrusyszyn, 1989). Evaluation of learning is just as complex a process. However, evaluation of affective behavior is more difficult than determining cognitive and psychomotor skill acquisition, because affective behaviors are not usually overt and clearly observable. Rather, these behaviors are less tangible and more challenging to measure. Bucher (1991) and Maier-Lorentz (1999) suggest using the Likert scale as a means of discovering learner attitudes relative to particular learning experiences.

## The Psychomotor Domain

The *psychomotor domain* is known as the "skills" domain. Learning in this domain involves acquiring fine and gross motor abilities with increasing complexity of neuromuscular coordination to carry out physical movement such as walking, handwriting, manipulation of equipment, or carrying out a procedure. Psychomotor skill learning, according to Reilly and Oermann (1990) "is a complex process demanding far more knowledge than suggested by the simple mechanistic behavioral approach" (p. 81). For development of psychomotor skills to take place, there must be integration of the other two domains of learning as well. The affective component conveys recognition of the value or worth of the skill being learned; the cognitive component relates to knowing the principles, relationships, and processes in carrying out the overt physical movement. Although all three domains are involved in demonstrating a psychomotor competency, the psychomotor domain can be examined separately and requires different teaching approaches and evaluation strategies (Reilly & Oermann, 1990). In contrast to the cognitive and affective domains, psychomotor skills are easy to identify and measure because they include primarily overt movement-oriented activities that are relatively easy to observe.

Psychomotor learning, including perceptual-motor tasks, can be classified in a variety of ways (Harrow, 1972; Simpson, 1972; Moore, 1970; Dave, 1970). Simpson's system seems to be the most widely recognized as relevant to client teaching. Objectives in this domain, according to Simpson (1972), are divided into seven levels as listed and described in the following section.

### Levels of Psychomotor Behavior

*Perception* (1.00–1.99): ability of the client to show sensory awareness of objects or cues associated with some task to be performed. Cues relevant to a situation are attended to, symbolically translated, and selected to guide action, gain insight, and receive feedback. This level involves reading directions or observing a process with attention to steps or techniques inherent in a process.

*Set* (2.00–2.99): ability of the learner to exhibit readiness to take a particular kind of action, such as following directions, through expressions of willingness, sensory attending, or body language favorable to performing a motor act (perception is a prerequisite behavior).

*Guided response* (3.00–3.99): ability of the learner to exert effort via overt actions under the guidance of an instructor to imitate an observed behavior with conscious awareness of effort. Imitating may be performed hesitantly but with compliance to directions and coaching (perception and set are prerequisite behaviors).

*Mechanism* (4.00–4.99): ability of the learner to repeatedly perform steps of a desired skill with a certain degree of confidence, indicating mastery to the extent that some or all aspects of the process become habitual. The steps are blended into a meaningful whole and are performed smoothly with little conscious effort (perception, set, and guided response are prerequisite behaviors).

*Complex overt response* (5.00–5.99): ability of the learner to automatically perform a complex motor act with independence and a high degree of skill, without hesitation and with minimum expenditure of time and energy; performance of an entire sequence of a complex behavior without the need to attend to details (perception, set, guided response, and mechanism are prerequisite behaviors).

*Adaptation* (6.00–6.99): ability of the learner to modify or adapt a motor process to suit the individual or various situations, indicating mastery of highly developed movements that can be suited to a variety of conditions (perception, set, guided response, mechanism, and complex overt response are prerequisite behaviors).

*Origination* (7.00–7.99): ability of the learner to create new motor acts, such as novel ways of manipulating objects or materials, as a result of an understanding of a skill and developed ability to perform skills (perception, set, guided response, mechanism, complex overt response, and adaptation are prerequisite behaviors).

Table 10–4 lists verbs commonly used in writing psychomotor-level behavioral objectives.

### Examples of Behavioral Objectives in the Psychomotor Domain

*Guided response level:* "After watching a 15-minute video on the procedure for self-examination of the breast, the client will perform the exam on a model with 100% accuracy."

*Set level:* "Following demonstration of proper crutch walking, the patient will attempt to crutch walk using the correct three-point gait technique."

Another taxonomic system for psychomotor learning proposed by Dave (1970) is also based on behaviors that include muscular action and neuromuscular coordination. Reilly and Oermann (1990) suggest that this taxonomy allows teachers to acknowledge the multivariant characteristics of psychomotor behavior and to focus on the orderly process of neuromuscular development over time of student nurses in academic programs. They support this taxonomy to measure competence in performance within educational programs because it stresses accuracy over speed and recognizes that levels of skill attainment can be achieved and refined over a period of months due to the infrequency of students using certain skills in practice. Objectives in this domain, according to Dave (1970), are divided into five levels:

*Imitation* (1.0–1.99): At this level, observed actions are followed. The learner's movements are gross, coordination lacks smoothness, and errors occur. Time and speed required to perform are based on learner needs.

*Manipulation* (2.0–2.99): At this level, written instructions are followed. The learner's coordinated movements are variable, and accuracy is measured based on the skill of using written procedures as a guide. Time and speed required to perform vary.

*Precision* (3.0–3.99): At this level, a logical sequence of actions is carried out. The learner's movements are coordinated at a higher level, errors are minimal and relatively minor. Time and speed required to perform remain variable.

*Articulation* (4.0–4.99): At this level, a logical sequence of actions is carried out. The learner's movements are coordinated at a high level, and errors are limited. Time and speed required to perform are within reasonable expectations.

*Naturalization* (5.0–5.99): At this level, the sequence of actions is automatic. The learner's movements are coordinated at a consistently high level, and errors are almost nonexistent. Time and speed required to perform are within realistic limits, and performance reflects professional competence.

These taxonomic criteria for the development of psychomotor skill competency suggest that accuracy should be stressed before the speed at which a skill is acquired (Reilly and Oermann (1990). The levels of psychomotor behavior, no matter which taxonomic system is used, require the general and orderly steps of *observing, imitating, practicing,* and *adapting.*

**Teaching of Psychomotor Skills** When teaching psychomotor skills, it is important for the educator to remember to keep skill instruction separate from a discussion of principles underlying the skill (cognitive component) or a discussion of how the learner feels about carrying out the skill (affective component). Psychomotor skill development is very egocentric and usually requires a great deal of concentration as the learner works toward mastery of a skill. It is easy to interfere with psychomotor learning if the teacher asks a knowledge (cognitive) question while the learner is trying to focus on the performance (psychomotor response) of a skill. For example, while a staff member is learning to suction a patient, it is not unusual for the teacher to ask, "Can you give me a rationale for why suctioning is important?" or "How often should suctioning be done for this particular patient?" These questions demand a cognitive response during the psychomotor performance.

As another example, while the patient is learning to self-administer parenteral medication, the teacher may simultaneously ask the patient to cognitively respond to the question, "What are the actions or side effects of this medication?" or "How do you feel about injecting yourself?" These questions demand cognitive and affective responses during psychomotor performance. Although a teacher frequently intervenes with questions in the midst of a learner's performing, it is definitely an inappropriate teaching technique. What the educator is doing, in fact, is asking the learner to demonstrate at least two different behaviors at the same time. This technique can result in frustration and confusion, and ultimately it may result in failure to achieve any of the behaviors successfully. Questions related to the cognitive or affective domain should take place before or after the learner's practicing of a psychomotor skill (Oermann, 1990).

In psychomotor skill development, the ability to perform a skill is not equivalent to learning a skill. Performance is a transitory action, while learning is a more permanent behavior that follows from repeated practice and experience (Oermann, 1990). The actual learning of a skill requires practice to allow the individual to repeat the performance time and again with accuracy, coordination, and out of habit. Practice does make perfect, and so repetition leads to perfection and reinforcement of the behavior. The riding of a bicycle is a perfect example. When one first attempts to ride a bicycle, movements tend to be very jerky, and the act requires a great deal of concentration. Once the skill is learned, bicycle riding becomes a smooth, automatic operation that requires minimal attention to the details of fine and gross motor movements acting in concert to allow the learner to achieve the skill of riding a bicycle. Some behaviors that are learned do not require much reinforcement, even over a long period of disuse, whereas other behaviors, once learned, need to be rehearsed or relearned to perform them at the level of skill once achieved.

The amount of practice required to learn any new skill varies with the individual, depending on many factors. Oermann (1990) and Bell (1991) have addressed some of the more important variables:

*Readiness to learn:* The motivation to learn affects the degree of perseverance exhibited by the learner in working toward mastery of a skill.

*Past experience:* If the learner is familiar with equipment or techniques similar to those needed to learn a new skill, then mastery of the new skill may be achieved at a faster rate. The effects of learning one

skill on the subsequent performance of another related skill is known as *transfer of learning* (Gomez & Gomez, 1984). For example, if someone already has experience with downhill skiing, then learning cross-country skiing should come more easily and with more confidence because the required coordination and equipment are similar. To use an example in teaching healthcare skills, if a family member already has experience with aseptic technique in changing a dressing, then learning to suction a tracheostomy tube using sterile technique should not require as much time to master.

*Health status:* Illness state or other physical or emotional impairments in the learner may affect the time it takes to acquire or successfully master a skill.

*Environmental stimuli:* Depending on the type and level of stimuli as well as the learning style (degree of tolerance for certain stimuli), distractions in the immediate surroundings may interfere with skill acquisition.

*Anxiety level:* The ability to concentrate can be dramatically affected by how anxious someone feels. Nervousness about performing in front of someone is particularly a key factor in psychomotor skill development. High anxiety levels interfere with coordination, steadiness, fine muscle movements, and concentration levels when performing complex psychomotor skills. It is important to reassure learners that they are not necessarily being "tested" during psychomotor skill performance. Reassurance and support reduce anxiety levels related to the fear of not meeting expectations of themselves or of the teacher.

*Developmental stage:* Physical, cognitive, and psychosocial stages of development all influence an individual's ability to master a movement-oriented task. Certainly, a young child's fine and gross motor skills as well as cognitive abilities are at a different level than those of an adult. The older adult, too, will likely exhibit slower cognitive processing and increased response time (needing longer time to perform an activity) than younger clients.

*Practice session length:* During the beginning stages of learning a motor skill, short and carefully planned practice sessions and frequent rest periods are valuable techniques to help increase the rate and success of learning. These techniques are thought to be effective because they help prevent physical fatigue and restore the learner's attention to the task at hand.

Performing motor skills is not done in a vacuum. The learner is immersed in a particular environmental context full of stimuli. Learners must select those environmental influences that will assist them in achieving the behavior (relevant stimuli) and ignore those that interfere with a specific performance (irrelevant stimuli). This process of recognizing and selecting appropriate and inappropriate stimuli is called *selective attention* (Gomez & Gomez, 1984).

Motor skills should be practiced first in a laboratory setting to provide a safe and nonthreatening environment for the novice learner. Gomez and Gomez (1987) suggest also arranging for practice sessions to be done in the clinical or home setting to expose the learner to actual environmental conditions. This technique is known as "open" skills performance learned under changing and unstable environments. In addition, research findings indicate that progress in mastery of a psychomotor skill can be accomplished just as effectively through self-directed study as with teaching in a structured laboratory situation (Love, McAdams, Patton, Rankin, & Roberts, 1989). Yoder (1993) found that computer-assisted interactive video (CAIVI) resulted in

a greater amount of transfer of cognitive learning than did linear video for the performance of psychomotor skills in a clinical setting. Yoder reported that three types of transfer learning occur: *self-transfer* (repetition of learning), *near transfer* (occurs in situations that are very similar), and *far transfer* (occurs in situations that are very different). Application of psychomotor skills in the clinical arena is a type of far transfer.

More recently, Miracle (1999) summarized research findings on educational strategies and innovations for teaching psychomotor skills to nursing students and suggested that the limited and mixed findings of research studies warrant further investigation on methods to teach kinesthetic skills. In any event, contact with the teacher during practice sessions is an important element for successful psychomotor learning. Although educator workload necessitates finding cost-effective and time-efficient ways to teach skill development, mediated instruction should not be used as a substitute, only a supplement, for instructor input (Baldwin, Hill, & Hanson, 1991).

In addition to using demonstration and return demonstration, mediated instruction, and self-directed study as teaching methods for psychomotor learning, mental imaging (also known as mental practice) has surfaced as a viable alternative for teaching motor skills. Research indicates that learning psychomotor skills can be enhanced through use of imagery. Mental practice is similar to the type of practice athletes use when preparing to perform in a sports competition (Eaton & Evans, 1986; Doheny, 1993; Bachman, 1990; Miracle, 1999).

Another hallmark of psychomotor learning is the type and timing of the feedback given to learners. Psychomotor skill development allows for immediate feedback such that learners have an idea on the spot of the results of their performance. During skill practice, learners receive *intrinsic feedback* that is generated from within the self, giving them a sense of or a feel for how they have performed. They may sense that they either did quite well or that they felt awkward and need more practice. In addition, the teacher has the opportunity to provide *augmented feedback* by sharing with learners an opinion or conveying a message through body language about how well they performed (Oermann, 1990). The immediacy of the feedback, together with the self-generated and teacher-supplemented feedback, makes this a unique feature of psychomotor learning. Performance checklists, which can serve as guides for teaching and learning, are also an effective tool for evaluating the level of skill performance.

An important point to remember is that it is all right to make mistakes in the process of teaching or learning a psychomotor skill. If the teacher makes an error when demonstrating a skill or the learner makes an error during return demonstration, this is the perfect teaching opportunity to offer anticipatory guidance: "Oops, I made a mistake. Now what do I do?" Unlike cognitive skill development, where errorless learning is the objective, in psychomotor skill development a mistake made represents an opportunity to demonstrate how to correct an error and to learn from the not-so-perfect initial attempts at performance. The old saying, "You learn by your mistakes," is most applicable to psychomotor skill mastery.

Thus learning is a very complex phenomenon. It is clear that the cognitive, affective, and psychomotor domains, although representing separate behaviors, are to some extent interrelated. Movement-oriented activities require an integration of related knowledge and values (Oermann, 1990). For example, the performance of a psychomotor skill often requires a certain degree of cognitive knowledge or understanding of information, such as the scientific principles underlying a practice or why a skill is important to carry out. Also, there may be an affective component to performing the movement dimension for the psy-

chomotor behavior to be integrated as part of the learner's overall experience and ability to attain the ultimate goal of independence in self-care or practice delivery.

## ▪ DEVELOPMENT OF TEACHING PLANS

After mutually agreed-upon goals and objectives have been written, it should be clear what the learner is to learn and what the teacher is to teach. Predetermined goals and objectives serve as a basis for developing a *teaching plan*. Organizing and presenting information in the format of an internally consistent teaching plan require skill by the nurse educator. Developing an action plan to achieve the goals and objectives set forth requires a determination of the actual purpose, content, methods and tools, sequence, timing, and evaluation of instruction. The teaching plan should clearly and concisely describe the various elements of the education process.

The three major reasons for constructing teaching plans are:

1. To force the teacher to examine the relationship among the steps of the teaching process to ensure a logical approach to teaching, which can serve as a map for organizing and keeping instruction on target.

2. To communicate in writing and in an outline format exactly what is being taught, how it is being taught and evaluated, and the time allotted for accomplishment of the behavioral objectives. As such, not only is the learner aware of and can follow the action plan, but, just as importantly, other healthcare team members are informed and can contribute to the teaching effort with a consistent approach.

3. To legally document that an individual plan for each learner is in place and is being properly implemented. Also, the existence of current teaching plans is essential evi-

dence required by healthcare agencies and organizations to satisfy mandates for institutional accreditation.

Teaching plans can be presented in a number of different formats. No matter which format is chosen, all the various elements of the teaching process should be included. A complete teaching plan consists of eight basic parts (Ryan & Marinelli, 1990):

1. The purpose
2. A statement of the overall goal
3. A list of objectives (and subobjectives, if necessary)
4. An outline of the related content
5. The instructional method(s) used for teaching the related content
6. The time allotted for the teaching of each objective
7. The instructional resources (materials/tools) needed
8. The method(s) used to evaluate learning

The major criterion for judging a teaching plan is whether it facilitates a relationship between its parts. A sample teaching plan format is shown in Figure 10–1. This format is suggested because the use of columns allows the educator, as well as anyone else who is using it, to see all the parts of the teaching plan at one time and provides the best structure for monitoring internal consistency of the plan. A different format can be used to meet institutional requirements or the preference of the user, but all parts must be included for the teaching plan to be considered comprehensive and complete.

When constructing a teaching plan, the educator must be certain, above all else, that internal consistency exists within the plan (Ryan & Marinelli, 1990). A teaching plan is said to be internally consistent when all eight parts of the plan are related to one another and when the domain for learning in any objective is integrated in the overall purpose and goal for teaching. Internal consistency requires adherence to two major aspects of the plan. The first aspect ensures that the domain of learning in any objective that is written is reflected across the elements of the teaching plan, from the purpose all the way through to the end process of evaluation. The following example is adapted from Ryan and Marinelli's (1990) self-study module on *Developing a Teaching Plan*:

*For example:* If the educator has decided to teach to the psychomotor domain, then the goal, objectives and subobjectives, related content, and so on should be reflective of the psychomotor domain.

*Purpose:* To provide the client with the information necessary for monitoring blood glucose.

*Goal:* The client will demonstrate the ability to test for blood glucose on a regular basis.

*Objective:* Following a 20-minute teaching session, the client will be able to use a reagent strip, Chemstrip bG, to determine blood glucose level with 100% accuracy.

*Subobjective:* The client will be able to assemble all equipment necessary to test for blood glucose using a reagent strip without assistance.

The purpose, goal, objective, and subobjective are reflective of the psychomotor domain and, thus, the content, instructional method(s), instructional resource(s), time allotment, and evaluation method(s) should be appropriate to the domain as well and are therefore internally consistent. The decision about what domain should be the focus of a teaching plan must be made prior to developing the plan and should remain consistent throughout the plan. Thus, if the purpose and goal are written with a focus on just the cognitive domain, then the objectives (and subobjectives) and the remaining five parts should be reflective of the cognitive domain. If the purpose and goal are written for the accomplishment of a skill set that

| Objectives and Subobjectives | Content Outline | Method of Instruction | Time Allotted (in min.) | Resources | Method of Evaluation |
|---|---|---|---|---|---|
| | | | | | |

PURPOSE:

GOAL:

FIGURE 10–1    Sample Teaching Plan

includes more than one domain, then the teaching plan should reflect objectives, content, methods of teaching, and methods of evaluation in these different domains (see Figure 10–2).The overall design of the teaching plan must match whatever domain(s) of learning have been selected, as identified below:

| Domain | Teaching Design |
| --- | --- |
| Cognitive | Topic-centered |
| Affective | Feeling-centered |
| Psychomotor | Performance-centered |

The second aspect of internal consistency identified by Ryan and Marinelli (1990) is related to the content to be presented. The educator must determine the complexity and detail of the material that is to be taught depending on the data obtained during assessment of the learner, such as the client's readiness to learn, learning needs, and learning style, as well as other factors such as the resources and time available for teaching and learning.

The amount and depth of information to be taught depend on the learning level of the client. The focus for teaching a low-level learner would be to concentrate on the "need to know" information to ensure that a skill can be performed safely. By comparison, a high-level learner can handle and may desire additional "nice to know" information. Whoever the client may be, the content to be taught for each objective must be directly related to the objective. If subobjectives are included in the plan, then the same rule applies; that is, the content to be taught for each subobjective is directly related to the subobjective.

The method of instruction chosen also should be appropriate for the information being taught. If, for example, the purpose is to teach a client to self-administer medication from an asthma inhaler (psychomotor domain), perhaps some discussion will be necessary and relevant to meet the underlying cognitive aspects of psychomotor skill development, but the primary method of teaching should nevertheless be demonstration and return demonstration. Conversely, lecture and programmed instruction are appropriate teaching methods if the purpose of teaching, for example, is to impart knowledge of what constitutes a low-fat diet (cognitive domain).

The time set aside for the teaching and learning of each objective and subobjective must be specified. How much time is needed for instruction and acquisition of a skill depends on learner attributes, the type and complexity of the behavior, the depth of content, and the resources to be used to supplement teaching and assist with learning. Each teaching session should be no more than 20 to 30 minutes in length. In this period of time, one or more objectives may be accomplished or partially accomplished. Additional teaching sessions may be required for the learner to attain expected outcomes.

The resources to be used should appropriately match the content and teaching methodology. If the purpose is to teach breast self-examination, for example, then written or audiovisual materials or an anatomical model of the breast would be useful instructional tools. It is also important for the educator to keep in mind what resources would be an appealing, comfortable, and convenient medium for the learner. A variety of resources may be necessary to maintain the learner's attention and to serve as reinforcers of information. An important consideration is the literacy level of the learner. Giving a low-literate person technical reading materials will merely frustrate and confuse the learner and defeat the plan for teaching. Conversely, it is possible that giving too simple material to a highly literate person may lead to boredom and inattention to instruction.

Finally, the method of evaluation should match the domain in which learning is to take place. For example, if the behavioral objective is for the learner to be able to identify (cognitive) three major symptoms of an impending heart attack, then the evaluation method must test that knowledge by requiring the learner to state, list, or circle (or some other cognitive term) three of the most important symptoms of a heart attack. Evalu-

PURPOSE: To provide patient with information necessary for self-administration of insulin as prescribed

GOAL:    The patient will be able to perform insulin injections independently according to treatment regimen

| Objectives | Content Outline | Method of Instruction | Time Allotted (in min.) | Resources | Method of Evaluation |
|---|---|---|---|---|---|
| Following a 20-minute teaching session, the patient will be able to: | | | | | |
| Identify the five sites for insulin injection with 100% accuracy (cognitive) | Location of five anatomical sites Rotation of sites | 1:1 instruction | 2 | Anatomical chart | Post-testing |
| Demonstrate proper techniques according to procedure for drawing up insulin from a multidose vial (psycho-motor) | Accepted technique according to procedure<br><br>Reading syringe unit dose markings | Demonstration Return demonstration | 5 | Alcohol sponges Sterile SQ needles and insulin syringes Multidose vial of sterile water | Observation of demonstration |
| Give insulin to self in thigh area with 100% accuracy (psychomotor) | Procedure for injecting insulin SQ at 90-degree angle using aseptic technique | Demonstration Return demonstration | 10 | Human model SQ needle and syringe Multidose vial of sterile water Alcohol sponges | Observation of return demonstration |
| Express any concerns about self-administration of insulin (affective) | Summarize common concerns Exploration of feelings | Discussion | 3 | Video Written handouts | Question and answer |

FIGURE 10–2    Completed Teaching Plan for Self-Administration of Insulin

ation methods must measure the desired learning outcomes to determine if and to what extent the learner achieved the expectations for learning.

In summary, just as with a nursing care plan, all elements of a teaching plan need to "hang together." The goal must be reflective of the purpose, the objectives depend on and must derive from the goal, the instructional content depends on and must be derived from the objectives, the teaching methodology depends on and must be related to the content, and so forth. If, for instance, content outlined in the plan is not related to any of the objectives, then the content is either unnecessary or another objective must be written as a basis for including the extra content. Likewise, if a teaching plan has no content relative to a particular stated objective or subobjective, then additional content must be included or the objective or subobjective eliminated, if appropriate. Also, during the teaching process, if the learner indicates in some way an interest in or demonstrates a need for knowing more than the original plan addressed, then the plan should be revised accordingly. Whether a plan is adhered to or revised, it must, above all else, reflect internal consistency. (See Figure 10–2 for a sample teaching plan.)

## ▚▚▚ USE OF LEARNING CONTRACTS

The concept of *learning contracts* is a relatively new but increasingly popular approach to teaching and learning that can be implemented with any audience of learners—patients and their families, nursing staff, or nursing students. In the strictest sense, a contract is a formal legal agreement governing the terms of a transaction over a specified period of time between two or more parties (O'Reilly, 1994). In education, a learning contract is defined as a written (formal) or verbal (informal) agreement between the teacher and the learner that delineates specific teaching and learning activities that are to occur

within a certain time frame. A learning contract is a mutually negotiated agreement, usually in the form of a written document drawn up by the teacher and the learner, that specifies what the learner will learn, how learning will be achieved and within what time allotment, and the criteria for measuring the success of the venture (Keyzer, 1986; McAllister, 1996).

Inherent in the learning contract is the existence of some type of reward for upholding the contractural agreement (Wallace & Mundie, 1987). For patients and families, the reward may be recognition of their success in mastery of a task that facilitates moving closer to independence in self-care and a higher quality of life. For staff nurses, the reward might be having the privilege granted to practice in a chosen setting or at an advanced level. For nursing students, the reward might entail being allowed continued progression through a program of study. Rewards may be tangible, such as a certificate or award in recognition of successful attainment of an outcome, or intangible, such as outward praise from the teacher or an intrinsic sense of satisfaction in accomplishing a predetermined goal.

Contract learning has been introduced in education as an alternative and an innovative approach to structuring a learning experience that embodies the principles of adult learning (Knowles et al., 1998). The origin of contract learning is derived from humanistic theory that acknowledges the person as an autonomous being whose efforts are continuously aimed at self-determination and self-actualization. The central view of the humanistic educational theory is that knowledge is a process, not a product (Mazhindu, 1990). As such, according to Kreider and Barry (1993), contract learning emphasizes how a body of knowledge will be acquired (process plan), not how a body of knowledge will be transmitted (content plan). Learning contracts are considered to be an effective teaching strategy for empowering the learner because they emphasize self-direction, mutual negotiation, and mutual evaluation of established competency levels. A number of terms have been used to describe this approach, such as *independent learning, self-directed learning,* and *learner-centered* or *project-oriented learning* (Lowry, 1997; Waddell & Stevens, 2000; Chan & Wai-tong, 2000).

Knowles et al. (1998) describe the purpose of using learning contracts, the steps to developing a learning contract, and the guidelines for the implementation of learning contracts. Years of research on adult learners have revealed time and again that "what adults learn on their own initiative, they learn more deeply and permanently than what they learn by being taught" (Knowles et al., 1998, p.211). The imposed structure of traditional education—that is, telling learners the objectives they need to work toward, what resources they are to use, how and when to use those resources, and how their accomplishments will be evaluated—conflicts with the psychological need by adults to be self-directing. Being told what, how, and when to learn something may lead to resistance, apathy, or withdrawal by the learner. This does not mean that adult learners do not need guidance or that they do not want structure or specifics, but rather that they often desire flexibility for learning and they want to be involved in decision making when it comes to planning, implementation, and evaluation of their learning.

Learning contracts stress shared accountability for learning between the teacher and the learner. The method of contract learning actively involves the learner at all stages of the teaching–learning process, from assessment of learning needs and identification of learning resources to the planning, implementation, and evaluation of learning activities. Because learning contracts are a unique way of presenting information to the learner and are the essence of an equal and cooperative partnership, they challenge the traditional teacher–client relationship through a redistribution of power and control. Allowing learners to negotiate a contract for learning shifts the control and emphasis of the learning experience from a traditionally teacher-centered focus to a learner-centered focus. Active involvement of the learner increases feelings of commitment and fosters accountability for self-directed learning (Wallace & Mundie, 1987; Knowles et al., 1998).

The purpose of learning contracts is to encourage active participation by the learner, improve teacher–client communication, and enhance learner expressiveness and creativity. Learning contracts, whether formal or informal, can be used to facilitate personal development of the learner. In the case of staff and student nurses, this approach to learning can enhance professional development as well. Learning contracts serve as a vehicle for fulfilling the internal needs of the learner and the external needs of an organization (Keyzer, 1986). Learners have an opportunity to change behavior and reach their human potential through an approach that fosters choice and growth-promoting independence and allows for self-paced learning. Clearly defined expectations reduce learner anxiety, decrease frustration, increase levels of personal satisfaction, encourage the development of self-directed learning habits, increase the rate and quality of learning, and provide a defined basis for evaluation of the learner. Learning contracts also can be used to facilitate discharge of patients to the home setting. In complex cases involving the care of a patient by a large number of multidisciplinary team members, a contract provides cohesion and an excellent communication tool between the patient, family caretakers, and the healthcare team (Cady & Yoshioka, 1991). The major advantage of contract learning is that it provides structure while simultaneously offering the flexibility required to meet the various learning needs of individuals (Wallace & Mundie, 1987; Mazhindu, 1990).

## Components of the Learning Contract

A complete learning contract includes the following four major components (Wallace & Mundie, 1987):

1. *Content*—specifies the precise behavioral objectives to be achieved. Objectives must clearly state the desired outcomes of learning activities. Negotiation between the educator and the learner determines the content, level, and sequencing of objectives according to learner needs, abilities, and readiness.

2. *Performance expectations*—specify the conditions under which learning activities will be facilitated, such as instructional strategies and resources.

3. *Evaluation*—specifies the criteria used to evaluate achievement of objectives, such as skills checklists, care standards or protocols, and agency policies and procedures of care that identify the levels of competency expected of the learner.

4. *Time frame*—specifies the length of time needed for successful completion of the objectives. The target date for completion should reflect a reasonable period in which to achieve expected outcomes depending on the learner's abilities and circumstances.

In addition to these four components, it is important to include the terms of the contract. Role definitions describe the teacher–learner relationship with respect to clarifying the expectations and assumptions about the roles each will play. The educator is responsible for coordinating and facilitating all phases of the contract process. In the case of nursing staff and student nurse learning, the educator plays a major role in the selection and preparation of preceptors and acts as a resource person for both the learner and the preceptor. (See Figure 10–3 for a sample learning contract.)

---

Name of Learner: _____

Name of Educator: _____

Name of Preceptor (if applicable): _____

Date of Contract Negotiated: _____

Terms of Contract: _____

_____

| Objectives | Activities | Evaluation | Target Date | Completion Date |
|---|---|---|---|---|
| Lists congnitive, affective, and psychomotor behaviors mutually agreed on and intended to be achieved | Lists teaching-learning strategies and resources to be used to achieve the objectives | Lists the criteria to be used to measure learning demonstrated | Lists a realistic time frame for achievement of expected outcome | Specifies the dates that each objective is accomplished |

Signatures: _____ (Learner) _____ (Educator)_____ (Preceptor)

FIGURE 10–3  **Sample Learning Contract**

## Steps to Implement the Learning Contract

Knowles et al. (1998) described the steps involved in developing a learning contract with any adult learner. Wallace and Mundie (1987) also outlined the steps to implement a learning contract, although they specifically addressed the implementation of contract learning with regard to the orientation of new staff nurses. The following steps apply to establishing and carrying out a learning contract for any type of learner:

**Step 1** *Determine specific learning objectives.* Encourage the learner to identify his or her learning needs and what the learner wants to be able to do within an allotted time frame.

**Step 2** *Review the contracting process.* It is vital that learners have a complete understanding of what contract learning is all about as well as their role in the process. Because learning contracts have not been widely used until recently, most people are unfamiliar with this teaching–learning strategy.

**Step 3** *Identify the learning resources.* Introduce the learner to instructional resources available, such as self-study materials and audiovisual tools.

**Step 4** *Assess the learner's competency level and learning needs.* The entire process of negotiation of a contract is based on the learner's current abilities and learning needs. The educator initiates the assessment of the learner and collects data primarily through interview, observation, and pretesting to formulate objectives.

**Step 5** *Define roles.* Before planning learning experiences and negotiating a contract, the roles of the learner and the educator must be clearly established regarding expectations of each.

**Step 6** *Plan the learning experiences.* Determine the content, learning resources to be used, the skills that must be demonstrated, and the amount of time to pursue learning through assisted or self-study to meet the predetermined objectives.

**Step 7** *Negotiate the time frame.* Based on appropriate sequencing of behaviors, from simplest to most complex, establish a target date for completion of each objective.

**Step 8** *Implement the learning experience.* Take into consideration individual variations in the level of ability to do self-directed study and any other variables that may play a factor in completion of the specified learning activities. For patients, progress in learning may be influenced by changes in their health status. For staff nurses, the constant pressures of providing patient care services may place constraints on the time available for educational activities. For any learner, the education process is influenced by readiness to learn and how well the information to be learned is organized and communicated.

**Step 9** *Renegotiate.* The type and level of complexity of behavioral objectives and the target dates set forth for accomplishing these objectives may be renegotiated at any point along the continuum of the learning experience to meet the needs of the learner. Adults may change their notions about what they want to learn, how they want to learn it, and how long it will take to achieve objectives, so they should be encouraged to revise their contract as it is being carried out.

**Step 10** *Evaluate.* Periodic (formative) and final (summative) evaluation of the learner's progress and the actual learning experience itself is a shared responsibility between the learner and the educator. Preestablished performance criteria, agreed on prior to the initiation of the learning process, serve as the means to ascertain achievement of outcomes based on predetermined and prenegotiated behavioral objectives.

**Step 11** *Document*. Evidence of achievement of learning objectives is determined jointly by the learner and the educator (and preceptors if used for nursing staff and students). When an objective is satisfactorily met according to written performance expectations, each party cosigns the date completed in the appropriate column. (See Figure 10–4 for an example of a completed learning contract.)

# THE CONCEPT OF LEARNING CURVE

*Learning curve* is a term commonly used to describe how long it takes for a learner to acquire a knowledge, attitude, or motor skill. It also implies the level of difficulty for the learner in achieving an outcome. Although the term is used frequently, very loosely, and sometimes incorrectly (because it really applies only to psychomotor skill acquisition) by nurse educators, a search of the nursing and allied health literature indicates that there is no documentation of what is meant by the term or how the concept can be applied in the

---

Name of Learner: _____

Name of Educator: _____

Name of Preceptor (if applicable): _____

Date of Contract Negotiated: _____

Terms of Contract: Employee will increase work efficiency at place of employment by 20% within 2 months

| Objectives | Activities | Evaluation | Target Date | Completion Date |
|---|---|---|---|---|
| Improve time management and organizational skills to increase productivity by 20% | Read articles and books on topic<br><br>Interview three managers on how to organize work and manage time<br><br>Observe a productive colleague for one day, noting techniques used | Report on knowledge acquired<br><br>Performance of productivity observed with feedback from observer | | |

FIGURE 10–4   **Completed Learning Contract**  SOURCE: Adapted from Knowles et al. (1998), p. 213–245.

education of patients, professional staff, or students. To understand the learning curve concept as it relates to the process of teaching and learning, one must refer to educational psychology literature. Cronbach (1963) defined a learning curve specifically as it relates to psychomotor skill development as "a record of an individual's improvement made by measuring his ability at different stages of practice and plotting his scores" (p. 297).

The theoretical learning curve is a schematic used to summarize many features of learning, which according to Cronbach (1963) is divided into six stages (see Figure 10–5):

1. *Negligible Progress:* Initially very little improvement in score is detected. This "prereadiness" period is when the learner is not ready to perform the entire task, but relevant learning is taking place, such as developing attention, manipulation, and perceptual skills. This period can be rela-

tively long in young children who are developing physical and cognitive abilities as well as in older adults who may have difficulty in making key discriminations.

2. *Increasing Gains:* The rate of learning increases as the learner grasps the essentials of the task. Scores rise rapidly as the learner becomes aware of cues to attend to, goals to attain, or ways to effectively organize responses. Motivation may account for rapid gains when the learner has interest in the task, receives approval from others, or experiences a sense of pride in discovering the ability to perform.

3. *Decreasing Gains:* The rate of improvement slows. In this period of refinement, the slowing of task mastery is inevitable as practice does not produce such steep gains. Learning occurs in smaller increments of response as the learner incorporates changes by using cues to smooth out performance.

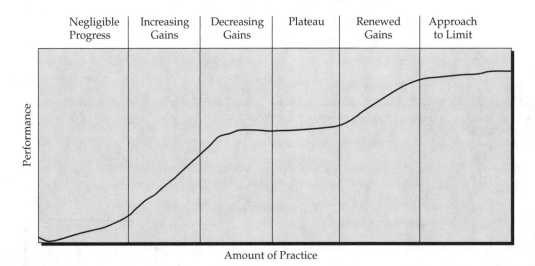

FIGURE 10–5   **A Schematic Learning Curve** SOURCE: Adapted from Cronbach (1963). *Educational Psychology*, 2nd ed., New York: Harcourt, Brace & World, p. 299.

4. *Plateau:* No substantial gains are made. This "leveling off" period is characterized by a negligible rate of progress in level of performance but further gains are possible. During this stage, the learner is making small adjustments, such as modifying subskills, reducing dependence on mediators, and correcting responses to more remote cues. Plateaus are not observed in all instances, and the very idea of a "period of no progress" is considered false. Gains in skills can occur even though overall performance scores remain stable.

5. *Renewed Gains:* The rate of performance again rises if further gains are possible. If additional progress can be made after the plateau period has ended, it usually is due to growth in physical development, renewed interest in the task, a response to challenge, or the drive for perfection.

6. *Approach to Limit:* Progress at this point becomes negligible. The ability to perform has reached its potential. The "limit" is a hypothetical stage only because there is never certainty that a learner cannot improve further. Just as with a performer who has broken a world record, he or she may at some point be able to exceed that top score.

Individual learning curves are characterized by irregularity (see Figure 10–6) and are often unlike the smooth theoretical curve. Fluctuations in performance can be attributed to changes in such factors as focus, interest, energy, ability, situational circumstances, or favorable/unfavorable conditions for

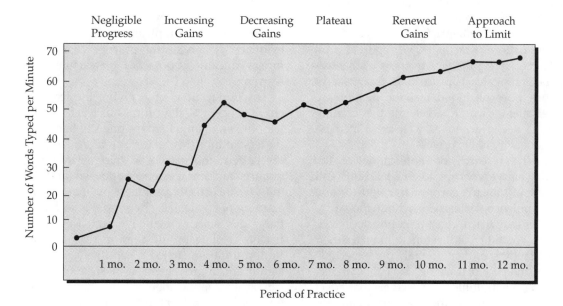

**FIGURE 10–6**  **Learning Curve During One Year of Typing Practice**  SOURCE: Adapted from Cronbach (1963). *Educational Psychology*, 2nd ed., New York: Harcourt, Brace & World, p. 303.

learning (Cronbach, 1963; Barker, 1994; Gage & Berliner, 1998).

The concept of learning curve has been heavily applied to business and industry to measure employee productivity, which, in turn, has a direct effect on cost of labor, the time it takes to manufacture a product or deliver a service, the quality of the product or service, and the pricing of goods and services. The concept has been broadened to be used in other fields of activities, as the cost of doing repetitive tasks generally decreases as experience is gained.

The learning curve (also sometimes referred to as the *experience curve*) is a phenomenon that can be applied to the analysis of learning that occurs by any individual or groups of individuals. McCray and Blakemore (1985) note that the learning curve "is basically nothing more than a graphic depiction of changes in performance or output during a specified time period" (p. 5). A learning curve shows the relationship between practice and performance of a psychomotor skill and provides a concrete measure of the rate at which one or more people learn a task. In many situations, a pattern of learning (improvement) follows a very productive pattern. Kratzer (1995) reported on a study measuring the effectiveness of mentoring beginning teachers in their first year of practice. She concluded that the mentorship model offers a way to accelerate the learning curve of new teachers as well as to increase their longevity in the profession.

Nursing research on application of the learning curve concept to the teaching and learning of patients and nursing staff (or any other audience of learners whom the nurse educator may teach) must be conducted. Such studies would help educators to improve their understanding of the "normal" or "expected" pattern and pace of learning, assist them in recognizing the multitude of variables that affect the length of time and the ease or difficulty for any given learner to achieve an intended outcome, and aid them in choosing appropriate educational interventions based on evidence of the different stages of practice required by the learner for improvement in skill development. Research could answer such questions in patient and staff education as the following:

- Can a learning curve be shortened given the characteristics of the learner, the situation, or the task at hand?

- Why is the learning curve steeper, more drawn out, or more irregular for some learners than for others?

- Can we predict the learning curves of our patients or nursing staff depending on their educational or experiential backgrounds?

- What can we do from an educational standpoint to influence the pace and pattern of learning that may result in earlier or more complete achievement of expected outcomes?

- How can the learning curve concept be applied to improve staff performance, thereby increasing work satisfaction and productivity, decreasing costs of care, and improving the quality of care?

These are just a few of the questions that research could attempt to answer to provide evidence as a basis for practice changes in nurse educator approaches to teaching and learning.

The implications of applying the learning curve concept to the process of teaching and learning are many. Perhaps one key benefit to understanding this concept is to realize that the pattern and pace of learning is irregular, not even and linear as once supposed (and still may be incorrectly assumed by many). The learning of any task is often rapid after an initial slow start, inevitably decreases, then reaches a plateau, and then increases again, until a limit is reached when likely no more significant improvement in mastery of a skill can be achieved. Understanding this phenomenon will help educators adjust their expectations or deal with their frustrations when different paces and patterns of learning occur in individuals as they attempt to master any psychomotor skill.

Awareness that learning is not linear and that the amount of practice needed to improve performance is variable can also be shared with learners to reduce their expectations and frustrations when mastering a skill. For example, a patient who is undergoing rehabilitation to learn how to walk again following a stroke or injury may easily become discouraged with the progress he or she is making toward the achievement of a goal because gains in the learning may slow down or the patient may experience a time at the beginning or in the middle of the curve when he or she seems not to be learning at all. Educators can realistically support the learner if they understand the pace and pattern of skill development.

## SUMMARY

The major portion of this chapter focused on differentiating goals from objectives, preparing accurate and concise objectives, classifying objectives according to the three domains of learning, and the teaching of cognitive, affective, and psychomotor skills using appropriate instructional interventions. The writing of behavioral objectives as to type and complexity is fundamental to the education process. Goals and objectives serve as a guide to the educator in the planning, implementation, and evaluation of teaching and learning.

Assessment of the learner is a prerequisite to formulating objectives. Prior to selecting the content to be taught and the methods and materials to be used for instruction, there must be a clear understanding of what the learner is expected to be able to do. Appraisal should be based on a mutual determination between the educator and the client as to what needs to be learned, under what conditions learning can best occur, and the teaching and evaluation methods most preferred. Objectives setting must be a partnership effort by the learner and the educator for any learning experience to be successful and rewarding in the achievement of expected outcomes.

This chapter also outlined the development of teaching plans and learning contracts. Teaching plans provide the blueprint for organizing and presenting information in a coherent manner. Above all else, a teaching plan must reflect internal consistency of its parts. Learning contracts are an innovative and unique alternative to structuring a learning experience based on adult learning principles. Contracts are designed to provide for self-directed study, thereby encouraging active involvement and accountability on the part of the learner. The communication of desired behavioral outcomes and the mechanisms for accomplishing behavioral changes in the learner are essential elements in the decision-making process with respect to both teaching and learning. The concept of learning curve is applicable to the process of teaching and learning and must be explored from the research perspective to yield findings for the practice of evidence-based teaching.

## REVIEW QUESTIONS

1. What is the difference between the terms *educational* or *instructional objectives* and *behavioral* or *learning objectives*?
2. What two (2) major factors distinguish goals and objectives from one another?
3. What is the definition of the terms *goal* and *objective*?
4. Why do some educators argue against the use of behavioral objectives?
5. What are five (5) advantages of using behavioral objectives that justify the importance of writing clear and concise statements of expected behaviors?

6. What are the three (3) major characteristics that should be included in every written behavioral objective?
7. What eight (8) mistakes are commonly made when writing behavioral objectives?
8. What are the three (3) domains of learning?
9. Which levels of behavior, according to the taxonomic form of hierarchy, are considered the most simple and the most complex in the cognitive, affective, and psychomotor domains?
10. Why is it important for the educator to remember to keep psychomotor skill instruction separate from the cognitive and affective components of skill development?
11. What five (5) factors or variables influence the amount of practice required to learn any new skill?
12. What are the eight (8) basic components of a teaching plan?
13. Why are learning contracts an increasingly popular approach to teaching and learning?
14. What are the four (4) major components of a learning contract?

## REFERENCES

American Nurses Association. (1995). *Nursing's Social Policy Statement.* Washington, DC: Author.

American Nurses Association. (2001) *Code of Ethics for Nurses with Interpretative Statements.* Washington, DC: Author.

American Nurses Association. (1998). *Standards of Clinical Nursing Practice*, 2nd ed. Pub. No. 9801. Washington, DC: Author.

Andrusyszyn, M. A. (1989). Clinical evaluation of the affective domain. *Nurse Education Today, 9*(2), 75–81.

Arends, R. I. (1994). *Learning to Teach*, 3rd ed. New York: McGraw-Hill.

Babcock, D. E. & Miller, M. A. (1994). *Client Education: Theory and Practice.* St. Louis: Mosby–Year Book.

Bachman, K. (1990). Using mental imagery to practice a specific psychomotor skill. *Journal of Continuing Education in Nursing, 21*(3), 125–128.

Baldwin, D., Hill, P., & Hanson, G. (1991). Performance of psychomotor skills: A comparison of two teaching strategies. *Journal of Nursing Education, 30*(8), 367–370.

Barker, L. M. (1994). *Learning and Behavior: A Psychobiological Perspective.* New York: Macmillan College Publishing Company.

Bell, M. L. (1991). Learning a complex nursing skill: Student anxiety and the effect of preclinical skill evaluation. *Journal of Nursing Education, 30*(5), 222–226.

Bloom, B. J., Englehart, M. S., Furst, E. J., Hill, W. H., & Krathwohl, D. R. (1956). *Taxonomy of Educational Objectives: The Classification of Educational Goals, Handbook 1: Cognitive Domain.* New York: David McKay.

Bucher, L. (1991). Evaluating the affective domain. *Journal of Nursing Staff Development, 7*(5), 234–238.

Cady, C. & Yoshioka, R. S. (1991). Using a learning contract to successfully discharge an infant on home total parenteral nutrition. *Pediatric Nursing, 17*(1), 67–70, 74.

Chan, S. W. & Wai-tong (2000). Implementing contract learning in a clinical context: Report on a study. *Journal of Advanced Nursing, 31*(2), 298–305.

Cronbach, L. J. (1963). *Educational Psychology*, 2nd ed. New York: Harcourt, Brace, & World.

Cummings, C. (1994). Tips for writing behavioral objectives. *Nursing Staff Development Insider, 3*(4), 6, 8.

Dave, R. (1970). *Psychomotor Levels in Developing and Writing Objectives.* Tucson: Educational Innovators Press.

Doheny, M. O. (1993). Mental practice: An alternative approach to teaching motor skills. *Journal of Nursing Education, 32*(6), 260–264.

Durbach, E., Goodall, R., & Wilkinson, K. (1987). Instructional objectives in patient education. *Nursing Outlook, 35*(2), 82–83, 88.

Eaton, S. L. & Evans, S. B. (1986). The effect of nonspecific imaging practice on the mental imagery ability of nursing students. *Journal of Nursing Education, 25*(5), 193–196.

Ellis, C. (1993). Incorporating the affective domain into staff development programs. *Journal of Nursing Staff Development, 9*(3), 127–130.

Ferguson, L. M. (1998). Writing learning objectives. *Journal of Nursing Staff Development, 14*(2), 87–94.

Gage, N. L. & Berliner, D. C. (1998). *Educational Psychology,* 6th ed. Boston: Houghton Mifflin.

Gomez, G. E. & Gomez, E. A. (1984). The teaching of psychomotor skills in nursing. *Nurse Educator, 9*(4), 35–39.

Gomez, G. E. & Gomez, E. A. (1987). Learning of psychomotor skills: Laboratory versus patient care setting. *Journal of Nursing Education, 26*(1), 20–24.

Gronlund, N. E. (1985). *Stating Objectives for Classroom Instruction,* 3rd ed. New York: Macmillan.

Haggard, A. (1989). *Handbook of Patient Education.* Rockville, MD: Aspen.

Harrow, A. J. (1972). *A Taxonomy of the Psychomotor Domain: A Guide for Developing Behavioral Objectives.* New York: David McKay.

Keyzer, D. (1986). Using learning contracts to support change in nursing organizations. *Nurse Education Today, 6*(8), 103–108.

Knowles, M. S., Holton, E. F., & Swanson, R. A. (1998). *The Definitive Classic in Adult Education and Human Resource Development,* 3rd ed. Houston: Gulf Publishing.

Krathwohl, D. R., Bloom, B. J., & Masia, B. B. (1964). *Taxonomy of Educational Objectives: The Classification of Educational Goals. Handbook II: The Affective Domain.* New York: David McKay.

Kratzer, C. C. (April 1995). *Reflective Practice in a Community of Beginning Teachers: Implementing the STEP Program.* University of California, Los Angeles, Graduate School of Education and Information Studies. Paper presented at the Annual Meeting of the American Educational Research Association, San Francisco.

Kreider, M. C. & Barry, M. (1993). Clinical ladder development: Implementing contract learning. *Journal of Continuing Education in Nursing, 24*(4), 166–169.

Love, B., McAdams, C., Patton, D. M., Rankin, E. J., & Roberts, J. (1989). Teaching psychomotor skills in nursing: A randomized control trial. *Journal of Advanced Nursing, 14*(11), 970–975.

Lowry, M. (1997). Using learning contracts in clinical practice. *Professional Nurse, 12*(4), 280–283.

Mager, R. F. (1997). *Preparing Instructional Objectives,* 3rd ed. Atlanta, GA: Center for Effective Performance.

Maier-Lorentz, M. M. (1999). Writing objectives and evaluating learning in the affective domain. *Journal for Nurses in Staff Development, 15*(4), 167–171.

Mazhindu, G. N. (1990). Contract learning reconsidered: A critical examination of implications for application in nurse education. *Journal of Advanced Nursing, 15*(1), 101–109.

McAllister, M. (1996). Learning contracts: An Australian experience. *Nurse Education Today, 16*(3), 199–205.

McCray, P. & Blakemore, T. (1985). *A Guide to Learning Curve Technology to Enhance Performance Prediction in Vocational Evaluation.* Menomonie, WI: Research and Training Center, Stout Vocational and Rehabilitation Institute, School of Education and Human Services, University of Wisconsin–Stout.

Menix, K. D. (1996). Domains of learning: Interdependent components of achievable learning outcomes. *Journal of Continuing Education in Nursing, 27*(5), 200–208.

Miracle, D. J. (1999). Teaching psychomotor skills in simulated learning labs. Chapter 3 in K. R. Stevens & V. R. Cassidy, *Evidence-Based Teaching: Current Research in Nursing Education.* Boston: Jones and Bartlett.

Moore, M. R. (1970). The perceptual-motor domain and a proposed taxonomy of perception. *Audio Communications Review, 18,* 379–413.

Napholz, L. & McCanse, R. (1994). Interactive video instruction increases efficiency in cognitive learning in a baccalaureate nursing education program. *Computers in Nursing, 12*(3), 149–153.

Oermann, M. H. (1990). Psychomotor skill development. *Journal of Continuing Education in Nursing, 21*(5), 202–204.

O'Reilly, D. (1994). Communication and effective learning: Negotiated study and learning contracts. *Nursing Times, 90*(9), I–viii.

Reilly, D. E. & Oermann, M. H. (1990). *Behavioral Objectives: Evaluation in Nursing,* 3rd ed. Pub. No. 15-2367. New York: National League for Nursing.

Richards, B. & Vicary, J. R. (1985). The affective domain in health occupations education. *Nursing Management, 16*(7), 52–54.

Rinne, C. (1987). The affective domain: Equal opportunity in nursing education. *Journal of Continuing Education in Nursing, 18*(2), 40–43.

Ryan, M. & Marinelli, T. (1990). *Developing a Teaching Plan*. Unpublished Self-Study Module, College of Nursing, State University of New York Health Science Center at Syracuse.

Schoenly, L. (1994). Teaching in the affective domain. *Journal of Continuing Education in Nursing, 25*(5), 209–212.

Simpson, E. J. (1972). The classification of educational objectives in the psychomotor domain. In M. T. Rainier (ed.), *Contributions of Behavioral Science to Instructional Technology: The Psychomotor Domain*, 3rd ed. Englewood Cliffs, NJ: Gryphon Press, Prentice-Hall.

Waddell. D. L. & Stephens, S. (2000). Use of learning contracts in a RN-to-BSN leadership course. *Journal of Continuing Education in Nursing, 31*(4), 179–184.

Wallace, P. L. & Mundie, G. E. (1987). Contract learning in orientation. *Journal of Nursing Staff Development, 3*(4), 143–149.

Yoder, M. E. (1993). Computer use and nursing research: Transfer of cognitive learning to a clinical skill: Linear versus interactive video. *Western Journal of Nursing Research, 15*(1), 115–117.

## CHAPTER 11

# Instructional Methods

*Kathleen Fitzgerald*

## KEY TERMS

instructional strategy
instructional method
lecture
group discussion
one-to-one instruction
demonstration
return demonstration

gaming
simulation
role-playing
role-modeling
self-instruction
computer-assisted instruction
distance learning

## OBJECTIVES

After completing this chapter, the reader will be able to

1. Define the term *instructional method*.
2. Explain the various types of instructional methods.
3. Describe how to use each method effectively.
4. Identify the strengths and limitations of each method.
5. Discuss the variables that influence the selection of a method.
6. Recognize strategies to enhance teaching effectiveness.
7. Explain how to evaluate the method(s) used.

After an excellent presentation, have you ever heard someone comment, "Now, there is a born teacher!"? This comment would seem to indicate that effective teaching comes automatically. In reality, teaching effectively is a learned skill. Development of this skill requires knowledge of the educational process, including the instructional methods available and ways to use them with a variety of learners and settings. Stimulating and effective learning experiences are designed, not accidental.

*Instructional strategy* is the overall plan for a learning experience. It involves the use of one or several methods of teaching, and it encompasses both the content and the process that will be used to achieve the desired outcomes of instruction (Rothwell & Kazanas, 1992). *Instructional methods* are the techniques or approaches the teacher uses to bring the learner into contact with the content to be learned. *Methods* are a way, an approach, or a process to communicate information, whereas *instructional materials* or *tools* are the actual vehicles by which information is shared with the learner. Some examples of methods are lecture, group discussion, one-to-one instruction, demonstration and return demonstration, gaming, simulation, role-playing, role-modeling, self-instruction modules, computer-assisted instruction, and distance learning techniques. Books, videos, and posters are examples of materials and tools. It is important to draw this distinction between the terms *methods* and *tools*, because they are often used interchangeably by educators and not dealt with as distinctly separate entities, which they should be, when planning an educational activity.

This chapter will review the types of instructional methods available and consider how to choose and use them efficiently and effectively. It will also identify the strengths and limitations of each method, the variables influencing the selection of various techniques, and ways to evaluate the methods used to improve the delivery of instruction.

Throughout, examples will be drawn from a variety of learners, such as the person in a wellness program trying to stop smoking, the patient learning how to self-manage his or her diabetes, and the staff nurse learning to coordinate a cardiac arrest, because the nurse is expected to teach a variety of learners in a variety of settings.

## TYPES OF INSTRUCTIONAL METHODS

When learners know what is expected of them, it has been claimed that they learn regardless of the methods or tools used for teaching (Haggard, 1989). However, the teacher functions in a vital role by providing guidance and support for learning. In addition, the influence of appropriate methods to meet the needs of learners should not be underestimated. There is no one perfect method for all learners and learning experiences. Whatever the method chosen, it will usually be most effective if it is used in conjunction with other techniques and tools to enhance learning. Even though a teacher may use one method predominately, that single method is rarely adhered to in a pure fashion and is really a combination of various methods. For example, the lecture may be used as the primary format, with opportunities for question and answer periods and short discussion sessions being interspersed throughout the lecture period.

Decisions about which methods to use will be based on such variables as how active the learner is or wishes to be and how much control the teacher chooses to exert over the learning experience. Audience size, diversity (e.g., age, educational background, culture), preferred learning style, and the setting for teaching are also important considerations.

Instructional methods can be categorized in many ways. The rationale for the classification reflects whether the learner's role is active or passive, the technique is student- or instructor-centered, or the focus is on content versus process knowledge. For the purposes of this discussion, traditional teaching methods, with which most people are familiar, will be examined first, followed by nontraditional methods of instruction. The traditional methods include lecture, group discussion, one-to-one instruction, demonstration, and return demonstration. These methods tend to have more teacher input and control during encounters with the learner than do the less traditional formats, which include gaming, simulation, role-playing, role-modeling, self-instruction activities, computer-assisted instruction, and distance learning. In the nontraditional approaches, teachers act more as designers and facilitators than as verbal presenters and givers of information. Both traditional and nontraditional methods can be used either with the individual learner or with groups of learners.

## TRADITIONAL METHODS

### Lecture

*Lecture* can be defined as a highly structured method by which the teacher verbally transmits information directly to groups of learners for the purpose of instruction. It is one of the oldest and most often used methods. The word lecture comes from the Latin term "lectura," which means to read. The lecture method has been much maligned in recent years, but if a lecture is well organized and delivered effectively, it can be a very useful method of instruction (Haggard, 1989).

In its purest form, the lecture format allows for only minimal exchange between the teacher and the learner, but it can be an effective method of teaching in the lower-level cognitive domain to impart content knowledge. It is useful to demonstrate patterns, highlight main ideas, or present unique ways of viewing information. Lecture is an efficient, cost-effective method for getting large amounts of information across to a large number of people all at the same time as well as within a rel-

atively reasonable time frame. For example, the lecture might be used to introduce an agency's mission statement to new staff orientees or to explain diabetes mellitus to a group of laypeople. It should not be used, however, to give people the same information that they could read independently at another time and place. It is the lecturer's expertise, both in theory and experience, that can substantially contribute to the learner's understanding of a subject.

Lecture is also useful in providing foundational background information as a basis for subsequent group discussions and is a means to summarize data and current research findings not available elsewhere (Boyd, Gleit, Graham, & Whitman, 1998). In addition, the lecture can be easily supplemented with handout materials and other audiovisual aids.

With respect to its limitations, the lecture method is ineffective in influencing affective and psychomotor behaviors. It does not provide for much stimulation of learners, and there is little opportunity for learner involvement. Rather, learners are passive recipients of the information being presented. The focus, instead, is very instructor-centered, and thus the most active participant is frequently the most knowledgeable one—the teacher.

Because the lecture does not account for individual differences in background, attention span, or learning style, all learners are exposed to the same information regardless of their ability or need. This is particularly evident in patient groups, where cognitive abilities and stages of coping with some topics vary widely. This diversity within groups makes it difficult and challenging, if not impossible, for the teacher to effectively target the needs of all learners in the audience.

Although the lecture method is considered cost-effective, cost-effectiveness should not be determined just by calculating the teacher–student ratio of contact hours during class. Teacher preparation time, number of times the material needs to be presented, and the follow-up time used to individualize learning and evaluate outcomes must also be taken into account.

Despite the limitations of this method, there are specific strategies to strengthen the effectiveness of a lecture. Each lecture should include an introduction, body, and conclusion.

During the introduction, learners should be presented with an overview of the behavioral objectives pertinent to the lecture topic, along with an explanation as to why these objectives are significant. Engage learners' attention by conducting an informal survey or stating the objectives as questions that will be answered during the body of the lecture. Use humor and your personality to help establish rapport with your audience. If the occasion is one of a series of lectures, you need to make a connection with the overall subject and the topic being presented as well as its relationship to previous topics covered and the lectures that will follow.

The next portion of the lecture is the body, or the actual delivery of the content. Careful preparation is needed so that the important aspects are covered in an accurate, logical, cohesive, and interesting manner. Examples should be used throughout to enhance the salient points you wish to make, but extraneous facts and redundant examples should be edited so as not to reduce the impact of your message. Because the lecture format tends to be very passive for learners, you can enhance the effectiveness of your presentation by mixing it with other instructional methods, such as discussion or question and answer sessions.

Use of audiovisual materials, such as a video, overhead projections, or slides, can also add variety to your presentation. The widespread availability of graphics software makes it easy to enhance your presentation, but you should follow some general guidelines. Do not put all your content on slides; instead, focus on the key concepts to supplement your presentation. Use the largest font possible, fewer than 25 words per slide, and color and graphics when appropriate. Color

should have a high level of contrast between background and text if you plan to lecture in a large room with bright lights. Graphics are very useful when you are presenting large amounts of numerical data (Evans, 2000). Make sure that all audiovisual equipment is functional and that you know how to use it before beginning the lecture. A technical malfunction will be disconcerting for both you and your audience.

If you are nervous or inexperienced, practice before a mirror, a video camera, or a constructive colleague. Outline key points of your presentation on index cards, overhead projections, or slides. Reading a printed copy of the entire presentation is exceedingly boring to your audience. Vary your presentation style and tone of voice to avoid monotony. Move around the stage or room. Your enthusiasm, expertise, and interest in the topic can also be used to capture and hold the group's attention. Be sure to keep within the time allotted to you. Lectures of long duration will result in loss of attention and boredom on the part of the learner.

The final section of the lecture format is the summary or conclusion. At this juncture, review the major concepts presented. It is very important that your lecture not exceed the prescribed time so that you do not have to end abruptly because time has run out.

Try to leave some leeway for questions and summary information. If you are using a microphone in a large group, be sure to repeat the questions so the rest of the audience can hear them. If time runs short, state that you will be able to answer only a few queries but invite immediate follow-up by meeting with interested individuals alone or in a smaller group or by suggesting relevant readings.

## Group Discussion

*Group discussion*, by definition, is a method of teaching whereby learners get together to exchange information, feelings, and opinions with one another and with the teacher. Discussion is one of the most commonly employed instructional techniques. The activity is learner-centered and subject-centered. Group size can vary, but most group discussion techniques can be used with as few as 3 people and as many as 15 to 20 people. Group discussion is an effective method for teaching in both the affective and cognitive domains.

The most important element on which to focus is the preset behavioral objectives when using this method. These objectives are the learning goals of the interaction and should be presented at the beginning of each session. Careful adherence to them will prevent the discussion from becoming an aimless wandering of ideas or a forum for the strongest group member to expound on his or her opinions and feelings. The teacher's role is to act as a facilitator in keeping the discussion focused and in tying points together. The instructor must be well versed in the subject matter to field questions, to move the discussion along in the direction intended, and to give appropriate feedback.

Teacher involvement and control of the process vary with the needs of the group. Group discussion requires the teacher to be able to tolerate less structure and organization than other traditional methods such as lecture or one-to-one instruction. The group must have some knowledge of the content before this method can be effective; otherwise, the discussion will be based on "pooled ignorance." An experienced group of staff may need little input while they work out a complex patient problem. A new group of patients or family members with little understanding of a topic will need to access information directly from the teacher or another source before they can knowledgeably participate in problem-solving integral to the discussion process. The teacher's responsibility is to make sure that every member of the group has interpreted information correctly, because failure to do so will lead to conclusions based on faulty data. For this reason, patient groups need to be prescreened. While diversity within a group is beneficial, a large range in literacy skills, states of anxiety, and experiences with acute and chronic conditions may lead to difficulty in meeting any one member's needs.

Abruzzese (1996) suggests some group learning techniques that require preparation by staff prior to the activity but are good vehicles for active learning. Debates offer teams with opposing views the opportunity to present each side of the issue and help staff consider both perspectives. Seminars are small discussion groups in which each member reads an assignment and considers questions prior to the activity so that all learners can actively participate in the discussion. The case study approach offers an opportunity to thoroughly discuss a patient and related health problems.

It is important for the teacher to maintain the trust of the group. Everyone must feel safe and comfortable enough to express his or her point of view. Respectful attention and tolerance toward others should be modeled by the teacher and required of all group members. Of course, this consideration does not preclude correcting errors or disagreements. A clear message must be given that while personal opinions may be debatable, the inherent value of what each member has to say and the member's right to participate is guaranteed.

The major advantage of group discussion is that it stimulates learners to think about issues and problems and to exchange their own experiences, thereby making learning more active. It provides opportunities for sharing of ideas, receiving peer support, fostering a feeling of belonging, giving guidance, and reinforcing previous learning. Discussion is effective in assisting learners to identify resources and to internalize the topic being discussed by helping them to reflect on its personal meaning (Brookfield & Preskill, 1999). Active learning leads to greater retention of information (Haggard, 1989).

The group discussion method is economically beneficial from a time-efficiency perspective. Teaching people in groups rather than individually allows the teacher to reach a number of learners at the same time. With healthcare costs rising, this method should be considered as an efficient and effective method to teach groups with similar objectives, such as preparation for childbirth or cardiac bypass surgery. Through group work, members share common concerns and receive reinforcement from one another. The idea that "we're all in the same boat" or "if you can do it, I can do it" serves to stimulate motivation for learning as a result of peer support.

Group size, a major consideration in group teaching, should be determined by the purpose or task to be accomplished (Boyd et al., 1998). Although a large group has the potential for greater diversity because members will vary in experiential and knowledge background, there will be less chance for everyone to participate and for individual needs to be met (Anderson, 1990). Arnold and Boggs (1989) suggest that a group size of six to eight members is ideal to achieve diversity of ideas and yet allow for balanced interaction among members. Larger groups can be broken down into smaller units to promote greater interaction by all members and to better attend to the skill development of each individual.

Group discussion has proved particularly helpful to patients and families dealing with chronic illness. It offers a forum in which to share content information for cognitive growth as well as an opportunity to learn self-efficacy. This increase in confidence levels of patients and families increases their ability to handle an illness (Lorig & Gonzalez, 1993). The process helps people learn how to respond to situations, improve their coping mechanisms, and explore ways to incorporate needed changes into their lives. Group discussion is most effective during the accommodation stage of psychological adjustment to chronic illness, because the interactions help reduce isolation and foster identification with others who are in similar circumstances (Fredette, 1990). Group discussion also benefits other types of learners. For example, following a panel presentation by persons living with AIDS, a discussion session was an effective way to break down the negative stereotypes on the part of some healthcare workers (Peters & Connell, 1991).

The opportunity afforded all members to be active participants is the major benefit of group discussion, but this method can also lead to difficulties if one or two members tend to dominate the discussion or digress from the objectives. Shy learners may refuse to become involved or may need a great deal of encouragement to participate, while digressing or dominating learners may need to be tactfully redirected in a manner that lessens their influence on the group without damaging the trust of other group members. Harsh or sarcastic treatment resulting in insults breaks down the relationship between the teacher and the learners as well as relationships among learners, which creates an environment unsuitable for learning. One helpful approach is to tell the group at the beginning of the session that the goal is to hear from all members by asking for their input and points of view during the actual discussion period. Persons who digress should be requested to hold questions that can be handled privately until the end of class because these inquiries are important but unique to their circumstances. The discussion method may prove especially difficult and disconcerting for the novice teacher when faced with a group whose members do not easily interact.

From a financial perspective, it must be noted that group discussion requires the teacher's presence during each session to act as facilitator and resource person. Also, it often takes more time to transmit information via this method than other methods such as lecture. In addition, third-party payment for some types of group patient education programs may be difficult to obtain when the traditional fee-for-service reimbursement is not available. However, these programs may be economically valuable in preventing hospitalization or reducing time in acute care. Documenting these benefits based on measurable outcomes is very important.

## One-to-One Instruction

In *one-to-one instruction*, the teacher delivers individual instruction designed specifically for a particular learner. It is an opportunity to communicate ideas and feelings primarily through oral exchange, although nonverbal messages can be conveyed as well. This method should never be a lecture delivered to an audience of one to meet the teacher's goals. Instead, the experience should actively involve the learner and be based on his or her unique learning needs.

One-to-one instruction begins with an assessment of the learner and the mutual setting of objectives to be accomplished. One part of the assessment process that has been found to be very important is to determine at which stage of change the person is regarding a problem behavior such as smoking and to then tailor the interventions to that stage (Prochaska, DiClemente, Velicer, & Rossi, 1993).

Change is characterized by five stages (Prochaska, DiClemente, & Norcross, 1992):

1. *Precontemplation*. In this stage, there is no intention to change within the next six months. People do not fully realize there is a problem so they are resistant to change.

2. *Contemplation*. In this stage, people realize that a problem exists and are considering change but have not taken action. People in this stage are considering change in the next six months but are still struggling with the pros and cons.

3. *Preparation*. In this stage, people combine the intention to change with some beginning action. They intend to take action in the next month and have unsuccessfully taken action in the last year.

4. *Action*. In this stage, people actually modify their problem behavior. People in this stage have altered their behavior for a period ranging from one day to six months. This stage requires a large time commitment and energy expenditure.

5. *Maintenance*. In this stage, there is a continuation of the behavior change. People are working to prevent relapse and consolidate the new behaviors and have been successful for more than six months.

This model is generalizable across a broad range of behaviors, including but not limited to, smoking cessation, weight control, avoidance of high-fat diets, safer sex, and exercise initiation (Proschaska et al., 1994).

The nurse's interactions with learners should focus on helping them through the stages of change. In the precontemplation stage, it is important to provide information in a nonthreatening manner to help the learner become aware of the negative aspects or consequences of the behavior. In the contemplation stage, the nurse should support the decision making for change by identifying benefits, considering barriers to the change, and making suggestions for dealing with these obstacles. During the preparation stage, the goal is to support the move to action. Contracting with small, realistic, and measurable goals, information on effective ways to achieve the change, and support to think positively will help at this point. The action stage calls for support as the person actually practices the behavior change. It is critical to encourage positive thinking to prevent relapse, point out the benefits of each achievement, and help the learner monitor his or her behavior change by implementing strategies such as a food diary. Last is the maintenance stage, where continued encouragement and support are important (Saarmann, Daugherty, & Riegel, 2000).

One-to-one instruction can be tailored to meet objectives in all three domains of learning. For example, teaching an individual to give insulin would address both the cognitive and psychomotor domains. Coaching an expectant mother so she feels she has enough control in using the techniques learned in birth preparation classes is an example of instruction primarily in the affective domain.

Mutual goal setting by teacher and learner is very important. It has been proved that patient education and counseling in chronic illness will result in better outcomes when the learner plays an active role in discussing alternatives and in setting the objectives and goals for learning (Kaplan et al., 1989).

Contracting, which clearly spells out the roles and expectations of both teacher and learner, is one effective way to facilitate mutual goal setting. Contracts should be written in specific terms and evaluated by both participants (see an explanation of learning contracts in Chapter 10). Whenever teaching is done on a one-to-one basis, instructions should be specific and followed by immediate response from the learner and feedback from the teacher. Allowing learners the opportunity to state their understanding of information gives the teacher an opportunity to evaluate the extent of learning. Also, communicating to learners what further information is forthcoming allows them to connect what they have just learned with what they will be learning. For example, the nurse teaching a patient about hypoglycemia might say, "Now that you understand what causes low blood sugar, we will talk about how to tell when you have it and what to do if you experience it after discharge."

The process of one-to-one instruction involves moving learners from repeating the information to applying what they have learned. In the preceding example regarding hypoglycemia, you might give the person a hypothetical situation as close to the patient's lifestyle as possible and let the person work through how to respond to it. In this type of simulation, a potentially threatening situation can be presented in a nonthreatening manner (Boyd et al., 1998). For instance, you might ask a busy executive who has diabetes how he would respond to feeling shaky and sweaty at 2:00 P.M. on a day when a meeting runs late and he misses lunch. Be sure to clearly state that this scenario is not a test but rather a "dress rehearsal" for life situations. You can change the scenarios with further questioning to help learners plan how they could prevent such situations in the future. This technique gives learners a chance to use the information at a higher cognitive level. It also gives the nurse educator a chance to evaluate learning in a nonthreatening manner.

With the one-to-one method of instruction, questioning is an excellent technique. It can be used to involve learners as active participants in the learning process and to give feedback on their progress to the instructor. Questions can be matched to the cognitive objectives. For example, for the knowledge level, you might ask "What is the next step?" in a procedure.

For the higher level of synthesis, you might ask a nurse to plan how he or she would respond to an angry family member (Abruzzese, 1996). Questioning should not be interpreted by the learner as a test of knowledge but rather as a way to exchange information and stimulate thinking.

Two problems can occur with questioning. Questions can be too ambiguous such that the learner does not know what you are asking, or they can contain too many facts for the person to process effectively (House et al., 1990). Watch your learner's nonverbal reactions, and rephrase the question if you detect either of these problems. If the learner seems confused, it is helpful to state that perhaps you did not ask the question in a clear manner. This technique will guard against the learner feeling guilty or becoming discouraged if a question was incorrectly answered.

It is important to give learners time to process information and respond to your questions. Sometimes teachers are uncomfortable waiting in silence for an answer or are impatient and attempt to correct an answer before learners complete their responses. Questioning will be ineffective as a technique when learners are not given enough time to process information. Preliminary interruption may further interfere with a learner's thinking process and create a tense atmosphere.

Many nurse educators conduct individualized teaching of other nurses or student learners in the clinical setting. Clinical instruction is not a discrete instructional method but rather a very complex setting in which to teach experientially. A variety of methods other than one-to-one instruction can be used. Role-modeling, demonstration, return demonstration, and discussion are but a few. One-to-one instruction may be part of orientation, student preceptorship, or a continuing education activity. The learner is singularly guided in the actual practice setting, which may be a hospital, mental health center, home of a patient, or any other setting in which nursing care is delivered. Each learning experience needs specific objectives that are tailored to the individual's needs. These objectives should be known to both the instructor and the learner.

The "Performance-Based Development System" was designed to determine a newly hired nurse's competency (del Bueno, Griffin, Burke, & Foley, 1990). This structured assessment of an individual's competency is completed before planning of clinical experiences. Very focused clinical activities can then be planned with the staff nurse, nurse educator, and clinical manager.

Preceptors who assume clinical teaching roles may need to be taught how to teach effectively because they are usually expert cli-

nicians but may not necessarily be expert teachers. Workshops and coaching sessions may be an effective way to accomplish this task. Evaluation is difficult, especially when there is difficulty separating the learning phase from the testing phase. This is the difference between formative and summative evaluation. Formative evaluation is done during the learning phase to mark learner progress and give feedback for growth. Summative evaluation is the testing phase and a final assessment; it includes assessment of patterns rather than single events.

One-to-one instruction has many advantages. The major benefit is the ability to individualize teaching. This method is an ideal intervention for initial assessment and continued evaluation of the learner in all three domains of learning. It is especially suitable for teaching those who are educationally disadvantaged or who have been diagnosed with low-level literacy skills or learning disabilities. The teaching can be paced and the content tailored to meet individual needs. Understanding of content can be determined on a regular ongoing basis followed by immediate feedback from the teacher.

The major drawback of one-to-one instruction is the isolation of the learner from others who may have similar needs or concerns. Learners are deprived of the opportunity for identification with others through the sharing of ideas, thoughts, and feelings with those who may be in like circumstances. New staff nurses being oriented to an agency or patients recently diagnosed with cancer can benefit from group interaction that allows them to explore mutual concerns.

Caution in using the one-to-one method also must be exercised to avoid having learners feel "put on the spot" because they are the only ones who are the object of teaching—the sole focus of attention. The educator, too, must be careful in the use of questioning because learners may interpret this technique as a "test" of their knowledge and skills. In addition, it is not unusual for the educator to make the mistake of cramming too much information into each session, which can result in the learner feeling overwhelmed and anxious.

Economically, one-to-one instruction is a very labor-intensive method and should be well tailored to make the expense worthwhile in terms of learner outcomes. One-to-one teaching of patients and families is often an inefficient approach to learning because the educator is reaching only one person at a time. Clinical orientation of staff and students and continuing education for staff development are vital but costly when carried out on a one-to-one basis. The cost comes in payroll dollars and in short-term nonproductivity of the employee being oriented (del Bueno et al., 1990).

## Demonstration and Return Demonstration

It is imperative to begin by making a clear distinction between the methods of demonstration and return demonstration. *Demonstration* is a method by which the learner is shown by the teacher how to perform a particular skill. *Return demonstration* is the method by which the learner attempts to perform the skill with cues from the teacher as needed. These two methods require different abilities by both the teacher and the learner. Each is effective in teaching psychomotor domain skills. Both may also enhance cognitive and affective learning—for example, when helping someone develop interactive skills to be used in crisis intervention or assertiveness training.

Prior to giving a demonstration, learners should be informed of the purpose of the procedure, the sequential steps involved, the equipment being used, and the actions expected of them. Equipment should be tested beforehand to ensure that it is complete and in working order. For the demonstration method to be employed effectively, the learners must be able to clearly see and hear the steps being taught. Therefore, the demonstration method is best suited to teaching individuals or small groups. The use of a big screen or multiple screens for video presentations of demonstrations can allow larger groups to more easily visualize detail.

Watching a demonstration can be a passive activity for learners, whose role is to observe the teacher presenting an exact performance of the required skill. The demonstration can be enhanced by the teacher slowing the actual timing of the demonstration and exaggerating some of the steps (de Tornyay & Thompson, 1987) or breaking lengthy procedures into a series of shorter steps. In the process of demonstrating a skill, it is important to explain why each step needs to be carried out in a certain manner. The performance should be flawless, but the teacher should take advantage of a mistake to show how errors can be handled. Used correctly, an error may increase rapport with some learners. However, too many mistakes disrupt the mental image that the learner is forming.

When demonstrating a psychomotor skill, if possible, work with the exact equipment that the learner will be expected to use. This consideration is particularly important for novice learners. For instance, the novice patient or family member who is learning to administer tube feedings at home will be anxious and frustrated if taught the use of one pump in the hospital when another type is used after discharge. Often the learner is too inexperienced to see the skill pattern and instead will handle each pump as a separate task. The seasoned staff nurse, on the other hand, will find it easier to transfer what is already known about tube feeding pumps if called on to learn to use a newly purchased pump from a different manufacturer.

Return demonstration should be planned to occur close to when the demonstration was given. It may be necessary to do some anxiety reduction prior to the beginning of the learner's performance because the opportunity to return demonstrate may be viewed by the learner as a test and may lead to the expectation of a perfect performance for the first time around. Once a learner recognizes that the teacher is a coach and not an evaluator, the climate will be less tense and the learner will be more comfortable in attempting to practice a new skill. Stress the fact that it is expected that the initial performance will not be perfect. In addition, allowing the learner to manipulate the equipment before being expected to use it may help to reduce anxiety levels. Some patients may experience an increased level of anxiety when faced with learning a new skill because they identify the need to learn a skill in relation to their illness. For example, a young woman learning to care for a venous access device may be very anxious because of the diagnosis of cancer that has necessitated use of the device.

When the learner is giving a return demonstration, the teacher should remain silent except for offering cues when necessary or briefly answering questions. Learners may be prompted by a series of pictures or coached by a partner with a checklist. Casual conversation or asking questions should be avoided because they merely serve to interrupt the learner's thought processes and interfere with efforts to focus on mentally imprinting the procedure while performing the actual task. Breaking the steps of the procedure into small increments will give the learner the opportunity to master one sequence before attempting the next. Praising the learner along the way for each step correctly performed will reinforce behavior and give the learner confidence in being able to successfully accomplish the task in its entirety (Haggard, 1989). Emphasis should be on what to do, rather than on what not to do.

Practice should be supervised until the learner is competent enough to perform steps accurately. It is important that the initial skill pattern be correct before allowing for independent practice. High-risk skills should be practiced first on a model prior to actual clinical application. Learners will need a varying amount of practice to become competent, but once they have acquired the skill, they can then practice on their own to increase speed and proficiency. A critical care nurse, for example, will probably need little practice with a new IV pump that is similar to others already mastered. In contrast, a patient learning to manipulate a pump for home IV therapy may need many practice sessions.

It is very important to plan return demonstration sessions close enough together that the learner does not lose the benefit of the last practice session. As with demonstration, the equipment for return demonstration needs to exactly match that used by the instructor and expected to be used by the learner.

Learners also will require help in compensating for individual differences. If you as the instructor are right-handed and the learner is left-handed, perhaps sitting across from each other would be more helpful than sitting adjacent to one another. The person with difficulty seeing the increments on an insulin syringe may need a magnifying device to facilitate accurate performance of a skill.

These methods actively engage the learner through stimulation of multiple visual, auditory, and tactile senses. The opportunity afforded for mental rehearsal of procedures being demonstrated prior to actual return demonstration has been associated with increased performance levels (Haggard, 1989). Repetition of movement and constant reinforcement of practice are the mainstays of successful learning in the psychomotor domain. Overlearning through extended practice instills confidence on the part of both the teacher and the learner that the skill will be competently performed and will be retained for a longer period of time.

Although the cliché "practice makes perfect" is quite true, demonstration and return demonstration sessions are very time-consuming and require plenty of time to be set aside for teaching as well as learning. These methods are expensive because of the necessity of keeping the size of the group small and the need for individual supervision during follow-up practices. There are some ways to reduce the cost of this method. If the audience comprises a homogeneous group of health professionals who need yearly CPR review, demonstration can be via videotape. Return demonstration can initially be performed with a partner supervising the competency of the skill. However, the final evaluation of staff competency must be carried out by an expert to ensure the accuracy of learning. The cost of obtaining, maintaining, and replacing equipment must also be calculated. Expenses can be reduced by reusing equipment if it will not interfere with the accuracy, safety, or completeness of the demonstration/return demonstration.

## ■ NONTRADITIONAL METHODS

### Gaming

*Gaming* is an instructional method requiring the learner to participate in a competitive activity with preset rules. These activities do not have to reflect reality, but they are designed to accomplish educational objectives. The goal is for the learners to win a game by applying knowledge and rehearsing skills previously learned. Gaming is fun with a purpose. It promotes retention of information by stimulating learner enthusiasm and increasing learner involvement. Games can be devised or modified for individual or group learning. More complex games require the learner to use problem solving and critical thinking strategies. This method adds variety to the learning experience and is excellent for dull or repetitious content that requires periodic review.

Games can be placed anywhere in the sequence of a learning activity (Joos, 1984)—as a device to introduce a topic, check learner progress, or summarize information. This instructional method is primarily effective for improving cognitive functioning but can also be used to enhance skills in the psychomotor domain and to influence affective behavior through increased social interaction (Robinson, Lewis, & Robinson, 1990). Rowell and Spielvogle (1996) also used an infection-control game as a needs assessment to determine whether a knowledge deficit among staff was contributing to rising rates of Methicillin Resistant Staphylococcus Aureus (MRSA). They had staff members identify violations of effective infection-control practices in a mock isolation room. Participants completed and turned in an answer sheet, then proceeded to an answer station. Not only did staff have an opportunity to test themselves and correct wrong information, but participants also provided information to plan future education programs.

In gaming, the teacher's role is that of a facilitator. At the beginning of a game, the group needs to be told the objectives and the rules. Any materials needed to play a game are distributed, and the various teams are assigned. Once the game starts, the teacher needs to keep the flow going and interpret the rules. The game should be interrupted as seldom or as briefly as possible so as not to disturb the pace (Joos, 1984). When the game is completed, winners should be rewarded. Prizes do not have to be expensive because their main purpose is to acknowledge achievement of learners in a public manner (Robinson et al., 1990).

At the finish of the game, the teacher should conduct a debriefing session focusing on educational content and evaluating the gaming experience. Learners should be given a chance to discuss what they learned, ask questions, receive feedback regarding the outcome of the game, and offer suggestions for improving the process.

Games may be either purchased or designed. Well-known commercial games such as "Trivial Pursuit," "Bingo," "Monopoly," or "Jeopardy" have the advantage in that their formats can be modified, the equipment is reusable for many topics, and many players already have familiarity with the rules of play. Word searches, crossword puzzles, treasure hunts, and card and board games are also flexible in format and can be developed inexpensively and with relative ease. Be sure to pilot games prior to widespread use. Some examples of games are a word search for foods that are known to elevate serum potassium used with patients with end-stage renal disease (Robinson et al., 1990) (Figure 11–1), and "Emergency Pursuit," which has content that is related to emergency situations that might occur on a medical-surgical unit. It uses a question and answer format, with two teams of staff nurses competing against each other (Schmitz, MacLean, & Shidler, 1991).

Computer games, although much more expensive, are becoming increasingly available and are a popular option for many learners. Gaming is a method particularly attractive to children, who enjoy the challenge of learning through playlike activity. An interactive video game was used for young people from ages 8 to 16 with Type 1 diabetes. The game modeled the daily challenges of self-care. Participants were told to play the game as much or as little as they wished. By the end of the six-month trial, there was a 77% drop in diabetes-related urgent care as well as an increase in diabetes-related self-efficacy in communication with parents about diabetes and in self-care. Players were engaged in learning in a simulation game that was fun (Lieberman, 2001).

FIGURE 11–1    **Sample Word Search Game for Patients**  SOURCE: Reprinted with permission of the American Nephrology Nurses Association, publisher, *ANNA Journal*, Volume 17/Number 4 (August 1990), page 307.

To participate, learners must have the ability and background knowledge sufficient to play the game. Games should be exciting and challenging enough to stimulate learner interest but not so difficult or competitive as to result in frustration, inability to succeed, or the avoidance of this learning opportunity (Walts, 1982).

It is particularly important to remember that games, whether purchased or self-developed, must serve the purpose of helping the learner accomplish the predetermined behavioral objectives. Are people learning while they are having fun? Bays and Herman (1997) tested students who learned the same content but through different methods. One group was taught with gaming and the other with lecture. When the students took the same test at the conclusion, no significant difference was found between the two groups.

Along with its advantages, the gaming method has some limitations. Gaming can create a competitive environment that may be threatening to some learners. The group size must be kept small so that all members can participate. The room must be more flexible than a traditional conference room or classroom to be set up in different clusters for teamwork. The noise level may be higher and the requirements more physically demanding than many other methods. Not all learners may be able to participate if they are restricted by a disability. Lewis and colleagues (1989) designed a game suitability checklist that is helpful in determining if gaming is a viable alternative to meet the objectives for learning (Figure 11–2).

---

### GAME SUITABILITY CHECKLIST

| Criteria | Yes | No |
|---|---|---|
| • Does the game meet the program objectives? | _____ | _____ |
| • Can the game be completedwithin the time allotted? | _____ | _____ |
| • Is the size and layout of the room conducive to the game? | _____ | _____ |
| • Will the available participants meet the minimum number required for the game? | _____ | _____ |
| • Do staff members have the time and interest to design or adapt games? If not, are funds available to purchase games? | _____ | _____ |
| • If the game requires equipment or supplies, are they readily available? | _____ | _____ |
|    a. Are resources or funds available to design or purchase needed materials? | _____ | _____ |
|    b. Does the game require replacement of materials following each use? | _____ | _____ |
| • Does the game require preparation or cleanup time? | _____ | _____ |

**FIGURE 11–2   Game Suitability Checklist** SOURCE: Lewis et al. (1989). Reprinted with permission from *The Journal of Continuing Education in Nursing.*

Economic considerations include the cost of purchasing the game and the time taken by the instructor to design, pilot, and update the material. Some types of gaming also require the instructor to be present each time that the game is played.

## Simulation

*Simulation* is a method whereby an artificial or hypothetical experience is created that engages the learner in an activity that reflects real-life conditions but without the risk-taking consequences of an actual situation (Rystedt & Lindström, 2001). Participants can try out their problem-solving, interactive, and psychomotor skills. A simulation provides realistic learner involvement in a "real-life" situation with consequences determined by variables inherent in the situation (Abruzzese, 1996). Simulations are effective for teaching higher-level learning in the cognitive domain as well as promoting the attainment of psychomotor and affective skills.

In actual use, there is overlapping between games, simulations, and role-playing because all three teaching methods require active participation on the part of the learner in dealing with concrete, realistic learning experiences. All are experiential learning methods that call for the learner to choose an action and see the consequences. They are effective in facilitating problem solving, attitude change, and preparation for anticipated events (Rorden, 1987). It is important to have a discussion with learners after use of these experiential methods to facilitate analysis of the experience.

When planning a simulation, it is most effective if the learning experience is made to resemble real life as much as possible but in a nonthreatening way. The activity should challenge the decision-making ability of the learner. This can be done by the imposition of time constraints, provision of realistic levels of tension, and use of actual equipment or other important features of the environment in which the specific skill will be performed. For example, a scenario could be developed to help parents of a baby with sudden infant death syndrome work through how to handle a situation when the monitor signals respiratory difficulty in their infant. Another example would be when a staff nurse is learning to respond to a chest trauma victim in an emergency room setting and is expected to make an assessment rapidly and set up a chest tube drainage system with accuracy and speed. All of these actions will take place while the nurse is pretending to interact with other team members and a very frightened patient.

An effective use of simulation would need to include as many aspects of these complex processes as possible to determine whether the learner has the necessary skills to do the activity correctly. Simulation should be followed by a debriefing session (de Tornyay & Thompson, 1987). It should include discussion of events that happened during the experience, the decisions made, the actions taken, the consequences of the choices, the possible alternatives, and suggestions for improvement in skill performance. Simulation provides the opportunity for anticipatory learning.

There are many types of simulations. A written simulation uses a case study to which the learner responds. Staff nurses, for example, may be asked to describe how they would handle a staff communication problem or manage a physiologically complex patient in the critical care environment. Clinical simulations can be set up to replicate complex care situations such as a mock cardiac arrest. One innovative program creates a mock code in a room on a pediatric unit with a mannequin. An experienced nurse is a "buddy" or a coach for the inexperienced nurse who is "running" the code. This simulation allows the novice to practice these skills in a nonthreatening situation with immediate feedback. Participants report that this simulation helps them validate their thinking and allows for ongoing "think-ing out loud" to ask questions they might not ask otherwise (Cuda, Doerr, & Gonzales, 1999)

Models are frequently used in simulation to teach both patients and nurses. For instance, a patient or a nurse may be taught to change a venous access device dressing on a torso model. A peer, instructor, or trained individual may act as a patient in an effective and economical method to teach certain non-invasive skills. An exciting new technology is high-fidelity whole-body patient simulators that reproduce in a life-like manner the car-diovascular, respiratory, urinary, and neuro-logical systems. Some models even have the ability to respond to selected drugs. This resource is limited by its cost, however (Lupien & George-Gay, 2001). Computers can be used to present simulated situations whereby information as well as feedback is given to learners in helping them to develop decision-making skills.

A growing phenomenon related to use of simulation is the learning laboratory. In this environment, staff and patients can easily access models, computers, tapes, videos, and other equipment for use in practicing various skills. For example, a staff member may request an audiotape with heart sounds to practice this assessment. The role of the instructor is that of facilitator. Nursing staff report that the learning laboratory is a non-threatening environment in which to learn (Jeska & Cosgrove, 1992). This type of labora-tory has also been used on college campuses for nurses reentering the workforce. These returning students claim the learning labora-tory is a stimulating and helpful approach to updating their skills. Following this simulated experience, they have increased self-confi-dence when returning to the workforce (Wood, 1994). Many of the same models and equipment employed for simulation exercises in the laboratory setting can also be used to train patients or family providers in such skills as transfer techniques, sterile proce-dures, and urinary catheter care. Even though the equipment for simulation remains perma-nently assigned to the learning center, efforts should be made to make the equipment portable so that it may be used on hospital units, in outpatient clinic settings, or in home settings.

Simulated experiences should be followed with the actual experience as soon as possible. The simulation is never exactly the same as the real experience for which one is preparing and, therefore, the learner will need help with the transfer of skills learned in a simulated experi-ence to the actual situation. In the future, vir-tual reality has the potential to narrow the dis-tance between simulation and real life.

Limitations of this instructional method are that it can be expensive and very labor-inten-sive in many cases. Simulation can be made more cost-effective by reuse of supplies and by teaching a higher volume and a more diverse population of learners (Jeska & Cosgrove, 1992). Findings suggest that the modern learn-ing laboratory, in particular, is an approach that will help nursing education to function both more efficiently and more effectively in the future (Kleinknecht & Hefferin, 1990).

## Role-Playing

*Role-playing* is a method by which learners participate in an unrehearsed dramatization. They are asked to play assigned parts of a character as they think the character would act in reality. This method is a technique to arouse feelings and elicit emotional responses in the learner. It is used primarily to achieve behavioral objectives in the affective domain.

Role-playing differs from simulation, where learners are rehearsing behaviors or roles that they will need to master and apply in real life. For example, the patients in a dia-betes self-management education program will need to practice behaviors such as select-ing foods from a restaurant menu and setting their insulin pumps for the correct bolus of insulin because these are self-management skills that they are trying to master. In role-playing, on the other hand, the learner is not mastering a role with plans to use it but rather to develop understanding of other people. The nurse attending an education program, for instance, may wear an insulin pump containing saline and select the appropriate foods to "see how it feels" to have to be aware of these issues rather than for the purpose of mastering the techniques.

The responsibility of the teacher is to design a situation with enough information for learners to be able to assume character roles without actually giving them a script to follow. Occasionally, people are assigned to play themselves to rehearse desired behavior, or the instructor takes a part to act as a positive role model for the learners. Most often, however, the teacher designates members in a group to play the part of someone else, and then they pretend to be that person for the duration of the exercise. Participants do and say things that they perceive the actual person would do, say, and feel. The purpose is to help learners see and understand a problem through the eyes of others. In other words, it gives them a chance to "walk in someone else's shoes." For example, children may use role-playing with puppets to explore their responses to such illnesses as asthma (Ramsey & Siroky, 1988). When professional caregivers take the place of patients, this role reversal helps to sensitize staff to the care they deliver to their patients.

For role-playing to be employed effectively, the teacher must be sure that the group has attained a comfort level that allows each member to feel secure enough to participate in a dramatization. This method should never be used with learners in the beginning of a group session encounter. Members need time to establish a rapport with one another as well as with the instructor, or else learners may feel embarrassed or self-conscious about playing a part. All learners should be given an assignment.

Those who are actual participants need to be informed about the role they are to portray so they can effectively develop the appropriate actions. Those who are designated as observers require specific instructions about what to attend to during the role-playing session.

Role-playing is best done in small groups so that all learners can actively take part as players or as observers. Active participation by learners is particularly important during the postactivity discussion or debriefing session. Because this method is most effective for learning in the affective domain, all participants need to discuss how they felt and share what they observed to gain insight into their understanding of interpersonal relationships and their reactions to role expectations or conflicts.

Role-playing can be used in conjunction with other instructional methods, but such a combination requires careful planning as to the sequential placement of this strategy and the important points to be captured during the dramatization period. This method offers an opportunity for the learner to explore feelings and attitudes. Role-playing has the potential for bridging the gap between understanding and feeling, thereby narrowing the role distance between and among clients and professionals (Redman, 2001).

One major drawback in using this instructional method is the tendency by some participants to overly exaggerate the roles to which they have been assigned. If they become too dramatic, the part loses its realism and credibility. This approach also has limitations when participants are uncomfortable in their roles and therefore are unable to develop the roles sufficiently. Despite these disadvantages, when role-playing is planned and carried out well, it is an effective technique to help learners change feelings or attitudes.

## Role-Modeling

The use of self as a role model is often overlooked as an instructional method. Learning from *role-modeling* is called identification and emanates from socialization theories that explain how people acquire new behaviors and social roles. Nurse educators have many opportunities to demonstrate behaviors and attitudes they would like to instill in learners, whether they be patients, family members, nursing staff, or students. The competency with which you perform a skill, the way you interact with others, the personal example you set, and the enthusiasm and interest you convey about a subject or problem all can influence learners' motivation levels and the extent to which they perform a desired behavior. Role-modeling does influence attitudes and is a significant factor in achieving behavior change in the affective domain. "Actions speak louder than words" is a popular saying relevant to the use of self as a role model (de Tornyay & Thompson, 1987).

## Self-Instruction Activities

*Self-instruction* is a method used by the teacher to provide or design instructional activities that guide the learner in independently achieving the objectives of learning. Each self-study module usually focuses on one topic, and the hallmark of this format is independent study. The self-instruction method is effective for learning in the cognitive and psychomotor domains, where the goal is to master information and apply it to practice. Self-study can also be an effective adjunct for introducing principles and step-by-step guidelines prior to demonstration of a psychomotor skill. This method is sometimes difficult to identify as a singular entity because of the variety of terms used to describe it, such as "mini-course," "self-instructional package," "individualized learning activities," and "programmed instruction" (de Tornyay & Thompson, 1987). For the purposes of this discussion, the term *self-instruction* will be used and is defined as a self-contained instructional activity that allows learners to progress by themselves at their own pace (Abruzzese, 1996).

Self-instruction modules come in a variety of forms including, but not limited to, workbooks, study guides, work stations, videotapes, Internet modules, and computer programs. They are specifically designed to be used independently. The teacher serves as a facilitator–resource person to provide motivation and reinforcement for learning. This method requires less teacher time to "give" information, and each session with the learner is intended to meet individual needs.

Some learners and teachers resist the self-instructional method because it appears to depersonalize the teaching–learning process (de Tornyay & Thompson, 1987). This is not necessarily true. Communication can still occur between the teacher and the learner, but the focus of instruction is different. The amount of time for direct interaction is more limited than with other so-called traditional methods of teaching. This method adheres to the principles of adult education whereby the learner assumes responsibility for learning and is self-directed.

A self-instruction module is carefully designed to achieve preset objectives by bringing learners from diverse knowledge and skill backgrounds to a similar level of achievement prior to undertaking the next step in a series of learning activities. For example, during orientation to an agency, there may be a self-study module on pharmacology prior to staff nurses' attending mandatory medication administration classes. A self-instructional activity can be made available to educate all staff on new infection-control practices in an agency. Patients can learn breast self-examination or cardiopulmonary resuscitation techniques by using specifically prepared self-study materials. Self-instruction modules should be piloted with a small group before use with larger groups to confirm their suitability for the intended learners (Schmidt & Fisher, 1992).

Each self-instruction module needs to contain the following elements:

1. *An introduction and statement of purpose,* which generally include a table of contents, the terminal objectives, the intent of the module, and directions for its use.

2. *A list of prerequisite skills* that the learner needs to have to use the module.

3. *A list of behavioral objectives,* which are clear and measurable statements describing which skills the learner is expected to acquire on completion of the unit.

4. *A pretest* to diagnostically determine whether the learner needs to proceed with the module. Some learners may demonstrate mastery in the pretest and can move on to the next module. Other learners will get a sharper focus on their areas of weakness and may decide to seek additional preparation prior to beginning the module.

5. *An identification of resources and learning activities,* which specifies the equipment needed, such as videotapes, slides, or written materials, and outlines the actual learning activities that will be presented. Objectives are given to direct the learner, followed by material presented in small units of discrete information called frames. The total length of a well-designed module is kept relatively short so as not to dampen the motivation to learn. How the material is presented will vary with the objectives and the resources available. For example, information may be given via programmed instruction or through a series of readings on the principles of conflict resolution. This is followed by a video presentation of a relevant case with the requirement that the learner write a response to what has been read and observed.

6. *Periodic self-assessments,* which provide feedback to the learner throughout the module. The user is frequently able to do periodic self-assessments prior to moving on to the next unit. This allows the learner to decide whether the previous information

has been processed sufficiently enough to progress further.

7. *A post-test* to evaluate the learner's level of mastery in achieving the objectives. If the learner is aware that a post-test needs to be completed, this requirement encourages paying attention to the information. Keeping a record of final outcomes is helpful in both staff and patient education as documentation of competency, as proof that standards were met, and for the purpose of planning for continuing education.

Modules can be made readily accessible to learners along with any resources that are needed to complete the self-study program. Inherent in this method of teaching are the advantages of self-pacing, active learning, the chance to review and reflect on information, the ability to get frequent feedback, and a mechanism to prove mastery of material accomplished in a particular time frame. Self-instruction represents an attractive alternative to traditional classroom and group learning methods in the rapidly changing healthcare environment. Hospitals and community agencies are not able to "release" staff in large numbers for continuing education programs that are rigidly timed. This constraint conflicts with the need to share information on the newest advances and documentation of continuing competence of staff.

Self-instruction modules are excellent choices for annual training updates in selected topics or skills that require periodic review to determine competency (O'Very, 1999). One example is a series of stations with different activities related to IV competency. One station contains an infusion pump, another a model of an arm with various complications, and yet another allows nurses to practice calculations (Markiewicz & Wells, 1997).

The Internet also offers some continuing education self-instruction modules. Nurse practitioners have been educated regarding "low back pain" and "common dermatological problems in primary care" with interactive, realistic case studies. E-mail links to faculty can facilitate communication (Hayes, Huckstadt, & Gibson, 2000).

Self-instruction modules have been found to be cost-effective because they are designed to be used by large numbers of individuals with minimal and infrequent revisions. It may be less time-consuming and more efficient to purchase, rather than produce, a self-instruction module if the information presented in a commercial product is appropriate for the target audience. An example of the method's effectiveness in helping learners achieve objectives is a study that compared the use of programmed instruction and traditional classroom methods to teach nurses how to protect themselves from occupational exposure to hepatitis B virus and human immunodeficiency virus (HIV) (Goldrick, 1989). Self-instruction was found to be efficient because it took half the time to present the information than it would using classroom instruction. It was also effective because nurses who learned through programmed instruction scored higher on the post-test than did nurses who attended a lecture, regardless of their pretest scores, experiential backgrounds, or educational levels.

The use of self-instruction is limited with learners who have low literacy skills, which would impede their ability to read or comprehend information as presented. Also, learners with visual and hearing impairments, low levels of motivation, a tendency to procrastinate, or little experience with learning by self-pacing will have difficulty with this method (de Tornyay & Thompson, 1987). Self-study also may be boring if this method is overused with the same population with no variation in the activity design.

## Computer-Assisted Instruction

*Computer-assisted instruction* (CAI) is an individualized method of self-study using computers to deliver an educational activity. CAI allows learners to proceed at their own pace with immediate and continuous feedback on their progress as they respond to a software program. Most computer programs assist the learner in achieving cognitive domain skills but can also be used to master psychomotor behaviors and to change attitudes. Computers integrated with color, sound, and video motion are a type of CAI known as interactive videodisc (IAVD) or computer-assisted video instruction (CAVI). This type of instruction is more expensive because of the multimedia applications.

CAI software encompasses a variety of approaches, such as drill and practice, tutorial, simulation, and basic problem solving (Anderson, 1992). An example of a drill and practice type of application would be a program on drug calculations that teaches by continued repetition of exercises. Tutorials usually present new information to the learner such as instruction on basic or advanced anatomy and physiology principles. Clinical simulations hold great promise for teaching because learners with background knowledge and experiences are exposed to the requirements of data collection and decision making to test their skills in artificial but realistic clinical situations under very low-risk conditions. An example would be a simulation program challenging the clinical responses of nursing staff to cardiac dysrhythmias. Problem-solving software allows the learner to develop the process of seeking solutions to situations presented.

Computer games, also referred to as *edutainment* (educational software disguised in a game format), introduce content or involve the process of competition in the application of strategies for decision making toward attaining a goal. They are an enjoyable and effective way to teach specific cognitive, psychomotor, and affective skills (Green & Brightman, 1990). Lieberman (2001) reports that children and adolescents improved their self-care after engaging in interactive games related to smoking prevention, asthma, and diabetes. The players actively engaged in an appealing game that was a simulation of self-care and prevention strategies.

Computer programs can also evaluate learning. One complex type of testing is known as computerized adaptive testing (CAT). CAT presents test items and scores each response made, and then the computer decides what the next item will be based on the previous response by the learner (Halkitis & Leahy, 1993). Nursing students are using this type of testing to take their state nursing licensing examinations.

The most valuable aspect of CAI is that it actively involves the learner in the learning process and instruction is individualized to meet learner needs. The student can set the pace, spend as much time on a subject as needed for mastery, and do so in a private, nonjudgmental environment (Anderson, 1992). Computer programs have enormous possibilities for teaching fundamental as well as advanced skills. The computer is a reliable, attentive, and tolerant drill and practice partner (Green & Brightman, 1990). CAIs offer consistent presentation of material and round-the-clock accessibility. They are a time-efficient and effective instructional method that reduces student–teacher ratios (McAlindon & Smith, 1994). It has been demonstrated that CAI assists the learner in the achievement of educational objectives in about one-third the time required by traditional methodologies. This instructional method not only saves time but also accommodates different types of learners. With its extensive branching capacity, it provides multiple self-assessment opportunities to allow slow learners to repeat lessons as many times as necessary, while quick-to-grasp users can advance more rapidly or test out of a program (Armstrong, 1989).

The limitations of CAI are that it is labor-intensive if self-composed, and this type of instructional design is not a widespread skill among nurse educators (Whiteside et al., 1990). In addition, selection of CAI materials may present difficulty to the educator who is not experienced with this type of technology. Consultation with a nursing informatics specialist is suggested for educators who need to be updated on the use of and possibilities for CAI application to patient and staff education. *Nursing informatics* is an area of specialization that weds nursing education and practice with information and computer sciences. Postel (1993) suggests review criteria for educators to make the best use of limited informatics personnel and to employ the instructional and clinical expertise of other staff members. Authoring software systems are available to assist instructors in designing CAIs.

There is also concern that computer instruction depersonalizes the learning process. Nontraditional methods should not be taken to mean that the teacher is unavailable for guidance in learning. This technology simply delivers content, which allows more time for the nurse educator to concentrate on the personal aspects of individual reinforcement and ongoing assessments of learning. Because CAI requires self-motivation, this instructional method may not be adequate for learners who have an external locus of control and who need human interaction to learn best (Poston, 1993).

Evidence suggests that nurses have a slightly positive attitude toward computers (McAlindon & Smith, 1994; Scarpa et al., 1992), which will surely increase as nurses as well as the general public become more familiar with this relatively new technology. An effective approach for introducing this type of instruction would be to mix it with other methods of instruction.

Economic considerations remain a real concern because both the hardware and the software for computer instruction can be expensive. The future, however, portends enormous possibilities for widespread use of this method in institutions and agencies for purposes of patient and staff education. For example, CAIs have been used with good patient acceptance for both pre- and postoperative instruction on joint replacement (Tibbles et al., 1992). This instructional method has also been useful in teaching hospital staff nurses the concepts of quality improvement (McAlindon & Smith, 1994). The prediction is that someday soon multimedia systems for learning will be commonplace in educational settings around the globe (Green & Brightman, 1990).

## Distance Learning

*Distance learning* is a telecommunications approach to instruction using video technology to transmit live or taped messages directly from the instructor to the viewer. It is becoming more popular as an instructional technique for staff development, continuing education programs, and student learning in academic settings. Distance learning is made possible by network technology. It is particularly advantageous for cognitive domain instruction when the goal is to get information to a wide variety of people located at great distances from one another. It is an ideal way to transmit current information without incurring the cost and time in traveling needed to meet face-to-face with the expert delivering the instruction (Kaihoi, 1987).

The delivery format used with teleconferencing allows for one-way video and audio information to be sent via satellite, microwave, or ground telephone line from one place to another. It can become interactive for the learner when teleconferencing is set up to allow for call-in questions via regular telephone. Because this format can reach large audiences, it is a relatively inexpensive approach to teaching. The limitation to this delivery format is that the teacher and learner are physically removed from each other, and it can become a lecture-type, one-way interaction session if no telephone hookup is available for interactive question and answer periods.

Newer technology has overcome some of the limitations of older one-way delivery formats. University of Kentucky Center for Rural Health (UKCRH) has been using interactive video technology (IAV) since 1991 for instruction of both undergraduate and graduate students. Two-way IAV transmits voice, graphics, and full-motion video. Voice-activated microphones are fastened to student desks to facilitate communication. This format is not a lecture delivered to a camera, so the instructor needs specific skills and support to effectively use this delivery format. UKCRH has demonstrated mastery of the barriers of this format. The center staff's expertise and the motivation of their students has led to a very low dropout rate of 2.6% over five years. Some of the recommendations from their experience with this form of distance learning follow (Ware, Oleniski, Cole, & Pray, 1998):

- Provide course materials to the remote site well in advance of the class. Lecture notes and other materials can be placed on the World Wide Web.

- Use graphics experts to aid in the design of materials specifically for this medium.

- Present an early class at the remote site to meet students "face to face." Have an off-site facilitator at each class.

- Begin and end classes by letting students ask questions and voice concerns.

- Encourage interaction by using discussions, debates, and/or case studies. Give students extra time to respond to or ask questions if there is a audio delay. Balance the interactions with students at the remote site and the local site.

- Have on-line office hours.

- Train instructors to use the technology effectively prior to use.

- Be sure the system technician understands your needs before class begins. Have technical support available at all times and at all sites.

• Have a plan and contact numbers for technical failures.

As large healthcare networks develop, this method may be useful for staff development and for patient education in a multicenter network.

Distance has also been eliminated as a barrier through access to the Internet. This network provides the learner with ready access to a vast array of resources such as databases and human expertise in a variety of fields. This global resource is limited only by the learner's inquiry skills and energy. In the rapidly changing world of health care, there will be increasing reliance on this source for both clinicians and consumers. (See Chapter 13 for information on how to evaluate Internet sites.)

The Internet can also be a source for patient or consumer information in both English and other languages. But how accurate and readable is the information for the consumer? Berland et al. (2001) evaluated health information on the Internet regarding breast cancer, depression, obesity, and childhood asthma in both English and Spanish. They looked at accessibility, quality, and reading level. Their findings indicate that access to information was inefficient when using search engines and simple key phrases. Only half of the topics that expert panels thought important for consumers were covered more than minimally on English-language sites. This problem was even worse on Spanish-language sites. The reading level was also high. English sites required at least a tenth-grade reading level on most sites and, with one exception, the Spanish sites required at least a ninth-grade reading level.

Table 11–1 summarizes the general characteristics of instructional methods.

## SELECTION OF INSTRUCTIONAL METHODS

The process of selecting an instructional method requires a prior determination of the behavioral objectives to be accomplished and an assessment of the learners who will be involved in achieving the objectives. Also, consideration must be given to available resources such as time, money, space, and materials to support learning activities. The teacher is also an important variable in the selection and effectiveness of a method.

Teachers are at different levels on the novice-to-expert continuum, and how seasoned they are influences their choices of instructional methods. An expert skilled at facilitating small-group discussion may be a novice in the design and selection of CAI. A nurse may be an expert clinician but have only limited experience and effectiveness in the teaching role. Nurses are expected to teach but may not have adequate time, inclination, energy, or capability for developing the quality and variety of instruction necessary. Teaching is a skill that can be developed in formal academic settings, in continuing education programs, or through guidance by an expert peer mentor.

Teachers are likely to focus on a particular method because it is the one they feel most comfortable using without considering all the criteria for selection. There is no one right method, because the best approach depends on many variables, such as the audience, the content to be taught, the setting in which teaching–learning is to take place, and the resources at your disposal. Nevertheless, the ideal method for any given situation is the one that best suits the learner's needs, not your own. If you are a novice, begin instruction with very familiar content so that you can focus on the teaching process itself and feel more confident in trying out different techniques and instructional materials. Ask questions of learners and peers in the evaluation process to ascertain whether the method chosen was appropriate for accomplishing the behavioral objectives and meeting the needs of different learners in terms of their learning styles and readiness to learn.

Narrow (1979) emphasized the importance of periodically examining your role as a

**TABLE 11–1  General characteristics of instructional methods**

| Methods | Domain | Learner Role | Teacher Role | Advantages | Limitations |
|---|---|---|---|---|---|
| Lecture | Cognitive | Passive | Presents information | Cost-effective<br>Targets large groups | Not individualized |
| Group discussion | Affective<br>Cognitive | Active—if learner participates | Guides and focuses discussion | Stimulates sharing ideas and emotions | Shy or dominant member<br>High levels of diversity |
| One-to-one instruction | Cognitive<br>Affective<br>Psychomotor | Active | Presents information and facilitates individualized learning | Tailored to individual's needs and goals | Labor-intensive<br>Isolates learner |
| Demonstration | Cognitive | Passive | Models skill or behavior | Preview of "exact" skill/behavior | Small groups needed to facilitate visualization |
| Return demonstration | Psychomotor | Active | Individualizes feedback to refine performance | Immediate individual guidance | Labor-intensive to view individual performance |
| Gaming | Cognitive<br>Affective | Active—if learner participates | Oversees pacing<br>Referees<br>Debriefs | Captures learner enthusiasm | Environment too competitive for some learners |
| Simulation | Cognitive<br>Psychomotor | Active | Designs environment<br>Facilitates process<br>Debriefs | Practice "reality" in safe setting | Labor-intensive<br>Equipment costs |
| Role-playing | Affective | Active | Designs format<br>Debriefs | Develops understanding of others | Exaggeration or under-development of role |
| Role-modeling | Affective<br>Cognitive | Passive | Models skill or behavior | Helps with socialization to role | Requires rapport |
| Self-instruction | Cognitive<br>Psychomotor | Active | Designs package<br>Gives individual feedback | Self-paced<br>Cost-effective<br>Consistent | Procrastination<br>Requires literacy |
| Computer-assisted instruction | Cognitive | Active | Purchases or designs program<br>Provides individual feedback | Immediate and continuous feedback<br>Private<br>Individualized | Costly to design or purchase<br>Must have hardware |
| Distance learning | Cognitive | Passive | Presents information<br>Answers questions | Targets learners who are at varying distances from expert | Lack of personal contact<br>Accessibility |

teacher and assessing the factors of energy, attitudes, knowledge, and skills, which influence the priority you assign to teaching and the ability to teach effectively. The following is a summary of her suggestions.

At any given point in time, your energy level will be influenced by both psychological and physical factors, such as the amount of satisfaction you derive from your work, the demands and responsibilities of your professional and personal life, and the state of your health. Your feelings toward the learner also influence the enthusiasm you bring to the teaching–learning situation. If you feel drawn to the learners because you find them interesting or you are concerned or anxious about their situation, then teaching will most likely be a satisfying experience. If, on the other hand, the learners are demanding or display inappropriate behavior, you may feel negatively toward them and find the teaching–learning encounter more difficult and less fulfilling. You can develop the ability to accept individuals without necessarily approving of their behavior.

Another factor to consider is your comfort with and confidence in the nature of the subject matter to be taught. If you find certain content to be stressful to teach because you lack relevant knowledge or skills, then additional study and practice to increase your understanding of the subject will likely relieve your stress and apprehension, allowing you to function more effectively in the teaching role. If you have difficulty communicating with learners about what you may consider sensitive material, such as sexual behavior, mental illness, abortion, birth defects, disfigurement, terminal illness, and the like, it would be important for you to examine your own feelings, seek support from colleagues, and use resources to help create an effective teaching approach. If the teaching–learning process is to be a partnership, not only is it crucial to assess the learner but it is equally important to assess yourself as the teacher. Often teachers

fail to take into account their own circumstances and needs.

## EVALUATION OF INSTRUCTIONAL METHODS

An important aspect of evaluating any instructional program is to assess the effectiveness of the method. Was the choice selected as effective, efficient, and appropriate as possible? There are five major questions to ask yourself that will help you to decide which method to choose or if the method selected should be revised or rejected:

1. *Does the method help the learners to achieve the stated objectives?* This question is the most important criterion for evaluation—if the method does not facilitate accomplishing the objectives, then all the other criteria are unimportant. Examine how well matched the method is to the learning domain of the predetermined objectives. Will the method expose learners to the necessary information and training to learn the desired behaviors?

2. *Is the learning activity accessible to the learners you have targeted?* Accessibility includes such issues as when information is presented, the location and setting in which teaching takes place, and the availability of resources and equipment to deliver your message. Patients and family members need programs to be offered at suitable times and accessible locations. For example, childbirth preparation classes scheduled during the daytime hours likely would not be convenient for expectant couples who are working.

3. *Is the method efficient given the time, energy, and resources available in relation to the number of learners you are trying to reach?* To teach large numbers of learners, you will have to choose a method that can accommodate groups, such as lecture, discussion sessions, or role-playing, or a method that

can reach many individuals at one time, such as the use of various self-instructional formats or CAI.

4. *To what extent does the method allow for active participation to accommodate the needs, abilities, and style of the learner?* Active participation has been well documented as a way to increase interest in learning and the retention of information. Evaluate how active learners want to be or are able to be in the process of gaining knowledge and skills. No one method will satisfy all learners, but adhering to one method will exclusively address the preferred style of only a segment of your audience.

5. *Is the method cost-effective?* It is vital to examine the cost of educational programs to determine whether similar outcomes might be achieved by using less costly methodologies. In this era of cost containment, insurers want their monies invested in patient programs that yield the best possible outcomes at the lowest price as measured in terms of preventing illness and injury, minimizing the severity and extent of illness, and reducing the length of hospital stays and readmissions. Healthcare agencies want the best staff nurse performance with the most reasonable use of resources and the least amount of time taken away from actual practice.

## ▆ INCREASING EFFECTIVENESS OF TEACHING

Excellent teachers have one thing in common—a passion to keep improving their abilities. One does not "arrive" at being an expert teacher. The drive toward excellence is an ongoing process that continues throughout the teacher's entire professional life. What constitutes creative teaching? What personal attributes does the creative teacher possess? The following are techniques, not listed in any particular order, that creative teachers use to enhance the effectiveness of verbal presentations. In addition, some general principles for teaching are also put forth that can be used by all teachers.

## Creative Techniques to Enhance the Effectiveness of Verbal Presentations

*Present information enthusiastically.*   The teacher who comes across as invested in the material excites the learner to identify with the subject at hand. No matter how well a lesson is planned or how clearly it is presented, if it is delivered in a dry and dull monotone, it will likely fall on deaf ears (Cunningham & Baker, 1986). Try to vary the quality and pitch of your voice, use a variety of gestures and facial expressions, change position if necessary to make direct and frequent eye contact with everyone in the group, and demonstrate an ardent interest in the topic to attract and fascinate an audience. The enthusiastic teacher is aware that an energetic attitude is contagious and enticing. However, one must exercise caution in overusing body language and overt actions because mannerisms can be distracting and can adversely affect learning.

*Include humor.*   Many creative teachers use humor as a technique to grab, arouse, and maintain the attention of the learner. Appropriate humor can help establish a rapport with learners by humanizing the teacher. Humor does not necessarily require the teacher to tell jokes, and joke telling should not be attempted if this is not a skill one possesses. Furthermore, the teacher should avoid making someone the object of humor if it results in a "put-down." Humor establishes an atmosphere that allows for human error without embarrassment and encourages freedom and comfort to explore alternatives in the learning situations. Humor is a means to reduce anxiety when dealing with sensitive material, to provide poignant examples of everyday life experiences, and to reinforce traditional teaching methods (Freitas et al., 1991).

*Exhibit risk-taking behavior.* Creative teachers are willing to develop exercises in which many variables can lead to any number of possible outcomes. They use this technique to encourage learners to reach their own conclusions about controversial issues. Regardless of the outcome, creative teachers are prepared to deal with uncertainty. Exercises that allow learners freedom to experiment and express their ideas focus more on the process than on the result (Freitas et al., 1991).

*Deliver material dramatically.* Creative teachers seek ways to engage the learner emotionally by using surprise, controlled tension, or ploys. The teacher uses strategies that connect the educational material directly to the learner's life experiences so that information is made more understandable and relevant. Learners may be asked to participate in simulations, games, or role-playing to act out a part, live an experience, or test their capacities. These activities involve the learner and can leave a profound, lasting impression that can be recalled vividly and can be drawn upon when faced with a real situation. This technique engages learners by arousing their emotions (Freitas et al., 1991).

*Choose problem-solving activities.* Whether the learners are staff members or patients, the creative teacher recognizes that learners need to be immersed in activities to help them develop problem-solving skills. In today's world, professionals must have the ability to identify both patient and system problems by searching and sorting data, uncovering problems, and finding solutions. Increasingly, they are expected to work with interdisciplinary teams to determine and implement solutions to healthcare problems. Learning activities must be designed to help these nursing staff members and students develop critical thinking and collaborative skills. Patients, especially those with chronic conditions, need problem-solving skills to know how to respond to changes demanded by their condi-

tion. What should they do differently on a "sick day," or what constitutes an emergency? Patients and families need more than just low-level cognitive information to make adjustments in their lives. The teacher must therefore devise and orchestrate opportunities that challenge learners to critically analyze situations as well as support the learner in exploring possible alternative situations. The creative teacher encourages brainstorming sessions and supports the testing out of possible answers by the more nontraditional methods of teaching.

*Serve as a role model.* The creative teacher constantly seeks new information by keeping abreast of current research, theories, and issues in clinical practice for application relevant to the teaching situation. Expanding one's own knowledge base gives credence to what is taught and gains the confidence of learners in the teacher's expertise. A commitment to lifelong learning transmits an important value to others of their need for continuous personal or professional development. As part of the creative teacher's repertoire of behavior, role-modeling is an effective way to facilitate learning. Teachers are seen as credible role models when they are actively engaged in scholarly activities, are experienced in the field, and have advanced credentials to teach complex skills. The believability of a role model is greatly affected by the values displayed and the congruence demonstrated between what the teacher says and does (Babcock & Miller, 1994). If the learners regard the behavior of the creative teacher as desirable, they will likely imitate that behavior, which they perceive as eliciting positive effects (Narrow, 1979).

*Use anecdotes and examples.* The creative teacher uses stories, tales, and examples of incidences and episodes to illustrate points. Anecdotes, whether amusing, alarming, sad, or anger-provoking, are valuable in driving a point home, clarifying a topic under discussion, or helping someone better relate to an issue. Use examples to reinforce the learning principle that simple representations can assist the learner to grasp complex ideas. Using examples relevant to past experiences and the knowledge base of learners helps them identify and connect in a concrete way with the material being taught.

*Use technology.* Creative teachers use technology to broaden and add variety to the opportunities for teaching and learning. They continue to increase the level of their own skills by taking advantage of the advances in technology to introduce and coach others in new ways of learning. They recognize that the sophisticated use of technology is a primary skill that will be needed for educational programs of the future. The use of different types of technology assists the teacher in helping learners meet their individual needs and styles of learning. Technology has the potential for making the teaching–learning process more convenient, accessible, and stimulating. Creative teachers are future-oriented. A mastery of technological skills assures their ability to teach in innovative and eclectic ways to prepare students for learning into the twenty-first century.

## General Principles for All Teachers

*Give positive reinforcement.* Educational research is replete with examples of the effects of positive reinforcement on learning. Acknowledging ideas, actions, and opinions of others by using words of praise or approval, such as "That's a good answer," "I agree with you," and "You have a very good point," or using nonverbal expressions of acceptance, such as smiling, nodding, or a reassuring pat on the back, will encourage learners to participate more readily or try harder to improve their performance. Rewarding even a small success can instill satisfaction in the learner. Reproval, on the other hand, will dampen motivation and cause learners to withdraw.

A powerful incentive is to ask learners to share their experiences with others. In a group, it is important to recognize the contributions of each member rather than focus primarily on the more aggressive learner or high achiever. What constitutes positive reinforcement for one individual may not suffice for another, as rewards are closely tied to value systems. The quantity of reinforcement will also vary in its effectiveness from one individual to another. A small amount of praise can have a strong effect on the learner who is not used to succeeding, whereas significant praise may be relatively ineffective for a consistently high achiever. The effects of reinforcement are also transitory. An incentive that works for a learner at one time may not work well at another time.

Positive reinforcers, in the form of recognition, tangible rewards, or opportunities, should closely follow the desired behavior (de Tornyay & Thompson, 1987). The clearer the correlation between the desired behavior and the reward, the more meaningful the reinforcement will be.

*Project an attitude of acceptance and sensitivity.* The ease with which teachers conduct themselves, the willingness to receive and answer questions, the simple courtesies extended, and the responsiveness demonstrated toward an audience set the tone for a friendly, warm, and receptive atmosphere for learning. If you exhibit self-confidence and self-respect, the learner in turn will feel comfortable, confident, and secure in the learning environment. If you come across as believable, trustworthy, considerate, and competent, you help to put your audience at ease, which serves as an invitation for them to learn. When you exercise patience and sensitivity with respect to age, race, culture, and gender, this projects an acceptance of others, which serves to establish a rapport and opens up the avenues of communication for the sharing of ideas and concerns. People will learn better in a comfortable and supportive environment. Not only is it important that the physical environment be conducive to learning, but the psychological climate should also be respectful of learners and focused on their need for an atmosphere of support and acceptance. Teachers must have a clear view of their role as facilitators and expert coaches and avoid acting as controlling disseminators of information.

*Be organized and give direction.* Excellent discussions, meaningful experiences in role-playing, or successful attempts at self-study are examples of teaching that do not happen by accident. They are the result of hours of skilled preparation, careful planning, and organization, which allow the learner to stay focused on the objectives. Material should be logically organized, objectives clearly defined and presented up front, and directions given in a straightforward, specific, and easily understood manner. Instructional sessions should be relatively brief so as not to overload the learner with too much detail and extraneous content. "Need to know" information should take precedence over the "nice to know" information to ensure that enough time is allotted for the essentials. Regardless of the method of instruction used, the attention span of the learner waxes and wanes over time, and what is learned first and last is retained the most (Ley, 1972). Audiovisual materials selected to supplement various methods of teaching should clarify or enhance a message. Advance organizers should be used to structure information and assist the learner in identifying the subject to be presented and in what order.

*Elicit and give feedback.* Feedback should be a reciprocal process. It is a strategy to give information to the learner as well as to receive information from the learner. Both the teacher and the learner need to seek information about the quality of their performance. Feedback should be encouraged during and at the end of each teaching–learning encounter as well as at the completion of an educational

program. It can take the form of either verbal or nonverbal responses to a situation.

Feedback that learners receive can be subjective or objective. Subjective data, whether physiological or psychological, come from within the learners themselves. People sense how they are reacting to a situation. Internally, they usually know how well they performed or how they feel by their own responses, such as fatigue, anxiety, disinterest, or satisfaction. Learners are able to compare their own performance to what they expect of themselves or what they think others expect of them. Objective data come to the learners from the teacher, who measures their behavior based on a set of standards or criteria and who gives them an opinion on the progress they have made. To get feedback, the learner might ask, "How well did I do?", "Am I on track?", "Did I do all right?", or "What do you think?"

Feedback to the teacher is equally important because the effectiveness of teaching depends to a great extent on the learners' reactions. Whether positive or negative, verbal or nonverbal, feedback enables you to determine if you should maintain or modify your approach to teaching. Feedback indicates whether to proceed, take time to review or explain, or cease instruction altogether for the moment. The teacher should be direct in eliciting feedback from the learners by asking questions such as "Did I answer your questions?", "Is this clear?", "Do you need me to explain it further?", or "What more can I help you with?" The teacher should also be sensitive to nonverbal expressions such as a nod, a smile, a look of bewilderment, or a frown indicating an understanding or lack thereof.

Feedback is neutral unless it is compared with established norms, preset criteria, or past behavior. How much someone learned, for example, is meaningless unless compared to what the person knew previously or how the person stacks up against other learners under similar conditions. Feedback, either positive or negative, is needed by both the learner and the teacher. Praise reinforces behavior and increases the likelihood the behavior will continue. Constructive criticism tends to redirect behavior to conform with expected norms. Labeling someone's personality as cooperative, smart, stubborn, unmotivated, or uncaring is harmful, but it is helpful to label someone's performance to give that person specific information for improving, correcting, or continuing the behavior (Narrow, 1979).

*Use questions.* Questioning is one of the means for both the teacher and the learner to elicit feedback about performance. If the teacher is skillful in the use of questioning, it serves multiple purposes in the teaching–learning process. Questions help to clarify or substantiate concepts, assess what the learner already knows about the topic, stimulate interest in a new subject, or evaluate the learner's mastery of the predetermined objectives.

Babcock and Miller (1994) identified three types of questions that can be used to elicit different types of answers. The first type of question is known as a factual or descriptive question. It begins with words such as *who, what, where,* or *when* and asks for recall-type responses from the learner. Factual questions such as "Which foods are high in fat?" or "Whom should you call if you run out of medication?" elicit straightforward facts. Descriptive questions take a more open-ended approach, such as "What kinds of exercise do you get daily?", "What problems do you have with activities of daily living?", or "What are the signs and symptoms of infection?", and require a more detailed and organized response from the learner.

The second type of question involves clarifying questions that ask for more information and help the learner to convey thoughts and feelings. Such questions might include "What do you mean when you say . . . ?" or "I'm not sure I understand exactly what you are expressing."

The third type of question, known as a high-order question, requires more than

memory or perception to answer by asking the learner to make inferences, establish cause and effect, or compare and contrast concepts. Examples include "Why does a low-salt diet help to control blood pressure?" or "What do you think will happen if you don't take your medication?" or "What do you see as the advantages and disadvantages in following the treatment plan?" After asking questions, a period of silence may occur, which can be uncomfortable for both the teacher and the learner. Anxiety over silence may be reduced by encouraging the learner to think about the answer before responding. In a group, this strategy also allows all participants to have a chance to think through their responses to the questions, which gives them the opportunity to make more thoughtful and deliberate responses. Questioning helps the teacher appropriately pace the material being presented and arrive at an evaluative judgment as to the progress the learner is making in the achievement of the behavioral objectives.

*Know your audience.* The effectiveness of teaching will be severely limited when the choice of instructional method is based on the interest and comfort level of the teacher and not on the assessed needs of the learner (Freitas et al., 1991). Use methods that match the topic rather than the teacher's personality. Most teachers have a preferred style of teaching and tend to rely on that approach regardless of the content to be taught. Skilled teachers adapt themselves to a teaching style appropriate to the subject matter, setting, and various styles of the learners. Flexibility is their hallmark in tailoring the instructional design to the unique needs of each population of learners. Be willing to use a variety of teaching methods to provide the best possible experience for achievement of objectives.

*Use repetition and pacing.* Repetition, if used with discretion, is a technique that strengthens learning. It reinforces learning by aiding in the retention of information. If overused, repetition can lead to boredom and frustration because you are repeating what is already understood and remembered. If used deliberately, it can assist the learner in focusing on important points and keep the learner on track. Repetition is especially important when presenting new or difficult material. The opportunity for repeated practice of behavioral tasks is called skill inoculation. Repetition can take the form of a simple reminder, a review of previously learned material, or the continued practice of a skill. Assessing the learner's understanding will help you to use repetition effectively.

Pacing refers to the speed at which information is presented. Some self-instruction methods of teaching, such as programmed instruction, allow for individualized pacing so that learners can proceed at their own speed, depending on their abilities and style of learning. Other methods of group learning require the teacher to take command of the rate at which information is presented and processed. Many factors determine the optimal rate of teaching, such as previous history with learning, attention span, the domain in which

learning is to take place, the learner's eagerness and determination to obtain a reward or attain a goal, the degree of progress in learning, and the learner's ability to cope with frustration and discomfort. Keeping in touch with your audience will help you to pace your teaching so that it is slow enough for assimilation of information, yet fast enough to maintain interest and enthusiasm (Narrow, 1979).

*Summarize important points.* Summarizing of information at the completion of the teaching–learning encounter gives a perspective on what has been covered, how it relates to the objectives, and what you expect the learner to have achieved. Summarizing also reviews key ideas to instill information in the mind and helps the learner to see the parts of a whole. Closure should be used at the end of one lesson before proceeding to a new topic.

Summary reinforces retention of information. It provides feedback as to the progress made, thereby leaving the learner with a feeling of satisfaction with what has been accomplished.

## SUMMARY

This chapter has presented all of the major traditional and nontraditional methods of instruction. An in-depth review of the various instructional methods highlighted the means for effective use, addressed the specific domains for learning, and compared the advantages and limitations of each approach. Emphasis was given to the importance of taking into account the learner characteristics, behavioral objectives, teacher characteristics, and available resources prior to selecting or designing any of the vast array of methods at the teacher's disposal. In many instances, guidelines were put forth to assist nurse educators in planning and developing their own instructional activities. In addition, the major questions to be considered when evaluating the effectiveness of instructional methods were assessed in detail. Lastly, but equally as

important as selecting the right method, were the strategies a creative teacher uses as well as the general principles all teachers should use to effectively communicate with learners.

What must be stressed are the inherent qualities of each method and the fact that no one method is better than another. The effectiveness of any method depends on the purpose for and the circumstances under which it is used. Nurses in the role of educators are urged to take an eclectic approach to teaching by avoiding reliance on any one particular method and by using a combination of teaching methods to accomplish the objectives for learning while at the same time meeting the different needs and styles of each and every learner. Multisensory stimulation is best for increasing the acquisition of skills and the retention of information.

## REVIEW QUESTIONS

1. How is the term *instructional method* defined?
2. Which instructional methods are considered to be traditional and which are considered to be nontraditional?
3. What are the strengths and limitations of lecture, group discussion, and one-to-one as instructional methods?
4. Which instructional methods encourage active participation by the learner?
5. Which instructional methods are best for learning cognitive skills? Psychomotor skills? Affective skills?
6. What instructional methods isolate the learner from others who may have similar needs/concerns?
7. What is meant by the term "pooled ignorance" and in which method does this likely occur?
8. What are the six (6) variables that influence the selection of any method of instruction?
9. What major questions should you ask yourself when evaluating the effectiveness of any instructional method?
10. Which question posed in Question 9 above is considered to be the most important criterion for evaluation?
11. What is the difference between factual/descriptive questions, clarifying questions, and high-order questions?
12. What are the techniques that creative teachers use to enhance the effectiveness of teaching?
13. Are teachers born or made? Explain.
14. What quality do all expert teachers have in common?

## REFERENCES

Abruzzese, R. S. (1996). *Nursing Staff Development: Strategies for Success*, 2nd ed. St. Louis: Mosby–Year Book.

Anderson, J. M. (1990). Health care across cultures. *Nursing Outlook, 38*, 136–139.

Anderson, S. K. (1992). *Computer Literacy for Health Care Professionals*. Albany, NY: Delmar.

Armstrong, M. L. (1989). Orchestrating the process of patient education. *Nursing Clinics of North America, 24*, 597–604.

Arnold, E. & Boggs, K. (1989). *Interpersonal Relationships*. Philadelphia: Saunders.

Babcock, D. E. & Miller, M. A. (1994). *Client Education: Theory and Practice*. St. Louis: Mosby–Year Book.

Bays, C. & Hermann, C. (1997). Gaming versus lecture discussion: Effects on students' test performance. *Journal of Nursing Education, 36*(6), 292–294.

Berland, G, Elliot, M., Morales, L., Algazy, J., Kravitz, R., Broder, M., Kanouse, D., Munoz, J., Puyol, J-A., Lara, M., Watkins, K., Yang, H., & McGlynn, E. (2001). Health information on the Internet—Accessibility, quality, and readability in English and Spanish. *Journal of the American Medical Association, 285*(20), 2612–2621.

Boyd, M. D., Gleit, C. J., Graham, B. A., & Whitman, N. I (1998). *Health Teaching in Nursing Practice: A Professional Model*, 3rd ed. Stamford, CT: Appleton and Lange.

Brookfield, S. D. & Preskill, S. (1999). *Discussion as a Way of Teaching: Tools and Techniques for Democratic Classrooms*. San Francisco: Jossey-Bass.

Cuda, S., Doerr, D., & Gonzalez, M. (1999). Using facilitators in mock codes: Recasting the parts for success. *Journal of Continuing Education in Nursing, 30*(6), 279–283.

Cunningham, M. A. & Baker, D. (1986). How to teach patients better and faster. *RN, 49*(9), 50–52.

del Bueno, D. J., Griffin, L. R., Burke, S. M., & Foley, M. A. (1990). The clinical teacher as a critical link in competence development. *Journal of Nursing Staff Development, 6*, 135–138.

de Tornyay, R. & Thompson, M. A. (1987). *Strategies for Teaching Nursing*, 3rd ed. New York: Wiley.

Evans, M. (2000). Polished, professional presentation: Unlocking the design elements. *Journal of Continuing Education in Nursing, 31*(5), 213–218.

Fredette, S. L. (1990). A model for improving cancer patient education. *Cancer Nursing, 13*, 207–215.

Freitas, L., Lantz, J., & Reed, R. (1991). The creative teacher. *Nurse Educator, 16*(1), 5–7.

Goldrick, B. A. (1989). Programmed instruction revisited: A solution to infection control inservice education. *Journal of Continuing Education in Nursing, 20*, 222–227.

Green, P. & Brightman, A. J. (1990). *Independence Day: Designing Computer Solutions for Individuals with Disabilities*. Olm Park, Allen, TX: Apple Computer.

Haggard, A. (1989). *Handbook of Patient Education*. Rockville, MD: Aspen.

Halkitis, P. N. & Leahy, J. M. (1993). Computer adaptive testing: The future is upon us. *Nursing & Health Care, 14*, 378–384.

Hayes, K., Huckstadt, A., & Gibson, R. (2000). Developing interactive continuing education on the Web. *Journal of Continuing Education in Nursing, 31*(5), 199–203.

House, B. M., Chassie, M. B., & Spohn, B. B. (1990). Questioning: An essential ingredient in effective teaching. *Journal of Continuing Education in Nursing, 21*, 196–201.

Jeska, S. B. & Cosgrove, K. (1992). Education centers: Which features are best? *Journal of Nursing Staff Development, 8*, 109–113.

Joos, I. R. M. (1984). A teacher's guide for using games and simulation. *Nurse Educator, 9*(3), 25–29.

Kaihoi, B. H. (1987). Implementing use of learning resources in our technical age. In C. E. Smith (ed.), *Patient Education: Nurses in Partnership with Other Health Professionals* (pp. 189–232). Philadelphia: Saunders.

Kaplan, S. H., Greenfield, S., & Ware, J. E. Jr. (1989). Assessing the effects of physician–patient interactions on the outcomes of chronic disease. *Medical Care, 27*(Suppl. 3), S110–S127.

Kleinknecht, M. K. & Hefferin, E. A. (1990). Maximizing nursing staff development: The learning laboratory. *Journal of Nursing Staff Development, 6*, 219–224.

Lewis, D. J., Saydak, S. J., Mierzwa, I. P., & Robinson, J. A. (1989). Gaming: A teaching strategy for adult learners. *Journal of Continuing Education in Nursing, 20*, 80–84.

Ley, P. (1972). Primacy, rated importance, and recall of medical statements. *Journal of Health and Social Behavior, 13*, 311–317.

Lieberman, D. (2001). Management of chronic pediatric diseases with interactive health games: Theory and research findings. *Journal of Ambulatory Care Management, 24*(1), 26–38.

Lorig, K. & Gonzalez, V. M. (1993). Using self-efficacy theory in patient education. In B. Gilroth (ed.), *Managing Hospital-Based Patient Education* (pp. 327–337). Chicago, IL: American Hospital Publishing.

Lupien, A. & George-Gay, B. (2001). High fidelity patient simulation. In Lowenstein, A. & Bradshaw, M. (eds.) *Fuszard's Innovative Teaching Strategies in Nursing*, 3rd ed. (pp. 134–148). Gaithersburg, MD: Aspen Publication.

Markiewicz, T. & Wells, N. (1997). Mundanatories no more. *Journal of Continuing Education in Nursing, 28*(2), 88–90.

McAlindon, M. N. & Smith, G. R. (1994). Repurposing videodiscs for interactive video instruction: Teaching concepts of quality improvement. *Computers in Nursing, 12*, 46–56.

Narrow, B. (1979). *Patient Teaching in Nursing Practice: A Patient and Family Centered Approach*. New York: Wiley.

O'Very, D. (1999). Self-paced: The right pace for staff development. *Journal of Continuing Education in Nursing, 30*(4), 182–187.

Peters, F. L. & Connell, K. M. (1991). Incorporating the affective component into an AIDS workshop. *Journal of Continuing Education in Nursing, 22*, 95–99.

Postel, N. (1993). Guidelines for the evaluation of instructional software by hospital nursing departments. *Computers in Nursing, 11*(6), 273–276.

Poston, I. (1993). How to develop computer assisted instruction programs. *Nursing & Health Care, 14*, 344–349.

Prochaska, J., DiClemente, C., & Norcross, J. (1992). In search of how people change—Applications to addictive behaviors. *American Psychologist, 47*(9), 1102–1114.

Prochaska, J., DiClemente, C., Velicer, W., & Rossi, J. (1993). Standardized, individualized, interactive, and personalized self-help programs for smoking cessation. *Health Psychology, 12*(5), 399–405.

Prochaska, J., Velicer, W., Rossi, J., Goldstein, M., Marcus, B., Rakowski, W., Fiore, C., Harlow, L., Redding, C., Rosenbloom, D., & Rossi, S. (1994). Stages of change and decisional balance for 12 problem behaviors. *Health Psychology, 13*(1), 39–46.

Ramsey, A. M. & Siroky, A. S. (1988). The use of puppets to teach school age children with asthma. *Pediatric Nursing, 14*, 187–190.

Redman, B. K. (2001). *The Practice of Patient Education*, 9th ed. St. Louis: Mosby.

Robinson, K. J., Lewis, D. J., & Robinson, J. A. (1990). Games: A way to give laboratory values meaning. *American Nephrology Nurses Association Journal, 17*, 306–308.

Rorden, J. W. (1987). *Nurses as Health Teachers: A Practical Guide*. Philadelphia: Saunders.

Rothwell, W. J. & Kazanas, H. C. (1992). *Mastering the Instructional Design Process: A Systematic Approach*. San Francisco: Jossey-Bass.

Rowell, S. & Spielvogle, S. (1996). Wanted: "A few good bug detectives." A gaming technique to increase staff awareness of current infection control practices. *Journal of Continuing Education in Nursing, 27*(6), 274–278.

Rystedt, H. & Lindström, B. (2001). Introducing simulation technologies in nurse education: A nursing practice perspective. *Nurse Education in Practice, 1*(3), 134–141.

Saarmann, L., Daugherty, J., & Riegel, B. (2000). Patient teaching to promote behavior change. *Nursing Outlook, 48*(6), 281–287.

Scarpa, R., Smeltzer, S. C., & Jasion, B. (1992). Attitudes of nurses toward computerization: A replication. *Computers in Nursing, 10*, 72–79.

Schmidt, K. L. & Fisher, J. C. (1992). Effective development and utilization of self-learning modules. *Journal of Continuing Education in Nursing, 23*, 54–59.

Schmitz, B. D., MacLean, S. L., & Shidler, H. M. (1991). An emergency pursuit game: A method for teaching emergency decision making skills. *Journal of Continuing Education in Nursing, 22*, 152–158.

Tibbles, L., Lewis, C., Reisine, S., Rippey, R., & Donald, M. (1992). Computer assisted instruction for preoperative and postoperative patient education in joint replacement surgery. *Computers in Nursing, 10*, 208–211.

Walts, N. S. (1982). Games and simulations. *Nursing Management, 13*(2), 28–29.

Ware, S., Oleninski, R., Cole, C., & Pray, M. (1998). Teaching at a distance using interactive video. *Journal of Allied Health, 27*(3), 137–141.

Whiteside, M. F., McCulloch, J., & Whiteside, J. A. (1990). Helping hospital educators and clinical nurse specialists learn to use and develop computer assisted instruction. *Journal of Continuing Education in Nursing, 21*, 113–117.

Wood, R. Y. (1994). Use of the nursing simulation laboratory in reentry programs: An innovative setting for updating clinical skills. *Journal of Continuing Education in Nursing, 25*, 28–31.

## CHAPTER 12

# Instructional Materials

*Diane S. Hainsworth*

## CHAPTER HIGHLIGHTS

General Principles

Choosing Instructional Materials

The Three Major Components of Instructional Materials

    Delivery System

    Content

    Presentation

Types of Instructional Materials

    Written Materials

    Demonstration Materials

    Audiovisual Materials

Evaluation Criteria for Selecting Materials

## KEY TERMS

instructional materials

delivery system

realia

illusionary representations

replica

analogue

symbol

audiovisual materials

learner, media, and task characteristics

## OBJECTIVES

After completing this chapter, the reader will be able to

1. Differentiate between instructional materials and methods of instruction.

2. Identify the three major variables (learner, task, and media characteristics) to be considered when selecting, developing, and evaluating instructional materials.

3. Cite the three components of instructional materials required to effectively communicate educational messages.

4. Discuss general principles applicable to all types of media.

5. Identify the multitude of audiovisual tools—both print and nonprint materials—available for patient and professional education.

6. Describe guidelines for development of printed materials.

7. Analyze the advantages and disadvantages specific to each type of instructional medium.

8. Evaluate the type of media suitable for use depending on the characteristics of the audience, seating, preference, resources available, nature of the subject, and characteristics of the learner, such as age, literacy level, and sensory deficits.

9. Identify where educational tools can be found.

10. Critique tools for value and appropriateness.

11. Recognize the supplemental nature of media's role in patient education.

Whereas instructional methods are the approaches or processes used for instructor–client communications, instructional materials are the resources and tools used as vehicles to help communicate the information. Often the terms *instructional strategy, instructional design,* and *teaching technique* serve to describe both the methods and the materials used in teaching. Instructional materials are tangible substances and real objects that provide the audio and/or visual component necessary for learning. Many of them can be manipulated. They stimulate a learner's senses and may have the power to arouse emotions. They help the teacher make sense of abstractions and simplify complex messages (Babcock & Miller, 1994).

In this chapter, the term *instructional materials,* also referred to as tools and aids, includes both print and nonprint media that are intended to supplement, rather than replace, actual teaching. The selection and development of materials used for teaching form a complex component of the educational process, yet the means by which information is communicated to the learner is often not considered in depth (Weston & Cranston, 1986). Thus, a discussion of media goes hand in hand with a consideration of methods because of the need to expand the teacher's understanding of the full potential that a broad knowledge of media brings to instructional methods.

The purpose of instructional media is to help the nurse educator deliver a message creatively and clearly. The advantage of a multimedia approach for teaching is that it may assist learners in gaining increased awareness and skills as well as retaining more effectively what they learn (Rankin & Stallings, 2001). In addition, instructional materials stimulate the learners' bodily senses, help clarify abstract or complex concepts, add variety to the teaching–learning experience (Babcock & Miller, 1994), reinforce learning, and potentially bring realism to the experience, saving time and energy on the part of both the teacher and the learner. Research indicates that the use of audiovisual aids does, indeed, facilitate learning (Haggard, 1989; Rankin & Stallings, 2001).

Considering such factors as the time constraints on healthcare professionals as a result of increased workloads, the decreasing length of patient hospital stays, the increase in patient acuity, the alternative healthcare settings in which education is now delivered, and shrinking resources for educational services, to name a few, the nurse educator must look for ways to supplement teaching and provide alternative approaches to educating learners.

This chapter provides an overview of the process for selecting, developing, using and evaluating instructional materials. A systematic approach is taken to examine various types of instructional media with an eye to matching their use to the particular characteristics of learners and to specific topics and situations. The advantages and disadvantages of media types will be discussed. Although the choice of which instructional materials to use often depends on availability or cost, whatever materials are selected should enhance the expected learning. This chapter is intended to inform nurse educators about various media options and allow them to make informed choices regarding appropriate instructional materials that fit the learner, that will accomplish the learning task, and that will affect the motivation of the learner. Whether nurses educate patients and families or other healthcare professionals, the same principles apply in making selection decisions about the type of instructional materials to use for teaching.

## GENERAL PRINCIPLES

Before selecting or developing media from the multitude of available options, you should be aware of the following general principles regarding the effectiveness of audiovisual tools:

- The teacher must be familiar with media content *before* a tool is used.

- Print and nonprint materials do change learner behavior by influencing a gain in cognitive, affective, or psychomotor skills.

- No one tool is better than another in enhancing learning. The suitability of any particular medium depends on many variables.

- The tools should complement the instructional methods.

- The choice of media should be consistent with subject content and match the tasks to be learned to assist the learner in accomplishing predetermined behavioral objectives.

- The instructional materials should reinforce and supplement—not substitute for—the educator's teaching efforts.

- Media should match the available financial resources.

- Instructional aids should be appropriate for the physical considerations and the learning environment, such as the size and seating of the audience, acoustics, space, lighting, and display hardware (delivery mechanisms) available.

- Media should complement the sensory abilities, developmental stages, and educational level of the intended audience.

- The message imparted by instructional materials must be accurate, valid, authoritative, up-to-date, state-of-the-art, appropriate, unbiased, and free of any unintended messages.

- The media should contribute meaningfully to the learning situation by adding diversity and additional information.

## CHOOSING INSTRUCTIONAL MATERIALS

Many important variables must be considered when choosing instructional materials. The role of the nurse educator goes beyond the dispensing of information only; it also involves skill in the designing of and planning for instruction. Learning can be made more enjoyable for both the learner and the teacher if the educator knows what instructional materials are available, as well as how to select and use them so as to enhance the teaching–learning experience. Knowledge of the diversity of instructional tools and their appropriate use will enable the teacher to make education more interesting, challenging, and effective for all types of learners. With current trends in healthcare reform, educational strategies to teach patients will need to include instructional materials for health promotion and illness prevention among well persons, as well as instructional materials for health maintenance and restoration for ill persons.

Making appropriate choices of instructional materials depends on a broad understanding of three major variables: (1) characteristics of the learner, (2) characteristics of the media that make them suitable for achieving the objectives of the task, and (3) characteristics of the task to be achieved (Frantz, 1980). A useful mnemonic for remembering these variables is LMAT: **L**earner, **M**edia, **a**nd **T**ask.

1. *Characteristics of the learner:* As variables in the learner are known to influence learning, it is important to "know your audience" so as to choose media that best suit their needs. You must consider the learners' perceptual abilities, physical abilities, reading abilities, motivational levels (locus of control), developmental stages, and learning styles.

2. *Characteristics of the media:* The nurse educator has the opportunity to choose from a wide variety of media, print and nonprint, to enhance methods of instruction. Nonprint media include the full range of audio and visual possibilities. An enormous variety of educational materials is available. The tools selected are the form through which the information will be communicated. No single medium is most effective. Therefore, the educator must be flexible, sometimes combining a multimedia approach.

**3.** *Characteristics of the task:* Task characteristics are defined by the predetermined behavioral objectives. The task to be accomplished depends on identification of the learning domain and the complexity of behavior required by the task.

## THE THREE MAJOR COMPONENTS OF INSTRUCTIONAL MATERIALS

Whatever instructional method is used, decisions will also have to be made regarding the media necessary to help communicate information. The delivery system (Weston & Cranston, 1986), content, and presentation (Frantz, 1980) are the three major components of media that should be kept in mind when evaluating print and nonprint materials for potential instruction.

### Delivery System

The *delivery system* is both the physical form of the materials and the hardware used to present the materials. For instance, a person is the delivery system for a lecture. This lecture might be embellished through other delivery systems, such as the use of overhead transparencies or slides (physical form), and a projector (hardware). Videotapes (physical form) in conjunction with VCRs (hardware) and computer programs (physical form) in conjunction with the computer (hardware) are other examples.

The delivery system is independent of the content of the message. The choice of the delivery system is influenced by the size of the intended audience, the pacing or flexibility needed for delivery, and the sensory aspects most suitable to the audience.

### Content

The content, or message, is the actual information that is communicated to the learner, which might be on any topic from sexuality to educational psychology. When selecting media, the nurse educator must consider several aspects:

- Is the information presented accurately?
- Is the medium chosen appropriate to convey particular content?

For example, audiotapes can be a very appropriate tool for teaching content related to the cognitive or affective domain but not a good tool for teaching a psychomotor skill. Content relative to psychomotor behavior might be better served with printed pamphlets, videos, or the use of real equipment for demonstrations.

- Is the readability of the materials appropriate for the audience to accomplish a given task?

The more complex the task, the more important it is to write clearly understandable instructions at a level suitable to the learner. Readability of any printed materials is enhanced through the use of illustrations or the rewriting of instructions in simple, succinct language (see Chapter 7).

### Presentation

Frantz (1980) describes presentation as those variables that affect the way in which the content or message to be learned is delivered. Weston and Cranston (1986) state that the form of the message is the most important consideration for selecting or developing instructional materials, a consideration that is frequently ignored. They describe the form of the message as occurring along a continuum from concrete (real objects) to abstract (symbols).

**Realia**   Weston and Cranston (1986) term the most concrete form of stimuli that can be used to deliver information as *realia*. For example, an actual woman demonstrating breast self-examination is the most concrete example of realia. Because this form of presentation might be less acceptable for broad teaching situations, the next best choice would be a model, which has many characteristics of reality, including three-dimensionality, without the accompanying embarrassment for the learner. The message is less concrete, yet using a model as an instructional medium allows for an accurate presentation of information with near-maximal use of the learners' perceptual abilities. Further along the continuum of realia is a video presentation of a woman performing breast self-examination. The learner could still learn accurate breast self-examination this way, but the aspect of dimensionality is absent. The message becomes less concrete and more abstract.

**Illusionary Representations**  Many realistic cues, including dimensionality, are missing from this category of instructional materials. Moving or still photographs and audiotapes projecting true sounds are good examples of illusionary representations, as are representations through drawings and graphs (Weston & Cranston, 1986). They are less concrete and more abstract, but the instructional advantages of illusionary media are that these forms can offer learners experiences to which they might otherwise not have access because of such factors as size, location, or expense. Examples, such as pictures of how to stage decubitus ulcers or audiotapes of how to discriminate between normal and various abnormal lung sounds, although more abstract in form, do to some degree resemble realia.

**Symbolic Representations**  Numbers and words, symbols written and spoken that are used to convey ideas or represent objects, are the most common form of instruction, yet are the most abstract types of messages (Weston & Cranston, 1986). Audiotaped presentations, written texts and handouts, and the use of blackboards are just a few examples of messages delivered in symbolic form. The chief disadvantage of symbolic representations stems from their lack of concreteness and the potential need to tailor their form and content to the cognitive abilities and limitations of

learners. For that reason, their use should be limited with young children, learners from different cultures, learners with low literacy skills, and cognitively and sensory impaired individuals.

When making decisions about how to best accomplish teaching objectives, the nurse educator must carefully consider these three components of instructional materials. The various delivery systems available, the content or message to be conveyed, and the form in which information will be presented are all important choices. A wide range of options among various media are available. Remember, no one type of media provides a clear advantage over another in promoting acquisition of knowledge; at the same time, the mere acquisition of knowledge does not guarantee that the learner will learn. It is important to keep in mind the supplemental nature of instructional materials. In other words, nurse educators must know how to select the tools that will best complement and support their teaching efforts for a particular audience and that will emphasize the key points to accomplish the behavioral objectives.

## TYPES OF INSTRUCTIONAL MATERIALS

### Written Materials

Handouts, leaflets, books, pamphlets, brochures, and instruction sheets are the most widely employed and most accessible type of media used for teaching. Although printed teaching materials have been described as "frozen language" (Redman, 2001), written materials are, nonetheless, the most common form of teaching tool.

The use of printed materials offers some distinct advantages. The greatest virtue of written materials is that they are available to the learner as a reference for information when the nurse educator is not immediately present to answer questions or clarify information. Also, printed materials are widely used at all levels of society, so this type of media is acceptable and familiar to the public. In addition, enormous varieties of materials are available through commercial sources and are easily obtainable, usually at relatively low cost, for distribution by educators. They often come in convenient forms, such as pamphlets, which are portable and usually contain concise amounts of information. In recognition of significant cultural and ethnic shifts in the general population, printed materials in languages other than English, such as Spanish, are becoming more widely available. Their ready availability makes written materials especially useful for learners who prefer reading as opposed to receiving messages in other formats. The speed at which materials are read may be controlled by the reader, which is an asset for comprehension of complex concepts and relationships. Content may also be altered to target specific audiences.

The disadvantages of printed materials include the fact that they are the most abstract form of reality, possibilities for immediate feedback are limited, and the proper reading level is essential to realize their full usefulness. A large percentage of materials are written at too high a level for comprehension. Learners with low literacy skills or those persons who are visually or cognitively impaired may not be able to take full advantage of written materials, and illiteracy negates the use of printed materials altogether. Doak, Doak, Friedell, and Meade (1998) concluded that individuals with low literacy skills understand less healthcare advice and are less likely to take timely actions to reduce their health risks.

**Commercially Prepared Materials**   A wealth of commercially prepared brochures, posters, pamphlets, and patient-focused texts is currently available. Whether they enhance the quality of learning is an important question for nurse educators to consider when trying to evaluate these products for content and presentation. Examining the factuality of material

presented is very important because commercial products may or may not be produced in collaboration with health professionals (Foster, 1987). Attention must also be paid to the cognitive level at which materials are aimed. For example, Foster described a preoperative instruction booklet advertised as appropriate for children of all ages that depicted animal caretakers of a child. Because very young children tend to interpret what they see concretely, they might believe that real animals would be caring for them and could become frightened. For that reason, this particular booklet was clearly inappropriate for such a broad audience.

Several factors must be considered when reviewing commercial materials for possible use (Foster, 1987):

- Who produced the item? Was there any input from healthcare professionals?

- Can the item be previewed? The educator should have an opportunity to examine the accuracy and appropriateness of content to ensure that the item will provide the target group with the information needed.

- Is the price of the teaching tool consistent with its educational value? Getting across an important message effectively may justify a higher cost outlay, especially if the tool can be used with large numbers of learners, but simple printed sheets may do the job just as well and at less expense. Another cost consideration is how quickly the information will become outdated.

The advantage of using commercial materials is their ready availability. Using commercially prepared materials is certainly less time-consuming and often cheaper for educators than designing their own instructional materials. For instance, the American Heart Association produces many fine booklets on cardiac and stroke education for patients and families that cost 50 cents or less when bought in bulk. An educator would need to spend hours researching, writing, and copying materials to create information packets of equal quality.

The disadvantages of using commercial materials may include issues of cost, accuracy and adequacy of content, and readability of the materials. Some educational booklets are expensive to purchase and impractical to give away in large quantities to learners. The American Parkinson's Disease Association produces a number of fine but costly booklets, and an educator might encourage learners to buy their own rather than provide them for free. Also, the actual usability of commercially prepared instructional materials for particular learners must be evaluated on an individual basis because the level of readability might be a problem for some, and the content might not completely and accurately cover all the information the learner needs to know.

**Self-Composed Materials** Educators may choose to write their own instructional materials for several reasons, which might include cost saving or the need to tailor content to specific audiences.

Advantages to composing your own materials are many. By writing your own materials, you can tailor the information to fit your own institution's policies, procedures, and equipment. You can build in answers to those questions asked most frequently by your patients, highlighting points considered especially important by physicians or other healthcare professionals. Tailoring your written materials to reinforce specific oral instructions will enhance their efficacy and gives you the opportunity to clarify difficult concepts by using multifaceted approaches that work well for getting the message across (Haggard, 1989; Brownson, 1998).

The following example illustrates this point nicely. Using teacher-generated instructional materials, Rice and Johnson (1984) found that groups of patients receiving specific instructions were more likely to follow directions and required less oral teaching time than groups of patients receiving general or nonspecific instructions.

Doak et al. (1998) outlined specific suggestions for tailoring information to help patients want to read and remember the message and to act on it. These authors describe *tailoring* as personalizing the message so that the content, structure, and image fit an individual patient's learning needs. Writing the patient's name on the cover, and opening a pamphlet with a patient and highlighting the most important information as it is verbally reviewed, are two examples. Studies by Campbell et al. (1994) and Skinner, Strecher, and Hospers (1994) support the efficacy of tailored instruction over nontailored messages in achieving reading, recall, and follow-through in health teaching.

There are, of course, disadvantages to composing your own materials. You need to exercise extra care to ensure that materials are well written and laid out effectively, which can be a time-consuming endeavor. Many tools written by patient educators are too long, too detailed, and written at too high a level for the target audience (Haggard, 1989). If you find this skill difficult to master, it may be easier to use commercially prepared tools or to follow the simple guidelines below.

Boyd (1987) pointed out that accuracy of content is a very important factor in written patient education materials, but that another very important factor is patients' ability to read and understand the materials. Nurse educators are expected to enhance their methods of teaching with audiovisual materials, but few have ever had formal training in the development and application of written materials. Boyd (1987), Haggard (1989), Doak, Doak, and Root (1996), and Brownson (1998) suggest the following guidelines for writing patient education materials with clarity and completeness:

- Make sure the content is accurate and up-to-date.

- Organize the content in a logical, step-by-step fashion so learners are being informed adequately but are not being overloaded. Prioritize the content to address what they "need to know" first. Content that is "nice to know" can be addressed with less immediacy or emphasis.

- Make sure the information succinctly discusses the *what*, *how*, and *when*. Do not overwhelm the reader with large amounts of information. Follow the KISS rule: Keep it simple and smart. Avoid giving detailed rationales because they may unnecessarily lengthen the written information. Try to integrate information that you think the learners need to know with information they want to know. For instance, patients need to know how to turn, cough, and deep breathe after surgery, but they will also want to know when they can eat. This material can best be handled by putting the information into a question-and-answer format or by dividing the information into subheadings according to the nature of the content.

- Regardless of format, avoid medical jargon whenever possible, and define any technical terms in layman's language. Sometimes it is important to expose patients to technical terms because of complicated procedures and ongoing interaction with the medical team, so careful definitions can minimize misunderstandings. Be consistent in words used.

- Find out the average grade in school completed by the targeted patient population, and write the patient education materials two to four grade levels below that level. Follow guidelines for decreasing reading level (see Chapter 7). Employing a readability level appropriate to the audience cannot be emphasized enough.

- Keep words and sentences short and to the point. Write in a conversational style.

- Write in the active voice. For example, "Clean the wound with soap and water" is more directive and effective than "It is important to keep the wound clean."

- Use the second person *you*, instead of the third person.

- Present the most important information first by making the first sentence of a paragraph be the topic sentence.

- Use adequate spacing, which is more restful to the eye.

- Do not use all-capital letters because words in capitals are much more difficult to read than words printed with lowercase letters.

- Use advance organizers, such as outlines, to set the frame of reference for the learner.

- Build in reviews at the end of written materials to reemphasize key points.

In addition to the guidelines for clarity and completeness in constructing written materials, format and appearance are equally important in motivating learners to read the printed word. If the format and appearance are too detailed, learners will feel overwhelmed, and instead of attracting the learners, you will discourage and repel them (Figure 12–1). To avoid common pitfalls in writing good instructional tools, follow these important tips (Doak et al., 1996):

- Allow plenty of white space, including double spacing, generous margins, indentation of important points, and highlighting or setting off of key statements.

- Do not put too much written information in the document.

- Use illustrations to break up blocks of print and to reinforce important information in the text.

- Note that a clear, concrete line drawing may be just as or more effective than a photograph or an elaborate piece of artwork.

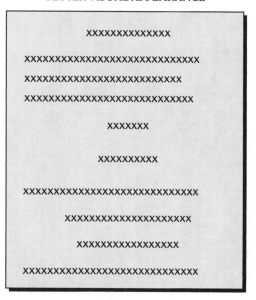

CLUTTERED APPEARANCE        BETTER VISUAL APPEARANCE

FIGURE 12–1    **Inadequate versus Adequate Appearance and Formatting**

- Always state things in positive, not negative, terms. Never illustrate incorrect messages. For example, depicting a hand holding a metered-dose inhaler in the mouth not only incorrectly illustrates a drug delivery technique (Weixler, 1994) but reinforces that message by its visual impact alone (Figure 12–2 illustrates the correct way to use an inhaler).

As a way of evaluating the effectiveness of self-composed materials, Boyd (1987) suggests interviewing a few patients with different educational levels and asking them for reactions to the materials you write. Computerized readability formulas for writing patient education handouts are also available (see Chapter 7). Baker (1991) offers specific suggestions for writing easily readable handouts, including examples of original and rewritten text. As a further point of interest, Houts et al. (1998) describe a study that demonstrated significant efficacy with the use of pictographs in enhancing recall of spoken medical instruction in nonliterate populations.

**Evaluating Printed Materials**    When evaluating printed materials, the following considerations should be kept in mind.

Nature of the audience    What is the average age of the audience? Certain age groups learn better with one type of media than another. For instance, older adults tend to prefer printed materials that they can read at their leisure. Children like short printed materials with many illustrations.

What is the preferred learning style of the particular audience? Printed materials with few illustrations are poorly suited to patients who not only have difficulty reading but also do not like to read. Representations of information in the form of graphs and charts can be included with the content of printed materials for those who are visual and conceptual learners.

Shake vigorously.

Hold upright with cap off.

Hold inhaler 1 to 2 inches from mouth. Breathe out.

Press down on inhaler. Breathe in slowly (3 to 5 seconds).

Hold breath 10 seconds, then repeat puffs.

FIGURE 12–2    Diagram Illustrating Proper Technique for Inhaler Use

Older learners, in particular, like handouts. With this group, written materials are most effective when combined with oral presentations, especially on a one-to-one basis. However, vision deficits are common with older adult patients, and short-term memory may be a problem for comprehension. Having materials that can be reread at their own convenience and pace can reinforce earlier learning and minimize confusion over treatment instructions. Lengthy materials are less problematic for older learners, who frequently have enough time and patience for reading educational materials. Diagrams should be explicit. Examples should relate to activities relevant to the audience's lifestyle. Advice for dealing with problems should be explicit. To accommodate those individuals with vision impairments, use a large typeface and lots of white space in printed materials. Separate one section from another with ample spacing and highlight important points (Haggard, 1989).

*Literacy level required*  The effectiveness of patient education materials for helping the learner accomplish instructional objectives can be totally undermined if the materials are written at a level beyond the comprehension of the learner. A study of patients' reading abilities in a public hospital by Glazer-Wald-man, Hall, and Weiner (1985) found that only 40% of their sample could read at the sixth-grade level. A cross-sectional survey in two urban, public hospitals by Williams et al. (1995) revealed a high proportion of patients who were unable to read and understand basic medical instructions, including directions for taking medications, follow-up appointments, and informed consent forms for medical procedures. The Joint Commission on Accreditation of Healthcare Organizations mandates that health information must be presented in a manner that can be understood by patients and family members. This requirement underscores the importance of screening potential educational tools to be used as adjuncts to various teaching methods. A number of formulas (e.g., Fog, SMOG, Flesch, Fry) are available for determining readability (see Chapter 7 and Appendix A). Boyd's (1987) guidelines, listed previously, are helpful in reducing the reading level of materials you write yourself.

*Linguistic variety available*  Linguistic variety refers to choices of printed materials in different foreign languages, which may be limited because duplicate materials in more than one language are costly to publish and not likely to be undertaken unless the publisher antici-pates a large demand. The growth of the His-panic population in the United States has pro-moted increasing attention to the need for Spanish-language teaching materials. For instance, organizations such as the American Heart Association, the Parkinson's Disease Association, and the National Institute for Head Trauma have begun providing Spanish- and English-language versions of their most widely used printed materials. Regional dif-ferences exist, so there may be more availabil-ity of Asian-language materials on the West Coast and more Spanish-language materials in the Southwest and Northeast than in other parts of the country.

*Brevity and clarity*  In education, as in art, simpler is better. Remind yourself of the KISS rule: Keep it simple and smart. Address the critical facts only. What does the patient *need* to know? Choose words that explain *how*; the *why* can be filled in by a lec-ture or discussion. Including rationales in handouts lengthens materials unnecessarily (Haggard, 1989). Remember—ideally, in-structional materials will be supplements to learning.

Figure 12–3 provides a good example of a clear, easy-to-follow instructional tool used to teach an asthma patient how to determine when a metered-dose inhaler is empty. Using simple graphics and minimal words, it guides the learner through the procedure with very little room for misinterpretation and is suit-able for a wide range of audiences.

As another example, Hanafin (1993) described a pamphlet called *The 5-Minute Teaching Series*, which was designed for brief in-service topics at the Minneapolis Veterans Affairs Medical Center. Each topic is printed on a single, brightly colored 8 1/2-by-11-inch paper folded into thirds. On the inside of the pamphlet is information about the topic being covered; the outside flaps emphasize particu-larly important aspects of the topic. Develop-ment of content for this teaching series is

Full                1/2 Full              Empty

FIGURE 12–3    **Examples of a Clear, Easy-to-Follow Instructional Tool for an Asthma Patient**

based on adult learning principles. Topics chosen are problem related and immediately applicable to nursing care interventions. These pamphlets are easily distributed, are cost-effective, and have been used to meet a variety of learning needs.

*Layout and appearance* The appearance of written materials is crucial in attracting learners' attention and getting them to read the information. If the potential tool has too much wording, with inadequate spacing between sentences and paragraphs, small margins, and numerous pages, the intended learner may disregard it under the impression that it is much too difficult and too time-consuming to read. Figure 12–4 illustrates an example of this problem. Figure 12–5 illustrates an improved version of the same material.

Doak et al. (1996) point out that allowing plenty of white space is the most important step that should be taken to improve the appearance of written materials. This means double-spacing, leaving generous margins, indenting important points, using bold characters, and separating out key statements with extra space. Inserting a graphic in the middle of the text can break up the print and may be

visually appealing, as well as providing a mechanism for reinforcing textual information. Redman (2001) states that pictorial learning is better than verbal learning for recognition and recall. For subjects that lend themselves to concrete explanations, this is especially true. An example used earlier in this chapter is teaching the psychomotor task of using a metered-dose inhaler (see Figure 12–2). More abstract topics, such as teaching communication skills, rely heavily on written information in combination with use of demonstration.

*Opportunity for repetition* Written materials can be read later, again and again, to reinforce your teaching. This consideration is especially important when you are not there to answer questions. Thus it is an advantage if materials are laid out in a question-and-answer format. If you are writing your own materials, be mindful of the need to keep them current, and update them against changing patient populations.

*Concreteness and familiarity* Using the active voice is more immediate and concrete. For example, "Shake the inhaler very well three times" is more effective than "The inhaler should be shaken thoroughly" (Figure 12–6).

**DYSPHAGIA**
(Swallowing and Chewing Disorder)

**Major Risk:** Aspiration Pneumonia

Telltale Clues:
1. Dysarthria (difficulty articulating words)
2. Decreased tongue mobility
3. Facial weakness
4. Decreased gag reflex
5. Weak or hoarse cough
6. Coughing or choking during or after meals
7. Pockets of food in mouth
8. Wet or gurgly voice quality

Diagnosis based on: Modified Barium swallow or Bedside Evaluation
by qualified speech pathologist

Common Etiologies (causes):
CVA, traumatic brain injury, cerebral palsy, ALS, myasthenia
gravis, multiple sclerosis, muscular dystrophy, Parkinson's,
spinal cord dysfunction, head and neck cancers, COPD, confused
patients, encephalitis.

Nursing Diagnosis: Potential for Injury (Aspiration), related to
impaired swallowing secondary to _____

Nursing Interventions:
1. HOB up > 30 degrees AAT.
2. Feed in upright position (approx. 90 degrees), neck
slightly flexed forward (chin tucked).
3. Supraglottic diet, unless otherwise ordered.
4. Suction equipment on standby AAT.
5. Dentures in for meals, when applicable.
6. If unilateral facial weakness, place food on unaffected side.
7. Small bites, chew food well.
8. Patience. Allow plenty of time to eat.
9. No straws, unless individually evaluated.
10. Check mouth for residual food after each swallow.
11. Leave in upright position 30 minutes after meal.

FIGURE 12–4    **Example of a Poorly Formatted Teaching Tool**

Also, the importance of using plain language instead of medical jargon cannot be overstated. Byrne and Edeani (1984), Estey, Musseau, and Keehn (1994), and Lerner, Jehle, Janicke, and Moscati (2000) surveyed knowledge of medical terminology among hospital patients and determined that inadequate patient understanding of common medical terms used by healthcare providers could be a significant factor in noncompliance with medical regimens by patients. The studies indicated that patients understood medical terms at a lower rate than health professionals expected.

### DYSPHAGIA
(Swallowing and Chewing Disorder)

**Major Risk: Aspiration Pneumonia**

Major Causes in Neuroscience Patients:
   Stroke, SLD, Myasthenia Gravis, MS, Parkinson's Disease,
   Spinal Cord Injury, Confusion

Important Clues:
   1. Difficulty articulating words
   2. Weak tongue movement
   3. Facial droop one side
   4. Decreased gag reflex
   5. Weak or hoarse cough
   6. Coughing or choking during or after meals
   7. Wet or gurgly voice quality

Most Important Nursing Interventions:
   1. Head of bed up greater than 30 degrees at all times.
   2. Feed in upright position with chin tucked in slightly
   3. Suction equipment on standby at all times.
   4. Supraglottic diet, unless otherwise ordered.
   5. If face weak on one side, place food on unaffected side.
   6. Small bites, chew food well.
   7. Patience. Allow plenty of time to eat.
   8. Check mouth for food after each swallow.
   9. Leave in upright position 30 minutes after meal.

FIGURE 12–5   **Example of a Properly Formatted Teaching Tool**

### STEPS FOR CORRECT INHALER TECHNIQUE

   1. Shake the container well.
   2. Remove cap and hold inhaler upright.
   3. Hold the inhaler 1 to 2 inches from mouth.
   4. Tilt head back slightly, and breathe out fully.
   5. Press down on the inhaler and start to breathe in slowly.
   6. Breathe in slowly (3 to 5 seconds) and deeply to pull medication
      deeper into the lungs.
   7. Hold breath for 10 seconds to hold the medicine in the lungs.
   8. Take a few normal breaths.
   9. Repeat puffs as directed.

FIGURE 12–6   **Example of Instructions Written in the Active Voice**

| TABLE 12–1   Advantages and disadvantages of printed materials | |
| --- | --- |
| Advantages | Disadvantages |
| Always available<br>Rate of reading is controllable by the reader<br>Complex concepts can be explained both fully and adequately<br>Procedural steps can be outlined<br>Verbal instruction can be reinforced<br>Learner is always able to refer back to instructions given in print | Impersonal<br>Limited feedback; absence of instructor lessens opportunity to clear up misinterpretation<br>Passive tool<br>Highly complex materials may be overwhelming to the learner<br>Literacy skill of learner may limit effectiveness |

SOURCE: Adapted from Hinkle, Albanese, & McGinty, 1993.

In summary, self-designed or commercially produced printed teaching materials are widely used for a broad range of audiences. They vary in literacy demand levels and may be found written in several languages. Table 12–1 summarizes their major advantages and disadvantages.

## Demonstration Materials

Demonstration materials include many types of nonprint media, such as models and real equipment, as well as displays, such as posters, diagrams, illustrations, charts, bulletin boards, flannel boards, flip charts, chalkboards, photographs, and drawings. All represent unique ways of communicating messages to the learner. These aids primarily stimulate the visual senses but can combine the sense of sight with touch and sometimes even smell and taste. From these various forms of demonstration materials, the educator can choose one or more to complement teaching efforts in reaching predetermined objectives. Just as with written tools, these aids must be accurate and appropriate for the intended audience. Ideally, these media forms bring the learner closer to reality and actively engage him or her in a visual and sometimes participatory manner. As such, demonstration tools are useful for cognitive, affective, and psychomotor skill development. The major

forms of demonstration materials—displays and models—will be discussed in detail.

**Displays** Displays can be permanently installed or portable. They have been referred to as static instructional tools because they are usually stationary and unchanging (Haggard, 1989), but that does not imply that they are immovable or unalterable. Some demonstration materials, such as posters (discussed later in more detail), are tools that can effectively achieve teaching objectives and vividly represent the essence of relationships between objects with or without the presence of the teacher. Other tools, such as chalkboards and flip charts, usually require an instructor to directly assist in the flow and interpretation of information being depicted. Displays, such as chalkboards, signs, white markerboards, flip charts, bulletin boards, and flannel boards, are found in almost any educational setting and are useful for a variety of teaching purposes. They can advertise events, convey simple or quick messages about healthcare issues, and clarify, reinforce, or summarize important topics and themes.

The proverbial chalkboard and flip charts and the more recent white markerboard are particularly helpful in delivering information. These tools are most useful during brainstorming sessions in formal classes or group discussions. You can use them spontaneously to make drawings or diagrams (with contrasting colored chalk or markers if you wish) or to jot down ideas generated from participants while you are in the process of teaching. You can add, correct, or delete information quickly while the learners are actively following what you are doing or saying. These board devices are excellent in promoting participation, keeping the learners' attention on the topic at hand, and noting and reinforcing the contributions of someone else. They are flexible tools that provide opportunities for the teacher, in an immediate and direct fashion, to organize data, integrate ideas, perform on-the-spot problem solving, and compare and contrast various points of view. Unlike some other types of visuals, these display tools allow learners to see parts of a whole picture while assisting the teacher in filling in the gaps.

Babcock and Miller (1994) list guidelines for use of chalkboards and white markerboards. The most important points include using legible and discernible lettering, being sure to step aside and face the audience after putting notations on the board to maintain contact with the audience and allowing learners to copy the message, and enlisting a good note-taker to capture a creative design or record an idea before the board is erased.

How sophisticated a display is depends on the budget available to produce it, as well as the detail you desire and the creativity you put into getting the message across (Haggard, 1989). On one end of the continuum, you might have a simple illustration with print and line graphics, like Figure 12–3, which can be used to teach asthmatics how to tell when a metered-dose inhaler is empty or full. A more sophisticated display might be used to help teach the same content with colored photos, three-dimensional objects, and more sophisticated graphics and print.

Displays can be an effective way of achieving learning outcomes, although they may be time-consuming to use or prepare and, like

models, sometimes expensive to purchase (Haggard, 1989). However, computer technology has made it easier to create attractive, up-to-date, and impressive displays as well as to revise ones already made (Bushy, 1991).

The following are some advantages of displays as teaching tools:

- A quick way to attract attention and get an idea across
- Flexible (especially if made for easy modification)
- Portable (Many posters can be folded for storage and unfolded for mounting. Some blackboards and bulletin boards are on rollers.)
- Reusable
- Stimulate interest or ideas in the observer
- Can change or influence attitudes
- Purchasable, and depending on the educator's budget, many can be made. Figure 12–7 shows an "Aspiration Precautions" sign made by an educator to be displayed for use by nurses over patients' beds on a stroke unit.

Some of the disadvantages of displays include the following:

- Take up a lot of space
- Time-consuming to have prepared, and for that reason tend to be reused again and again, which increases the risk of their becoming outdated
- May be overused—they need to be used as supplements to learning, not as an end in themselves
- Unsuitable for large audiences if information is to be viewed simultaneously
- Cannot present large amounts of information at one time
- Not good for teaching psychomotor skills when movement needs to be demonstrated
- Get too cluttered when too much information is placed on them

**ASPIRATION PRECAUTIONS**

1. HOB up > 30 degrees AAT.
2. Feed in upright position (approx. 90 degrees), neck slightly flexed forward (chin tucked).
3. Supraglottic diet, unless otherwise ordered.
4. Suction equipment on standby AAT.
5. Dentures in for meals, when applicable.
6. If unilateral facial weakness, place food on unaffected side.
7. Small bites, chew food well.
8. Patience. Allow plenty of time to eat.
9. No straws, unless individually evaluated.
10. Check mouth for residual food after each swallow.
11. Leave in upright position 30 minutes after meal.

FIGURE 12–7   **Example of a Sign Designed for Display in a Stroke Unit**

- May be ignored if posted too long or poorly arranged

- If permanently mounted on a large backing, difficult or impossible to transport

- The symbolic nature of the message may be misunderstood, a problem that underscores their importance as supplements to learning

Some displays, such as posters, are essentially hybrids of print and nonprint media because they heavily employ the written word as well as graphic illustration. Because of the increasing use of two-dimensional posters as a legitimate and reasonable alternative to more formal presentations for conveying information (Duchin & Sherwood, 1990; Moneyham, Ura, Ellwood, & Bruno, 1996; Thurber & Asselin, 1999), this type of display tool will be discussed in more detail here. Posters have become an important educational strategy, particularly as a mode to disseminate information less formally in classrooms and in clinical settings to patients and their families, as well as at educational seminars and research meetings to educate staff and students.

As a visual aid, posters can be used as an independent source of information or in conjunction with other modalities. Some critics view the poster as a passive instructional medium, but this conjecture can easily be disputed because reading and recall require involvement on the part of the learner. Inherent in the design, the message conveyed by a poster is brief, constant, and interactive with the audience (Duchin & Sherwood, 1990). Because the primary mode of the poster is visual stimulation, it must be designed to attract attention (Flournoy, Turner, & Combs, 2000). Effective posters leave a mental image long after they are seen. This mental image is a cue to the viewer to recall the message. Much like a bumper sticker you see on a car in front of you while driving, effective poster displays can potentially leave lasting impressions that are easily recalled at some future date.

The advantage of posters is that they can be used as a cognitive stimulator, as a way to reinforce and synthesize information, and as an ongoing instructional resource. Their value derives from the repetition, individual pacing, and availability of the message across various settings (Duchin & Sherwood, 1990; Bach, McDaniel, & Poole, 1994; Hayes & Childress, 1999; Thurber & Asselin, 1999). Posters serve as an important teaching tool to help bring about a change of behavior by adding knowledge, reinforcing skill, or appealing to attitudes. By forcing content brevity and using eye-catching imagery, a message can be conveyed quickly and simultaneously to an audience in a variety of settings. Posters can also be used with individuals and small groups to transmit or reinforce information with or without the teacher present. They are relatively inexpensive to produce. With practice, an educator can become skilled at putting together effective posters in an efficient and timely way.

The disadvantage of posters is that the content is static and, therefore, may become quickly dated. If the same poster is kept around too long, the potential audience begins to disregard its message. The key to a poster's effectiveness lies in its planning and design. Bushy (1991) states that "good ideas do not speak for themselves . . . a good poster display cannot rescue a bad idea, but a poor one can easily sink the best idea . . ." (p. 11). She puts forth important aesthetic considerations when preparing and evaluating poster presentations specifically for research purposes. Duchin and Sherwood (1990) and Bach et al. (1994) also provide guidelines for developing attractive, simple, yet effective posters that include considerations of content, audience needs, and settings. Both Bushy (1991) and Duchin and Sherwood (1990) refer to the application of design elements such as color, spacing, graphics, lettering, and borders required to create presentations that not only catch the eye but also persist in memory. Duchin and Sherwood (1990) further point out that effective imagery can take the form of graphic designs or photographs. Great artistic skill is not required. Simple pictures, such as schematics, outlines, and stick figure drawings, work well and can be created using colored pencils, markers, or construction paper. The ability of a poster to influence behavior or increase awareness can be greatly enhanced by careful consideration of content, audience, and design elements.

Because aesthetic appeal is critical in capturing learners' attention, the following tips,

adapted from Bushy (1991), Bach et al. (1994), Duchin and Sherwood (1990), and Haggard (1989) should be adhered to when making and critiquing a poster for use as a teaching tool:

- Use complementary (opposite-spectrum) color combinations, taking into consideration the three color aspects of hue (wavelength of the light spectrum), saturation (purity of color), and value (brilliance of color). Two colors clash when they are close to each other in these three elements. See Duchin and Sherwood (1990) for a discussion of the use of color in posters.

- One color should make up as much as 70% of the display. No two colors should be used in equal proportions, and a third color should be used only to accent or highlight printed components such as titles, subheadings, or credits. Too many colors make the design appear cluttered and complicated.

- Because a picture is worth a thousand words, graphics should be used to break up blocks of script or lettering.

- Use simple, high-quality (but not necessarily sophisticated or ornate) drawings or graphics that can be easily interpreted.

- Balance script with white space (or another background color) and graphics to add variety and contrast.

- Use high-quality photographs with colored borders and of different contours, widths, and shapes.

- Convey the message in common, straightforward language, avoiding jargon and unfamiliar abbreviations or symbols.

- Adhere to the KISS principle (keep it simple and smart) when using words to decrease length, detail, and crowding. Simplicity and neatness attract attention.

- Be concise; do not repeat. Include only essential information, but be sure the message is complete.

- Keep objectives in mind for the focus of this display tool.

- Be sure content is current and free of spelling, grammar, and mathematical errors.
- Add textures by using a variety of paper and fabrics.
- Make titles catchy and crisp, using 10 words or less (no longer than two lines) and lettering large enough to read from a distance of at least four to six feet.
- Use a title or introductory statement that orients readers to the subject.
- Logically sequence the written and graphic components.
- Use letter-quality script or laser print instead of dot matrix if using computer-generated type.
- Letters should be straight and at least one inch in height. Avoid using all-capital letters except for very short titles and labels.
- Use arrows, circles, or directional lines to merge the parts to achieve correct focus, flow, sequence, and unity.
- Achieve balance in visual weight on each side by positioning information around an imaginary central axis running vertically and horizontally.
- Handouts can be used to supplement, highlight, and reinforce the messages conveyed by the poster.
- If a poster is to be transported, use durable backboards and overlays (Styrofoam, heavy cardboard, lamination, or acrylic sprays).

Bushy (1991) has devised a 30-item poster appraisal tool (R-PAT) to further assist nurses in critiquing posters specifically designed for research. This tool can be modified for use in preparing and evaluating posters as tools for educational purposes.

The ability of a poster to influence behavior or expand awareness can be greatly enhanced by careful consideration of its content, intended audience, and design elements. The poster for AIDS awareness (Figure 12–8) is a stunning example. The interaction of the viewer with the message is the key to a poster's success. This AIDS awareness poster and the World War I poster "Uncle Sam Wants YOU!" are examples of the element of visceral connection between viewer and message that linger in memory.

Computers and printers have opened the door to very professional-looking productions of posters by almost any user. Software programs such as Print Shop Deluxe and Canvas are frequently used for these purposes.

**Models** Models are three-dimensional instructional tools that allow the learner to immediately apply knowledge and psychomotor skills by observing, examining, manipulating, handling, assembling, and disassembling objects while the teacher provides feedback (Rankin & Stallings, 2001). In addition, these demonstration aids encourage learners to think abstractly and give them the opportunity to use many of their senses (Boyd et al., 1998). Whenever possible, the use of real objects and actual equipment is preferred, but a model is the next best thing when the real object is not available, accessible, or feasible, or is too complex to use. The three specific types of models used for teaching and learning are replicas, analogues, and symbols. To differentiate the three types of models, Babcock and Miller (1994) suggest associating a replica with the word *resemble*, an analogue with the term *act like*, and a symbol with the words *stands for*.

A *replica* is a facsimile constructed to scale that resembles the features or substance of the original object. The dimensions of the reproduction may be decreased or enlarged in size to make demonstration easier and more understandable. A replica of the DNA helix is an excellent example of a model used to teach the complex concept of genetics. Replicas can be examined and manipulated by the learner to get an idea of how something looks and works. They are excellent for teaching psychomotor skills because they give the learner an opportunity for active participation

## Last night Jennifer had a fatal accident.
## She just doesn't know it yet

FIGURE 12–8    **Example of an Effective Poster for AIDS Awareness**

through hands-on experience. Not only can the learner assemble and disassemble parts to see how they fit and operate, but the pace of learning can also be controlled by the learner (Babcock & Miller, 1994).

Replicas are used frequently by the nurse educator when teaching anatomy and physiological processes. Models of the heart, kidney, ear, eye, joints, and pelvic organs, for example, allow the learner to get a perspective on parts of the body not readily viewed without these teaching aids. Resuscitation dolls are a common type of replica used to teach the skills of cardiopulmonary resuscitation. Breast self-examination is another topic best taught to wide audiences through the use of a model. Pinto (1993) assessed training and mainte-

nance of breast self-examination skills. The high incidence of deterioration in breast self-examination skills led her to evaluate approaches for improving maintenance. Learners who regularly refreshed their skills using demonstration models as instructional tools were more likely to maintain regular and effective use of the technique than learners who did not.

Using inanimate objects first is a technique educators can use to desensitize learners before doing injections or procedures on themselves or other human beings (Haggard, 1989). Teaching a diabetic how to draw up and inject insulin can best be accomplished by using a combination of real equipment and replicas. Patients first draw up sterile saline in real syringes, then practice injecting oranges, and progress to a model of a person before actually injecting themselves.

For lessons aimed at psychomotor learning, skills checklists can be used as a mechanism for evaluating whether the message has been incorporated by the learner (Grier, Owens, Peavy, & Pelt, 1991). These checklists are easily used in observation of return demonstrations. Simulation laboratories, for example, use this evaluation method frequently. Sims (1992) describes "Demonstration Day" in a neonatal unit, which had stations for chest tube care, umbilical artery catheter placement, exchange transfusion, metabolic screening and rhythm strips, and code arrest. Using various models, this demonstration day offered a chance to provide hands-on practice to all new staff nurses as well as an annual review of seasoned nurses.

The second type of model is known as an *analogue* because it uses analogy to explain something by comparing it to something else. Unlike replicas, analogue models can be used effectively to explain and represent dynamic systems (de Tornyay & Thompson, 1987). An analogue performs like the real object because it has the same properties as the dynamic system under consideration. Mechanical devices such as extracorporeal and dialysis machines are good examples of analogues. Although they do not look like the actual anatomy of a person, these pieces of artificial equipment perform similar physiological functions of the heart, lungs, and kidneys. Another popular analogue is the use of a computer model to see how the human brain functions (Babcock & Miller, 1994).

The third type of model is a *symbol*, which is used more frequently in a teaching situation. Words, mathematical signs and formulas, diagrams, musical notes, cartoons, stick figures, and traffic signs are all examples of symbolic models that convey a message to the receiver through imaging, convention, or association. As Babcock and Miller (1994)

point out, the meaning of words as symbols to convey concepts and ideas can vary depending on the language familiar to the one giving the message or the one receiving it. Symbols, such as international signs, are increasingly being used in multilingual or multicultural areas. However, abbreviations common to healthcare personnel, such as NPO, PRN, and PO, should be avoided when interacting with consumers because they may not be familiar with these acronyms.

The advantage of models is their usefulness when the real object is too small, too large, too expensive, too complex, unavailable, or a potential source of difficulty for learners. Models also allow learners to practice acquiring new skills without compromising themselves in practicing self-care activities or risking damage to valuable equipment (Haggard, 1989). Learners become more actively involved, and the application of knowledge and skills is immediate, as is the feedback from the instructor. These tools are especially attractive and useful for the kinesthetic learner who prefers the hands-on approach to learning. A vast array of models can be purchased from commercial vendors at varying prices (some for free) or improvised by the teacher. Models do not need to be expensive or elaborate to get concepts and ideas across (Rankin & Stallings, 2001).

In terms of their disadvantages, some models may not be suitable for the learner with poor abstraction abilities or for visually impaired audiences, unless each individual is given the chance to tangibly appraise the object using other senses. Also, some models can be fragile and others very expensive, like the Resusci-Annie doll used to teach cardiopulmonary resuscitation. Many are bulky to store and difficult to transport. Unless models are very large, they cannot be observed and manipulated by more than a few learners at any one time. This difficulty can be overcome by using team teaching and by creating different "stations" at which to arrange the replica for demonstration purposes (Babcock & Miller, 1994).

| TABLE 12-2   Advantages and disadvantages of demonstration materials | |
| --- | --- |
| Advantages | Disadvantages |
| Brings the learner closer to reality through active engagement | Content may be static, easily dated |
| Useful for cognitive reinforcement and psychomotor skill development | Can be time-consuming to make |
| Effective use of imagery may impact affective domain | Potential for overuse |
| Many forms are relatively inexpensive | Not suitable for simultaneous use with large audiences |
| Opportunity for repetition | Not suitable for visually impaired learners or for learners with poor abstraction abilities |

Table 12–2 summarizes the advantages and disadvantages of demonstration materials.

## Audiovisual Materials

Technology has changed the traditional approach to teaching. Nowhere is this shift more evident than in the audiovisual arena. *Audiovisual materials* support and enrich the educational process by stimulating the learner's visual and auditory senses, adding variety to the teaching–learning experience, and instilling visual memories, which have been found to be more permanent than auditory memories (de Tornyay & Thompson, 1987). Some visual aids, such as pictures and diagrams as demonstration materials, have been around since antiquity. Only relatively recently, however, has technology allowed for application of sophisticated audiovisual tools for purposes of instructing and learning. They are exceptional aids because many can influence all three domains of learning by promoting cognitive development, stimulating attitude change, and helping to build psychomotor skills. Audiovisuals have been known to increase retention of information by combining what we hear with what we see.

Because we live in an increasingly technological age, educators have to be aware of what audiovisual tools are available, how tools potentially and actually affect the ability to learn, and how to effectively and efficiently implement the various tools at our disposal. When and to what extent we should use them to augment teaching depend on many variables, not the least of which is the educator's comfort level and expertise in operating these technological devices. We assume that all educators are oriented to the use of audiovisual aids. This is not necessarily true, however, especially in light of the newness of some of the technology, such as computer-assisted instruction. Also, it should not be forgotten that some learners may have difficulty orienting to the newer modes of learning or have physical or cognitive limitations that may preclude the use of some types of audiovisual tools.

As with any teaching aids, audiovisuals must be carefully previewed for accuracy and appropriateness of content. Another major concern affecting which media you choose will depend on budgetary resources available for the purchase or rental of hardware equipment and software programs. It is extremely costly, in terms of time and money, as well as technologically demanding to self-produce audiovisual instructional materials. Thus, three issues (Smith, 1987) must be addressed:

1. Technical feasibility: technical expertise, professional and repair service support, equipment fit and replacement

**2.** Economic feasibility: budgetary allowance and justification of cost

**3.** Social/political acceptability: learner's willingness to use, impersonality of machines, acceptance by institutional administrations

There are many nonprint media whose primary mode of presentation is visual or audio or a blend of these two forms. Audiovisual materials can be categorized into five major types: projected, audio, video, telecommunications, and computer formats. Most of these learning resources are popular devices common to the general public. Others, like the computer, have only recently been applied to education; for this reason, learners are not as accustomed to receiving information via this type of media.

Kaihoi (1987) conducted a thorough review of many such learning resources for implementation into health education in our technological age. The following is a summary of the various types of audiovisual tools available for teaching.

**Projected Learning Resources**   The category of projected media, the best known of all audiovisual formats, includes slides, overhead transparencies, and computer outputs and video that can be projected on a screen. These media types are most frequently used with audiences of various sizes but can also be effective tools for teaching individuals.

*Slides*   There exist both conventional slide shows that appear static as slides are advanced one by one manually and newer slide/sound programs that change slides automatically in a rapid, synchronous manner to simulate motion. Slides have many advantages. For example, they offer the instructor a great deal of flexibility. They are inexpensive both to purchase and to make. Out-of-date material can readily be redone and replaced. Slides also can be easily rearranged and added to the original sequence. Close-ups can be made for a look at important details. During a slide presentation, it is easy to go backward to review information for purposes of reinforcing or clarifying a point. They can enhance an oral presentation by adding visual dimensions to the narration. Slide cassettes and projectors are portable, can fit into small rooms for viewing, and are easily stored. Most importantly, learners can start and stop equipment by themselves. Slides are excellent for conveying a message because they are an attractive mode for learning at all ages and facilitate retention and recall. Slides can capture real situations and can be personalized or tailored to meet specific audience needs.

The biggest disadvantage is that conventional slides must be shown in darkness for best visibility. With the lights lowered, the teacher can lose eye contact with the audience, and learners are less likely to ask questions or raise concerns when in the dark. A screen and projector setup must be available. Because slide equipment is manufactured by so many companies, you must be sure the carousel and projector being used are compatible. Careful composition of the slides is needed to avoid clutter or complex visuals that are boring or too difficult for the viewer to assimilate. In addition, slide programs take time to prepare and may not be appropriate for those with vision impairment.

Haggard (1989) suggests the following special considerations when preparing slides:

- Illustrate one idea per slide.

- Keep images simple by using clear pictures, symbols, or diagrams. Put long lists of words or complex figures on handouts that supplement the slides.

- Avoid distorted images by keeping the proportion of height to width at 2:3.

- Use large, easily readable, and professional-looking lettering.

- Use a 35-mm camera and slide film for photographing.

Microsoft's computer-generated software program, PowerPoint, is rapidly replacing conventional slides for instruction. Power-Point slides are easy to design, economical to produce, and an impressive medium by which to share information with a large or small audience. The program allows for flexi-bility to make changes in the slides whenever necessary as well as flexibility during the presentation to repeat slides or skip slides to move ahead to other content. Brown (2001) suggests the following important tips on how to employ this innovative tool productively:

- Use this medium to generate interaction between the teacher and the learner rather than as a tool that provides an outline of content to be followed for presenting infor-mation only in a traditional lecture format.

- On various slides, leave out some points to be made or ideas that should be included so that the learner must figure out what may be missing. This omission encourages critical thinking by the audience.

- Open a blank slide and type in the main points as they emerge from interactive discussion.

- Use text sparingly on each slide to keep details to a minimum by including no more than six points about any one idea per slide and limiting the word count to approxi-mately six words per point.

- Use contrasting but bold complementary col-ors so the text of each slide is clearly visible.

- Be sure the print size on each slide is large enough for the audience to read with ease at a distance. The Floor Test is one simple method to determine appropriate print size. That is, can you read a printout of the slide placed on the floor in front of you when in a standing position?

- Minimize or avoid animated text, sounds, and fancy transitions, which can serve to distract the reader from the message being conveyed.

- Keep unity of design from slide to slide by using a master slide as a template.

- Provide students with handouts of the slides (three slides per page) for purposes of note taking.

- The maximum number of slides to be pro-jected for teaching should be no more than one to two slides per minute to avoid pre-senting too much content in a given period of time. It is important to provide time for cognitive processing that allows learners to internalize the concepts being presented and to give learners a chance to discuss content and ask questions.

PowerPoint slides must be used judiciously to avoid overuse and abuse of this medium as a tool for effective teaching and learning.

*Overhead transparencies*  This medium is fre-quently used for teaching in a variety of set-tings, both in the classroom and for large con-ference presentations. Its advantages are many. Large numbers of people can see the projected images at one time while informa-tion is being explained. This medium is a par-ticularly useful tool to stimulate group discus-sion. Overheads share some of the same qualities of slides, such as the ability to isolate single facts, ideas, or themes. They also can be used to enlarge images. The biggest advan-tage from a teaching standpoint is that they can be shown in lighted rooms. They are also inexpensive to produce or purchase. Dia-grams and figures can readily be photocopied and made into transparencies. Multiple trans-parencies can be overlaid to illustrate changes in the content of teaching material.

Transparencies can be black-and-white or color. Use of colored acetates or colored felt pens provides contrast to images and lettering to enhance important teaching points. Color is known to attract attention and help differenti-ate information for better retention and recall (Cooper, 1990).

| TABLE 12–3    Advantages and disadvantages of projected learning resources | |
| --- | --- |
| Advantages | Disadvantages |
| Most effectively used with groups<br>May be especially beneficial for hearing-<br>  impaired, low-literate patients<br>Good for teaching skills in all domains | Lack of flexibility due to static content for some<br>  forms<br>Some forms may be expensive<br>Requires darkened room for some forms<br>Requires special equipment for use |

Among the disadvantages of overhead transparencies are the need for both specialized equipment for projection and the support of verbal feedback. For this reason, they are more conducive for use in a classroom than for purposes of individual self-instruction. The projector itself is awkward to transport, and the noise given off by the fan of the machine can be distracting in a small room. It is essential that finished transparencies be viewed ahead of time for an assessment of their readability, specifically related to the size of the lettering. Usually letters 1/4-inch high or letters that can be read at a distance of 10 feet before projection are sufficient for easy reading (Haggard, 1989). Note also that too much content on an overhead transparency will decrease its efficacy as a teaching tool.

Babcock and Miller (1994) recommend the following helpful guidelines for the use of overhead projectors and transparencies:

- Do not block the audience's view of the screen by standing in front of the machine. This common error can best be solved by making a habit of sitting or standing to the side to avoid interference with the projected image.

- Turn the projector off when you have finished referring to the transparency so as to keep the learners' attention on you and away from what is being projected. Constant use of the machine is also distracting because of the fan noise.

- Keep the message on the transparency simple. Use handouts to cover complex information as a supplement to your message.

- Display only one point at a time by masking the rest with a piece of paper if you have listed several ideas on one transparency. This approach allows listeners to focus on what you are saying and gives them time for note taking.

- Use a screen large enough for the audience to read the information projected.

- Use a light-colored blank wall if a screen is unavailable or too small.

- Pull the projector closer or farther away from the screen to change the size of the projection.

- Use tinted film to reduce glare of light.

- Use colored pens to help organize information or make specific points.

- Use overlays to help illustrate complex or sequential ideas. Note, however, that too many overlays can make the picture fuzzy.

Table 12–3 summarizes the advantages and disadvantages of projected learning resources.

**Audio Learning Resources**  Audio technology, although it has existed for a long time, has not been used to any great extent for educational purposes until recently. For years, it has been a useful tool for the blind or for those with serious visual or motor impairment. With significant advances in audio hardware and software and a turn away from the purely commercial use of this technology, however, audiotapes, compact discs (CDs), and radio have become more popular tools for teaching and learning. They can be used to relay many different types of messages, can help learners who benefit from repetition and reinforcement, and are well suited for those who enjoy or prefer auditory learning. They are also useful adjuncts for teaching illiterate persons.

*Audiotapes*   A very popular format today is the cassette tape. Use of this medium by educators has been growing. The biggest advantage of cassettes is their practicality. They are small, portable, inexpensive, simple to operate, and easy to prepare or duplicate; required recorders are also inexpensive. The audiotape recorder can be a powerful tool to augment other teaching methods by providing the listener with the opportunity to review previously heard information, to receive taped feedback from instructors, or to hear information available from no other source (Haggard, 1989). A good example of the latter is recorded lung sounds, which allow comparison between normal and abnormal breathing.

Cassettes are now available on a variety of health topics, from stress reduction to programs to stop smoking, and can be prepared specifically to meet the needs of a learner by reinforcing facts, giving directions, or providing support. As an example, Hagopian (1996) describes effective use of audiotapes for increasing knowledge and self-care behaviors of persons undergoing radiation therapy. If the tapes are self-made, the learner derives much comfort from hearing your familiar voice and reassuring words. This tool is used extensively by Excelsior College, a nursing external degree program of independent study, to provide direct feedback to students on the results of their examinations. Fredette (1984) described the use of audiotapes for

process recordings as a way to individualize clinical instruction for nursing students.

Information can be listened to at the leisure of the learner and reviewed as often as necessary. They can be used almost anywhere, such as the home, office, clinic, or hospital setting, and can be listened to while simultaneously driving a car or fixing a meal, thus filling in what normally would be considered wasted time. Developing a sizable library of tapes is well within the capability of most instructors thanks to this medium's low cost and easy storage. Pictures, diagrams, and printed handouts can accompany these instructional tools to fit the needs of a variety of learners.

The disadvantages of using audiotapes are few. The biggest drawback is that because audiotapes address only one sense—hearing—they cannot be used for hearing-impaired individuals. Also, some learners may become easily distracted from the information being presented unless they have visuals to accompany the tapes. There is also no opportunity for interactive feedback between the listener and the speaker. As with any medium, audiotapes should be used only as supplements to the various methods of instruction.

*Radio*   The radio has tremendously affected all of our lives for many years and is the oldest form of audio technology. Due to its commercial nature and appeal to mass audiences, it has typically been used more for pleasure than for education. In recent years, the medium of radio has been exploited by both public and private radio stations, which have begun airing community service and medical talk shows for public education on health issues. These programs are helpful in delivering a message, and, because of the convenience and popularity of radio as a communication tool, they could become more useful as vehicles in teaching and learning.

The disadvantage of radio relates to the difficulty of consistently delivering information

| TABLE 12–4   Advantages and disadvantages of audio learning resources | |
| --- | --- |
| Advantages | Disadvantages |
| Widely available | Relies only on sense of hearing |
| May be especially beneficial for visually impaired, low-literacy patients | Some forms may be expensive |
| May be listened to repeatedly | Lack of opportunity for interaction between instructor and learner |
| Most forms very practical, cheap, small, and portable. | |

on major topics to general as well as specific populations. The nurse educator has little control over the variety and depth of topics discussed or how regularly one listens to a program, and the general nature of radio programs is not tailored to meet individual needs. Unlike audiotapes, radio does not allow the opportunity for repetition of information. However, because of its widespread use and versatility, it has the potential for becoming a major source for important and useful healthcare information, especially if air time is funded by private foundations or sponsored by special groups or agencies dedicated to health teaching.

*Compact discs*   This modern form of media has replaced traditional vinyl record albums and in many instances is rapidly replacing traditional audiotapes. The major advantage of CDs is their superior fidelity, which does not deteriorate over time. Other advantages and disadvantages of CDs are similar to those of audiotapes, except for the fact that not as many people or institutions have the recording hardware or the computer capability to accommodate the use of this tool. However, the versatility of CDs for application to education is currently growing at a rapid rate in academia and will certainly affect patient and staff education in the near future. As with all technological advances over time, the cost is becoming very reasonable, and the hardware availability for healthcare education will increase in the near future.

Table 12–4 summarizes the advantages and disadvantages of audio learning resources.

**Video Learning Resources**   Videotapes, along with videotape recorders and television sets as electronic devices with which to view the tapes, have become commonplace in homes and healthcare settings. Camcorders and video cameras to make tapes are also owned by many people and institutions. People are becoming more accustomed to receiving information via this medium, and health educators are using it extensively for teaching in a variety of settings. Videotapes are one of the major nonprint media tools for enhancing patient/family, staff, and student education because tapes can be simultaneously entertaining and educational.

The major disadvantage of this medium is that the quality of videotapes, like audiotapes, can deteriorate over time. For this reason alone, VHS, the analog version of audio and visual projection combined, will be replaced by the newer DVD technology. DVDs (digital video discs), which incorporate the sound quality of CDs and video images by way of digital technology, have incredible archival qualities similar to CDs that allow for long-term storage and use. Unlike videotapes and audiotapes, DVDs will not deteriorate. Once used for entertainment purposes only, these discs are now gaining a wider audience in the field of higher education. Today, DVDs are being used to integrate PowerPoint slides and video images for classroom presentations by faculty on college and university campuses. In the not too distant future, this technology is expected to serve as an instructional tool for patient and staff education. The market for this innovative technology will increase as the cost of the software becomes more reasonable, as the hardware becomes more commonplace, and as educators become more well versed in using this new form for instruction.

Over the last few years, healthcare facilities have begun to use videotapes to develop patient education materials and broadcast them over in-house televisions. Its convenience and flexibility allow an educator to use the VCR for individual patient teaching situations as well as for large groups. Role-modeling of particular behaviors, attitudes, and values may be demonstrated powerfully through this medium. As an example, Daroszewski and Meehan (1997) effectively used videotaped role-playing as a staff development strategy for updating pain management skills of experienced nurses. An innovative variation on the use of videotaped role-playing for hospital staff was used by Henderson and Cumming (1997), who created and played two humorous characters, Olga and Bertha, to demonstrate the intricate discharge planning needs of a young single mother and her dependent mother.

Videotapes are a good means to promote discussion because they can capture real-life situations. This technique may be used as a teaching tool for nurse educators because its use as a critiquing instrument may provide direct feedback regarding learners' performances of complex interpersonal and psychomotor skills (Nielsen & Sheppard, 1988; Blank-Reid & Kaplan, 1996). Minnick, Peterson, and Krawczak (1988) described such use of audiovisual modeling to improve the teaching skills of baccalaureate nursing students. It has been especially beneficial for students with high performance anxiety and to convey teaching–learning principles to large groups in nonclinical settings. Blank-Reid and Kaplan

(1996) described use of video recordings of trauma resuscitations in the emergency department as an opportunity for education, research, and quality improvement. Their article provides a very useful outline for proper equipment setup, video storage, and disposal that could be adapted for many other settings. Couchman (1995) used videotaping and conversational analysis to educate staff working with people with learning disabilities. In a study investigating the use of videotaping to help nurses maintain and enhance their skills, Hill, Hooper, and Wahl (2000) were able to demonstrate improved performance and learner satisfaction.

The usefulness of videotape derives from its flexibility as a tool for instruction. The combination of color, motion, different angles, and sound enhances learning through visual as well as auditory senses. Videotaping has become very inexpensive, although whether the recorder is rented or owned by the user is a cost factor (Sternberger & Freiburger, 1996). The ready portability of recorders allows access to learning situations unavailable elsewhere. Williams, Wolgin, and Hodge (1998) wrote an extremely informative article that detailed steps for creating educational videotapes and identifying advantages of video instruction.

The disadvantage of purchased tapes is that they may be beyond the viewers' level of understanding, inappropriate for learner needs, or too long. The attention spans of learners vary, and the ideal length of tapes in most instances should be limited to 15 to 20 minutes. To avoid the possibility of creating a "talking head" effect, the operator of the recorder needs to be knowledgeable in the use of motion picture technology. Use of close-ups, dramatization of situations, and angle effects are not in the usual repertoire of many nurse educators. Scheduling for videotape viewing must take into account unit routines and the importance of repeat viewing opportunities (Nielsen & Sheppard, 1988).

| TABLE 12–5 Advantages and disadvantages of video learning resources | |
|---|---|
| Advantages | Disadvantages |
| Widely used educational tool | Viewing formats limited depending on use of |
| Inexpensive, for the most part | VHS or DVD |
| Uses visual and auditory senses | Some commercial products may be expensive |
| Flexible for use with different audiences | Some purchased materials may be too long or |
| Powerful tool for role-modeling, demonstration, | inappropriate for audience |
| teaching psychomotor skills | |

If you are planning to do your own videotapes, Haggard (1989) suggests striving for network-quality production by using the following guidelines:

- Write a script for the program. Rehearse thoroughly.

- Consider hiring a video technician on a per diem basis. This may be time- and cost-effective.

- For a small budget, a single camera with zoom capacity should be used. A larger budget may allow hiring a professional to edit the final product.

- Always be mindful of the program's objectives to avoid being seduced by the glamour of the process.

- Keep the program short. The longer the video, the more risk of losing viewer interest. Five to 15 minutes is ideal.

Table 12–5 summarizes the advantages and disadvantages of video learning resources.

**Telecommunications Learning Resources**
Telecommunications is a means by which information can be transmitted via electrical energy from one place to another in a sense that is meaningful for the person receiving it. This form of media includes television and telephone and its related modes of audio and video teleconferencing and closed-circuit, cable, and satellite broadcasting. Telecommunications devices have allowed messages to be sent to many people at the same time in a variety of places at great distances.

*Television* The television, ubiquitous in American homes, has been used for many years as an entertainment tool. Today, there are more televisions than telephones in private residences. The TV is also well suited for educational purposes and has become a popular teaching–learning tool in homes, schools, businesses, and healthcare settings. The power to influence cognitive, affective, and psychomotor behavior is well demonstrated by television commercials, whose messages are simple, direct, and variously repetitive to effectively influence the behavior of intended audiences.

Cable TV is legally obligated to provide public access programming by offering channels for community members to air their own programs. Health education, if placed on the cable system, can be seen in any home hooked up to cable. The advantage of this option is that distribution of programs is relatively inexpensive. The disadvantage is that one cannot control who is watching, and this medium cannot serve as an interactive question-and-answer experience unless call-in phone lines are provided.

Closed-circuit TV allows for education programs to be sent to specific locations, such as patient rooms or staff units. The learner can request a particular program at any given time, much like a guest in a hotel can choose from a variety of movies day and night. This

| TABLE 12–6    Advantages and disadvantages of telecommunications learning resources | |
| --- | --- |
| **Advantages** | **Disadvantages** |
| TV program distribution is relatively inexpensive to wide audiences | Complicated to set up interactive capability |
| Telephone is relatively inexpensive, widely available | Expensive to broadcast via satellite |

telecommunications technology requires programs to be played intermittently or continuously, with program availability clearly advertised. Because the learner controls program viewing, the nurse educator must follow up to answer questions and determine whether learning has, in fact, occurred.

Satellite broadcasting, a newer form of telecommunications, can reach far more distant locations, and a number of programs can be carried at any one time. Because of its expense, not many institutions send health information via this mode, but many receive it. More types of satellite systems are being developed such that this form of communication for educational purposes will become possible in the near future on a worldwide basis.

Heidenreiter (1995) described use of video teleconferencing for continuing education and staff development as one strategy for maintaining quality and viability of continuing education programs in a time of tight budgets. In addition, several health networks, such as Lifetime, broadcast to cable companies and hospitals.

*Telephones*   It is almost impossible to imagine being without the telephone as a daily tool. Americans have come to depend on it as a fundamental means of communication. It is not surprising, therefore, that the telephone can be used effectively for education. In recognition of this fact, many healthcare associations have begun to provide telephone services with messages about disease treatment and prevention. The American Cancer Soci-

ety, for example, has established a toll-free number for the public to obtain short taped messages about various types of cancer. Hospitals, too, have set up call-in services about a variety of health-related topics and sources for referral. The advantage is that these services are relatively inexpensive and can be operated by someone with minimal medical knowledge because the taped message contains the substance of the content. Another advantage is that this type of service is available in most cases around the clock. The disadvantage is that there is no opportunity for questions to be answered directly.

Telecommunications as an instructional tool is becoming increasingly popular and sophisticated. Many hospitals and healthcare agencies have already established hot-line consumer information centers, which are manned by knowledgeable healthcare personnel so that information can be personalized and appropriate feedback can be given on the spot. The Poison Control hot line is a good example of the use of this medium.

Table 12–6 summarizes the advantages and disadvantages of telecommunications learning resources.

**Computer Learning Resources**   In our technological society, the computer has changed our lives dramatically and has found widespread application in industry, business, schools, and homes. The computer can store large amounts of information, and is designed to display pictures, graphics, and text. The presentation of information can be changed depending on user input.

Although computer technology is a fairly recent addition to the educational field, it is becoming very common, especially with the rapid increase of computer literacy among students, professionals, and the general public. There is a great deal of evidence that computer-assisted instruction (CAI) promotes learning in primarily the cognitive domain. More research needs to be done to establish its usefulness to change attitudes and behaviors or promote psychomotor skill development. Retention is improved by an interactive exchange between the learner and the computer, even though the instructor is not actually present. CAI simulates the feedback of a face-to-face exchange between individuals. For instance, the computer game NumberMaze, developed by Great Wave Software for the Macintosh, was designed to teach math at a variety of skill levels. Instructions can be selected that will present more word problems or more numerical problems to learners at a pace of their own choosing. The game's changeability makes it endlessly challenging and new to the user.

CAI has many advantages. The ability to individualize instruction to the learner on a moment-by-moment basis is one unique feature of CAI. Lessons can be varied readily, and the learner controls the pace. With no time constraints, the learner can move as quickly or as slowly as desired to master content without incurring penalties for mistakes or performance speed. An instructor can easily track the level of understanding of the learner. Because the computer has the ability to ask questions and analyze responses, it can perform ongoing assessment of the learner and alter the content, pace, and examples presented. Computers can be programmed to provide feedback to the educator regarding the learner's grasp of concepts, the speed of learning, and those aspects of learning that need reinforcement.

The interactive features of this medium also provide for immediate feedback to the learner.

Many software packages are available from a wide variety of sources. Even costly packages may be cost-effective if the potential audience is large (Gillespie & Ellis, 1993). Time efficiency is a major advantage of CAI, in that the teacher has more time to devote to teaching other tasks not taught via computer, such as affective and psychomotor skills (Boyd et al., 1998). In addition, the content of CAI programs is consistent for all learners because they are exposed to the exact same information. Computers are also valuable tools for those with aphasia, hearing impairment, or learning disabilities (see Chapter 9 on special populations).

The major disadvantage of CAI is that both hardware and software can be quite expensive, making it infeasible for some learning situations. In most cases, programs must be purchased because they are too time-consuming and too complex for the educator to develop. Even if someone has programming skills, it can take up to 500 hours to produce 1 hour of instructional material (Boyd et al., 1998). In addition, lack of computer literacy or a comfort level with computers may be a barrier to some learners and even some nurse educators. As Boyd et al. (1998) further point out, many older adults are computer shy or computer illiterate. However, this situation is beginning to change, as computers become more of a household item. Unfortunately, people with reading problems will likely have major difficulty making sense of the information on the screen (see Chapter 7 on literacy). In addition, learners with physical limitations, such as arthritis, neuromuscular disorders, pain, fatigue, paralysis, or vision impairment, may find computer use difficult if not impossible (see Chapter 9 on special populations). Moreover, it should not be forgotten that the computer is a machine, so the learner is necessarily deprived of the personal, compassion-

| TABLE 12–7    Advantages and disadvantages of computer learning resources | |
|---|---|
| Advantages | Disadvantages |
| Interactive potential promotes quick feedback, retention of learning<br>Potential database enormous<br>Instruction can be individualized to suit different types of learners or different paces for learning<br>Time-efficient | Primarily promotes learning in cognitive domain; less useful in changing attitudes and behaviors or promoting psychomotor skill development<br>Both software and hardware are expensive, therefore less accessible to a wide audience<br>Must be purchased—too complex and time-consuming for most educators to prepare<br>Limited use for many elderly, low-literate learners, and those with physical limitations |

ate, one-to-one interaction that only a teacher can provide to facilitate learning. Because of the independent nature of the computer learning experience, it is not very suitable for nondirected or poorly motivated learners. Lack of access to computers may be a barrier, even for the computer-literate learner. Although the market for computer software has skyrocketed, only a relatively small percentage of programs have dealt with patient education to date, and the quality of the products is uneven (Gillespie & Ellis, 1993).

More recently, the growth of the Internet has opened new doors for learners to gain access to libraries and to direct learning experiences, which can include on-line discussions with educators at great distances from the learner. Use of the Internet is not restricted to any age group. Anyone with a computer and access to on-line technology can make use of this tremendous resource (see Chapter 13 on technology in education).

Table 12–7 summarizes the advantages and disadvantages of computer learning resources.

### EVALUATION CRITERIA FOR SELECTING MATERIALS

Choosing the right tools for patient education calls for judgment on the part of the nurse educator, who must take into consideration the *learner*, the *task*, and the *media* available to help achieve learning objectives. Decisions may need to be made on an individual basis or for large groups, depending on the size and characteristics of the audience. There may be multiple objectives. Not only must the educator consider the media available in general, but different objectives may best be reached with different teaching materials.

Both the learning objectives and the domains of learning in which instruction must occur will dictate the most appropriate materials. Discenza (1993) states that the method for selection of instructional materials is the same, regardless of the domain of learning. Selection is based on the ability of materials to help with the instruction of a given behavioral objective. Materials should not be selected before the objectives are set. Discenza also states that evaluation of media involves evaluating the content, the instructional design, the technical production of the instructional material, and the packaging. Figure 12–9 depicts Discenza's checklist for selecting and evaluating instructional materials.

Written materials are one of the most important tools available in comprehensive patient education. They can be used for direct

|  | Yes | No |
|---|---|---|
| A. Content | | |
| Is the content valid? | | |
| Relevant? | | |
| Currant? | | |
| Is the purpose of the program stated? | ___ | ___ |
| Are instructional objectives given? | ___ | ___ |
| | ___ | ___ |
| B. Instructional Design | ___ | ___ |
| Are the ideas and information presented logically? | ___ | ___ |
| Is the format of the program appropriate for the audience? | | |
| Does the Instructor actively engage the learner? | | |
| Is there evidence of formative evaluation? | ___ | ___ |
| Is summative evaluation material provided? | ___ | ___ |
| | ___ | ___ |
| C. Technical Production | ___ | ___ |
| Is the visual material sharply focused and clear? | | |
| Is the image composition clear and uncluttered? | | |
| Is the text legible at the maximum viewing distance? | ___ | ___ |
| Is the audio clear and intelligible? | ___ | ___ |
| Is there any distracting background noise? | ___ | ___ |
| Is the pace of the narration appropriate for the audience? | ___ | ___ |
| | ___ | ___ |
| D. Packaging | | |
| Is the material available in a format for which equipment is available? | | |
| Is descriptive information provided? | ___ | ___ |
| Is a User's Guide provided? | ___ | ___ |
| Has the instructional material won any awards? | ___ | ___ |

FIGURE 12–9   **A Checklist for Selecting and Evaluating Instructional Materials**   SOURCE: David J. Discenza (1993). A systematic approach to selecting and evaluating instructional material. *Journal of Nursing Staff Development, 9*(4), 198. Reprinted by permission of J.B. Lippincott Company.

learning and as reinforcement for oral and audiovisual presentations. An evaluation of readability is essential when selecting print media that will best enhance a given audience's learning (see Chapter 7 on literacy). Pastore and Berg (1987) and Doak et al. (1996) offer practical advice for developing and evaluating written patient education materials. Their recommendations focus on needs assessment of audience, consideration of readability (including formatting and readability formulas), patient and staff reviews of materials, and agency approval.

Remember to consider the predetermined behavioral objectives. Ask yourself, Which materials will best support the teaching to meet these objectives with this audience? Also, remember that active is best, real is best, and instructional materials should be used only to support the learning.

Table 12–8 provides a helpful, easy-to-use reference for selection of media.

## Table 12–8   Effectiveness of teaching tools and methods

| Mode of Learning | Retention | Media | Methods |
|---|---|---|---|
| Reading | Learners retain 10% of what they read. | Leaflets, books, brochures, flip charts, chalkboards, instruction sheets | Self-instruction |
| Hearing | Learners retain 20% of what they hear. | Audiotapes, telephones | Lectures, discussion |
| Watching | Learners retain 30% of what they see. | Silent films, displays, photos, pictures, posters, cartoons, drawings | Demonstration, self-instruction |
| Watching and hearing | Learners retain 50% of what they see and hear. | Movies (films), TV, videotapes, slides, overheads, models | Lecture or demonstration |
| Watching and speaking | Learners retain 70% of what they see and talk about. | Audiovisual media | Group discussion, 1:1 verbal interactions, demonstrations |
| Speaking and doing | Learners retain 90% of what they talk about and do. | Interactive media | Demonstration, return demonstration, gaming, role-playing |

SOURCE: Adapted from Heinich et al. (1992).

## SUMMARY

This chapter discussed the major categories of instructional materials and answered questions about how to select media from a range of possible options as well as how to evaluate their effectiveness. Nurse educators are expected to be able to make these choices every day, whether it be to meet the needs of an individual learner or to design a large educational program to satisfy a broader, more diverse group. In this chapter, the importance of considering characteristics of the learner, the media, and the task when choosing instructional materials was emphasized. The supplemental nature of teaching materials was also stressed, as well as the need to keep the teaching objectives and behavioral objectives in focus when selecting these materials as adjuncts to instruction.

When using print and nonprint media, it is crucial that nurses alert patients to watch for specific points of information. This effort individualizes content by helping patients focus on what is particularly important to them. After viewing any instructional materials, make yourself available to learners to answer questions or provide opportunity for cognitive practice on what they have seen or read. Audiovisual programs that can be taken home and that have accompanying reference materials on which patients can jot notes and write questions can be effective in engendering patient involvement and retention.

The major categories of print and nonprint media were reviewed in full. Where appropriate, examples of effective teaching tools were contrasted with examples of less effective instructional aids. Finally, comprehensive evaluation criteria were presented to assist the educator in selecting appropriate tools for purposes of teaching and learning.

Print media include both commercially prepared and self-composed materials. The problem of matching literacy level and cognitive level of learners to instructional tools is relevant to both types of media. The major advantages of printed tools are that they are widely available, that patients are able to refer back to these materials for review at any time and at their own pace, and that they have potential for reinforcing explanations of complex concepts. Disadvantages include the limited opportunity for learner–educator feedback. For some learners, literacy level and complexity of information may be significant barriers to full utilization of printed tools. This chapter contains several guidelines that should be useful to educators in selecting or developing printed materials appropriate to both the audience and the task.

Demonstration materials include many types of nonprint media, such as models, real equipment, diagrams, charts, flip charts, posters, photographs, and drawings. They may exploit the senses of sight, touch, smell, and even taste. They are especially useful for cognitive and psychomotor skill development and may even influence the affective domain through creative imagery. Other advantages include bringing the learner closer to reality through active engagement and the opportunity for repetition. The major disadvantage of demonstrations is the potential for static con-

tent or overuse, as demonstrations are often time-consuming to prepare and the educator may be reluctant or unable to revise these materials frequently. In addition, these materials are not suitable for large audiences, visually impaired learners, or individuals with poor abstraction abilities. Guidelines for selecting demonstration media were presented in this chapter.

Audiovisual materials are the fastest growing category of instructional tools. Their ability to stimulate learners' visual and auditory senses enhances their power to actively engage learners and increase retention of information. Many audiovisual tools can influence all three domains of learning by promoting cognitive development, stimulating attitude change, and helping to build psychomotor skills.

This chapter examined the five major categories of audiovisual tools: projected, audio, video, telecommunications, and computer formats. The discussion included audience appropriateness, expense, and convenience of use. Comprehensive guidelines for selecting and developing audiovisual materials were presented. The principal advantages and disadvantages of the five categories were also described. Learners with low literacy skills may benefit from most categories of these media except computer formats. Visually impaired learners may be limited to audio materials, while hearing-impaired learners may do well with projected, video, computer, and some forms of telecommunications.

## REVIEW QUESTIONS

1. How do instructional materials differ from instructional methods?
2. What are five (5) general principles regarding the effectiveness of audiovisual tools?
3. What are the three (3) major variables to consider when selecting, developing, and evaluating instructional materials?
4. What are the three (3) primary components of media to be kept in mind when evaluating

appropriateness of audiovisual materials for instruction?
5. Which instructional materials are examples of illusionary representations?
6. Why are numbers as well as oral and written words known to be the most abstract forms of messages?
7. What factors must be considered when reviewing commercially prepared print materials for use in instruction?

8. What are six (6) of the eleven (11) guidelines to be followed for writing patient education materials with clarity and completeness?

9. Why are format and appearance equally as important as clarity and completeness in constructing written materials?

10. What are some examples of demonstration materials? Of audiovisual materials?

11. What is the difference between projected learning resources and audio learning resources?

12. What are the major advantages and disadvantages of computer learning resources?

13. Why is the statement true that instructional materials should not be selected before behavioral objectives are determined?

14. Which two (2) modes of learning are most effective for the retention of information? Why?

## REFERENCES

Babcock, D. E. & Miller, M. A. (1994). *Client Education: Theory and Practice.* St. Louis: Mosby–Year Book.

Bach, C. A., McDaniel, R. W., & Poole, M. J. (1994). Posters: innovative and cost-effective tools for staff development. *Journal of Nursing Staff Development, 10*(2), 71–74.

Baker, G. C. (1991). Writing easily-read patient education handouts: A computerized approach (review). *Seminars in Dermatology, 10*(2), 102–106.

Blank-Reid, C. A. & Kaplan, L. J. (1996). Video recording trauma resuscitations: A guide to system set-up, personnel concerns, and legal issues. *Journal of Trauma Nursing, 3*(1): 9–12.

Boyd, M. D. (1987). A guide to writing effective patient education materials. *Nursing Management, 18,* 56–57.

Boyd, M. D., Gleit, C. J., Graham, B. A., & Whitman, N. J. (1998). *Health Teaching in Nursing Practice: A Professional Model,* 3rd ed. Stamford, CT: Appleton & Lange.

Brown, D. G. (March 2001). *Judicious PowerPoint.* www.syllabus.com.

Brownson, K. (1998). Education handouts: Are we wasting our time? *Journal of Nurses in Staff Development, 14*(4), 176–182,

Bushy, A. (1991). A rating scale to evaluate research posters. *Nurse Educator, 16*(1), 11–15.

Byrne, T. J. & Edeani, D. (1984). Knowledge of medical terminology among hospital patients. *Nursing Research, 33*(3), 178–181.

Campbell, M. K., DeVellis, B. Strecher, V. J., Ammerman, A. S., DeVellis, R. S., & Sandler, R. S. (1994). Improving dietary behavior: The effectiveness of tailored messages in primary care settings. *American Journal of Public Health, 84,* 783–787.

Cooper, S. S. (1990). Teaching tips, one more time: The overhead projector. *Journal of Continuing Education in Nursing, 21*(3), 141–142.

Couchman, W. (1995). Using video and conversational analysis to train staff working with people with learning disabilities. *Journal of Advanced Nursing, 22,* 1112–1119.

Daroszewski, E. B. & Meehan, D. A. (1997). Pain, role play, and videotape: Pain management staff development in a community hospital. *Journal of Nursing Staff Development, 13*(3), 119–124.

de Tornyay, R. & Thompson, M. A. (1987). *Strategies for Teaching Nursing,* 3rd ed. Albany, NY: Delmar.

Discenza, D. J. (1993). A systematic approach to selecting and evaluating instructional materials. *Journal of Nursing Staff Development, 9*(4), 196–198.

Doak, C. C., Doak, L. G., Friedell, G. H., & Meade, C. D. (1998). Improving comprehension for cancer patients with low literacy skills: strategies for clinicians. *CA–Cancer Journal for Clinicians, 48*(3), 151–162.

Doak, C. C., Doak, L. G., & Root, J. H. (1996). *Teaching Patients with Low Literacy.* Philadelphia: J. P. Lippincott.

Duchin, S. & Sherwood, G. (1990). Posters as an educational strategy. *Journal of Continuing Education in Nursing, 21*(5), 205–208.

Estey, A., Musseau, A., & Keehn, L. (1994). Patient's understanding of health information: A multihospital comparison. *Patient Education and Counseling, 24,* 73–78.

Flournoy, E., Turner, G., & Combs, D. (2000). Innovative teaching: Read the writing on the wall. *Dimensions of Critical Care Nursing, 19*(4), 36–37.

Foster, S. D. (1987). Are commercial patient education materials right for you? *MCN: American Journal of Maternal Child Nursing, 12*(4), 287.

Frantz, R. A. (1980). *Selecting Media for Patient Education. TCN/Education for Self-Care.* Rockville, MD: Aspen.

Fredette, S. L. (1984). Individualized clinical teaching via the tape recorder. *Image, 16*(3), 80–83.

Gilliespie, M. O. & Ellis, L. B. (1993). Computer-based patient education revisited (review). *Journal of Medical Systems, 17*(3–4), 119–125.

Glazer-Waldman, H., Hall, K., & Weiner, M. F. (1985). Patient education in a public hospital. *Nursing Research, 34*(3), 184–185.

Grier, E. C., Owens, C., Peavy, B. A., & Pelt, F. (1991). Use of a checklist to teach advanced technical skills. *Nurse Educator, 16*(5), 37–38.

Haggard, A. (1989). *Handbook of Patient Education.* Rockville, MD: Aspen.

Hagopian, G. A. (1996). The effects of informational audiotapes on knowledge and self-care behaviors of patients undergoing radiation therapy. *ONF, 23*(4), 697–700.

Hanafin, L. F. (1993). The 5-minute teaching series: Pamphlet designed for brief inservice topics. *Journal of Nursing Staff Development, 9*(4), 199–220.

Hayes, S. K. & Childress, D. M. (1999). Fairy tales of storyboarding. *Journal for Nurses in Staff Development, 15*(6), 260–262.

Heidenreiter, T. J. (1995). Using videoteleconferencing for continuing education and staff development programs. *Journal of Continuing Education in Nursing, 26*(3), 135–138.

Heinich, R., Malenda, M., & Russell, J. D. (1992). *Instructional Media and the New Technologies of Instruction,* 4th ed. New York: Macmillan.

Henderson, T. & Cumming, B. (1997). An innovative teaching strategy for staff development departments. *Journal of Nursing Staff Development, 13*(4), 183–188.

Hill, R., Hooper, C., & Wahl, S. (2000). Look, learn, and be satisfied: Video playback as a learning strategy to improve clinical skills performance. *Journal for Nurses in Staff Development, 16*(5), 232–239.

Hinkle, J. L., Albanese, M., & McGinty, L. (1993). Development of printed teaching materials for neuroscience patients. *American Association of Neuroscience Nurses, 25*(2), 125–129.

Houts, P. S., Bachrach, B., Witmer, J. T., Tringali, C. A., Bucher, J. A., & Localio, R. A. (1998). Using pictographs to enhance recall of spoken medical instructions. *Patient Education and Counseling, 35,* 83–88.

Kaihoi, B. H. (1987). Implementing use of learning resources in our technological age. Chapter 7 in C. E. Smith, *Patient Education: Nurses in Partnership with Other Health Professionals.* Philadelphia: Saunders.

Lerner, E. B., Jehle, D. V. K., Janicke, D. M., & Moscati, R. M. (2000). Medical communication: Do our patients understand? *American Journal of Emergency Medicine, 18*(7), 764–766.

Minnick, A., Peterson, L. M., & Krawczak, J. (1988). The effects of audiovisual modeling and reading on baccalaureate students' patient teaching. *Western Journal of Nursing Research, 10*(6), 766–777.

Moneyham, L., Ura, D., Ellwood, S., & Bruno, B. (1996). The poster presentation as an educational tool. *Nurse Educator, 21*(4), 45–47.

Nielsen, E. & Sheppard, M. A. (1988). Television as a patient education tool: A review of its effectiveness. *Patient Education and Counseling, 11,* 3–16.

Pastore, P. O. & Berg, B. K. (1987). The evaluation of patient education materials: Focus on readability. *Patient Education and Counseling, 9*(2), 216–219.

Pinto, B. M. (1993). Training and maintenance of breast self-examination skills. *American Journal of Preventive Medicine, 9*(6), 353–358.

Rankin, S. H. & Stallings, K. D. (2001). *Patient Education: Principles and Practice,* 4th ed. Philadelphia: Lippincott.

Redman, B. K. (2001). *The Practice of Patient Education,* 9th ed. St. Louis: Mosby.

Rice, V. H. & Johnson, J. E. (1984). Preadmission self-instruction booklets, postadmission exercise performance, and teaching time. *Nursing Research, 33*(3), 147–151.

Sims, S. (1992). Demonstration day: A unique way to learn. *Neonatal Network—Journal of Neonatal Nursing, 11*(1), 41–44.

Skinner, C. S., Strecher, V. J., & Hospens, H. (1994). Physician's recommendations for mammography: Do tailored messages make a difference? *American Journal of Public Health, 84*, 43–49.

Smith, C. E. (1987). *Patient Education: Nurses in Partnership with Other Health Professionals.* Philadelphia: Saunders.

Sternberger, C. S. & Freiburger, O. A. (1996). Faculty-produced videos: An educational resource. *Journal of Nursing Staff Development, 12*(4), 173–178.

Thurber, R. F. & Asselin, M. E. (1999). An educational fair and poster approach to organization-wide mandatory education. *Journal of Continuing Education in Nursing, 30*(1), 25–29.

Weixler, D. (1994). Correcting metered-dose inhaler misuse. *Nursing, 24*(7), 62–65.

Weston, C. & Cranston, P. A. (1986). Selecting instructional strategies. *Journal of Higher Education, 57*(3), 259–288.

Williams, A. V., Parker, R. M., Baker, D. W., Parikh, N. S., Pitkin, K., Coates, W. C., & Nurss, J. R. (1995). Inadequate functional health literacy among patients at two public hospitals. *Journal of the American Medical Association, 274*(21), 1677–1682.

Williams, N. H., Wolgin, C. S., & Hodge, C. S. (1998). Creating an educational videotape. *Journal for Nurses in Staff Development, 14*(6), 261–265.

## CHAPTER 13

# Technology in Education

*Deborah L. Sopczyk*

## CHAPTER HIGHLIGHTS

Health Education in the Information Age

The Impact of Technology on the Teacher and
   the Learner

Strategies for Using Technology in Healthcare
   Education

   The World Wide Web

   Healthcare Consumer Education and the World
     Wide Web

   Professional Education and the World Wide Web

The Internet

E-Mail

Electronic Discussion Groups

   Mailing Lists

   Usenet

   Other Forms of Online Discussion

Issues Related to the Use of Technology

Professional Education

   E-Learning

   Distance Education

## KEY TERMS

Information Age

consumer informatics

World Wide Web

Internet

information literacy

computer literacy

digital divide

e-learning

distance learning

## OBJECTIVES

After completing this chapter, the reader will be
able to

1. Describe changes in education that have
   occurred as a result of Information Age technology.

2. Define the terms *Information Age, consumer
   informatics, World Wide Web, Internet, information literacy, computer literacy, digital divide, e-
   learning,* and *distance learning.*

3. Identify ways in which the resources of the
   Internet and World Wide Web could be incorporated into healthcare education.

4. Describe the role of the nurse educator in using
   technology in client and staff education.

5. Recognize the issues related to the use of
   technology.

6. Discuss the effects that technology has had on
   professional education for nurses.

The end of the twentieth century gave witness to advances in technology that have changed the face of education. The birth of the Internet and the World Wide Web, the development of information technology, the wide-scale production of computers, the development of user-friendly software, and the educational applications that followed have all had profound effects on the way we learn and the way we teach (Heller, Ortos, & Crowley, 2000). Many adult learners can remember a time when writing a paper required traveling to the library to search a card catalog and spending countless hours looking through paper-based books and journals. Today, students have a world of information at their fingertips. Computers and the Internet have made it possible to get information from anyone, anywhere, anytime, within the blink of an eye. Educational technologies, once rare and highly desirable resources, have become commonplace, and both the on-site and distance learner now interact in a multidimensional learning environment. Like shiny new toys, educational technologies have captured the imagination of the world. At the same time, they have presented unlimited challenges and opportunities for educators and learners alike.

This chapter explores the challenges and opportunities resulting from the use of technology as they pertain to health and healthcare education by nurses and professional education for nurses. The use of technology in education has tremendous potential to increase access, to improve educational practices already in place, and to create new strategies that transform teaching and learning experiences for nurses and healthcare consumers. However, technology is not a magic solution that can be implemented without careful planning, monitoring, and evaluation. Although computer-based educational applications have become easier to use and require less technical skill than they did in the past,

the decision to use technology as part of an educational program is likely to have implications related to myriad issues, including access, cost, level of support, equipment, process, and outcomes.

It is important to remember that technology in education is a means to an end, not an end in and of itself. "Without hard questions about learning, technology is like an unguided missile" (Ehrmann, 1995). Although it has incredible power, without careful planning, technology may take you to a place you did not want to go and give results you had not anticipated or desired. Therefore, the nurse who uses technology to enhance learning must not only have a basic understanding of the technology itself, but also be able to integrate the technology into a plan that is based on sound educational principles.

This chapter is designed as an introduction to the use of technology in education. Because nurses provide both healthcare and professional education, it will address technology-based resources and strategies appropriate for use with clients and with nurses and other healthcare professionals. Although it is not intended to provide detailed instruction on the mechanics of computers and other types of hardware and software, the chapter will provide a basic overview of the technology involved and implications for the educator and the learner. Chapter 11 discusses the use of audiovisual materials in the classroom. Hence, this chapter will focus primarily on the Internet, the World Wide Web, and computer-based hardware and software applications that can be used to enhance learning with students in the classroom as well as with learners at a distance.

Before beginning this chapter, it is important to note that the Internet, the World Wide Web, and computer-based technologies are developing at a rapid pace that is accelerating with each new generation of discoveries and applications (Cetron & Davies, 2001). Because of this phenomenon, consumers are often advised that the computers they bought today are not likely to reflect the "state-of-the-art" technology tomorrow. The same caution must be given to readers of books on technology. Given the pace of technology and the development cycle of a textbook, it is impossible to capture all that is new and cutting-edge in the world of educational technologies in a textbook. Rather, this chapter is meant to serve as a starting point from which you can begin to investigate the educational technologies and resources available. Ideally, it will generate the interest and skill necessary for you to continue to search for new and exciting ways to integrate technology into your teaching and learning activities.

## HEALTH EDUCATION IN THE INFORMATION AGE

The use of technology in education is a reflection of what is happening on a much larger scale in our communities. Hence, it is useful to think of educational technology within the broader context of the environment in which we live and work. We are in a period of history often referred to as the *Information Age*. Mitchel and McCullough (1995) describe the Information Age as a place in time when sweeping advances in computer and information technology have transformed the economic, social, and cultural life of society. If you think about the many ways in which technology has changed the world we live in, it is clear that computers have become more than tools to make life easier—they have become part of our culture.

Computers have also become part of the culture of education. Computers are as common in the educational environment today as chalk and blackboards were in years past. Perhaps the most significant effect computers

have on our society and on education is related to their capacity to assist in the collection, management, transportation, and transformation of information at high speed. As a result of this newfound ability to handle information, we have experienced an "information explosion" and as a society we have increased both our use and our production of information of all kinds. As people living within this information-driven society, we not only benefit from the availability of information but are also challenged to keep up with the information that is bombarding us from all directions. Information and knowledge have become valuable commodities, and the ability to gather and evaluate information efficiently and effectively has become a twenty-first-century life skill.

How has the Information Age changed health education? Consider the following. As a result of technological advances, millions of miles of optical fiber, wire, and air waves now link people around the world to one another and to a vast array of Web-based information. In the United States alone, more than 104 million adults report having Internet access (Rainie & Packel, 2001). By the year 2010, 95% of the people in the industrialized world and half of those in the developing world are predicted to be online and wired for high-speed access (Cetron & Davies, 2001).

As nurses who are providing health and healthcare education, it has never been easier to reach our clients. For the first time, our health and healthcare messages can easily reach beyond local communities to a worldwide audience. Not only can we reach people, but we can also provide interactive learning experiences that extend far beyond what was even imaginable in recent past.

The use of Information Age technology has had such a dramatic influence on health education that a new and rapidly expanding field of study, *consumer informatics*, has emerged.

Also referred to as *consumer health informatics*, consumer informatics is defined as a discipline that "analyses consumers' needs for information, studies and implements methods of making information accessible to consumers, and models and integrates consumer preferences into medical information systems" (Eysenbach, 2000, p. 1713). Although much attention has been given to computer-based educational systems, consumer informatics is not restricted to computer-based programs and includes the study of a wide range of media that can be used to deliver health-related information.

The entire field of consumer informatics is growing rapidly. Schools such as the University of Maryland and the University of Virginia Health Science Center offer courses of study where healthcare professionals can gain knowledge and skill in using technology to meet the information needs of healthcare consumers. Organizations such as the American Medical Informatics Association (AMIA) have established task forces to identify the issues and explore the roles they might play in guiding the practice of professionals in the field (Kaplan & Brennan, 2001). Informaticians and healthcare professionals are conducting research on the use of technology in healthcare education to generate knowledge that will guide future educational endeavors.

An example of the work of consumer informatics can be found on the "Research Based Web Design and Usability Guidelines" Web site (*http://usability.gov/guidelines/index.html*) sponsored by the National Cancer Institute. This Web site contains guidelines that can be used in designing health-related Web sites. Not only are the guidelines provided here based on research studies and supporting information from the field, but ratings are also assigned to each guideline according to the strength of the evidence available. For example, a guideline that is given a rating of 5 is one that is supported by two or more research studies where hypotheses were

tested and the guideline was shown to be effective. A score of zero indicates that although the guideline may be routinely followed on Web pages, there is no evidence to support its effectiveness.

Despite the rapid growth of technology-based education programs and services, it is important to remember that electronic delivery of health information is in its infancy and there are still many issues that need to be resolved. One major area of concern is the limited oversight and control over the content that is posted on the Internet and World Wide Web, two of the major vehicles for delivering information to a global audience. Many people believe that the lack of censorship on the World Wide Web is a freedom of speech issue. However, healthcare professionals are concerned that consumers are making serious healthcare decisions based on information on the Web that has not been reviewed for accuracy, currency, or bias.

Recently, healthcare education and informatics professionals have begun to work together to develop "codes" to guide practice and safeguard healthcare consumers who use the educational information and services that are delivered via the World Wide Web and the Internet. For example, the Internet Healthcare Coalition, a non-profit group dedicated to quality healthcare information on the Internet, established the *e-Health Code of Ethics* to ensure confident and informed use of the health-related information found on the Internet (Internet Healthcare Coalition, 2000). The e-Health Code of Ethics is based upon the principles of candor, honesty, quality, informed consent, privacy, professionalism, responsible partnering, and accountability that are described in more detail in Table 13-1. The *e-Health Code of Ethics* is only one of several codes that have been established. Other codes have been established by the American Medical Association, and by representa-

## TABLE 13–1    Guiding principles of the *e-Health Code of Ethics*

**CANDOR**

- Disclose information about the creators/purpose of the site that will help users make a judgment about the credibility and trustworthiness of the information or services provided.

**HONESTY**

- Be truthful in describing products/services and present information in a way that is not likely to mislead the user.

**QUALITY**

- Take the necessary steps to ensure that the information provided is accurate and well supported and that the services provided are of the highest quality.
- Present information in a manner that is easy for users to understand and use.
- Provide background information about the sources of the information provided and the review process used to assist the user in making a decision about the quality of the information provided.

**INFORMED CONSENT**

- Inform users if personal information is collected and allow them to choose whether the information can be used or shared.

**PRIVACY**

- Take steps to ensure that the user's right to privacy is protected.

**PROFESSIONALISM IN ONLINE HEALTH CARE**

- Abide by the ethical code of your profession (e.g., nursing, medicine).
- Provide users with information about who you are, what your credentials are, what you can do online, and what limitations may be present in the online interaction.

**RESPONSIBLE PARTNERING**

- Take steps to ensure that sponsors, partners, and others who work with you are trustworthy.

**ACCOUNTABILITY**

- Implement a procedure for collecting, reviewing, and responding to user feedback.
- Develop and share procedures for self-monitoring compliance with the *e-Health Code of Ethics*.

SOURCE: Adapted from the Internet Healthcare Coalition. (2000). *e-Health Code of Ethics*. e-Health Ethics Initiative, 2000 at *http://www.ihealthcoalition.org/ethics/ehcode.html*.

tives of United States-based Healthdot.com organizations (Foubister, 2000).

Sophisticated technology will continue to make health and healthcare information more accessible and more meaningful to both healthcare consumers and healthcare professionals. Educators in all healthcare disciplines are identifying creative ways to use emerging technology to enhance the teaching–learning process. This trend is reflected in the nursing literature, where an increasing number of articles on uses of technology in professional and patient education can be found. It is important to note, however, that Information Age technology has done more than alter the way in which we teach. As Mitchel and McCullough

(1995) suggest in their definition of the Information Age, technology has and will continue to prompt dramatic, systemwide changes that will be evident in the roles played by nurses and clients, the relationships they establish, and the environments in which they interact.

## THE IMPACT OF TECHNOLOGY ON THE TEACHER AND THE LEARNER

Information Age technology has had a significant influence on educators and learners in all educational settings (Gross, 1999). Access to information bridges the gap between student and teacher. When information is widely available, the teacher is no longer the person who holds all of the answers or the individual who is solely responsible for imparting knowledge. Therefore, educators in the Information Age are becoming facilitators of learning rather than providers of information and are striving to create a collaborative atmosphere in their teaching and learning environments. As information becomes more and more accessible, the need for memorization becomes less important than the ability to think critically. Hence, educators in the Information Age are helping individuals to learn how to refine a problem, to find the information they need, and to critically evaluate the information they find. Healthcare education can and should follow a similar path. As educators, nurses must not only learn how and when to use technology, but also modify their educational approaches to be consistent with the needs of Information Age clients. Nurses must strive to be facilitators of learning and to create learning environments in which clients are encouraged and supported in their attempts to seek the information they need to achieve optimum health.

The Information Age has been witness to some dramatic changes in the behavior of healthcare consumers, making the role

changes discussed earlier inevitable. Technology and the increased accessibility to information it offers have empowered and enlightened healthcare consumers, encouraging them to form new partnerships with their healthcare providers (Kaplan & Brennan, 2001). Even those healthcare consumers who are reluctant to take on more responsibility for managing their own health care are moving in that direction as changes in the healthcare delivery system have forced them to assume more active roles. As a result, healthcare consumers in the Information Age are eager to learn about and make use of the many information resources available to them.

Today's healthcare consumers enter the healthcare arena with information in hand and are prepared to engage in a dialogue about their diagnoses and treatments. We can no longer assume that the clients we see in a hospital or clinic have little information other than what we have given them or that they haven't explored the treatment options available to them. Whereas healthcare consumers of the past were often isolated from others with similar diagnoses and dependent upon healthcare providers for information, today's consumers have the means to access networks of other patients and healthcare providers worldwide. Consumers who are being treated for healthcare problems can readily find detailed information about their diagnoses, treatments, and prognoses. Therefore, it is not surprising that the teaching needs of today's healthcare consumers and the expectations they hold for those who will be teaching them are changing. The role of the nurse educator has not been diminished, but it has changed. Nurses must now be prepared not only to use technology in education, but also to help clients access information, evaluate the information they find, and engage in discussions about the information that is available.

In addition to altering the educational needs and expectations of healthcare consumers, the Information Age has made a tremendous impact on professional education. Technology has given rise to a dramatic increase in educational opportunities for nurses and other healthcare providers. A 1999 survey of 281 colleges and universities, conducted by the American Association of Colleges of Nursing, found nearly 2,000 course offerings using distance education technology, a number that is expected to continue to grow in the twenty-first century (Potema et al., 2001). Nurses seeking advanced degrees and credentials can now study at colleges and universities offering distance education programs in a wide range of subject areas. Computers have made it possible to provide "anytime, anywhere" access to job training and continuing education. Virtual reality and computer simulation can provide opportunities to learn hands-on skills and develop competencies in areas such as diagnostic reasoning and problem solving. Like consumers, healthcare professionals in the Information Age can use the Internet and the World Wide Web as vehicles for sharing resources and for gaining access to the most current information in their fields of practice.

## STRATEGIES FOR USING TECHNOLOGY IN HEALTHCARE EDUCATION

### The World Wide Web

The technology-based educational resource that is familiar to most people is the World Wide Web. One merely has to turn on a television and hear the commercials for health-related Web sites or hear references to the Web on morning talk shows to appreciate its tremendous influence. A report produced by the Pew Foundation revealed that 52 million Americans, or more than half of all Americans with Internet access, have used the World Wide Web to obtain health-related information (Fox & Rainie, 2000). Healthcare consumers are bombarded with lures to the Web; once there, Web users can find anything from

videos of surgical procedures to sites where they can ask questions as well as receive information. The number of healthcare sites on the World Wide Web is difficult to capture with any accuracy, as new sites are being introduced on a daily basis. Nevertheless, it is estimated that more than 15,000 Web sites are devoted to healthcare issues and that they receive in excess of 22 million hits per month (Paris, 2001).

Having recognized the value of the World Wide Web, nurses and other healthcare educators are beginning to teach their clients how to use the Web to find the resources and healthcare information they need to become educated healthcare consumers. The nursing literature suggests that the Web is being incorporated into formal teaching plans for health and healthcare education with increasing frequency (Grandinetti, 2000; Leaffer & Gonda, 2000). Web pages designed to provide healthcare education are also being created by nurses as part of their outreach efforts to the community. Although healthcare information on the Web is a relatively new phenomenon, it has generated so much interest that several professional publications devoted to the topic have been initiated. For example, *The Interactive Health Care Report* was launched in 1999 to cover new developments in the world of digital healthcare information and to assist practitioners in keeping up with available resources on the World Wide Web. One feature found in the nursing journal *Computers in Nursing* is a listing and review of Web sites devoted to a particular health or nursing-related topic each month.

It is clear that the World Wide Web is an exceptionally rich educational resource for both professional and consumer use. However, despite people's familiarity with the Web, there is some confusion regarding terminology. Therefore, it may be helpful to clarify some commonly used terms.

From a technical perspective, the *World Wide Web* is a network of information servers around the world that are connected to the

Internet. The servers that make up the World Wide Web support a special type of document called a *Web page*. Web documents or Web pages are written using HTML (Hypertext Markup Language). In simple terms, the World Wide Web is a virtual space for information. More than 1 billion Web pages covering a wide range of topics can be found on the Web, displaying a variety of formats including text, audio, graphics, and, in some cases, video (Why-not.com, 2001). Links on a Web page allow the user to easily move from one Web page to another with the click of a mouse. A user moves around the World Wide Web by way of a *Web browser*, a special software program that locates and displays Web pages. Netscape Navigator and Microsoft Internet Explorer are examples of Web browsers. *Search engines* and *search directories* are computer programs that allow the user to search the Web for particular subject areas. Yahoo! is an example of a search directory, and Google is an example of a search engine. The Web is so large that any one search engine or directory will cover only a small percentage of the Web pages available (Pandia.com, 1999).

A common misconception is that the World Wide Web and the Internet are two names that describe the same entity. In fact, the Internet and the World Wide Web are related but different.

The *Internet* is a huge global network of computers established to allow the transfer of information from one computer to another. Unlike the World Wide Web, which was created to *display* information, the Internet was created to *exchange* information. The World Wide Web resides on a small section of the Internet and would not exist without the Internet's computer network. Conversely, the Internet could exist without the World Wide Web and, in fact, flourished for many years before the World Wide Web was ever conceived. Despite the immense size of both the Internet and World Wide Web, the two are relative newcomers to the world of technology. The Internet was originally commissioned in 1969 as a program of the Department of Defense, and the first experimental version of the World Wide Web was released only in 1989 (Howe, 2001). Since their inception, both the Internet and World Wide Web have grown dramatically in size and functionality.

Nurses or healthcare consumers need to go no farther than their computers if they wish to learn how to use the Internet or the World Wide Web. Getting into the Internet or the World Wide Web requires a computer with a modem or other telecommunication link and software to dial into an Internet Service provider (ISP). Once connected, it is simple to find a wide range of Web sites devoted to teaching Internet or World Wide Web navigation skills. With a properly worded command (e.g., "World Wide Web" and tutorial), a search engine will uncover a number of self-paced tutorials designed to teach novice or intermediate users the desired skills. Most search engines even provide guidance in creating commands that will elicit the information needed.

Knowledge of the World Wide Web is critical for nurses who work with and educate healthcare consumers for several reasons:

- Nurses will inevitably see an increase in the number of clients who enter the healthcare arena having already searched the Web for information. Familiarity with the type of information found on the Web will help direct the assessment of clients prior to teaching to identify the needs of the learner and to determine whether follow-up is necessary.

- The World Wide Web is a tremendous resource for both consumer and professional education. To use the Web effectively, nurses must possess information literacy skills and be prepared to teach these same skills to clients, including how to access the information on the Web and how to evaluate the information found.

- The World Wide Web provides a powerful mechanism for nurses to offer healthcare education to a worldwide audience. More and more health organizations are creating Web sites with pages dedicated to presenting healthcare information for consumers. Although nurses may not be responsible for actually creating the HTML document that will be placed on the Web, they may work with the Web site designers to develop the information it contains, evaluate the accuracy of the information presented, and interact with healthcare consumers who access the site.

The World Wide Web is a vital tool for nurses. It is mechanism for keeping up-to-date on professional and practice issues as well as a resource to be shared with clients. If it is to be used effectively, however, a plan to incorporate the World Wide Web into practice must be set in place.

## Healthcare Consumer Education and the World Wide Web

Preteaching assessment of a client in the Information Age must begin with questions about computer use. It is important to determine whether a client has a computer, has access to the Internet, is knowledgeable about using a computer, and has interest in using a computer to obtain information and resources regarding his or her health care. If a client does not have a computer but has interest in using one to access resources on the Web, places where he or she may access a computer should be discussed. Libraries, senior centers, and community centers commonly have computers with Internet access for public use and typically offer instruction and assistance for new users (Hendrix, 2000).

Clients who use computers should be asked about their use of the Web. A Pew Foundation study found that approximately 21 million Web users in the United States found information on the Web that either (1) influenced their decisions about how to treat an illness, (2) led them to ask questions, (3) led them to seek a second medical opinion, or (4)

affected their decision about whether to seek the assistance of a healthcare provider (Fox & Rainie, 2000). Because the Web can be so influential, it is important to determine that the information a client has found is accurate, complete, and fully understood. The World Wide Web contains information designed for both professional and consumer audiences. Healthcare consumers may not have the background necessary to comprehend professional literature and other types of information designed for healthcare professionals. When healthcare consumers do a search on a topic, they will access Web sites designed for them as well as for health professionals. Consumers should not be discouraged from accessing these sites, but nurse educators must help clients find information written for them at their level of readability and comprehension. A research study conducted by Graber, Roller, and Kaeble (1999) examined the readability level of medical information on the Web and found that many patient education materials are not written at a grade level that can be easily understood by the majority of the public (see Chapter 7 on literacy).

The Web also contains information that may be biased, inaccurate, or misleading. Because the Web has the potential to change so quickly, it is difficult to regulate. Even Web pages sponsored by physicians, nurses, and university medical centers have been found to contain inaccurate information and treatment recommendations (Kiernan, 1998; Paris, 2001).

Some clients may find that the Web has provided too much information, information they are not ready to handle or information they do not fully understand. For example, a patient newly diagnosed with a serious illness may be overwhelmed with the detailed information found on the Web regarding the course of the disease, prognosis, and treatment. Therefore, it is important to ask clients if they are using the Web to find health-related information and to explore the types of information they have found. Clients may or may not initially feel comfortable talking about information they have gathered. They may fear you will interpret their research as a lack of trust in your care. Some may be embarrassed to talk about information they do not fully understand. Others may be anxious about how to bring up information that conflicts with what they have been told or how they are being treated.

For these reasons, it is important to establish early in your relationships with clients that you are interested in talking with them about the information they have gathered from the Web or other resources they have available to them. Clients need to feel that you are open to discussing whatever information they find and that you are a partner in seeking the best information available. For clients who are being treated for a condition over an extended period of time, it is also important to continue the conversation about their Web searches throughout their treatment. Simply asking "Have you found any interesting information on the Web lately?" will keep the dialogue open and provide the nurse educator with the opportunity to respond to whatever questions or concerns they may have.

If possible, it is advantageous to conduct a teaching session in a place where there is computer access. Having a computer available during a teaching session can accomplish several goals. First, it will provide you with the opportunity to review Web-based information with the client. Not only can you introduce Web sites that are relevant to the client's needs, but you can also review some of the sites the client has been using. By reviewing the Web sites a client has been visiting, you can begin to determine the type and amount of information to which the client has been exposed, assess the client's knowledge, and identify areas where the client may have need for further teaching. You may also find information that needs further discussion. For example, a client may have visited a Web site that provides distressing information about side effects of treatment, prognosis, or disease progression. Looking at the site together will give you the stimulus to talk with the client about what he or she has discovered and do additional teaching if needed.

Another important advantage of reviewing Web sites with a client is that it provides a chance to teach clients information literacy skills. *Information literacy* is defined as "the ability to access, evaluate, organize, and use information from a variety of sources" (Humes, 1999). If clients are going to make use of the vast array of information on the Web, they must be able to find the information they are looking for, judge whether the information they find is trustworthy, and decide how they will use the information to meet their needs. Information literacy is different from *computer literacy*, the ability to use the necessary computer hardware and software (Association of Colleges and Research Libraries, 2000). A client who is information-literate knows how to find the information needed and can evaluate the information found for accuracy, currency, and bias.

Although healthcare consumers may not have the background knowledge to evaluate information to the same extent as a professional, they can be taught some simple steps to develop their information literacy skills and to help them begin to identify which Web sites are useful and which are problematic. These steps include the following:

1. *Reducing a problem or topic to a searchable command that can be used with a search engine or search directory.* If clients do not know how to narrow their topics or problems to a few words, they will be unable to find the information they desire or may be unable to broaden a search to find comprehensive coverage. Once the search command is identified, using a search engine or search directory is easy, especially if the help function available at most sites is used to solve problems.

2. *Categorizing Web pages according to their purpose.* A client should be taught to look for the person or organization responsible for the Web site and then place the Web

site into a category reflective of its purpose. For example, the purpose of a site created by a drug manufacturer could be categorized as marketing, sales, or promotion. Other categories could include, but are not limited to, advocacy, promotion, informational/news, personal, or instructional/tutorial.

3. *Identifying sources of potential bias that may influence the content or the manner in which the content is presented.* For example, an advocacy Web site is likely to present information that favors one side of a debate. A marketing or sales site will have a tendency to include information that is supportive of a particular product or service.

4. *Making a judgment as to the likelihood that the information found on the Web page is accurate and reliable.* Clients can be taught to look for the credentials of authors of reports or articles found on the Web, to see whether supportive data are provided, and to look at more than one site to see if they can find similar claims or suggestions. Some of the more reliable health-related Web sites have links to other sites such that the original site is not the sole source of information on a particular topic.

5. *Making a decision as to the completeness or comprehensiveness of the information presented.* Because clients may not have the background knowledge needed to quickly recognize when information is missing, they should be encouraged to look at more than one site when researching an area of interest. If you know that clients are using the Web to investigate a particular topic, you can help them to identify a list of things they should look for in articles or Web pages addressing the topic.

6. *Determining the currency of the information on a Web page.* Consumers need to know the importance of looking for a creation or modification date or other signs that the information on a Web site is up-to-date.

7. *Identifying resources to answer questions or verify assumptions made about the content of a Web page when necessary.* Healthcare consumers should be encouraged to check out information with their healthcare provider or other healthcare professional.

In years past, healthcare consumers were not encouraged to research healthcare topics but rather to rely on their healthcare providers for information. There were fears that clients would not understand the information they found or that they would find information they wouldn't be able to handle. Today, we have more confidence in the consumer's ability to manage his or her own health care. More and more nurses are empowering their clients by teaching and encouraging them to take advantage of the resources at their disposal. Nurses are using a variety of means to expose their clients to the resources on the Web. For example, nurses are placing computers in patient waiting rooms with appropriate Web sites set up in a "point and click" format (Klemm, Hurst, Dearholt, and Trone, 1999). Others are preparing teaching materials on how to use the Web and what to look for once there.

There are many reasons why teaching clients where to go on the Web to find information is good practice. Web-based information can be obtained quickly, and the cost of Internet access in the home is minimal. In fact, Internet access is even available for free in libraries and other community service organizations. Many healthcare consumers would benefit from having their questions answered quickly and inexpensively. For example, families with young children are likely to have frequent questions related to childhood illnesses, growth and development, and behavior problems and may not have the time or money to make a visit to the pediatrician. Senior citizens may have questions about the healthcare problems encountered with aging but may have difficulty getting to a healthcare provider because of transportation and financial issues. People with chronic illness may gain some sense of control over their lives when they are able to access information on the Web about their conditions. Healthy people may have many questions but few opportunities to talk with a health provider to get answers. Even when healthcare consumers do have the opportunity to meet with a healthcare provider, they often leave with unanswered questions. Sometimes they forget to ask, at times they are hesitant to ask, and in today's healthcare delivery system they may not be given sufficient time to ask the many questions that arise when people are dealing with health issues.

In the role of educator, the nurse can teach clients who access the Web to use it more effectively and can be proactive in encouraging others to give it a try. It may be helpful to compile lists of Web sites appropriate to the needs of different client populations. Table 13–2 provides examples of the various types of Web sites that are available for consumer use. As illustrated in Table 13–2, a variety of types of Web sites exist, from general sites covering a broad range of topics to sites with a specific focus or theme. Megaportals, or sites where health is just one of many topics covered, do exist, but are on the decline and being replaced with sites that focus on a single theme such as cancer (Kaplan & Brennen, 2001).

In selecting Web sites to share with clients, it is important that the nurse review them carefully. In recent years, multiple rating scales have been developed to assist in the evaluation of such sites. Most scales include criteria that address the accuracy of the content, design, and aesthetics of the site; disclosure of the authors; sponsors of the site; currency of information; authority of the source; ease of use; and accessibility and availability of the site (Kim, Eng, Deering, & Maxfield, 1999). Table 13–3 summarizes the questions that should be asked in evaluating a health-related Web site. Resource lists made up of quality sites will not only serve as references

for clients but also provide examples of the types of sites they should be accessing.

Finally, nurses can create Web sites to bring their healthcare messages to Web users around the world. Table 13–2 provides two examples of Web sites that exemplify the types of roles nurses can play to bring health information to various consumers via the World Wide Web. *Bandaids and Blackboards* is a creative site designed by a nurse to facilitate understanding of the problems faced by children growing up with healthcare problems. This site is thought-provoking rather than factual. The nurse who created it uses the words and drawings of children and parents to bring a real-life perspective to the thoughts, feelings, and experiences of growing up with illness. Bandaids and Blackboards teaches important messages about not being alone, about ways to solve common problems, and about what really matters to this population. *NetWellness*, another site in which nurses play a predominant role, is a very different site than Bandaids and Blackboards. NetWellness is an "electronic consumer health information service developed by the University of Cincinnati Medical Center and more than 35 community partners" (Hern, Weitkamp, Haag, Trigg, & Guard, 1997, p. 316). Nursing faculty at the University of Cincinnati, Ohio State University, and Case Western University assist in maintaining the site by responding to health consumer questions on the site's "Ask the Expert" feature and by providing information for the section of the site devoted to "Hot Topics."

A number of issues must be considered before engaging in health education via a Web site. Web sites have the potential to reach millions of users over an extended period of time. The healthcare consumers who use the Web have varying levels of sophistication. They may or may not know to check the dates on which the Web site was created and modified. Therefore, it is very important that the infor-

| TABLE 13–2 | Sample Web sites for healthcare consumers | | |
|---|---|---|---|
| Title | URL | Sponsor/Author | Description |
| Medline Plus | *www.nlm.nih.gov/medlineplus/* | National Library of Medicine | Example of a government site that provides access to extensive information about specific diseases/conditions, links to consumer health information from the NIH, dictionaries, lists of hospitals and physicians, health information in Spanish and other languages, and clinical trials. There is no advertising on this site. |
| Virtual Hospital | *http://www.vh.org/* | University of Iowa | Example of a university site created to help meet the information needs of healthcare providers and patients. The digital information provided is all dated and reviewed for quality and accuracy. |
| Aplastic Anemia and MDS International Foundation, Inc. | *http://www.aplastic.org/* | Aplastic Anemia and MDS International Foundation, Inc. | Example of a disease-specific Web site that provides a range of services, including free educational materials and access to a help line where consumer questions will be researched and answered. |
| National Center for Infectious Diseases Travelers Health | *http://www.cdc.gov/travel/index.htm* | Centers for Disease Control and Prevention | Example of a government site designed to provide a wide range of health-related information for travelers, including traveling with children, travelers with special needs, and specific disease information. |
| MayoClinic.com | *http://www.mayohealth.org* | Mayo Clinic | Example of a comprehensive hospital site that provides information as well as a variety of interactive tools to help healthcare consumers manage a healthy lifestyle, research disease conditions, and make healthcare decisions. Advertisement helps support this site. |
| Cancer Net | *http://wwwicic.nci.nih.gov/* | National Cancer Institute | Example of a government site devoted to all aspects of cancer. Provides both professional and consumer-oriented information and resources. |

*(continued)*

## TABLE 13–2    (continued)

| Title | URL | Sponsor/Author | Description |
|-------|-----|----------------|-------------|
| Bandaids and Blackboards | *http://www.faculty.fairfield.edu/fleitas/contents.html* | Nursing faculty members at Fairfield University | Site provides personal rather than factual information about growing up with health problems from the perspectives of kids, teens, and adults. |
| NetWellness | *http://www.netwellness.org/* | University of Cincinnati, Ohio State University, and Case Western Reserve University | Nonprofit consumer health Web site that provides high-quality information created and evaluated by medical and health professional faculty at several universities. |

**TABLE 13–3  Criteria for evaluating health-related Web sites**

**ACCURACY**

- Are supportive data provided?
- Are the supportive data current and from reputable sources?
- Can you find the same information on other Web sites?
- Is the information provided comprehensive?
- Is more than one point of view presented?

**DESIGN**

- Is the Web site easy to navigate?
- Is the site "Bobby Approved"?
- Is there evidence that care was taken in creating the site? Do the links work? Are there typos?
- Is the information presented in a manner that is appropriate for the intended audience?
- Do the graphics serve a purpose other than decoration?

**AUTHORS/SPONSORS**

- Are the sponsors/authors of the site clearly identified?
- Do the authors provide their credentials?
- Do the authors/sponsors provide a way to contact them or give feedback?
- Do the authors/sponsors clearly identify the purpose of the site?
- Is there reason for the sponsors/authors to be biased about the topic?

**CURRENCY**

- Is there a recent creation or modification date identified?
- Is there evidence of currency (e.g., updated bibliography reference to current events)?

**AUTHORITY**

- Are the sponsors/authors credible (e.g., is it a government, educational institution, or healthcare organization site versus a personal page)?
- Are the author's credentials appropriate to the purpose of the site?

mation on the site be accurate and updated as often as necessary. Depending on the topics covered, it may be necessary to include a disclaimer about the importance of checking with a healthcare provider.

If the site is interactive and the nurse will be responding to questions submitted by users of the site, liability issues must be carefully considered. Nurses who respond to questions from Web users are providing advice and guidance to people they do not see and cannot assess. Depending on the nature of the site, it may be advisable to include an attorney on the team to provide advice when needed (Hern et al., 1997). It is important to determine if there are relevant legal issues related to practice inherent in the activities of the nurse on the Web site. Although new technology has opened the door to many new and exciting opportunities, it has also raised many questions about *"telepractice"* and licensure. Because technology makes it so much easier than ever before to provide healthcare services to clients across state lines, the provision of nursing, medical and other types of technology-facilitated healthcare services to clients at a distance has been placed in the spotlight. Multistate licensure and other types of legislation have and will continue to be proposed and new practice guidelines are likely to be enacted.

Finally, the time commitment required to respond to questions from Web users cannot be underestimated. The nurse educators who respond to questions on NetWellness estimate a time commitment of 20–40 minutes for research and response to each question (Hern et al., 1997). They also suggest that it is important that daily coverage for an interactive Web site be maintained. Healthcare consumers will use the site 24 hours a day, 7 days a week. Therefore, if the site offers interactive features such as "Ask an Expert," it is important that questions be answered on a regular basis so that service is not interrupted for long periods of time.

## Professional Education and the World Wide Web

The World Wide Web provides unlimited resources for nurses to use in practice and in professional education and development. Web sites provide access to bibliographic databases, continuing education, on-line journals, and resources for patient teaching and professional practice. Sites established by nursing organizations and publishing companies serve as "resource centers" where nurses can find a wide range of information and services addressing any number of educational needs. Many of the informational sites on the World Wide Web provide both consumer and professional education. Some Web sites provide links on the home page directing users to either consumer or healthcare professional resources. Other sites do not attempt to discriminate and allow users to decide whether consumer material or professional literature is more appropriate to their needs.

It is impossible to list all of the educational opportunities for professionals found on the World Wide Web. The Web is constantly changing, with new sites being added and others being removed on a daily basis. Table 13–4 provides examples of the various types of Web sites that can be used by professional nurses and other healthcare professionals.

## ▬▬ THE INTERNET

The World Wide Web is merely a small component of a much larger computer network called the Internet. Although the Internet does not provide the eye-catching Web pages and the multimedia found on the World Wide Web, it does offer a wide range of services, many of which can be used to deliver health and healthcare education to clients. The Internet services most likely to be of interest to nurse educators include those that allow computer-facilitated communication. While the World Wide Web provides opportunities to send healthcare messages to large groups of people in the form of educational Web pages, the Internet can be used to enhance teaching by enabling individuals to communicate with one another and with groups of people via the computer. Electronic mail (e-mail), real time chat, and e-mail discussion or Usenet newsgroups have all been used to communicate with people about health and health care, some in very creative ways.

## E-Mail

A television commercial for a popular Web site was created to encourage women to log on to the Web site for answers to health-related questions. The commercial shows a woman speaking about all of the unanswered questions she has had following a visit to her healthcare provider. The woman in the commercial talks about the lack of time, the questions that she did not think about until after she got home, and her hesitancy to "bother" her healthcare provider with "silly" questions. Although this commercial did not involve a real patient, the message that was conveyed by this fictitious scenario is quite relevant. Despite the best efforts of healthcare professionals to provide needed information to consumers, time, stress, fear, lack of experience, and simple human dynamics may result in clients walking away from a visit to a healthcare provider with incomplete or inaccurate information. Sometimes questions come up only after clients go home and try to follow the instructions they have been given. At other times, they may misunderstand what is being taught or be afraid or hesitant to admit that they do not understand. Unless there is a mechanism in place for clients to contact the nurse with questions, the client is at risk for

**TABLE 13–4    Sample Web sites for healthcare professionals**

| Title | URL | Sponsor/Author | Description |
|---|---|---|---|
| Medline | *http://www.nlm.nih.gov/pubs/ factsheets/medline.html* | National Library of Medicine | Example of a government site providing access to a bibliographic database containing more than 11 million references to journal articles in the life sciences. |
| SchoolNurse.com | *http://www.schoolnurse.com/* | School Nurse Alert | Example of a commercial site devoted to school nursing. It contains a wide range of resources, including links of interest to school nurses, continuing education offerings, and a bibliographic search feature. |
| Speaker Kit on Lung Health in Minorities | *www.chestnet.org/minorities/* | American College of Chest Physicians | Example of a site that provides resources for education. This site contains a PowerPoint presentation that can be downloaded and used when presenting information to minority groups about lung health. |
| National Kidney and Urologic Diseases Information Clearinghouse | *http://www.niddk.nih.gov/health/ kidney/nkudic.html* | National Institutes of Health | One example of the kinds of disease-specific information that is available from the federally funded National Institutes of Health. It provides access to statistical data about kidney disease, free educational materials prepared at different reading levels, and access to a database of health education materials produced by health-related agencies of the federal government. |

*(continued)*

**TABLE 13–4** (continued)

| Title | URL | Sponsor/Author | Description |
|---|---|---|---|
| Gradschools.com | *www.gradschools.com* | Educational Directories Unlimited | Example of a commercial site that provides a wide range of information and services for students interested in graduate study. Campus-based and distance education nursing programs are among the more than 52,000 graduate programs listed in the site's database. |
| Auscultation Assistant | *http://www.wilkes.med.ucla.edu/intro.html* | University of California Medical Student | One example of the numerous Web sites devoted to teaching heart and breath sounds. This site provides information as well as audio clips of various heart and breath sounds. |
| NursingCenter.com | *http://www.nursingcenter.com/* | Lippincott, Williams & Wilkins | Example of a commercial site that was originally funded by a federal grant for the purpose of developing an interactive Web community for nurses. It contains a wide range of information and services about continuing education offerings, degree programs, and reference material. |

making a mistake that may have serious consequences. Simply telling clients to call if they have questions if often inadequate. A call to a busy office or clinic usually results in a call back and having to wait by the phone for an answer. Even calling hours can be problematic because they imply that the client is free to call at the designated hour.

E-mail offers a quick, inexpensive way to communicate with clients. It has the advantage of being *asynchronous*, which means that the message can be sent at the convenience of the sender and the message will be read when the receiver is online and ready to read it. Messages can be sent and responded to any time, day or night. E-mail is also a technology that is growing in popularity and use. It is estimated that 56 percent of all adults in the United States are online. Of those people who use the Internet, 93 percent use e-mail and spend an average of 4.2 hours per week engaged in e-mail and other Internet-based activities (Rainie & Packel, 2001).

Despite the fact that electronic mail can provide a simple and efficient way to do follow up with clients, nurses are just beginning to recognize its potential. To date, little has been written in the literature about ways in which nurses have used e-mail to communicate with clients. Some of the reasons nurses identify for not using e-mail include lack of instruction and support, limited access to computers, and preference for face-to-face communication (Hughes & Pakiesner, 2000). It should be noted that although there is little information about e-mail in the nursing literature, electronic communication has received much attention in the medical and general health literature.

E-mail is clearly a trend worth watching. In fact, in a discussion of health care in the twenty-first century, the National Institute of Medicine (2001) proclaimed that both patients and clinicians could benefit from improvements in timeliness through the use of Internet-based communication. Studies suggest that patients are interested in communicating with their healthcare providers via e-mail. One survey found that one-third of online health seekers would consider switching healthcare providers if they could communicate with them via e-mail (Kassirer, 2000). A recent editorial in *The New England Journal of Medicine* states that "e-mail has the potential to induce cultural changes in the delivery of care even more revolutionary than any restructuring going on today" (Paris, 2001, p. 15).

Given the opportunity e-mail provides for enhanced communication with clients, it is an approach worthy of further study by nurses. An e-mail message system gives clients who identify questions after they go home a chance to get answers from a reliable source familiar with their history. Clients who are not sure how to phrase a question or feel rushed when instructions are being given in a clinical setting have a chance to compose their thoughts at home and prepare an e-mail message. Also, from the nurse's perspective, an e-mail message system provides a simple way to check on clients to see whether they understood the instructions they were given and to respond to new questions that have arisen.

In some ways, an e-mail system is preferable to a voice messaging system. For clients who are anxious about asking questions, e-mail allows them all the time they need to gather their thoughts. In addition, clients do not have to remember the answers they are given by the nurse, as the e-mail message provides a written recording of the nurse's response. In contrast, many voicemail systems are time-limited. Clients are sometimes cut off in the middle of a voice message if the message is long or if clients are struggling to make themselves understood. Other clients may hesitate to leave a voicemail in the evening or night hours when they know no one is there to respond. However, by virtue of the way e-mail is designed, clients can feel comfortable sending messages at any time.

An e-mail message system is simple to implement. Client e-mail addresses need to be identified as part of the routine information-gathering process for new clients. Because e-mail addresses are likely to change, they need to be updated, just like telephone numbers, whenever a client visits the office, clinic, or other setting within the healthcare delivery system. It is a good idea to have more than one person be responsible for responding to e-mail messages, so that questions and concerns can be addressed even when a staff member is away due to vacation or time out of the office. One way to accomplish this goal is to have messages be sent to a mailbox rather than to an individual. Because more than one person can be given access to an electronic mailbox, continuous coverage can be established. If continuous coverage is not provided, it is important that clients know how long they can expect to wait to receive answers to their questions.

E-mail systems can be set up to serve a variety of purposes. If post-teaching follow-up is desired, e-mail offers one way for the nurse to initiate contact after the client has left the healthcare delivery system. The nurse can get in touch with the client via e-mail following a teaching session to convey interest in how he or she is doing with a medication regime, treatment, or other types of instructions given. The e-mail message could stress important points that were made during the teaching session—for example, "Remember to take your pill around the same time every day." An e-mail message could also be used to assess the client's understanding of what was taught. For example, a client might be asked: "What time of day have you decided to give your child his medication?" In all cases, the nurse should encourage the client to get in touch if questions remain. Any follow-up system will take time and commitment on the part of the organization. Time and resources must be allocated if the system is to work effectively.

An e-mail system can also be established as a mechanism to answer questions and exchange health-related information with clients who have received services at a particular healthcare organization. An "e-mail question box" can provide simple access to the nurse or other health educator who can serve as a reliable source of information. For this type of system to work, the e-mail address for the mailbox needs to be widely distributed and easy to remember. For example, a mailbox address such as *Questions@RDClinic.org* would be easy to remember because it includes the purpose of the mailbox and the name of the organization. The e-mail address can be placed on the bottom of written instructions, teaching materials, appointment cards, and other sources of communication with the client. A description of the service and instructions for use should also be distributed. For example, it may be helpful for clients to know who will be answering their questions, the types of questions that can be submitted, and the typical response time. Also, it is very important that clients understand that an e-mail message system is not intended to replace a visit or phone call when they need to see or talk with a healthcare provider about an immediate problem.

When sending e-mail messages, it is important to remember that electronic communication differs in several ways from face-to-face communication:

- Electronic communication lacks context. Without cues like facial expressions, tone of voice, and body posture, e-mail messages can appear cold and unfeeling. While *emoticons* (symbols like "smiley faces" used to express emotion) are commonly used by people who send e-mail messages, they may not be appropriate for all professional correspondences. However, a carefully constructed e-mail message can convey the intent of the sender.

- Although electronic communication is convenient, it may take longer in that the sender could wait hours or days before the message is received and answered. For this reason, it is very important that an e-mail response to a client question be clear and of sufficient detail so that it does not generate more questions that cannot be answered immediately.

- E-mail messages provide a written record. A printed copy can serve as a handy reference for a client, but it can also serve as documentation of inaccurate or inappropriate information. When responding to a client question, it is vital that the client's record be reviewed and that the response to the question be accurate and carefully thought out. Copies of the e-mail messages sent to clients should be placed in the client's record.

- Electronic communication can never be assumed to be private. Therefore, it is important that both nurses and clients understand that violations of privacy can occur in many ways. For example, clients who send e-mail messages from work may not be aware of the fact that their messages may be stored on servers and hard drives even after they have been deleted. In some cases, the employer may have legal access to this information (Kassirer, 2000). E-mail messages can also be easily forwarded. Therefore, the nurse should assume that the client may choose to share a response with others.

E-mail communication between nurse and client has tremendous potential to enhance teaching. However, despite the increased use of e-mail among the general population, it is important to remember that not every client has a computer, computer skills, or access to e-mail. A backup system such as voicemail should therefore be made available so that the needs of all clients will be met.

## Electronic Discussion Groups

The Internet provides many opportunities for clients and healthcare professionals to participate in electronic discussion groups with other people who share a common interest. In the case of health and healthcare education, common interests can focus on a particular healthcare problem such as cancer, a life circumstance such as death of a spouse, a health interest such as nutrition, or a professional issue such as nursing research. Although different types of electronic discussion groups are available, all share a common feature—the ability to connect people asynchronously from various locations via computer. People like electronic discussion groups because they are easy to use and are available 24 hours a day. Because electronic discussion involves "faceless" communication with strangers from all over the world, there is a sense of anonymity even when real names are used.

Electronic discussion groups fall into two main categories: those that distribute mail to individual subscribers and those that post messages in a way that make them accessible to group participants. In the first case, messages are sent to the individual; in the second case, the subscriber seeks out the messages that have been posted. Electronic discussion groups can be structured in many different ways. Some are moderated, whereas others have little or no oversight. Some electronic discussion groups have thousands of subscribers, whereas others are very small closed groups created for specific purposes.

For the nurse, electronic discussion groups can serve as either a vehicle for teaching or a learning resource to share with clients and other healthcare professionals. The nurse who chooses to create an electronic discussion group can use it to reach large or small groups of healthcare consumers or healthcare professionals from within the immediate vicinity or worldwide. For example, a number of electronic discussion groups have been created and moderated by nurses as a way to promote networking and information sharing among nurses within a particular specialty area. These groups are open to anyone who is interested and typically have memberships of several hundred people from countries around the world. In comparison, nurses in a hospital or clinic could choose to set up a small private electronic discussion group as a way to facilitate a journal club. Whether the group is large or small, the asynchronous nature of electronic discussion groups makes it possible for people to communicate with one another despite different time zones and work schedules.

Whether the nurse chooses to create an electronic discussion group or uses one already in existence, this form of online communication provides for a creative way to learn and to teach. The two major formats used to create electronic discussion groups, those that distribute mail (mailing lists) and those that post it (newsgroups), are discussed next.

## Mailing Lists

Automated mailing lists are one of the most common means of setting up an electronic discussion group. With an automated mailing list, people communicate with one another by sharing e-mail messages. The principle by which these groups work is simple. Individuals who have subscribed to the mailing list send their e-mail messages to a designated address, where a software program then copies the message and distributes it to all subscribers. Therefore, when a message is sent to the group, everyone gets to see it.

The most popular of these automated software programs is called "Listserv." In fact, the Listserv program is so commonly used that automated mailing lists are often referred to as "listservs." Other automated programs include Majordomo, Mailbase, and Listproc. Although some minor differences exist between these programs, essentially they all work in the same way.

Although mailing lists are owned or managed by an individual, much of the work

involved in running the list is automated by the software program used. Subscribers are given two e-mail addresses to use when interacting with the mailing list: one to use when posting messages to the entire group and another to use for administrative issues such as requests to stop mail for a period of time. Both functions—distributing messages and handling routine requests—are automated and handled by the software program rather than by a person. Subscribers must use the correct address and precisely worded commands when attempting to interact with the list because the computer program cannot problem solve. Upon enrolling, subscribers are sent directions and a list of properly worded commands that should be used when "communicating" with the software program. New subscribers are encouraged to save the instructions and refer to them as needed. Despite these precautions, new users frequently make mistakes. It is not uncommon to read messages from frustrated subscribers who cannot stop their mail because they are either posting to the wrong address or failing to use the correct command.

Listservs and other automated mailing groups are wonderful tools for the nurse when used as a means for delivering education to large numbers of people or when shared with clients and colleagues as a learning resource. Mailing lists are easy to use once a user understands how the system works and there are multiple free tutorials available on the Web to help. With more than 100,000 listservs and mailing lists available, it is possible to find an online group to cover almost any issue. The quality of the messages is usually very high in both health-related and professional mailing lists. Nurses who choose to create a group rather than to participate in an established one can learn to manage a large or small listserv without too much difficulty. However, it is helpful for list managers to have either the support of computer professionals in their institution or the knowledge and skill necessary to handle the routine computer issues that arise from time to time.

Listservs or mailing lists can be used effectively as a vehicle for education or information exchange with groups desiring education or information exchange over time. Because mailing lists facilitate group rather than individual communication, they work especially well with groups that are interested in collaborative learning or learning from the experiences of others. Mailing lists designed for professional audiences are good examples. Multiple lists or listservs are available covering everything from nursing history to nursing research to specific areas of nursing practice. Most lists are quite active and, at any given time, several discussion topics can be addressed by the group. Members post questions, ask advice, and comment on current issues. Relationships between active members are established over time, and group members come to count on others in the group for their counsel.

For these same reasons, listservs and other types of automated mailing lists have become popular as mechanisms for online support for health consumers (Bliss, Allibone, Bontempo, Flynn, & Valvano, 1998; Han & Belcher, 2001; Klemm, Reppert, & Visich, 1998). With the increased use of computers in the general population, an increasing number of people have turned to their computers to access information and resources that can help them deal with their health issues. As a result, the need for electronic discussion groups devoted to particular health problems was identified and online support groups were established. The Association of Cancer On-line Resources, Inc. (ACOR), has been a major player in the move to bring online support to healthcare consumers (Han & Belcher, 2001). This nonprofit organization devoted to assisting people with cancer has established more than 70 different online support groups since 1996, each devoted to a particular type of cancer or cancer-related problem. Its Web page states that

ACOR delivers almost 2 million messages per week to the almost 70,000 people who subscribe to one of its online groups (Association of Cancer On-line Resources, 2000). Memberships in the various groups range from about 25 people in the smaller groups to almost 2000 individuals in the larger groups.

Other individuals and organizations have established similar online groups covering a wide range of healthcare issues. Sometimes groups are started by individuals who have been unable to find the information and support they need in their home communities (Bliss et al., 1998). Others are started by advocacy groups interested in providing service to a particular group of people. In addition to the many public groups that have open enrollments, private groups can be established to meet the needs of a group of people associated with a specific healthcare provider or organization.

Online support groups are particularly relevant to a discussion of technology for education. In their study of the categories and themes that emerged from an analysis of the postings in an online support group for colorectal cancer, Klemm et al. (1998) found that "information giving and seeking" accounted for a major portion of the messages exchanged in the group. Han and Belcher (2001) surveyed subscribers of an online support group for parents of children with cancer and found that 76% of participants cited information giving and receiving as the main benefit of the online group. A review of the purposes and goals of several online support groups revealed education and information sharing as the reason for starting and maintaining a group.

The emphasis on information sharing in online support groups is not surprising. Many people join online support groups after they or their loved ones have been diagnosed with a serious illness. They come to the support group not only to receive reassurance and encouragement, but also to gather as much information as possible so that they can begin to make necessary decisions about treatment. By joining an online support group, they are turning to people who know what they are going through and who can give practical advice based on real-life experience. The desire to share the most current information is commonly what brings group members together, and a discussion of new treatments and other discoveries found in the literature is commonplace (Han & Belcher, 2001).

Nurses may wish to teach their clients about the benefits of online support groups, or, if an appropriate group is not available, nurses can start an online support group of their own. Online support groups may be especially helpful to people who find it difficult to leave home because of illness or care responsibilities. Clients who are unfamiliar with online communication should be reassured that there is no pressure for them to contribute to the discussion and that many people benefit just by reading the comments of others (Klemm et al., 1998). Clients who are insecure about their ability to express themselves in written format may find it helpful to initially compose their messages using a word processor so that they can take the time to think about what they want to say and use the spelling and grammar check function to edit their remarks. Clients who are unsure if an online support group will meet their needs should be encouraged to give one a try. There are no costs involved other than the cost of being online and there are no obligations to continue. Subscribers can withdraw from a group at any time.

Online support groups have some disadvantages that should be shared with clients who are thinking about joining a group. Most people who have participated in a listserv or other type of mailing list note that the volume of messages received each day can be problematic (Han & Belcher, 2001; Klemm et al., 1998). Some lists report an average of 50 or more messages per day. Experienced users

learn to sort messages and delete the unnecessary or irrelevant ones quickly. Others find requesting that messages be sent in digest form (all messages received in a day are combined and sent in one mailing) helps control the volume of e-mails received. In any case, the daily volume of messages initially can be overwhelming and may present a problem for people with low literacy levels or for people for whom English is a second language.

Clients should also be made aware of the fact that most online groups do not have a professional facilitator. Online groups are often run by someone who is interested in the health problem being discussed either because he or she has the condition or has a family member with the healthcare problem. As a consequence, inaccurate information may be shared and problems with group dynamics may not be addressed.

Finally, note that a phone line is often critical in the home when someone is seriously ill. Because many clients will connect to the Internet via the sole phone line into their homes, time spent on the computer may be a problem. Family members cannot call into the home when the client is online reading or responding to messages. If busy phone lines become a problem, it may help to go online at the same time every day and let significant others know that the phone will be unavailable at that time.

Although this chapter classifies online support groups as part of the category of automated mailing groups, it should be noted that online support groups take many forms. Many groups use the mailing list or listserv format described here. Others use a bulletin board format where messages are posted on a site where they can be reviewed by members of the group. Still others maintain a Web site that provides many avenues for communication, including scheduled and unscheduled chats, bulletin boards, mailing lists, and electronic newsletters. Regardless of the format, online support groups provide a mechanism for meeting the teaching and learning needs of many different client populations.

## Usenet

Another mechanism for facilitating online discussion is Usenet. Usenet is a global discussion system made up of a cooperative network of computers that distribute and archive messages posted to topic-specific electronic discussion groups called newsgroups. Although referring to Usenet newsgroups as electronic bulletin boards is technically incorrect, the analogy works well because newsgroups work in a manner similar to a bulletin board. People "post" messages to the newsgroup, and anyone who has access to a newsreader can then subscribe to the newsgroup and can read the messages that have been posted. Most Web browsers include "newsreading" software that make newsgroups accessible to large numbers of people worldwide.

There are thousands of Usenet newsgroups in existence, many of which are devoted to health topics. Similar to e-mail addresses and Web addresses (URLs), the names assigned to newsgroups follow a set of rules that define the group. A newsgroup name consists of several words or labels, each followed by a period—for example, *sci.med.diseases.lyme*. The first section of the name is the category and is the broadest label used in the newsgroup name. In the preceding example, the category "sci" indicates that this newsgroup falls under the broad category of science. Seven major categories are commonly used in Usenet newsgroup names as well as a number of alternative categories. The major categories include *comp* (computers), *misc* (miscellaneous), *sci* (science), *soc* (social or cultural), *talk* (debate-oriented), *news* (news network), and *rec* (recreation). In the example *sci.med.diseases.lyme*, each word that follows the major category "sci" narrows the focus. Therefore, this newsgroup falls under the category of science and is devoted to discussion of medical diseases—specifically, Lyme disease.

A review of the newsgroup *sci.med.diseases.lyme* revealed that it had more than 65,000 messages posted. The messages covered a variety of topics from advice on symptom control to requests for prayers for a loved one who was not doing well with the disease. A large percentage of the messages posted come from people who are either seeking information or sharing information about the disease and its treatment. Participants include people who have been diagnosed with Lyme disease, are caring for family members with the disease, or are healthcare professionals or others who were interested in the topic. Some of the subscribers are frequent contributors, whereas others are "lurkers" who log on and read messages but never post one of their own.

Usenet newsgroups are worthy of mention because, like Web sites and listservs, they are a source of health and healthcare information for both consumers and healthcare professionals. However, unlike health-related Web sites that are informational or educational in nature, newsgroups are designed to provide a venue for people to talk about health-related issues and to answer questions posted by members of the group. Therefore, the types of information found and the tone of the site are very different from those of sites on the World Wide Web. Healthcare consumers who are looking for specific information can expect to scroll through multiple messages posted to the newsgroup before finding the information they are seeking. Although the volume of messages is problematic for some, many people subscribe because they enjoy the interaction and like to read the various messages that have been posted. Unlike listservs that send newly posted messages to subscribers every day, newsgroups require that subscribers come to them whenever they want to read messages. Therefore, subscribers may be more episodic in their use of the system, which may affect the types of interactions that take place between subscribers.

Newsgroups may or may not be moderated, and the subscribers who post messages range from the very knowledgeable to the uninformed. Even moderated newsgroups that have a review mechanism in place are apt to have large numbers of messages that contain inaccurate information. The role of the newsgroup moderator is generally to keep the discussion relevant to the topic by eliminating messages that do not address the subject at hand. Moderator approval of a message simply means that the message can be posted. It does not mean that the moderator agrees with the message or that he or she has reviewed it for accuracy. Some newsgroups even use automated or "robotic moderation," which is a program that processes messages. This type of automated system may be programmed to screen for new users, certain phrases, or duplicate messages. Messages that are flagged by the program are then reviewed by an individual. It is important to note that automated systems do not assure accuracy, as the individual reviewing messages may not be a content expert.

When assessing a client's use of the Internet and World Wide Web, it is important to determine whether newsgroups are included in the client's list of online resources. Although clients may find newsgroups to be a source of support and practical information, they may also be a source of misinformation. Unlike Web sites where users can be taught some simple steps to evaluate the accuracy and currency of the information presented, the nature of the types of messages posted in a newsgroup makes them much more difficult to assess. Therefore, it is important for clients to understand the need to verify the information they receive from a newsgroup either by bringing questions to the nurse or by doing further research on the Web or in a library. Nurses who work with clients in a particular area of care may find it helpful to subscribe to relevant newsgroups to discover the types of messages that are being posted. Not only will

this exercise provide the nurse with data about the types of information clients are receiving, but it will also provide insight into the kinds of issues, concerns, and unanswered questions clients may have.

## Other Forms of Online Discussion

There are many other mechanisms by which online discussion can take place. Although listservs or mailing lists and Usenet newsgroups are two of the more common approaches to online discussion, others are worthy of mention. When choosing a method for teaching or exchanging information online, it is important to consider all of the options and select the method that is most appropriate for the content to be delivered and the audience to be targeted.

*Online forums, message boards, and bulletin boards* are systems that provide a way for people to post messages for others to read and respond to. They differ from newsgroups in two important ways. First, while newsgroups are found on the Internet and use e-mail as the means by which messages are sent to the group, online forums, message boards, and bulletin boards are found on a Web site. Because users of this type of discussion board are posting directly to the discussion board rather than indirectly via e-mail, many people may find this system easier to use. Second, although most discussion board-type forums require some system of registration, users can often select a user name of their choosing and e-mail addresses are not displayed. This added privacy is a boon to many people who are reluctant to share their names and e-mail addresses with strangers. Online forums, message boards, and bulletin boards for healthcare consumers and healthcare professionals can be found on many health-related sites on the World Wide Web.

*Chat* differs from e-mail and the other electronic communication modalities previously discussed in that it provides an opportunity for online conversation to take place in real time.

Although chat conversations take the form of text rather than audio, a chat session shares many features with a telephone conference call. In both scenarios, several people from different locations participate in a conversation at the same time. Both allow people to join or leave the session as needed. However, without adequate control systems in place, both chat and teleconferences can experience a number of communication problems, such as multiple ongoing conversations, lack of focus, and periods of silence.

There are many opportunities for clients and healthcare professionals to engage in online chats related to health issues. A search of the World Wide Web will uncover a vast array of scheduled chats where a particular topic is being discussed at a given time as well as ongoing chats where people are invited to stop in at any time to ask questions or engage in conversation with whomever happens to be in the chat room. For example, an award-winning Web site called MentalHealth.Net (*http://www.mentalhealth.net*) sponsors a wide range of scheduled chats for professionals, the general public, and persons dealing with mental illness. In addition to public chat rooms, many organizations sponsor chats for their own clients or staff as a way to offer ongoing educational programs or information exchange among groups.

When leading or facilitating a chat group, it is important to plan ahead. The discussion in a chat room can move quickly, and it is very easy to get so involved in the process of chatting that the content to be covered gets lost or forgotten. The following suggestions may help to organize a successful chat session:

- E-mail or post the purpose of the chat session several days in advance. If appropriate, include an agenda, assignments to be completed ahead of time, or other resources that participants will need to prepare for the session.

- Make a list of the discussion points to be covered during the session. The list should be well organized, easy to follow, and placed so that it can be easily seen during the chat. Chat sessions often move so quickly that there is little time for the facilitator to make sense of crumpled or scribbled notes.

- Depending on the topic and the experience of the facilitator, it may be appropriate to limit the number of participants. The larger the group, the more difficult the challenge of running a smooth and productive online chat.

- Sign on to the chat session early and encourage participants to do so as well. You want to be able to handle unexpected problems before the session begins.

- Watch the clock. Time in a busy chat session goes by quickly. If the chat was designed as a question and answer period, it may be helpful to ask people to e-mail important questions ahead of time so they are not forgotten.

- Help the group to follow the conversation taking place. It is easy for chat discussions to become disjointed or off-topic. When responding to a question, refer to the query and the person asking it—for example, "Karen asked about pain management. I think. . . ." If the group is losing focus, bring the participants back to the agenda and the points being discussed.

- Limit the amount of time spent discussing the detailed questions or concerns of one participant. If someone in the group needs individualized attention, suggest that they e-mail or call you after the chat has ended.

- If appropriate, ask participants who have not participated if they have any questions. Some participants choose not to make comments during a chat, which is acceptable. However, there may be others who were not quick enough to get their comments online and who have questions that need to be asked. A statement such as "Our conversation moved very quickly tonight so I want to give those who haven't had a chance some time to ask their questions" may slow down the conversation long enough for everyone to have an opportunity to contribute.

- Begin to wrap up the session about 10 minutes before the scheduled end time. Announce that there are 10 minutes left and ask for final questions or comments.

It may also help to prepare participants for the chat experience. Chat sessions can be overwhelming for new users. The following guidelines for chat participation should be shared with clients or colleagues who will be joining a chat session for the first time:

- Allow enough time before the chat starts to download software if it is needed. First-time users are often required to download software, called a chat client, before beginning. This software is typically offered as freeware or shareware on the Internet and is easy to install.

- Be prepared to choose a user name. Participants in public chats with strangers are often advised not to use their real names so as to protect their privacy.

- Keep comments short and to the point. If a user takes a long time to compose a message, the group may have moved on to an entirely new topic by the time the message gets posted.

- Be prepared for "chat lingo" in public chat rooms. Abbreviations like BTW (by the way) and emoticons (symbols that represent emotions such as ;) = winking) are commonly used.

- Do not worry about typos and grammar. Chat programs do not have spell checks and not everyone is an experienced typist. People who are frequent chat users learn to overlook spelling errors.

Chat works well as an online communication modality for many people. Clients who are homebound or isolated may benefit from having the opportunity to participate in education programs or to receive answers to their questions without leaving home. Likewise, many healthcare professionals would benefit from being able to access professional education that allows real-time discussion and dialogue. However, some limitations of chat must be considered. Because chat requires that people be online at the same time, scheduling conflicts and time-zone issues result in less accessibility than asynchronous forms of electronic discussion. Due to the fast pace of most chat discussions, it may be difficult for some clients to keep up with the dialogue. Clients with certain disabilities, clients who are ill, and clients with low literacy levels may find it difficult to participate if the group moves along quickly.

The future for electronic communication is exciting. The technology to add audio and video components to online conferencing is available and is becoming more refined and less expensive every day. Chat and other types of conferencing software are also becoming more sophisticated, allowing for more control and greater ease of use. It is likely that both audio and video online communication will be commonplace in the near future.

At this point in time, use of these new technologies remains limited in healthcare education for clients. Adding audio and video to electronic communication requires obtaining the hardware, software, and bandwidth necessary to support these enhancements. If we want to use technology to continue to reach clients in their homes, we need to think very carefully about cost and accessibility. The use of any technology should be based on its ability to support the goals and objectives of the learning program and should be appropriate for the widest range of users within the program's target audience (Ragan, 1999). For example, a video camera and software may cost only a few hundred dollars, but to some clients this amount is a great deal of money. Before asking our clients to purchase this equipment, we need to weigh its cost against the benefit it will bring to the educational encounter. In the case of videoconferencing, we need to think about the cost of the equipment, the quality of the video, and ways it could be used to meet the goals of the planned educational program. We also need to consider the negative effects of denying access to clients who cannot afford the added cost. As educators, we need to identify the least expensive, easiest to use, and most accessible technology that will work for the program in mind.

## ISSUES RELATED TO THE USE OF TECHNOLOGY

Despite the power of computer and Internet technology to enhance learning, the use of these technologies in healthcare education presents some unique challenges. Think for a moment about the many ways in which healthcare education differs from more traditional classroom education. The characteristics of the learners, the setting, and the access to hardware, software, and technological support are all likely to be different. Whereas traditional classroom education is likely to take place in a structured setting, healthcare education takes place in a wide range of settings, many of which are unstructured. Students who are part of an educational system are likely to have some access to the hardware, software, and technological support necessary for facilitating technology-based learning. By comparison, access to resources and support varies considerably among healthcare consumers and in healthcare organizations. Students in a classroom also often share many common characteristics related to age and ability, whereas clients in healthcare education programs may cover a wide range of ages, abilities, and limitations. As educators, nurses must be aware of the special issues involved in the use of computer and Internet technology in healthcare education and be prepared to make accommodations as needed.

One of the most widely publicized issues related to the use of computers and Internet technology is that of the *digital divide,* or the gap between those individuals who have access to information technology resources and those who do not. As a result of the digital divide, many healthcare consumers do not have the resources necessary to gain entry to computer- and Internet-based health education programs. Thus, although technology can increase access to healthcare education for some people, educators must be aware that large segments of the population will be denied access if attempts are not made to promote "digital inclusion." The first step in promoting digital inclusion is recognizing those groups who are at risk for limited access.

Studies conducted by the Pew Foundation and the U.S. National Telecommunication and Information Association have found that the factors determining the likelihood that someone will have access to information technology resources are age, income, race or ethnic origin, level of education, and ability (National Telecommunication and Information Association, 1999; Rainie & Packel, 2001). These studies revealed that those at risk for limited access included people older than 65, those with household incomes of less than $35,000, African Americans and people of Hispanic descent, adults who did not complete high school, and people with disabilities. For example, the studies found that 96% of the population with household incomes higher than $75,000 had computers and 83% had Internet access. In comparison, only 49% of people with household incomes of less than $30,000 had computers and only 35% had Internet access (Lenhart, 2000; Rainie & Packel, 2001). People with disabilities are less than half as likely to have Internet access, and more than half of the people with disabilities in the United States report never having used a computer (National Telecommunication and Information Association, 1999). Although the gap between computer ownership and Internet access between the white population and people of African American and Hispanic decent is diminishing, different levels of access still exist.

Lenhart (2000) categorizes the limited computer and Internet usage of people older than age 65 as the "gray gap." A Pew Foundation study found that as few as 15% of adults over the age of 65 had access to the Internet (Rainie & Packel, 2001). Those numbers increase slightly in the 50- to 56-year-old age group, largely because many people between these ages are still in the workforce (Lenhart, 2000). Despite the statistics, it would be a mistake to discount computer-delivered education as a possibility for the senior population. Studies have found wide diversity among older adults. While some seniors report believing that there is little reason for them to go online, others are taking the initiative to learn computer and Internet skills and are joining online communities (Alder, 1996; Lenhart, 2000). Although large numbers of older adults have only limited incomes, numerous government and private initiatives are available to provide free or low-cost computer and Internet access for the senior population. While some older adults have physiologic and neurologic problems that make computer use difficult, many other seniors enjoy good health and functionality.

Health and healthcare education is important to senior citizens, and computer- and Internet-based technology holds much promise for this segment of the population. Therefore, it is important that the nurse be prepared to support computer-based learning among older clients. The following interventions may be helpful in encouraging senior citizens to engage in computer-based learning activities:

- *Reinforce principles of ergonomics by making suggestions about equipment and posture that will minimize physical problems related to computer use.* Ergonomics is important for everyone, but is especially important for older adults who may have visual problems as well as arthritic changes in the neck, hands, and spine. Proper posture, correct positioning of the keyboard and monitor, adjusted screen colors and font size, a supportive chair, and a reminder to get up and walk around three to four times per hour will help older adults to avoid discouraging physical symptoms that may interfere with computer use.

- *Identify resources that will provide computer access and support in the senior citizen's home community.* Supply seniors with a comprehensive resource list containing places where free computer and Internet access is available, places where computer training is provided for seniors, and contact people who will assist if problems are encountered. In addition to public libraries and community centers, numerous projects nationwide are committed to digital inclusion for all segments of the population, including the older adult population. Many of these projects and resources can be identified on the Web. For example, SeniorNet (*http://www.seniornet.org*) is an organization created for the purpose of supporting computer use among senior citizens. One of the features on the SeniorNet Web site is a state-by-state listing of places where seniors can go for computer training.

- *Motivate older adults to use a computer by helping them to identify how the computer can meet their needs.* "Older people perform best when the task is relevant to their lives" (Hendrix, 2000, p. 66). It is important to talk to seniors about their needs and abilities. Find out how they like to learn, what kinds of things they enjoy doing, and what their healthcare needs are. Matching a computer program or Web site to the individual's unique circumstances will encourage computer use. For example, a senior who is caring for a spouse with cancer might enjoy an online support group if he or she enjoys interacting with and learning from the experiences of others. In this way, you will help to generate interest in learning how to use a computer for health education by starting at a place that piques the senior's interest.

* *Create a supportive and nonthreatening environment to teach older adults about using a computer for health education.* Seniors did not grow up with computers and may not have confidence in their ability to learn this new skill at this point in their lives. The language of computers may be seem foreign to them, so avoid jargon and define new terms. Pace your teaching according to their response. You may need to proceed slowly at first and provide opportunities for practice and for reinforcement of skills. Write the instructions down and go over them before the teaching session ends so that the senior client does not go home with unanswered questions.

Computers can open up a whole new avenue of support and information to older adults who are struggling with their own health problems and those of their partners. Seniors who enjoy good health can find resources to help them maintain their health and to become educated healthcare consumers. It is important that older adults be given the same opportunities to take advantage of the Information Age resources that are available to younger clients. The nurse can play a key role in promoting digital inclusion among this segment of the population.

People with disabilities make up another special population that may require additional planning before using technologies in health and healthcare education. Not only are people with disabilities less likely to have computer and Internet access than are members of the general population, but they may also have difficulty using hardware and software. The ability to use a computer without adaptive devices requires the fine motor coordination and mobility necessary to use a mouse and keyboard, the strength to sit and hold the head in an upright position, and the ability to comprehend information presented on the computer screen.

For example, individuals with visual impairments may have difficulty seeing text or graphics on a computer screen or performing tasks on the computer that require hand–eye coordination. When identifying obstacles related to visual impairments, it is important to think broadly and address the wide range of conditions that affect the way we see. Color blindness, which affects approximately 8% of all males and 0.5% of females, can cause significant problems for computer users if the Web site or software used does not display the correct color combinations, if the contrast between background and foreground is inadequate, and if color rather than text is used to convey directions.

Although hearing impairments cause fewer problems for computer users than visual impairments, some accessibility issues nevertheless need to be addressed. An individual with a hearing problem may not be able to hear the sounds that are often used as prompts when a wrong key is struck or when an e-mail message is delivered. Accessibility for individuals with hearing impairments will become a bigger issue in the future when it becomes easier to send audio signals across the Web and audio messages become more commonplace.

Despite the protections offered by the Americans with Disabilities Act and other federal legislation, accessibility issues on the Web and constraints with hardware and software persist. For example, many of the learning platforms used to deliver online courses are inaccessible to people with visual impairments. Federal legislation outlined in Section 508 of the Workforce Investment Act requires government agencies and institutions receiving government funding to make their Web sites accessible to people with disabilities. To date, only a small percentage of the required Web sites accommodate the disabled or have been approved by disability organizations (West, 2000).

Chapter 9 describes potential barriers and specific adaptations that can be employed to assist people who have disabilities to use computers. Nurses who use the Internet and the World Wide Web to teach also need to consider Web site design when creating or selecting Web sites that might be used by disabled learners. The World Wide Web contains multiple resources that can be used by Web designers or Web users to learn design principles for accessibility. For example, inserting the search command "color blindness" on a search engine will produce Web sites that explain color blindness, illustrate how various types of color blindness affect what might be seen on a Web site, describe good Web design principles for promoting accessibility, and provide tools that can be used to select color combinations that will not create barriers for individuals with color blindness.

One Web site of particular note is a site created by the Center for Applied Special Technology (CAST). CAST provides a free service called "Bobby" to assist Web page authors to identify and correct problems that could make their sites inaccessible to individuals with disabilities. Information on how to use Bobby, along with a database of approved Web sites, can be found at the Bobby Web site at *http://www.cast.org/bobby/*. Web developers who use Bobby to diagnose Web site problems and follow through by making the suggested revisions are encouraged to display a "Bobby Approved" icon on their sites. When searching the Web for sites to be used with clients, "Bobby Approved" sites should be given special consideration. However, it is important to keep in mind that Bobby approval is on the "honor system," as CAST does not have the resources to check for Web sites displaying the icon fraudulently.

## ▰▰ PROFESSIONAL EDUCATION

From work-site training to higher education, technology is making professional education more accessible and more meaningful for nurses. It is no longer necessary for nurses to quit working or to relocate to earn a higher degree. Technology has contributed to the growth of distance education programs at all levels in nursing. Likewise, technology is making it possible for nurses in the workplace to engage in a variety of educational activities designed to keep their practice current, to provide career mobility, and to enhance professional development.

### E-Learning

Technology has had such an impact on workforce training that it has given birth to a new industry and a new set of buzz words that define an Information Age approach to staff education. Professional development and training organizations have capitalized on the power of computer technology to provide businesses with learning solutions referred to as *e-learning*, an abbreviation for electronic learning. A study involving 300 interviews with representatives of business organizations in the United States and Canada revealed that more than 94% of the organizations were aware of e-learning, almost 50% had already implemented it, and another 33% had plans to do so within the next three years (Sofres, 2001). The survey also found that almost all of the organizations indicated that they had met or exceeded the benefits they anticipated as a result of implementing e-learning within their organizations.

Although no consensus of opinion has been reached on a precise definition for the term *e-learning*, there is some agreement that it involves the use of technology-based tools and processes to provide for customized learning anytime or anywhere. The emphasis in e-learning is on outcomes, with the goal of providing an individual with the information or practice opportunities required to perform a task or solve a problem at the point of need. E-learning has been well received in health care because it is cost-effective, promotes positive patient outcomes, and leads to greater staff satisfaction. The nature of the work of health care makes workforce training a critical issue, and e-learning appears to have provided a solution to the problem of keeping staff current in a world where new treatments and new techniques are always on the horizon.

What is the e-learning approach to workforce training in health care? First and foremost, e-learning provides learning opportunities at the point of need. In health care, this statement means that training is available 24 hours a day, 7 days a week. Because the point of need in health care is often related to patient care, e-learning must be structured in a way that it can be delivered on a clinical unit. Point-of-need training must also be efficient. In this era of nursing shortages and increasing complexity of care, such training must be provided in a way that it fits into the schedules of busy healthcare workers. Finally, e-learning in health care must be distributed so that it can be made available to people across any number of environments and situations. Many healthcare organizations have staff in a wide range of settings and locations. A centralized approach to training will not work well if it means that people have to travel to the staff education office for all training programs. However, it should be noted that most organizations view e-learning as a complement to traditional instructor-led training, rather than as a replacement for it (Sofres, 2001).

Multiple approaches to e-learning in health care are possible. Examples of some of the features of e-learning products that have proved attractive to healthcare organizations follow:

- E-learning training modules can be delivered via the World Wide Web. Web-based products are attractive because they are easily accessed in a variety of environments and situations. A computer workstation can easily fit into a clinical unit, and laptops can be carried into the field.

- E-learning can be delivered in small modules that can be completed in as little as 15 minutes. Many healthcare workers are unable to leave their work area for long periods of time. However, most can find 15–30 minutes in a given day, particularly if they do not have to leave the unit. Time permitting, staff can complete several modules in one sitting.

- E-learning programs can be customized at a variety of levels: the organization, the staff position, and the individual. Customization personalizes the program and helps to make it relevant to the individual and to the organization.

- E-learning programs can track completion and create a performance report for individual staff members.

- E-learning modules are interactive and reality-based. For example, a patient simulation can be created that allows the participant to manage the care of a virtual patient.

Nurses have many potential roles in the development and implementation of an e-learning program within an institution. As content experts, they may be hired by e-learning companies to create products designed to meet the needs of practicing nurses. Nurses within a healthcare organization may be in a position to work with the e-learning company by customizing the training package purchased and developing a plan for its implementation. Those who use the e-learning system can contribute to the program by completing the modules offered and submitting carefully thought-out evaluations of the products used. Staff training programs are important to the individual staff members, to the organization, and to the patients served. Every staff member has a responsibility to do what he or she can to ensure the success of the program.

## Distance Education

As a result of technological advances, distance education for nurses is flourishing in the twenty-first century (Potempa et al., 2001). This success was not always the case, however. When distance education programs were first introduced, they were quite controversial. For example, when the Regents External Degree Program was first created 30 years ago, many people felt that a distance model was inappropriate for nursing education. Today, the Regents External Degree Program, now Excelsior College, is one of the largest nursing programs in the world, with more than 11,000 nursing students enrolled in its associate, baccalaureate, and master's degree programs. Not only has the Excelsior program grown, but it has since been joined by countless other colleges and universities that offer a variety of distance education options for nurses seeking a college degree. In 1994, another milestone was reached in nursing education when Duquesne University in Pennsylvania opened the first online distance education program leading to a Ph.D. in nursing. With the opening of the Duquesne program, we now have a full range of distance options for nurses from the associate degree through the doctorate as well as post-baccalaureate and post-master's certificate programs in a number of specialty practice areas.

The term *distance learning* means different things to different people. Online courses, correspondence courses, independent study, and videoconferencing are just a few of the techniques that can be used to deliver education to students studying at a distance. The diversity of distance education programs in the United States reflects the myriad approaches that can be used to meet the needs of students who are separated from the traditional classroom setting. In all cases, distance education means that the teacher and the learner are separated from one another (American Association of Colleges of Nursing Task Force on Distance Technology and Nursing Education, 1999).

Although many methods are used to provide courses to students who are not in the same location as the teacher, online courses are growing at such a rapid pace that the Internet is becoming the primary vehicle for delivering distance education (Institute for Higher Education Policy, 2000). Some nursing programs are totally Internet-based, whereas others use a combination of on-site and Internet-based courses. Some nursing programs even include individual courses that incorporate a mix of classroom instruction and online discussion. It should be noted that online education is not restricted to higher education. Online continuing education programs are also available to nurses from a variety of sources.

Research has shown that distance education provides much more than a flexible approach to learning. Comparisons of students from distance education courses and from traditional classrooms have repeatedly found no significant difference in learning outcomes in these two settings (Russell, 1998). However, because distance education and particularly online education are still relatively new phenomena, the education community is still working hard to meet the many challenges associated with educating students who live and work at a distance. Several education organizations have developed guidelines and standards for distance education to assist faculty and to ensure program quality, including the American Council on Education, the National Education Association, the Commission on Higher Education of the Middle States Association of Colleges and Schools, and the Western Cooperative for Education Telecommunication (Institute for Higher Education Policy, 2000). Recognizing that distance education involves more than providing coursework, colleges and universities are also attempting to provide the support services necessary to ensure the success of the distance learner. For example, they are establishing online bookstores, online registration processes, virtual libraries, virtual student lounges, and online office hours with faculty.

Given the growth and development of online courses, it is likely that this teaching methodology will be incorporated into health and healthcare education as well. Nurses who are responsible for providing education for clients need to begin thinking about how online courses may fit into their programs.

Online courses not only provide learning activities and resources, but also facilitate teacher–learner and learner–learner interactions. Internet-based courses might work very well in areas such as parenting and diabetes education where there is an extended program of instruction and the need for group support.

## SUMMARY

This chapter focused on Information Age technology and its use in healthcare education. Specifically, the chapter discussed ways in which the World Wide Web and the Internet could be used by nurse educators to enhance health and healthcare education for consumers and healthcare professionals. The impact of technology on teachers and learners was addressed and special considerations for older adults and other client groups were identified. Trends in distance education for nurses were also explored.

Information Age technology has the potential to transform health and healthcare education. This powerful tool must be used thoughtfully and carefully, however. Education is about learning, not about technology. Technology is merely an enhancement, a vehicle to deliver educational programs and to promote learning. The benefits of technology-based education are numerous, as are the challenges for educators and learners. As nurses, we have a responsibility to learn to use this new tool to promote health in our clients and professional growth and development in ourselves. The future for health education looks very bright, and we can help to shape it by continuing to think creatively about how to use technology in education and by participating in research about its effectiveness.

## REVIEW QUESTIONS

1. What is the "Information Age" and how has it influenced education in general, healthcare education specifically, and healthcare consumers?

2. What Information Age skills are required by healthcare professionals and healthcare consumers?

3. Describe various standards that have been established to ensure quality on the World Wide Web and access by special populations?

4. What are the ways in which resources on the World Wide Web can be used as a health information resource for healthcare consumers and healthcare professionals?

5. What are the various ways in which the Internet can be used to facilitate electronic communication between and among nurse educators and healthcare consumers? What are the advantages and disadvantages of each?

6. When using computer resources with clients, which segments of the population require special considerations due to limited access or special needs? What are those considerations and how can they be addressed?

7. What is e-learning and what advantages does it offer in providing training in healthcare settings?

8. How has technology influenced professional and continuing education options for nurses?

## REFERENCES

Alder, J. (1996). *Older Adults and Computers: Report of a National Survey.* Retrieved from the World Wide Web, April 2001, at *http://www.seniornet.org/research/survey2.html.*

American Association of Colleges of Nursing Task Force on Distance Technology and Nursing Education. (1999). *White Paper: Distance Technology in Nursing Education.* Washington, DC: American Association of Colleges of Nursing.

Association of Cancer On-line Resources. (2000). *About ACOR.org.* Retrieved from the World Wide Web, May 2001, at *http://www.acor.org/about/index.html.*

Association of Colleges & Research Libraries. (2000). *Information Literacy Competency Standards for Higher Education.* Retrieved from the World Wide Web, April 2001, at *www.ala.org/acrl/ilintro.html.*

Bliss, J., Allibone, C., Bontempo, B., Flynn, T., & Valvano, N. (1998). Creating a Web site for online social support: Melanocyte. *Computers in Nursing, 16*(4), 203–207.

Cetron, M. J. & Davies, O. (2001). Trends now changing the world. *The Futurist, 35*(2), 27–40.

Ehrmann, S. C. (1995). Asking the right question: What does research tell us about technology and higher learning? *Change, 27,* 20–27. Retrieved from the World Wide Web, April 2001, at *http://www.learner.org/edtech/rscheval/rightquestion.html.*

Eysenbach, G. (2000). Clinical review. Recent advances: Consumer health informatics. *British Medical Journal, 320*(7251), 1713–1716.

Foubister, V. (2000). Developing rules for the Web. *Amednews.com.* Retrieved from the World Wide Web, October 2000, at *http://www.ama-assn-org/sci-pubs/amnews/pick_00/prsa0731.htm.*

Fox, S. & Rainie, L. (2000). The online healthcare revolution: How the Web helps Americans take better care of themselves. *Pew Internet and American Life Project: On-line Life Report.* Retrieved from the World Wide Web, April 2001, at *http://www.pewinternet.org/reports/toc.asp?Reports=26.*

Graber, M. A., Roller, C. M., & Kaeble, B. (1999). Readability levels of patient education material on the World Wide Web. *Journal of Family Practice, 48*(1), 58–61.

Grandinetti, D. A. (2000). Help patients surf the Net safely. *RN On-line, 63*(8), 51–63.

Gross, R. (1999) *Peak Learning: How to Create Your Own Lifelong Education Program for Personal Enlightenment and Professional Success.* New York: Putnam.

Han, H.-R. & Belcher, A. (2001). Computer-mediated support group use among parents of children with cancer—An exploratory study. *Computers in Nursing, 19*(1), 27–33.

Heller, B. A., Ortos, M. T., & Crowley, J. D. (2000). The future of nursing education: Ten trends to watch. *Nursing and Health Care Perspectives, 21*(1), 9–13.

Hendrix, C. (2000). Computer use among the elderly. *Computers in Nursing, 18*(2), 62–67.

Hern, M., Weitkamp, T., Haag, D., Trigg, J., & Guard, J. R. (1997). Nursing the community in cyberspace. *Computers in Nursing, 15*(6), 316–321.

Howe, W. (2001). *A Brief History of the Internet.* Retrieved from the World Wide Web, April 2001, at *http://www.walthowe.com/navnet/history.html.*

Hughes, J. A. & Pakiesner, R. A. (2000). Factors that impact nurses' use of electronic mail (e-mail). *Computers in Nursing, 17*(6), 251–259.

Humes, B. (1999). *Understanding Information literacy.* Office of Educational Research National Institute on Postsecondary Education, Libraries, and Lifelong Learning. Retrieved from the World Wide Web, October 2001, at *http://www.ed.gov/pubs/UnderLit/.*

Institute for Higher Education Policy. (2000). *Quality on the Line: Benchmarks for Success in Internet-based Distance Education.* Washington, DC: National Education Association.

Internet Healthcare Coalition. (2000). *e-Health Code of Ethics.* Retrieved from the World Wide Web, October 2001, at *http://www.ihealthcoalition.org/ethics/ehcode.html.*

Kaplan, B. & Brennan, P. F. (2001). Consumer informatics: Supporting patients as co-producers of quality. *Journal of the American Medical Informatics Association, 8*(4), 309–315.

Kassirer, J. P. (2000). Patients, physicians and the Internet. *Health Affairs, 19*(6), 115–123.

Kiernan, V. (1998). Study finds errors in medical information available on the Web. *Chronicle of Higher Education, XLIV:40,* A25.

Kim, P., Eng, T., Deering, M. J., & Maxfield, A. (1999). *Published Criteria for Evaluating Health-Related Web Sites: Review.* Retrieved from the World Wide Web, April 2000, at *http://bmj. org/cgi/contents/short/318/7184/647.*

Klemm, P., Hurst, M., Dearholt, S. L., & Trone, S. R. (1999). Cyber solace: Gender differences on Internet cancer support groups. *Computers in Nursing, 17*(2) 65–72.

Klemm, P., Reppert, K., & Visich, L. (1998). A non-traditional cancer support group: The Internet. *Computers in Nursing, 16*(1), 31–36.

Larkin, M. (1996). *Health Information Online.* U.S. Department of Health and Human Services. FD 96-1254.

Leaffer, T. & Gonda, B. (2000). The Internet: An underutilized tool in patient education. *Computers in Nursing, 18*(1), 47–52.

Lenhart, A. (2000).Who's not online: 57% of those without Internet access say they do not plan to log on. *Pew Internet and American Life Project: Online Life Report.* Retrieved from the World Wide Web, April 2001, at *http://www.pewinternet.org/ reports/pdfs/Pew_Those_Not_Online_Report.pdf.*

McKay, H. G., Feil, E. G., Glascow, R. E., & Brown, J. E. (1998). Feasibility and use of an Internet support service for diabetes self management. *The Diabetes Educator, 24,* 174–179.

Mitchel, W. J. & McCullough, M. (1995). *Digital Design Media: On-line.* Retrieved from the World Wide Web, September 2001, at *http://www.gds. harvard.edu/~malcolmDDM/DDMain.html.*

National Institute of Medicine, Committee on Quality of Health Care in America. (2001). *Crossing the Quality Chasm: A New Health System for the 21st Century.* Washington, DC: National Academy Press.

National Telecommunication and Information Association. (1999). *Falling through the Net: Toward Digital Inclusion.* Retrieved from the World Wide Web, April 2000, at *http://www.ntia. doc.gov/ntiahome/digitaldivide/.*

Pandia.com. (1999). *A Short and Easy Web Search Tutorial.* Retrieved from the World Wide Web,

April 2001, at *http://www.pandia.com/goalgetter/ index.html.*

Paris, J. J. (2001). Ethical issues in cybermedicine. *America, 184*(4), 15–22.

Potema, K., Stanley, J., Davis, B., Miller, K. L., Hassett, M. R., & Pepicello, S. (2001). Survey of technology use in AACN member schools. *Journal of Professional Nursing, 17*(1), 7–13.

Ragan, L. C. (1999). Good teaching is good teaching: An emerging set of guiding principles and practices for the design and development of distance education. *Cause/Effect, 22*(1), Retrieved from the World Wide Web, May 2001, at *http://www.educause.edu/ir/library/cem9915.html.*

Rainie, L. & Packel, D. (2001). More online doing more. *Pew Internet and American Life Project: Online Life Report.* Retrieved from the World Wide Web, April 2001, at *http://www.pewinternet.org/ reports/pdfs/PIP_Changing_Population.pdf.*

Russell, T. L. (1998). *The No-Significant Difference Phenomenon.* Retrieved from the World Wide Web, March 2001, at *http://www.cuda.teleeducation. nb.ca/nosignificantdifference/.*

Sofres, T. N. (2001*). E-learning in the United States and Canada Benchmark Survey.* Retrieved from the World Wide Web, June 2001, at *http://www.skillsoft.com/resources/white_papers/wh itepapers/tn_research.html.*

West, D. M. (2000). *Assessing e-Government: The Internet, Democracy, and Service Delivery by State and Federal Governments.* Retrieved from the World Wide Web, April 2001, at *http://www.brown.edu/Departments/Taubman_Center/polreports/egovtreport00.html #Executive Summary.*

Why-not.com. (2001). *World Wide Web User Statistics.* Retrieved from the World Wide Web, May 17, 2001, at *http://www.why-not.com/company/stats. htm.*

## CHAPTER 14

# Instructional Settings

*Virginia E. O'Halloran*

## CHAPTER HIGHLIGHTS

## KEY TERMS

instructional setting
healthcare setting
healthcare-related setting
non-healthcare setting

organizational factors
environmental factors
clientele factors

## OBJECTIVES

After completing this chapter, the reader will be able to

1. Recognize the trends in health care that are expanding opportunities and expectations of the nurse in the role of educator.

2. Classify the instructional setting in which the role of nurse as educator is played out.

3. Describe the factors that affect the nurse in the role of educator in each setting.

4. Select the preferred teaching strategies for each instructional setting.

Traditionally, the primary focus of nursing practice has been on the delivery of acute care in hospital settings. In recent years, however, the practice of nursing in community-based settings has experienced tremendous growth. The reasons for the shift in orientation of nursing practice from inpatient care sites to outpatient sites relate to the trends affecting the nation's healthcare system as a whole, such as cost-containment measures, regulatory mandates, public and private reimbursement policies, changing population demographics, advances in healthcare technology, an emphasis on wellness care, and increased consumer interest in health accompanied by demands for care options. In response to these trends, the domains of nursing practice have broadened to include a greater emphasis on the delivery of care in community settings such as homes, clinics, health maintenance organizations (HMOs), physicians' offices, public schools, and the workplace.

Because health education is an integral component of nursing practice and has become an increasingly important responsibility of nurses in all practice environments, it is imperative to examine the factors influencing the teaching–learning process in various settings where clients, well or ill, are consumers of health care. The chief difference in the delivery of nursing care in acute care and long-term care facilities versus community-based environments is not only in the health status of the client but also in the length of time and resources available for educational activities.

This chapter will

- Examine the trends in health care affecting the delivery of instruction in various settings.
- Classify instructional settings in which health teaching takes place.
- Present a comparative analysis of the variables affecting educational efforts within different practice environments.

- Recommend teaching strategies best suited for specific settings in which teaching and learning take place.

## EMERGING TRENDS IN HEALTH CARE

The major trends affecting the U.S. healthcare system come from healthcare economics coupled with advances in medical technology. As a result, patients are being discharged "quicker" and "sicker," with many of them receiving sophisticated treatment modalities outside the acute care environment. This has forced providers to cope with the challenge of delivering high-tech, complex care in less structured and at times less supportive community environments, with clients and their families having to assume increasingly more responsibility for the ongoing management of the medical regimen within their homes. Managed care, as part of the healthcare reform movement sweeping the country, has become a reality and is influencing the practice of nurses everywhere. Bridging the gap between inpatient services and community-based services has required all nurses to have greater involvement in client teaching for self-care management, discharge planning, and providing for continuing care (Redman, 2001; Rankin & Stallings, 2001; Boyd, Gleit, Graham, & Whitman, 1998).

With the increased focus on prevention, promotion, and independence in self-care activities, today's newly emerging healthcare system mandates the education of consumers to a greater extent than ever before. Opportunities for client teaching have become increasingly more varied in terms of the types of clients encountered, their particular learning needs, and the settings in which health teaching occurs. For health education to have a meaningful impact on the lives of others, nurse educators must have a sound understanding of the teaching–learning process to take advantage of the multitude of opportunities to educate consumers. They are also expected to be increasingly adept at identifying the type of content and instructional methodologies that most effectively and efficiently deliver the intended health messages. Additionally, nurses need to become knowledgeable about the Internet as a major source of information in the health education of clients (Desborough, 1999).

## CLASSIFICATION OF INSTRUCTIONAL SETTINGS

Although the professional literature contains a significant number of articles related to the practice of nursing in home health care, ambulatory care, school and occupational health care, and institutional care for the acutely and chronically ill, little attempt has been made by authors to comprehensively categorize settings specifically with respect to the nurse's role in patient/client education. Most of the major textbooks on patient education do not present a clear definition of instructional settings. Various authors refer to education taking place in a hospital, a client's home, a physician's office, or unit-based environments for cardiac care, kidney dialysis, or intensive care. Others identify location of practice by the level of service given such as acute, episodic, rehabilitation, or long-term care. Rankin and Stallings (2001) identify and define two general categories of communities—geographical communities and communities of interest—for community-based patient education programs. The implication is that these identified "areas" for practice serve a variety of clients with different educational needs requiring different assessment and teaching approaches (Rankin & Stallings, 2001; Redman, 2001; Boyd et al., 1998).

Graham and Gleit (1998) describe the teaching role of nurses from the perspective of community versus inpatient, labeling these various practice areas as *service settings*. Redman (2001) refers to specific and separate patient education practice areas to teach disease prevention, health promotion, and health maintenance and rehabilitation. She asserts that there has not developed an organized, coherent infrastructure for the delivery of patient education services. Cupples (1991) and Leckrone (1991) present data from various studies on the effectiveness of teaching in a variety of "situations," which they identify as settings. The consensus is that a "setting" is generally implied to be that place where health teaching occurs.

The setting for client and patient education is viewed by this author in a different manner than that presented by nurse educators in the past. An instructional setting is conceptualized on the basis of what relationship health education has to the primary function of the organization, agency, or institution within which it occurs. This approach is derived from the method used by Knowles (1964) and Schroeder (1980) to classify settings for adult education. Both of these experts in the field of adult education categorized instructional settings according to the extent to which education is a primary or secondary function of an agency, institution, or organization. For example, they define an academic institution as a setting whose primary purpose is education.

In this chapter, instructional settings are classified according to the primary purpose of the organization or agency that sponsors health education encounters. An *instructional setting* is an entity whose fundamental mission is to provide health care, to engage in activities related to health care, or to be involved primarily in activities unrelated to health care (Figure 14–1). Based on this perspective, three types of settings for the education of clients have been identified:

1. A *healthcare setting* is one in which the delivery of health care is the primary or sole function of the institution, organization, or agency. Hospitals, visiting nurse

## EXAMPLES OF INSTRUCTIONAL SETTINGS

Emergency Care Centers
Nurse Managed Centers
Surgery Centers
Physician Offices
Diagnostic Centers

**HEALTH-CARE SETTING**

Outpatient Clinics
HMOs
VNAs
Hospitals
Wellness Centers

**SHARED RESOURCES**
Staff
Facilities
Instructional Materials

Alzheimer's Associatioin
American Cancer Society
American Heart Association
Leukemia Society of America
Muscular Dystrophy
Association
Arthritis Foundation
American Lung Association
Head Injury Support Group

**HEALTH-CARE-RELATED SETTING**

**NON-HEALTH-CARE SETTING**

Shelters
Church Associations
Sheltered Workshops
Professional Associations
Senior Centers
PTAs
Military and Governmental Groups
Social/Civic Groups

Diabetic Club
Planned Parenthood
of America

Businesses
YMCAs/YWCAs
Schools

FIGURE 14–1   **Instructional Settings and Their Relationships**

associations, public health departments, outpatient clinics, extended-care facilities, health maintenance organizations, physician offices, and nurse managed centers are examples of organizations whose primary purpose is to deliver health care, for which health education is an integral aspect of the overall care delivered within these settings. Nurses function to provide direct patient care, and their role encompasses the teaching of clients as part of that care.

2. A *healthcare-related setting* is one in which healthcare-related services are offered as a complementary function of a quasi-health agency. Examples of this type of setting include the American Heart Association, the American Cancer Society, and the Mus-

cular Dystrophy Association. These organizations provide client advocacy, conduct health screenings and self-help groups, disseminate health education information and materials, and support research on disease and lifestyle issues for the benefit of consumers within the community. Education on health promotion, disease prevention, and improving the quality of life for those who live with a particular illness is the key function of nurses within these agencies.

3. A *non-healthcare setting* is one in which health care is an incidental or supportive function of an organization. Examples of organizations classified as being this type of setting include businesses, industries, schools, and military and penal institu-

tions. The primary purpose of these organizations is to produce a manufactured product or offer a non–health-related service to the public. Industries, for example, are involved in health care only to the extent of providing health screenings and nonemergent health coverage to their employees through a health office within their place of employment, making available instruction in job-related health and safety issues to meet Occupational Safety and Health Administration (OSHA) regulations, or providing opportunities for health education through wellness programs to reduce absenteeism or improve employee morale.

Thus, an instructional setting is an environment in which health education takes place to provide individuals with the opportunity to engage in learning experiences for the purpose of improving their health or reducing their risk for illness. It is best to select a broad definition of an instructional setting to enable nurses to consciously recognize the opportunities available for the teaching of those who are currently or potentially consumers of health care. Given that teaching is an important aspect of healthcare delivery, nurses engage clients of differing ages and at various stages along the wellness–illness continuum in health education activities, which can take place under a variety of circumstances, both formal and informal. Wherever and whenever teaching takes place, nurses need to recognize the importance of consciously applying the principles of teaching and learning to these encounters for maximum effectiveness in helping clients to attain and maintain optimal health.

Health teaching can occur during any encounter between a healthcare professional—in this case, the nurse in the role of educator—and another person or group seeking health-related information, regardless of the setting in which the information is shared.

The client who is the recipient of formal health teaching can be the patient who is ill, the patient's family members or significant others, or individuals or groups in the community who are presently well. Health teaching can also occur during impromptu or informal encounters between the nurse and anyone seeking health information.

Classifying instructional settings in which the nurse functions as educator provides a frame of reference through which to better understand the interrelationship between the components of the organizational climate, the target audience, and the resources within the environment influencing the educational tasks to be accomplished. The role and functioning of the nurse as client educator are affected differently by these components in each of the identified settings.

Approaching instructional settings from the perspective of these three components will assist the professional nurse responsible for teaching to gain insight into the common elements to be considered across settings as well as the unique factors associated with particular settings. Armed with this classification, the nurse educator can more accurately determine who the potential learner is, consider the circumstances under which learning is to take place, and understand the resources available, which can limit or dictate specific strategies for teaching, or conversely, allow for a diversity of teaching options for maximum effectiveness in learning. Each setting should be considered in terms of which factors have the greatest effects on it and how these factors influence the client, the nurse educator, and the teaching–learning process in the selected practice environment.

## FACTORS RELATED TO INSTRUCTIONAL SETTING

Before discussing the specific types of settings in which healthcare teaching can be carried out, it is necessary to acknowledge those common factors that can have a major impact on teaching and learning across settings. These variables, which positively or negatively influence the success of teaching strategies and the outcomes of learning in any particular situation, are classified into three main categories: *organizational*, *environmental*, and *clientele factors*. If any elements within these categories are insufficient or not conducive to the support of the teaching–learning process, they may act as barriers or obstacles that reduce the effectiveness of health education interventions by interfering with either the teacher's or the client's level of participation.

The following questions related to these factors must be taken into account when planning for the delivery of education programs in the various settings in which the nurse functions (Table 14–1). These elements will be specifically addressed later in the chapter as they apply to the discussion of particular settings.

## Organizational Factors

**1.** *What is the administrative perspective regarding health education?* The philosophy of the organization emanates from those who are in control of its operations. The attitude of the administration about the teaching of health information is of utmost importance to the success of educational endeavors. Administrative support influences the amount and types of resources available for education.

Within healthcare organizations and agencies, patient education carries an economic benefit because it is considered skilled care and is reimbursable by third-party payers in most instances. When patient education is a non–revenue-generating activity, the cost of educational interventions is balanced by a reduction in the incidence of illness, an improved quality of life, decreased rehospitalization, or overutilization of other services within the healthcare system (Shendell-Falik, 1990).

Within non-healthcare organizations, such as in occupational settings, employers can reduce their indirect healthcare costs by sponsoring health education programs that can decrease absenteeism and increase workers' safety and well-being. Because health insur-

| TABLE 14–1   Instructional settings, impacting factors, and teaching strategies | | |
|---|---|---|
| **Instructional Settings** | **Impacting Factors and Elements** | **Teaching Strategies** |
| Healthcare | Organizational | One-to-one instruction |
| Healthcare-related | Administrative perspective | Lecture |
| Non-healthcare | Time constraints | Group discussion |
| | Resources | Printed material |
| | Teaching expertise | Audiovisual materials |
| | Collegial support | Interactive media |
| | Environmental | Individual and group sessions |
| | External resources | Role-playing |
| | Structural characteristics | Simulated games |
| | Clientele | Situational problem solving |
| | Health status | Demonstration and return |
| | Nature of contact | demonstration |
| | Characteristics | |
| | Self-directedness | |
| | Educational need | |
| | Resources | |

ance premiums paid by employers are often determined by the health-risk level of their employees, these programs can offer employers an immediate, tangible financial reward for their efforts (Graham & Gleit, 1998). Thus, the value assigned by administrators to health education as a service to their clientele or employees, relative to the emphasis placed on other aspects of their operations, influences the development and provision of health education programs within an organization.

**2.** *How much time is allocated to the teaching of health information?* Regardless of the instructional setting, time is a valuable resource that exerts a major influence over the delivery of education to clients. The length of time a client remains in contact with the healthcare system for receipt of services is shrinking as a result of economic factors. Time for educational activities is often a scarce commodity within any organization but particularly in healthcare agencies, where the amount of contact time with patients is being further limited by organizational responses to external healthcare reforms, resulting in fewer nurses for the same number or more clients.

Although advances in technology have generally improved care, they also have reduced contact time by allowing patients to be discharged earlier from inpatient facilities to care for themselves at home. Early discharge requires patients to learn how to operate hightech equipment within time constraints imposed by the managed-care mandates of most HMOs and insurance providers. These same time constraints will force nurses in the role of educators to become more proficient when providing health education. Their focus must be on providing only essential information and skill development needed by the client during the recovery or convalescence period, prioritizing content that can be taught in shorter time frames, and selecting instructional methodologies that allow for more self-directed client involvement with less direct

educator presence. A concentrated effort must be made to use every available opportunity, no matter how brief, for client teaching and reinforcement of information across all levels of prevention including health promotion.

**3.** *To what extent are resources available to carry out educational endeavors?* Sufficient financial support is required to ensure adequacy of nursing staff, the purchase of needed audiovisual materials and instructional equipment, time to develop content-specific materials, and the provision of space for teaching. Adequate resources make possible the implementation of efficient and effective educational interventions. Without the required resources, information fails to be consistently provided, and the specific needs of clients go unaddressed. Teaching time can be decreased by combining the use of more standardized teaching materials with the sharing of resources among healthcare settings, thereby reducing bottom-line costs.

**4.** *Is the staff within the organization expert in the teaching role?* Although undergraduate nursing education may include principles of teaching and learning in patient education, a basic understanding is generally insufficient to prepare nurses to creatively integrate teaching into their demanding work schedules. In a healthcare environment, the informal reward system often recognizes physical care as more important than the teaching of self-care. Patient care is frequently viewed by nurses as a series of tasks rather than as an interactive process to support the development of new skills by the client. Furthermore, when staff nurses do teach, they often concentrate on presenting large amounts of didactic information rather than incorporating educational strategies that allow for skills training, family involvement, and opportunities to practice new skills in realistic situations.

The emphasis on improving cognitive skill levels rather than changing attitudinal or psychomotor behaviors reflects the fact that teaching efforts to meet cognitive needs are easier to deliver, are less time-consuming, and tend to involve a less threatening role for nurses (Zarle, 1989). The perspectives of nurses toward client education as well as their competencies with respect to their preparation for and experience with teaching must be evaluated in each environment. As more nurses become prepared at the baccalaureate level, with teaching, health promotion, and community experiences included as an integral part of their learning, future nurses will be better prepared for the client teaching role, whether it be in the acute care or community situation.

5. *What is the level of support from physicians and other colleagues?* Although a growing number of nurse educators are quite capable of identifying clients' learning needs and providing for the education to meet those needs, in healthcare settings physician support is imperative in providing for that education. Presently, Medicare and other third-party reimbursement will not be received if the service is not a direct order by a physician. Within healthcare organizations, instituting innovative client education approaches is facilitated when the support of physicians and other professional colleagues is present (Shendell-Falik, 1990). Good communication and positive relationships among colleagues are necessary to provide continuity of care, which includes patient education as one very important aspect of overall treatment.

## Environmental Factors

1. *What external resources are available within the environment to support and promote the educational process?* The services of consultants and specialists from other healthcare disciplines, such as dieticians, occupational therapists, physicians, physical therapists, speech therapists, and social workers, must be available to complement the efforts by nurse educators in helping clients to acquire skills needed to attain or maintain optimal wellness.

Members of the clergy and self-help groups may play a key role in assisting the client to adjust emotionally and socially to a difficult situation. Community-based organizations are often an excellent vehicle for disseminating information and providing a source of funding for client education services. The nurse's role is to facilitate and coordinate the interactions among these resources.

2. *What structural characteristics may stimulate or impede the development and use of educational programs?* Consideration must be given to location, travel time, space availability, costs, scheduling, and accessibility when designing a new program or continuing an existing one. The physical layout of a given area needs to be evaluated, with attention being paid to its adequacy for client privacy, low distraction potential, roominess, comfort, and ability to easily accommodate equipment related to the topics and skills being taught.

## Clientele Factors

1. *What is the health status of the client?* The client who is well most likely has a low or moderate state of anxiety and is therefore likely to be receptive to teaching and learning. For the patient who is acutely or chronically ill, however, symptom distress such as fatigue, discomfort, and anxiety, along with the client's and family's perceptions of the illness and support systems available, may adversely affect the person's ability to learn. For individuals who are hospitalized, the loss of personal control, lack of privacy, and social isolation can negatively affect their ability to actively participate in acquiring needed skills for self-care.

2. *What is the nature of the contact with the client over time?* Contact with the client is highly variable, depending on the situation. If the patient is hospitalized, the opportunity for frequent contact may be more concentrated, over a week or just a few days or even hours

in the case of same-day surgery units. The trend toward decreased lengths of stay means that nurses have less contact time in which to do the required teaching and patients are likely to be sicker and less receptive to educational interventions.

If care is being given in the home setting, the nurse's visits may be limited to only a half hour or so because of fee-for-service or insurance reimbursement regulations or the number of clients to be seen that day by the nurse. Repeated visits may be scheduled over a period of days or a few weeks, allowing opportunity for the nurse to establish an ongoing relationship with the patient and family and to pace the learning to the individual client situation. Ambulatory care provides for short and intermittent contacts, and the client may not consistently be cared for by the same nurse at every visit.

Rehabilitation settings, on the other hand, allow for extended contact in which to build rapport with the client and provide practice opportunities to learn self-care skills. In today's managed care climate, clients receive instruction across a continuum of care settings, requiring that attention be given to the coordination of teaching to guarantee that information is complete and the content presented and reinforced is similar.

**3.** *What are the developmental levels, language skills, age, literacy levels, disabilities, and cultural beliefs of the client?* For settings that serve special populations or multilingual, low-literate, or culturally diverse groups, education methods and materials must be specifically designed to meet the needs of these clientele (see Chapters 5, 7, 8, and 9). The nurse educator must determine the homogeneity and heterogeneity of the populations in different settings when planning educational strategies.

**4.** *How self-directed is the client in seeking information?* A major goal of education is to gain the compliance of the learner in carrying out treatment regimens and self-care activities. Research on locus of control suggests that internally oriented individuals prefer to maintain self-control and are likely to be health oriented, compliant with treatment regimens, and receptive to health teaching. Conversely, those with an external locus of control prefer to relinquish control to healthcare providers and present a challenge for the nurse educator in motivating them to attend educational sessions and actively participate in learning activities. This problem can become an even greater challenge to the health educator as the healthcare system demands more self-care responsibility from the client.

**5.** *How critical to the health and well-being of the learner is the educational content being presented?* If what is being taught is viewed as important information that can be used to help attain or maintain optimal health or reduce the likelihood of an emergency situation, then the clients' attention will be oriented to learning. If the learners do not see the relevance of the information to improving their lifestyle and health status, it is unlikely they will have much motivation for learning or participating in self-care (see Chapter 6).

**6.** *What resources are available to assist clients in achieving educational outcomes?* The clients' financial resources must be taken into account because they cannot be expected to follow a specific regimen of care if money to obtain the necessary equipment, medications, foods, or services prescribed is not available. Even healthy individuals who attend programs for promotion of health and disease prevention may not have the financial resources to carry through with all suggested lifestyle changes. Psychosocial resources, such as the presence of supportive family members or significant others, are most beneficial to the learning experience because they can reinforce the teaching–learning process and provide assistance with self-care activities for those less able for whatever reason.

## HEALTHCARE SETTING

The concept of a healthcare setting encompasses many types of institutions, organizations, and agencies, large and small, whose main focus is the delivery of patient care, with clients receiving patient education as a mandated part of their overall care. Some of these settings provide care on an inpatient basis, such as hospitals, nursing homes, and other extended- or skilled-care facilities. Others provide outpatient care in the home and community, such as visiting nurse associations (VNAs), health maintenance organizations, neighborhood health clinics, physicians' offices, and nurse managed centers. In addition, individual hospitals and large healthcare management networks own and operate smaller general or specialty-based units such as one-day surgery centers, outpatient clinics, and diagnostic and rehabilitation centers. Some of these units are found within hospitals, whereas others are physically located outside the organization as an extension of its services. They are commonly referred to as ambulatory and community outreach centers (Figure 14–1).

This broad spectrum of patient care services is associated with a wide range of sites in which nurses provide care and client education. In addition to providing patient care, these organizations or institutions are employing agencies. In this respect, they are like any other business entity in that they must conform to OSHA regulations and the required standards of various accrediting bodies and state licensing departments to provide workplace safety and health promotion instruction for all of their employees. They must also provide in-service education or staff development programs to maintain the practice competencies of their professional caregivers. Therefore, the responsibility of nurse educators in these healthcare settings is not only to teach patients, but also to instruct nursing staff and other personnel.

Teaching strategies incorporate a wide variety of instructional methods and tools to deliver content. They enhance the capacity of the learner to obtain, retain, and apply knowledge and skills. These techniques include such teaching methods as traditional lectures, group discussions, and simulated games as well as audiovisual materials (Table 14–1). Today's learners are most responsive to teaching strategies that employ stimulation of several senses and participatory learning exercises whenever possible (Green, 1998; Rankin & Stallings, 2001). Knowles (1983) predicted that by the end of the twentieth century, most educational services would be delivered electronically. The Internet abounds with health-related information which anyone can access. Nurses can use this technology in a variety of ways (see Chapter 13 on technology in education). They can, for example, create a Web page with information on criteria to evaluate reputable health information sources, develop hot links to specific recommended sites, or use online office hours or e-mail to communicate with discharged clients and their family caregivers (Desborough, 1999).

Nurses will need to be prepared to utilize this new technology in delivering health education. Computer-assisted instruction (CAI), interactive video programming, and virtual reality will soon be readily accessible in all settings. These strategies reduce the amount of direct contact time a nurse needs to spend providing education, allow for diverse learner needs, and provide for pacing, repetition, and flexibility of learning (Blackwood & White, 1991). The general content available in multimedia format can be used for initial instruction and repetitive learning for one or several learners at a time. It allows the nurse to use the limited time with the client to individualize instruction when needed. (For more details related to instructional methods and materials, see Chapters 11 and 12.)

Within the healthcare setting, a range of teaching situations require different strategies based on the characteristics of the clientele, their healthcare problems, and the type and extent of services the clients are receiving. A client on the inpatient unit and one in the outpatient clinic can be presented with some similar and some different strategies. Teaching strategies should be selected based on responses to the following four concerns:

- How much does the client need to know now and later?

- Is the information to be learned life-sustaining or general content that the client ought to know?

- To what degree will the client's physical and psychological condition interfere with knowledge acquisition and retention?

- How much teaching time and client contact over time are possible?

General care units, specialty units, outpatient units, community medical care centers, and physician offices all require teaching of clients. The strategies include one-to-one, lecture, and group discussions; brief, concise, printed instructions; and demonstration with return demonstration when necessary. The client situation will dictate whether teaching sessions need to be individual or group presentations. Teaching clients in a group should be selected whenever possible, because this approach uses staff time more effectively, is less costly, and affords the client an opportunity to have a shared experience. When the client situation is more individualized, such as on a same-day surgery unit, one-to-one teaching strategies need to be emphasized, along with the other modalities.

When contact with the client is expected to include multiple visits over time, such as in home care visits, outpatient clinics, HMO centers, and physician offices, then a multisensory approach is used, including films, videos, and take-home printed material, with staff accessible and actively engaging the clients in individualized discussions, clarification, and reinforcement of content after they have had the opportunity to view or read the materials or interact with the learning modules.

When more time is available and the health education involves more general care or ought-to-know content related to chronic conditions or lifestyle changes, then participatory learning strategies such as problem-solving situations, simulated games, and role-playing can be employed, with video films added for more varied sensory input and for repetition, so as to enhance understanding and retention of content. Charts or diagrams are a particularly helpful strategy to review content, to emphasize steps in a procedure, or to help clients learn the sequencing in an event (Breckon, Harvey, & Lancaster, 1985). Providing small increments of information over time is a better strategy when the learner's attention span is short, as when the client is a child, mentally disabled, an older adult, or very anxious.

Follow-up contact by phone should be included if discharge occurs immediately after the teaching session or contact with the client is brief, such as in an emergency care or same-day surgery center. The phone contact is used to evaluate the learning and to reinforce teaching as well as to assess physical status. A follow-up phone contact would also be used if the problems the client may encounter are likely to occur between the discharge time and the follow-up visit (Rankin & Stallings, 2001).

Instructional healthcare settings provide a wide variety of practice environments for the nurse educator, and a few will be described here. In reviewing the factors that affect the role of the nurse educator in large and small practice environments, an understanding will be gained regarding the clientele, environmental resources, and organizational characteristics of other similar but somewhat different practice environments that are not described here, yet are part of the instructional category of healthcare settings (Figure 14–1).

## Hospitals

Since the 1970s, patient education has been an integral part of hospitals. Organizational support and commitment of staff, resources, and time exist in hospitals for client health education and for the nurse as the primary provider of that education because mandates from accreditation and licensing bodies require it

(Simonds, 1973). The shortened hospital stay and the expansion of services into areas such as same-day surgery centers, hospital-based home care departments, cardiac rehabilitation centers, and hemodialysis centers are already increasing the emphasis on health education as part of the continuum of care. Continuity of care ensures that from admission through posthospital care, the patients have what they need in terms of treatment, medical equipment, knowledge, and skills to carry them to the end point of service, bridging the gap between acute inpatient service and less acute community service needed after rapid discharge, especially for older adults and those with chronic illnesses (Zarle, 1989). Patient teaching and the role of the nurse educator have become a more integral part of this system to identify and implement teaching plans needed to prepare clients for each phase of recovery. Accreditation standards that mandate patient education provide the impetus for the nurse educator role (Davidhizar, Bechtel, & Dowd, 1998).

**Organizational Factors**   Hospitals, like other large healthcare delivery systems or networks, are complex organizations that have a variety of organizational structures, with specialty units within the hospital or situated off-site in community centers. Although the nurse educator has organizational support, large organizational systems require formal, hierarchical communication among units, whether on or off premises, resulting in cumbersome negotiations when planning to establish an innovative patient education program or make changes in existing ones. Such an effort requires knowledge and application of change theory and involvement of interdisciplinary planning teams to ensure success (Rifas, Morris, & Grady, 1994; Shendell-Falik, 1990). Regardless of the size of the healthcare organization or the mandated regulations, it is often difficult to garner support of our medical colleagues for client education programs, and

this goal is often achieved only through persistent, lengthy, one-to-one discussions with key medical staff. Although sometimes difficult to obtain, their support is essential to comply with present insurance payment requirements. However, as consumers demand more information and healthcare systems require more self-care from clients, the client education component will become a more important part of the entire package of care delivered, with nurses providing it without specific medical orders.

The healthcare setting does not separate out the cost of patient teaching activities because many third-party payers do not currently pay for teaching, whether provided in the inpatient or outpatient unit. The future may see healthcare organizations being required to itemize separately patient or health education as well as many other items for the sole purpose of insurance reimbursement. The current state of financial reimbursement affects the setting in that no monies are specifically marked for this purpose and monies needed for patient education must come from the "common pot." The value placed by the organization on health education will determine the percentage of financial support that goes to such programs.

Nurse educators in these practice environments are restricted by many constraints imposed by organizational factors and are more traditionally bound by the established criteria to be met or required content to be taught. They may be limited by the monies or technical resources available to obtain or develop teaching materials or by the staff time allowed to prepare and deliver content. This constraint is especially applicable to outreach centers, which often operate on grant funds or time-limited financial support.

However, these detached services or specialty units often allow for a closer relationship to develop between physicians and nurses who provide care to clients, promoting a collegial, collaborative relationship through their joint efforts to meet patient education needs with less physician resistance evident. Teaching is still a less quantifiable, non–revenue-generating function, hampering its general acceptance and implementation in all ambulatory care situations. This is especially true for physician offices, where the nurse educator role is far less defined or developed and time for teaching is often underutilized (Hiss, Frey, & Davis, 1986).

The attitudes and value placed on client education by all involved, from administrators to staff-level nurses, can affect the quantity and quality of client education (DeMuth, 1989). The focus of care is still tasks and procedures, with seeing a high number of both scheduled and emergency clients within posted hours of operation taking priority and leaving little time for the nurse educator to engage in creative thinking to prepare or evaluate teaching plans, materials, or strategies. Client education must be a well-integrated activity with well-designed strategies and tools if it is to be a meaningful, worthwhile intervention. Planning ahead is essential, with input into yearly budgets to ensure that monies for client education activities and equipment are there, making what is needed become a reality in the year ahead.

Hospitals and their associated specialty units are more likely to have on staff nurse educators who oversee client education programs or who support less-prepared unit-level nurses in their teaching efforts. Unfortunately, these resources are not fully utilized, and a significant number of unit-level nurses remain inadequately prepared in the application of teaching–learning principles. They may not discriminate "need to know" from "nice to know" content to be taught, fail to assess what the clients perceive as important for them to learn about self-care, or lack sufficient knowledge regarding the aftercare situation for which the nurse needs to prepare the client (Bubela, Galloway, McCay, et al., 1990; Naylor & Shaid, 1991).

In general, these environments provide an opportunity for nurse educators to prepare extensively to meet the educational needs of the learners because they know the composition of the learning group, can anticipate their needs, and can individualize the educational plan using appropriate teaching strategies. Anticipated problems such as staff schedules and language or sensory disabilities of the learners can be discussed and solutions proposed ahead of time to make for a more successful learning situation, with fewer unanticipated difficulties arising in this type of setting.

For a variety of reasons, what clients learn in the hospital is not well recalled after discharge, necessitating reteaching by home care nurses. The patient education component of the system could be better organized, more efficient, and more effective if there were greater involvement and closer coordination among hospital-based patient educators, discharge-planning nurses, and home care nurses. It is essential to increase the standardization of content and teaching materials across units of patient care and to facilitate the development and implementation of teaching protocols for the more common acute and chronic health problems from the moment of admission through to discharge and subsequent home care, focusing on education for self-care as a major component to be addressed when planning for discharge. This effort would make possible cost-effective use of the nurse's teaching time and patient learning time, smooth the transition from acute to home care and from dependent to more independent client functioning, and include client education to ensure the quality of continuity of care and discharge planning.

Documentation in a healthcare setting is an important and integral component of the patient education activity, because it provides the basis for financial reimbursement of that portion of care. On one large metropolitan hospital's postpartum unit, a checklist is used to document standard teaching content for self and baby care. Every client is provided with the same content, which is noted on the checklist by the nurse who does the teaching. When home care nurses make the follow-up visit after discharge, they know what the clients have already been taught. Thus they can assess retention of that knowledge, reinforce it if necessary, and move on to other mutually agreed-on client education topics best taught in the home setting. Between the two experiences, the new mother will have received a total educational packet begun in the hospital and completed after discharge in the home (Smith, 1986).

For a number of years, both major and smaller community hospitals have used their nursing education departments creatively and fully by providing health promotion programs to the general community and many area businesses, such as offering free or fee-for-service cholesterol screening and weight management programs supported by small grants, or for a break-even cost. In the future, this area of practice for the nurse educator will expand and become a more profitable, revenue-generating endeavor in this healthcare setting, offering opportunities for collaboration and sharing of staff expertise, of facility space, and of instructional materials as well as meeting the general community's need for health promotion education provided by nurse educators.

**Environmental Factors** Resources, including consultants and specialists from all healthcare disciplines, are extensive and easily accessed in the hospital and large network practice environments. Even when the care delivery sites are off premises, the resources of the parent facility are available, with time and distance as the major barriers.

Specific teaching materials, such as pamphlets and videos, on standardized topics are often provided free through vendors that service healthcare settings. Closed-circuit TV

and freestanding TV/VCR units are commonly provided to any patient-occupied area. Classrooms or conference rooms are likely available but may need to be scheduled in advance if not dedicated for the sole use of patient education departments. Patient waiting areas, lounges, and patients' rooms are often used for small group or individualized client education sessions, providing an attractively furnished, comfortable environment and fostering inclusion of family or support persons in the sessions.

Even when space is available, the client's other medical care–related activities may take priority over scheduled patient education time because patient education is not viewed as having the same importance as other higher-cost interventions. The organization may not place as much value on the teaching component needed but rather focus more on the need to discharge the client as rapidly as possible, regardless of the client's psychological preparedness. In this instance, knowledge and skills for aftercare may be compromised.

Ambulatory care units such as same-day surgery centers, outpatient clinics, or emergency rooms process a high volume of clients in a brief time period, with major space and time constraints for care delivery including much needed client education presentations. A greater reliance on audiovisual and take-home printed materials coupled with follow-up phone calls to evaluate client status and teaching effectiveness is provided for client learning needs in those situations.

**Scenario** This is a same-day surgery unit of an ambulatory care center. Clients A and B are admitted for a diagnostic procedure. Client A is a schoolteacher, and Client B is a housewife with a limited understanding of English. The unit is fast-paced and dictated by schedules. Most clients have mild to moderate anxiety levels. The nursing staff must relate to many physicians and adhere to many protocols. The nurse–client encounters are brief, and the total length of stay for a client is less than 12 hours. Instructional encounters within this healthcare setting require brief, concise teaching of only key points. An explanation of the client's recovery process is done through use of a video individually viewed over a bedside TV. Staff are available to respond to client questions, to provide both verbal and written discharge instructions, and to make follow-up phone calls the next day to assess client status, evaluate learning, and provide additional teaching interventions. If the client has a vision problem or a language barrier, an audiocassette of instructions is provided for listening, with the audio and written instructions available in the more common languages. Current technology is used to provide postoperative clients with an e-mail address where they can ask questions or obtain general post-op care instructions if needed after they return home.

This setting dictates individual teaching strategies as a primary mode augmented with group presentations and multimedia materials whenever possible. Today, most same-day surgery centers use telephone follow-up after discharge to assess the client's condition and provide additional education.

The type and range of teaching strategies used in any instructional setting will be influenced by the value the organization places on client education, resources available to support the development and delivery of educational programs, and the characteristics of the clients to be served.

In most healthcare settings, the learning need is responded to more from the health provider's perspective and less from the client's viewpoint. For example, if it is decided that a newly diagnosed diabetic client needs to know how to test for blood sugar regularly and what the readings indicate, although the patient may not desire to learn that part of self-care first, the patient will be taught despite the probable lack of readiness to learn because discharge may be only a day away.

**Clientele Factors** The characteristics and needs of the clients serviced by large or small healthcare organizations and their specialty units dictate the specific content to be taught, the time and the amount of client teaching undertaken, and the most appropriate teaching strategies to be used. Clients admitted to these facilities are sicker and have higher anxiety levels due to the acute nature of their health problems at the time of contact with the setting, making them less receptive to learning. They may have one or more chronic illnesses, have a variety of compounding socially related issues such as homelessness or poverty, be newly diagnosed, or be at an advanced stage of illness.

Ambulatory care units such as outpatient clinics and emergency care centers see and treat clients for episodic conditions but have decreased opportunities for future encounters that might allow for more individualized health promotion and disease prevention–focused teaching. If clients return at a later point to one of the large or high-volume care areas, they will probably see a different nurse each time, reducing the possibility of continuity in client teaching. For these reasons, most teaching content should focus on the common concerns for the clients at whatever stage on the illness continuum they are, providing verbal and written information on signs and symptoms to report, medication or treatment regimens, and safety in self-care management (DeMuth, 1989).

Clients are oriented to receiving diagnostic procedures and treatments but not necessarily health education as an integral part of a visit to an ambulatory care facility. For clients to participate in the teaching–learning process as a part of their experience in ambulatory care, they must know ahead of time to expect health teaching as a component of their care, facilitating their readiness to learn at each visit.

The limited contact between the nurse and the client, for whatever reason, requires that this time be utilized to the fullest, with teaching sessions and reinforcement of information being woven into every patient contact. Hospitalized clients' acuity level makes them less receptive to learning, and the lack of an opportunity to apply the learning to their present condition makes retention difficult. Patients are not asked to self-medicate or do their own dressings while hospitalized and, therefore, are less likely to be skilled in these areas when discharged—unless the facility and the nurse educator have provided some realistic opportunities for application of self-care skills.

Although the ideal is to set up self-care units such as exist in New York University's Cooperative Care Model or the one at Newark Beth Israel Medical Center, that approach may not be financially possible for many hospitals. A smaller model like the Recuperative Skills Training Center at Sacramento's Kaiser Permanente Medical Center, where patients go to practice needed self-care skills, may be more feasible (Rifas et al., 1994). It is also possible to reorient staff nurses to "do less" and "teach more" by allowing able patients to do their own dressings with staff supervision or by providing group teaching sessions where patients on restricted diets select their daily menus with the teaching and guidance of the nurse educator and dietician. This approach is facilitated by the fact that the client in the hospital situation is narrowly focused on the disease condition with interest in treatments, side effects, medications, impact on lifestyle, and activities of daily living, with little concern being directed toward the general aspects of the disease or primary prevention components (Naylor & Shaid, 1991). Including the family or significant other in teaching sessions whenever possible will improve retention of content, increase support for the client, and enhance compliance with treatment regimens. Triad communication involves a third person who is assisting with daily care management decisions (Davidhizar & Rexroth, 1994).

One finds a wide range of demographic characteristics among today's clients. The nurse must therefore make a rapid, comprehensive assessment of each client's developmental level, language skill, literacy level, cultural and religious orientation, self-directedness, readiness to learn, and available support system. Regardless of the psychosocial readiness factors, the system mandates that the client be taught self-care with referral to home care for follow-up. Consequently, the nurse educator must select and prioritize the "must knows" from the "ought to knows" to accomplish the minimum teaching requirements. Many of the client characteristics and limited time frames for teaching are the same across most healthcare environments. However, the acuity of the clients, their anxiety level, and the number of contacts with the clients over time vary in each setting. To meet the learning needs in complex situations, clients with multiple health problems, life-threatening illnesses or complications, conditions requiring complex technical treatments, or multiple medication regimens should be identified as requiring more intense teaching that should begin as early as possible (Bubela et al., 1990).

Although large healthcare settings such as hospitals and their community-based units can more easily obtain reimbursable medical supplies and equipment or other support services, some items require out-of-pocket expenditures by the client with or without subsequent reimbursement, which may be an issue for older patients or others with fixed or limited income. These financial constraints may prevent compliance with health teaching.

Nurse educators need to be prepared for the wide variety of client characteristics and health-related elements encountered in the hospital setting that dictate learning needs. Nurses must revise the expectations of themselves, refrain from attempting to "teach it all," and adopt an abbreviated, efficient, and expeditious form of client education that meets the client's basic self-care needs (Phillips, 1999).

## Home Care

Home health care is one of the most rapidly growing practice settings, driven by early discharge and the need to provide acute and high-tech care as the client is shifted from hospital to home (Green, 1998). The home of today is the hospital of yesterday, with clients being maintained at home with skilled care until their next life-threatening episode brings them back to the hospital. Hospital administrators recognize that the home care clientele are fast replacing their shrinking hospital bed clients, and they welcome the opportunity to be involved in this area of community care through hospital-based home care units. At present, home care can be found within a variety of large and small healthcare organizations, such as VNAs, hospice associations, extended-care facilities, and large and small for-profit home care organizations. Some agencies provide home care for their own parent institutions as well as for other facilities that are not able to provide the home care directly but whose clients require these services, such as institutions outside the geographical area. If the parent organization is the more traditional hospital, for example, then teaching is influenced by factors related to that organization, its environmental resources, and its clientele.

**Organizational Factors**   When home care is a unit within a larger organization, it is committed to health education and will vary only somewhat based on individual philosophies or values of the facility. When the home care agency is a smaller independent agency or a for-profit unit, the organizational philosophy, value placed on client health education, scope of services provided, organizational structure, and legislative regulations will vary much more from agency to agency and influence to a much greater extent how much patient edu-

cation is provided, especially in today's money-driven system. For example, if the nurse's primary purpose for the visit is to oversee care and supervise home health aides in a long-term care program or a for-profit home care agency, then the nurse educator role focuses more on staff learning needs related to their care of the client and less on client-based learning needs regarding medications and treatments. Third-party payers, such as Medicare, in these instances will pay only for a nursing visit to reassess ongoing care needs and aide supervision once every few weeks in what is considered to be a more stable, chronic care situation. Thus, the type of home care agency and services rendered will directly affect the nurse educator by dictating the learner's identity, the nature of the educational content, and the time allocated for the teaching–learning session.

Documentation for client teaching in the home setting is essential in all instances regardless of the size of the organization because many insurance payers, such as Medicare, specifically look for teaching related to treatments and medications in nursing notes to support their reimbursement. Retrospective payment is being denied when these data are lacking, especially given that client education is often the primary purpose for home care services (Green, 1998). Time allotted for client visits, including client education activities, is becoming more limited by the increasing workload, with more cases to be seen each day as a result of reduced staffing and insurance reimbursement pressures.

The home care nurse is truly alone in the home environment, without colleagues to verify assessments or give assistance. Instead, these nurses must rely on theoretical knowledge, past experience, creativity, and often intuition to provide for the health education needs of their clients, where every home presents a different scenario. The positive side of this very different and solitary practice environment is that fewer "turf" issues arise than in other healthcare disciplines. Healthcare teaching for self-care management is an expected component of care, not in every instance requiring a physician order for implementation or reimbursement. If a client requires a dressing change daily, that activity is ordered by the physician; the nurse is then expected to teach the signs and symptoms of infection to be reported to the physician and teach the client or caregiver to do the dressing change, if possible, even though it was not specified by the physician's order. The home care nurse must be adept at rapid and comprehensive assessment of client learning needs for self-care management, prioritizing those learning goals that meet both the nurse's and the client's perceived needs. The nurse must be able to switch from the planned content of a teaching session to what the client wants or needs to learn, perhaps delaying intended objectives for learning until the next visit.

Because home care is one of the few practice areas less dramatically affected by healthcare industry restructuring, nurses are seeking such positions with little or no realization of the knowledge and skills required. While most hospital-based home care agencies and VNAs hire baccalaureate-prepared nurses, the smaller or for-profit agencies may not. Despite the educational preparation of the baccalaureate-degree nurse, few nurses are adequately prepared when it comes to patient education in complex client situations in the home. This problem has been specifically recognized. In response, an innovative partnership between the New York State Nurses Association and Pace University's Department of Continuing Education in Nursing has developed a program of classroom and clinical experiences to help transition nurses from shrinking acute care positions to home care nursing, enhancing their level of competency and feelings of comfort working within such a different practice environment (*Opening the door to home care,* 1995).

**Environmental Factors**  Home care nurses are permitted into clients' homes, as guests, interacting collaboratively with clients and caregivers, who are the primary decision makers in all aspects of their care. Home care provides an opportunity to see clients in their familiar surroundings, observe behavior that is more natural, determine the problems encountered in the home, and assess clients' perspectives on their illness and limitations now that they are in their own environment. The learning goals established must be mutually acceptable, and there is joint nurse/client responsibility and negotiation as part of the caregiving process (Davidhizar et al., 1998). For example, if the client does not wish to take narcotics for pain as prescribed, then through teaching and negotiation by the nurse, the client may agree to take the narcotic at bedtime and a non-narcotic analgesic with use of relaxation techniques taught by the nurse for daytime relief. The client has more freedom of choice in this setting. Health education needs must be prioritized based on the potential threats to health, the degree of client concern about a problem, and the ease of solution (Green, 1998).

The home can pose distractions that are not under the nurse's control and that are different for each home and client situation, unlike the hospital, where the environment of a patient unit or clinic is essentially the same. Disruptive family members, visitors, environmental noise, household pets, confined quarters, and inadequate or unfamiliar medical supplies and equipment are some of the distractions or impediments for the client and the challenges the nurse may encounter in the provision of health care in the home setting (Green, 1998). A client might have believed that he or she could do the dressing or injection taught in the hospital before discharge, but once home, reality sets in, and barriers within the home may interfere with the patient's ability to apply what had been learned earlier.

Most homes have TVs, VCRs, or cassette players and some have computers as potential instructional tools to present, support, or reinforce teaching content. Many teaching materials can be obtained from the parent facility, borrowed from other health facilities in the community, or provided from the nurse's own supplies to be brought into the home. The home care nurse has access to many of the same healthcare educational materials provided by healthcare vendors, much of which is free to healthcare professionals. With creativity and imagination, the nurse educator working in home care can develop a small library of teaching tools that address many of the common chronic illnesses or health problems, such as diabetes, cardiovascular disease, hypertension, chronic obstructive pulmonary disease, hip fractures, and cancer.

The nurse focuses on health education related to self-care management and can enlist the assistance of such professionals as dieticians, physical therapists, or speech therapists to provide their expertise while reinforcing the specialized content they offer at subsequent visits. Knowledge regarding area community agencies, self-help groups, and church-affiliated programs is essential to assist in providing specialized teaching materials, equipment, or financial and psychosocial support for the learning needs of clients, facilitating client compliance with the prescribed regimen.

**Clientele Factors** The clients in home care have the same requirements for needs assessment as do clients in hospital teaching situations. Clients in the home are less acutely ill, however. Most are chronically ill with multiple diseases and, although less anxious than hospitalized patients, they may still be fearful that the next symptoms might send them back to the acute care setting or that their lifestyle, quality of life, and level of independence will deteriorate as a result of their last acute care episode. Focusing on their educational needs related to these concerns will facilitate the teaching–learning process and ultimately achieve the self-care goals desired by the nurse and the client.

Client teaching in the home situation often needs to involve not only the client but also the primary caregiver or any other concerned family members who need health education information related to the client's care needs and condition (Green, 1998). The home care situation offers the opportunity for extended contact with the client and caregiver over time and a chance to evaluate the effectiveness of the teaching–learning process, enabling adjustments to be made as adaptation to levels of wellness occur. The degree of self-directedness in learning depends on the individual client and varies according to clients' views of their wants and needs. Because the home is their "turf," clients feel freer to question advice or teaching they receive, do things their way, and establish their own time schedules and priorities, all of which may prove challenging from the perspective of the nurse's teaching efforts. The nurse must be flexible and prepared for the unexpected, a hallmark of home care delivery. The goal is to maintain the client within the home and out of the acute or chronic care institutions for as long as possible through teaching self-care management skills. The focus of health teaching tends to be less on primary prevention or health promotion and more on secondary or tertiary levels of intervention. Teaching needs to be individualized, holistic, short-term, and often oriented toward chronic care. Client education is increasingly challenging because more high-tech equipment and greater acute care needs are being encountered in the home care situation than ever before, with increased responsibility for management being left to clients, family, neighbors, or unlicensed assistive personnel (Green, 1998).

Although the home situation allows for contact with clients over several visits, insurance payers are moving toward capitated care, further reducing the number of visits available for direct care and client education (Green, 1998). Nurses will need to be creative in accommodating the various teaching needs of clients, including aspects that may not be reimbursed, so as to meet client learning needs in a holistic, individualized manner.

Teaching strategies need to focus on priority content with brief explanations and easy-to-identify instructional guidelines; more detailed information and instructional materials may be offered at follow-up visits. A multisensory approach to presenting content is a helpful strategy for reinforcement and retention in the home situation, just as it is in all other situations. The use of more sophisticated interactive media in the home teaching situation is rapidly becoming more popular and should be applied to the fullest extent possible. For example, the nurse may take an educational video to the home for viewing with the client and family members during a teaching session, or a copy may be sent ahead to be viewed by the client in preparation for the visit and teaching session. Videotapes can be left in the home until the next visit for the client and family members to review for reinforcement of learning.

Myriad teaching strategies can be used with clients in home-based healthcare settings. Whenever hardware for audiovisual materials is unavailable, printed materials to supplement various methods of teaching may be likely substitutes. The selection of instructional strategies in this healthcare setting is dictated more by the client factors than by available resources and organizational factors, because health education and patient teaching are recognized and expected responsibilities of the nurse in these settings.

## ◼ HEALTHCARE-RELATED SETTING

Healthcare-related settings include voluntary, nonprofit agencies, organizations, and institutions, such as the American Lung Association, the American Heart Association, the American Cancer Society, and the Muscular Dystrophy Association (Figure 14–1); the major purpose of these entities is client advocacy, education, and/or research (Breckon et al., 1985). Health education may be the primary purpose of the organization, or it may have a secondary or equally valued advocacy or research goal. The educational services offered to the consumer by these agencies emphasize health promotion and disease prevention for the well public as well as maintenance and rehabilitation efforts to improve the quality of life for those who are living with a particular health problem.

In addition to responding to the needs of the general community, these organizations serve health professionals who are seeking up-to-date, reliable information either for the benefit of their patients or to enhance their own knowledge base. Relative to the primary concern of each of these organizations, they provide information on the latest research, treatments, or techniques available in their field of interest. Health education is viewed by these healthcare-related entities as a vehicle to further the general public's and the professional's knowledge regarding the magnitude and effects that a particular health problem or issue has on society as a whole.

The information provided by these organizations and agencies is narrowly focused on one topic area, which is the primary reason for their existence, and their clientele have similar learning needs driven by the motivation for a healthier heart or improved breathing, for example. Contact with these agencies is often initiated by clients, but they can also be referred by a provider to obtain the desired information or support services. Clients using these organizations' services tend to be less anxious than clients found in healthcare settings, are more self-directed in meeting learning needs, and seek information that is disease specific or involved with lifestyle changes such as smoking cessation.

Characteristic of these agencies is their single-minded focus on a specific health problem or issue, often with a fervor that can be all-consuming for their supporters. This narrow perspective influences their educational offerings, research initiatives, and client advocacy efforts. Thanks to their serious commitment to education about a specific identified health problem or issue, these associations are heavily involved in the development and dissemination of printed materials and audiovisual tools for purposes of teaching and learning.

As nonprofit organizations with limited funding sources, these agencies are primarily supported through individual charitable contributions and public or private grants. Some receive monetary allocations from community fundraising efforts, such as the United Way; others depend solely on direct public donations, potentially causing their resources and programs to wax and wane based on their current financial status. Many of their services are offered for free, although nominal fees are usually established for multiple copies of their printed materials because this system offers them a partial financial return to offset production costs. Because these associations heavily rely on printed materials as a medium through which to disseminate health information, the nurse as educator must be responsible for evaluating the literacy level and content of these materials to determine whether they are suitable for the intended audiences.

Many of the larger, well-supported organizations such as the American Cancer Society

and the American Heart Association have professional nurses on staff as paid employees or as voluntary members to develop health education materials, to plan and participate in programs such as conferences or health screenings, or to lead support groups. Teaching is a major responsibility of nurses functioning within agencies that operate in the healthcare-related setting. As referral sources, these agencies also exist to share informational materials and deliver educational services to augment and complement the resources of institutions and organizations belonging to the other healthcare or non-healthcare settings (Figure 14–1).

The teaching strategies used by nurses in the role of educators in this type of setting depend on the nature and size of the prospective audience as well as the learning situation. Instructional methods often involve group activities that stimulate active participation of the learner, such as discussion sessions, role-playing, and simulations augmented with audiovisual tools as effective means to involve the consumer. Health-screening encounters and telephone inquiries provide the opportunity for individual one-to-one teaching possibilities with a client. Although the emphasis for teaching is on health promotion and disease prevention with healthy individuals and groups, the nurse must also deal with ill clients who present while looking for information that can assist them in reaching optimal levels of functioning. Thus, the nurse working in this setting must demonstrate versatility and flexibility in the role as educator, employing a variety of teaching strategies to meet the needs and satisfy the demands of the various clients served by these community-based healthcare-related agencies.

## American Cancer Society

The American Cancer Society (ACS) is a well-known healthcare-related setting that focuses its activities and resources on the major health problem of cancer, providing information, research, advocacy, and programming. It uses nurses, other healthcare professionals, and non-healthcare individuals extensively as volunteers to meet the organization's goals at the local, regional, and national levels.

**Organizational Factors**  The American Cancer Society has national, regional, and local or satellite offices, a Web site (www.cancer.org.), a 24-hour hotline, educational pamphlets, textbooks, and a professional journal entitled *Cancer* as resources to service its professional and nonprofessional clients, as well as policymakers.

The various levels work closely together on national and individual local chapter programs. Programs, fundraising events, educational programs, and client services vary widely at the local level. The local chapters can select the national programs that are successful or delete those that are not, substituting their own options such as a gala dinner and silent auction event. The national office is used heavily as a major referral source for current information on area resources. It links client and services more efficiently and cost-effectively than in the past, when local chapters provided a wide range of similar services for clients and professionals. A phone call to any local or regional office will provide you with the national office's toll-free phone number for easy access to information and services. Patricia Steacy, the executive director of the ACS chapter for Cape Cod and the Islands, Massachusetts, provides some detailed information that is regional and locally specific (personal communication, July 9, 2001).

Local and regional offices have some form of paid director and limited clerical staff. All levels rely heavily on all types of professional and nonprofessional volunteers to organize and implement fund-raising and assist with implementing other local programs or events.

The national level works with other large healthcare-related organizations, such as the American Lung Association to lobby for legislation that limits access to tobacco by minors, benefiting their consumers.

**Environmental Factors**  ACS resources are limited but the local and regional chapters often partner with area hospitals, schools, and other community organizations to achieve program goals. For example, a local fundraising event entitled "Relay for life" uses the local school track to hold the event. Many of the local chapters engage in fundraising events, act as information brokers, and deal less with providing direct client services as they once did, such as conducting support groups or providing professional education workshops. Although donations are encouraged, the ACS provides all services and materials free to clients and professionals; its professional journal *Cancer* and textbooks do, however, carry a charge.

**Clientele Factors**  The clients who access the ACS are homogeneous, less anxious, and more self-directed in meeting their learning needs than those clients in healthcare settings. They are focused on learning all there is to know about cancer or using a selected service/program available. Even when national and local cancer awareness programs are presented, clients are self-directed in seeking out the program being provided, and selecting what they feel will benefit them the most. Clients' contact is highly variable. Some make a brief request for literature, participate in a screening or educational session, ask where wigs can be obtained, or attend a support group for weeks or months. Often these clients are more accepting of health education that focuses on health promotion and empowerment.

Nurses in this setting provide direct client education as they teach breast or testicular self-examination, provide one-to-one counseling and resource referral, moderate support groups, act as expert panel participants, and recruit other nursing colleagues to participate in screening programs and educating clients.

Since each chapter or local office provides a different scope of programming, the nurse in this setting needs to be prepared to educate clients directly or indirectly in a variety of programs to a greater or lesser degree.

## NON-HEALTHCARE SETTING

Included within the non-healthcare setting are organizations, institutions, or agencies whose primary purpose is anything other than health care and that voluntarily seek to provide health education or health care to their membership as a benefit or service. Of the three types of instructional settings under discussion, this type of setting includes the most varied kinds of organizations. Examples include industries; businesses; schools; YMCAs and YWCAs; community civic, social, and religious associations; senior centers; shelters for the homeless or abused; and others (Figure 14–1). Non-healthcare settings have clientele who vary widely in their educational needs and desires because they can be employees in industry or business, schoolchildren of various ages, parents in a parent–teacher organization, or members of all ages in civic or church groups. Some generalities can be applied to the members of these varied facilities in that most are an adult working population in need of educational programs covering a diverse group of topics—safety in the work environment, stress reduction, the importance of health screening for elevated blood pressure, lowering cholesterol or glucose levels, or health problems for which members are at risk, including controversial topics such as HIV.

Most institutions and organizations in the non-healthcare setting view health education

as a service to its members or a benefit for employees in the work environment. Employers see health education as a method for reducing the healthcare costs associated with unhealthy lifestyles or keeping absenteeism at a minimum. Nonwork settings that include civic, religious, or social organizations frequently view health education as meeting either the expressed need of its membership or the needs of the community as a whole. Those agencies and institutions that embrace a community perspective believe that improving the health of the public is everyone's responsibility. Health-related education in these organizations can range from a substantial commitment to a minimal interest on the part of the leadership in the health and well-being of their membership. Agencies and institutions within this setting will usually identify the topic that is to be provided, without detailing content, and provide the resources to accomplish the desired outcome by bringing in a nurse educator or other health professional to present the material to their members or employees. The nurse's responsibility for the health education encounter may be a brief one-session experience to meet a specific health need of a population of clients, or it can comprise a series of sessions occurring over an extended period of time.

Because this instructional setting encompasses a kaleidoscope of practice environments and populations, the attention here will focus on occupational health as one illustration of how the three factors of organization, resources, and clientele interact and influence on the client education role of the nurse.

### Occupational Health

Occupational health nurses compose the largest health specialty group employed in industry. They can be found in most large companies, providing for the healthcare needs of employees and working closely with management to expand their view of what constitutes health care in the workplace. In other instances, companies contract with hospitals or ambulatory care centers to provide services to meet their employees' healthcare needs, usually at a secondary level of prevention, such as through yearly health screenings, with little emphasis on activities promoting health or preventing disease. However, most industries are mandated by governmental regulations from OSHA to provide some level of safety or injury prevention programs, which may be presented by occupational health nurses. Occupational nurses in the role of educator have an opportunity to teach employers, to go beyond physical care of the ill or injured worker, to broaden their view of what encompasses the nurse's role, and to include health education for health promotion and disease prevention for the benefit of workplace wellness in providing health services to employees.

**Organizational Factors**  The attitude and perspective of company executive officers are major influences on what is made available to employees through their health programs. Management's understanding of its decision-making responsibility in providing healthcare services to employees, the scope of those services, and the way in which the health of employees affects the company's ability to meet its production goals will determine the organizational commitment of resources to the health education component of the occupational nurse's role. The size of the business or industry may dictate on the resources available to provide health-related education, but a positive view of health education by management will mean more programming even with limited resources. Here is where creative thinking and resource networking on the part of the nurse educator can make a real difference—by designing programs to provide health education at no cost, at a minimal

fee for service, or with cost sharing by the employers and employees.

Contracting with local hospitals or the American Lung Association, for example, for specific programs at a reduced or group rate for employees of area businesses may provide the expertise in a particular content area of health education that the occupational nurse is necessarily not prepared to offer. Networking, sharing expertise with nursing colleagues, and attending continuing education programs in work-site wellness programming can help the less prepared occupational nurse acquire the knowledge necessary to plan, implement, and evaluate health education programs at the workplace. Financial reimbursement from third-party payers for health education programs in non–health-related settings is indirect and minimal or nonexistent in most cases. However, some health insurance companies will provide free on-site wellness programs such as cholesterol screening, weight management, stress reduction, or healthy-back programs for their subscribers. Others will give financial rebates in the form of reduced premiums to employers or employees based on lower employee illness risk or employee participation in weight management or exercise programs, which foster healthy lifestyle behaviors. This commitment by insurers, although minimal at best, provides employers and employees with some tangible return for their investment in wellness programs.

The occupational nurse's activities are quite similar to those of the nurse in a physician's office. Episodic care is provided for minor on-the-job injuries or illnesses, with client education information regarding signs and symptoms of complications or safety precautions delivered via verbal or written format and specific to the problem presented. Organizations may or may not provide the nurse with time during the workday for assessing the health education needs of management and employees or for planning, implementing, and evaluating programs focused on health promotion and disease prevention in the workplace.

**Environmental Factors** The occupational health nurse has access to a variety of resources, usually within the limitations of the geographical area, such as consultation with other healthcare professionals and healthcare-related organizations such as the American Cancer Society, which can assist in providing health promotion materials or programming on or off premises. The health office, cafeteria, conference room, and reception area space can be creatively used to provide attractive, eye-catching health promotion literature at designated times during the year, such as during Diabetes Awareness Month, or throughout the year with changing monthly themes. Conference rooms or other suitable presentation areas are usually available within employing facilities and are often appropriate for health program presentations to small or large groups, but programming may need to be planned in advance to fit room availability. Standardized printed and audiovisual health education materials are available in limited or bulk quantity for free or for a nominal fee through healthcare product vendors, the Department of Health, or organizations such as the American Heart Association.

**Clientele Factors** The clients serviced by occupational health nurses include both management and employees, who are mostly a well adult population. Nevertheless, some clients will have lifestyle behaviors that put them at risk for diseases, will experience episodes of acute and chronic illness, could benefit from health promotion programs to reduce their risk factors, and need screening programs to detect the early stages of disease. The clients in this type of environment, as adult learners, are self-directed in seeking health education information. High anxiety levels usually do not interfere with the teaching–learning process in this setting. Often health education and promotion programs are offered at no charge to employee participants, who are then free to choose to attend or not attend. Motivating those less interested is a challenge for the nurse. Providing employee-requested programs on site, just before or after work hours or at lunchtime, is a strategy that can encourage and increase employee participation levels. Health education is more readily acceptable to clients when the programming meets their expressed interest and schedules and when information provided is appropriately matched to the client characteristics. The nurse can more readily foster health promotion with this group and empower these individuals to participate more fully in their own health care. In particular, the nurse has the opportunity to assist these healthcare consumers to learn how to search for and evaluate reliable, high-quality Internet health information sites (Lantier, 2001). (Chapter 13 provides information on how to evaluate Internet sites.)

**Scenario** You are the nurse in the health office of a moderate-sized corporation with access to multimedia resources. You provide a lending library of take-home videos, audio-cassettes, and printed materials on various health-related topics such as "Self-Care Management for Diabetics," "The Benefits of a Low-Fat, High-Fiber Diet," and "Understanding Label Reading for Sodium, Fat, and Fiber Content." You provide a health "topic of the month" series; cancer awareness is the topic for the current month. You have pamphlets on display in the lobby at the reception desk and an informational video playing in the health office waiting area on the topic. You provide several group teaching sessions for employees at various convenient times during the month. At these sessions, you demonstrate and provide opportunity for actual practice with models of breast self-examination for female employees, encouraging women and men alike to share what they learned with their spouses or significant others. In addition, you have arranged with the local hospital to provide baseline mammograms for interested female employees.

In the non-healthcare setting, the nurse as educator is free to select from a wide array of strategies that match the needs of the consumer for the achievement of behavioral outcomes. The instructional materials needed for support of educational efforts can be obtained through a variety of sources, such as healthcare-related organizations that offer up-to-date, reliable information. If the nurse is part of a healthcare organization that has been contracted to provide the health education program, then that organization will provide the necessary resources. The non-healthcare organization usually pays financial reimbursement to the provider of health education when these programs are subcontracted. Learning needs can be anticipated when the population being served is known and the educational events are planned in advance. The difficulty in this type of setting is that health programming is often requested only sporadically when triggered by a news event about a health risk or by other motivating environment factors specific to each situation.

These settings lend themselves well to standardized, prepackaged health education programming. A lending library of video- and audiotapes and a rack with printed materials are time-saving, cost-efficient, and motivating

teaching strategies for a population with varied health information interests and needs.

## SHARING RESOURCES AMONG SETTINGS

Professional nurses involved in client health education should use available opportunities to share resources among the three identified settings (Figure 14–1). Many already perform this service as printed or audiovisual materials are borrowed, rented, or purchased for small fees from area institutions, organizations, or agencies; nurse educators from healthcare or healthcare-related settings are contracted for or voluntarily provide health education programs to small and large groups in other healthcare, healthcare-related, or non-healthcare settings; and nurses from each category of setting collaborate on individual client situations or on major community health projects. The nurses from each of these settings can establish a health education committee in their community to coordinate health education programming, ensure effective use of all resources, and reduce duplication of efforts. The members of this committee can develop standardized health education content, delineate roles and services for each of the instructional settings, and share resources to provide a well-planned, comprehensive community program of health education for a wide spectrum of clients.

## SUMMARY

Classification of instructional settings for client or patient education offers a method for analyzing the role of the nurse as educator and for selecting teaching strategies that best fit the organizational climate, the resources available, and the clientele served. Instructional settings are classified according to the purpose of the organization, institution, or agency that provides or sponsors health instruction. Healthcare settings exist for the

primary purpose of providing direct patient care, with education occurring as an integral part of healthcare delivery services within the setting. Healthcare-related settings consist of voluntary agencies whose purposes are advocacy, research, and educating the general public as well as professionals regarding specific healthcare problems affecting society. Non-healthcare settings include institutions engaged in anything other than health care as their operational purpose, though they may choose to provide health education or health-care services as benefits to their membership or employees.

The factors that affect instructional settings are directly related to the organization that provides the education, the environmental resources available, and the clientele who are serviced by the health education program. These factors need to be assessed prior to engaging in health education activities or selecting teaching strategies appropriate for the instructional setting. As always, the learning needs and characteristics of the learners are the major determinants in choosing the teaching strategies to be used in any setting. These strategies are influenced to a lesser degree by the organizational and environmental factors associated with the particular setting. Teaching methods must be expanded to include multisensory, technologically advanced media to provide greater individualization and reach increasing numbers of clients. Even where organizational and environmental resources are limited, creative thinking and resourcefulness on the part of the nurse in the role of educator can expand the opportunities possible in any instructional setting to provide cost-effective client education that is well planned and comprehensive.

## REVIEW QUESTIONS

1. What are the seven (7) trends in health care expanding the opportunities and expectations of the nurse in the role of educator?

2. What are the three (3) classifications of instructional settings?

3. What are five (5) examples of organizations, institutions, or agencies identified as health-care settings?

4. What are five (5) examples of organizations, institutions, or agencies identified as health-care-related settings?

5. What are five (5) examples of organizations, institutions, or agencies identified as non-healthcare settings?

6. What is the concept upon which instructional settings are classified?

7. What are the three (3) major factors influencing instructional settings?

8. What are the preferred teaching strategies for each instructional setting?

## REFERENCES

American Cancer Society. Retrieved July 19, 2001, *www.cancer.org/eprise/main/docroot/aa/aa_o/AA_1_2_2000_Fact_Sheet*.

Blackwood, C. & White, B. (1991). Technology for teaching and learning improvement. In M. W. Galbraith (ed.), *Facilitating Adult Learning: A Transactional Process* (pp. 135–165). Malabar, FL: Kreiger.

Boyd M. D., Gleit, C. J., Graham, B. A., & Whitman, N. I. (1998). *Health Teaching in Nursing Practice: A Professional Model*, 3rd ed. Stamford, CT: Appleton & Lange.

Breckon, D. J., Harvey, R. J., & Lancaster, R. B. (1985). *Community Health Education: Settings, Roles and Skills*. Rockville, MD: Aspen.

Bubela, N., Galloway, S., McCay, E., et al. (1990). Factors influencing patients' informational needs at time of hospital discharge. *Patient Education Counseling, 16*(1), 21–28.

Cupples, S. A. (1991). Effects of timing and reenforcement of pre-operative education on knowledge and recovery of patients having coronary artery bypass graft surgery. *Heart and Lung, 20*(6), 654–660.

Davidhizar, R., Bechtel, G., & Dowd, S. B. (1998). Patient education: A mandate for health care in the 21st century. *Journal of Nuclear Medicine Technology, 26*(4), 235–241.

Davidhizar, R. & Rexroth, R. (1994). The benefits of triad communication in home health care. *Rehabilitation Nursing, 19*(6), 352–354.

DeMuth, J. S. (1989). Patient teaching in the ambulatory settings. *Nursing Clinics of North America, 24*(3), 645–654.

Desborough, K. (1999). Nursing on the 'net. *Canadian Nurse, 95*(3), 30–32.

Graham, B. A. & Gleit, C. J. (1998). Teaching in selected settings. In M. D. Boyd, B. A. Graham, C. J. Gleit, & N. I. Whitman (eds.). (1998). *Health Teaching in Nursing Practice: A Professional Model,* 3rd ed. (Chapter 3). Stamford, CT: Appleton & Lange.

Green, K. (1998). *Home Care Survival Guide.* Philadelphia: Lippincott.

Hiss, R. G., Frey, M. L., & Davis, W. K. (1986). Diabetes patient education in the office setting. *Diabetes Educator, 12*(3), 281–285.

Knowles, M. S. (1964). The fields of operations in adult education. In G. Jensen, A.A. Liveright, & W. Hallenbeck (eds.), *Adult Education: Outlines of an Emerging Field of University Study* (pp. 41–67). Washington, DC: Adult Education Association of the United States of America.

Knowles, M. S. (1983). How the media can make it or bust it in education. *Media and Adult Learning, 5*(2), 3–4.

Lantier, E. H. (2001). Evaluating health information on the Internet: Empowering consumers. *Journal of the New York State Nurses Association, 32*(1), 15–19.

Leckrone, L. (1991). Preparing your patient for surgery. *Nursing, 21*(7), 47–49.

Naylor, M. D. & Shaid, E. C. (1991). Content analysis of pre and post-discharge topics taught to hospitalized elderly by gerontological clinical nurse specialists. *Clinical Nurse Specialist, 5*(2), 111–116.

*Opening the door to home care.* (July 1995). Report, 1, 4.

Phillips, L. D. (1999). Patient education: Understanding the process to maximize time and outcomes. *Journal of Intravenous Nursing, 22*(1), 19–35.

Rankin, S. H. & Stallings, K.D. (2001). *Patient Education: Principles and Practices,* 4th ed. Philadelphia: Lippincott.

Redman, B. K. (2001). *The Practice of Patient Education,* 9th ed. St. Louis: Mosby.

Rifas, E., Morris, R., & Grady, R. (1994). Innovative approach to patient education. *Nursing Outlook, 42*(5), 214–216.

Schroeder, W. (1980). Typology of adult learning systems. In J. M. Peters (ed.), *Building an Effective Adult Education Enterprise* (pp. 41–77). San Francisco: Jossey-Bass.

Shendell-Falik, N. (1990). Creating self-care units in the acute care setting: A case study. *Patient Education Counseling, 15*(1), 39–45.

Simonds, S. K. (1973). President's committee on health education. *Hospitals, Journal of the American Hospital Association, 47,* 55–60.

Smith, L. F. (1986). New-parent teaching in the ambulatory care setting. *Maternal Child Nursing, 11*(4), 256–258.

Zarle, N. C. (1989). Continuity of care: Balancing care of elders between health care settings. *Nursing Clinics of North America, 24*(3), 697–705.

## CHAPTER 15

# Evaluation in Healthcare Education

*Priscilla Sandford Worral*

## CHAPTER HIGHLIGHTS

## KEY TERMS

assessment

evaluation

process (formative) evaluation

content evaluation

outcome (summative) evaluation

impact evaluation

program evaluation

evaluation research

## OBJECTIVES

After completing this chapter, the reader will be able to

1. Define the term *evaluation*.

2. Compare and contrast evaluation and assessment.

3. Identify purposes of evaluation.

4. Distinguish between five basic types of evaluation: process, content, outcome, impact, and program.

5. Discuss characteristics of various models of evaluation.

6. Describe similarities and differences between evaluation and research.

7. Assess barriers to evaluation.

8. Examine methods for conducting an evaluation.

9. Select appropriate instruments for various types of evaluative data.

10. Identify guidelines for reporting results of evaluation.

Evaluation is the process that can justify that what we do as nurses and as nurse educators makes a value-added difference in the care we provide. Evaluation is defined as a systematic process by which the worth or value of something—in this case, teaching and learning—is judged. Early consideration of evaluation has never been more critical than in today's healthcare environment. Crucial decisions regarding learners rest on the outcomes of learning. Can the patient go home? Can the nurse provide competent care? If education is to be justified as a value-added activity, the process of education must be measurably efficient and must be measurably linked to education outcomes. The outcomes of education, for the learner and for the organization, must be measurably effective.

Evaluation is a process within a process—a critical component of the nursing process, the decision-making process, and the education process. Evaluation is the final component of each of these processes. Because these processes are cyclical, evaluation serves as the critical bridge at the end of one cycle that guides direction of the next cycle.

The sections of this chapter follow the steps in conducting an evaluation. These steps include (1) determining the focus of the evaluation, including use of evaluation models; (2) designing the evaluation; (3) conducting the evaluation; (4) determining methods of analysis and interpretation of data collected; (5) reporting results of data collected; and (6) using evaluation results. Each aspect of the evaluation process is important, but all of them are meaningless if the results of evaluation are not used to guide future action in planning and carrying out educational interventions.

## EVALUATION VERSUS ASSESSMENT

While assessment and evaluation are highly interrelated and are often used interchangeably as terms, they are not synonymous. The process of *assessment* is to gather, summarize, interpret, and use data to decide a direction for action. The process of *evaluation* is to gather, summarize, interpret, and use data to determine the extent to which an action was successful. The primary differences between the two terms are those of timing and purpose. For example, an education program begins with an assessment of learners' needs. From the perspective of systems theory, assessment data might be called the "input." While the program is being conducted, periodic evaluation lets the educator know whether the program and learners are proceeding as planned. After program completion, evaluation identifies whether and to what extent identified needs were met. Again, from a systems theory perspective, these evaluative data might be called "intermediate output" and "output," respectively.

An important note of caution: Because you may conduct an evaluation at the end of your program, do not assume that you should plan it at this point in time. Evaluation as an afterthought is, at best, a poor idea and, at worst, a dangerous one. Data may be impossible to collect, be incomplete, or even be misleading. Assessment and evaluation planning should ideally be concurrent activities. Where feasible, use the same data collection methods and instruments. This approach is especially appropriate for outcome and impact evaluations, as will be discussed later in this chapter. "If only. . ." is an all too frequent lament, which can be minimized by planning ahead.

## DETERMINING THE FOCUS OF EVALUATION

In planning any evaluation, the first and most crucial step is to determine the focus of the evaluation. The focus then will guide evaluation design, conduct, data analysis, and reporting of results. The importance of a clear, specific, and realistic evaluation focus cannot be overemphasized. Usefulness and accuracy of the results of an evaluation depend heavily on how well the evaluation is initially focused.

Evaluation focus includes five basic components: audience, purpose, questions, scope, and resources (Ruzicki, 1987). To determine these components, ask the following questions:

1. For whom is the evaluation being conducted?

2. Why is the evaluation being conducted?

3. What questions will be asked in the evaluation?

4. What is the scope of the evaluation?

5. What resources are available to conduct the evaluation?

The *audience* comprises the persons or groups for whom the evaluation is being conducted (Ruzicki, 1987). These individuals or groups include the primary audience, or the individual or group who requested the evaluation, and the general audience, or all those who will use evaluation results or who might benefit from the evaluation. Thus the audience for an evaluation might include your patients, your peers, your supervisor, the nursing director, the staff development director, the chief executive officer of your institution, or a group of community leaders. When you report results of the evaluation, you will provide feedback to all members of the audience. In focusing the evaluation, however, first consider the primary audience. Giving priority to the individual or group who requested the evaluation will make focusing the evaluation easier, especially if results of an evaluation will be used by several groups representing diverse interests.

The *purpose* of the evaluation is the answer to the question, "Why is the evaluation being conducted?" The purpose of an evaluation might be to decide whether to continue a particular education program or to determine the effectiveness of the teaching process. If a particular individual or group has a primary interest in results of the evaluation, use input from that group to clarify the purpose.

An important note of caution: *Why* you are conducting an evaluation is not synonymous with *who* or *what* you are evaluating. For example, nursing literature on patient education commonly distinguishes among three types of evaluations: learner, teacher, and program. This distinction answers the question of *who* or *what* will be evaluated and is extremely useful for evaluation design and conduct. *Why* learner evaluation might be undertaken, for example, is answered by the reason or purpose for evaluating learner performance. Determining teaching or program effectiveness is another example of the purpose for undertaking evaluation.

An excellent rule of thumb in stating the purpose of an evaluation is: Keep it singular. In other words, state, "The purpose is. . . ," not "The purposes are. . . ." Keeping the purpose audience focused and singular will help avoid the all too frequent tendency to attempt too much in one evaluation.

*Questions* to be asked in the evaluation are directly related to the purpose for conducting the evaluation, are specific, and are measurable. Examples of questions are "To what extent are patients satisfied with the cardiac discharge teaching program?" and "How frequently do staff nurses use the diabetes teaching reference materials?" Asking the right questions is crucial if the evaluation is to fulfill the intended purpose. As will be discussed later in this chapter, delineation of evaluation questions is both the first step in selection of evaluation design and the basis for eventual data analysis.

The *scope* of an evaluation can be considered an answer to the question, "How much will be evaluated?" "How much" includes "How many aspects of education will be evaluated?", "How many individuals or representative groups will be evaluated?", and "What time period is to be evaluated?" For example, will the evaluation focus on one class or on an entire program; on the learning experience for one patient or for all patients being taught a particular skill? Evaluation could be limited to the teaching process during a particular patient education class or it could be expanded to encompass both the teaching process and related patient outcomes of learning. The scope of an evaluation is determined in part by the purpose for conducting the evaluation and in part by available resources. For example, an evaluation addressing learner satisfaction with faculty for all programs conducted by a staff development department in a given year is necessarily broad and long-term in scope and will require expertise in data collection and analysis. An evaluation to determine whether a patient understands each step in a learning session on how to self-administer insulin injections is narrow in scope and focused on a particular point in time and will require expertise in clinical practice and observation.

*Resources* needed to conduct an evaluation include time, expertise, personnel, materials, equipment, and facilities. A realistic appraisal of what resources are accessible and available relative to what resources are required is crucial in focusing any evaluation. Remember to include the time and expertise required to collate, analyze, and interpret data and to prepare the report of evaluation results.

Evaluation can be classified into different types, or categories, based on one or more of the five components described above. The most common types of evaluation identified include process, content, outcome, impact, and program evaluation. A number of evaluation models have been developed that help to clarify differences among these evaluation types as well as how they relate to one another (Abruzzese, 1978; Haggard, 1989; Koch, 2000; Puetz, 1992; Rankin & Stallings, 2001; Walker & Dewar, 2000).

## ▰▰▰ EVALUATION MODELS

Abruzzese (1978) developed the Roberta Straessle Abruzzese (RSA) Evaluation Model

for conceptualizing, or classifying, educational evaluation into different categories or levels. Although developed more than 20 years ago and derived from the perspective of staff development education, the RSA Model remains useful for conceptualizing types of evaluation from both staff development and patient education perspectives. A recent example of use of the RSA model is given by Dilorio, Price, and Becker (2001) in their discussion of the evaluation of the Neuroscience Nurse Internship Program at the National Institutes of Health Clinical Center.

The RSA Model pictorially places five basic types of evaluation in relation to one another based on purpose and related questions, scope, and resource components of evaluation focus (Figure 15–1). The five types of evaluation include process, content, outcome, impact, and program. Abruzzese describes the first four types as levels of evaluation leading from the simple (process evaluation) to the complex (impact evaluation). Total program evaluation encompasses and summarizes all four levels.

## Process (Formative) Evaluation

The purpose of *process or formative evaluation* is to make adjustments in an educational activity as soon as they are needed, whether those adjustments be in personnel, materials, facilities, learning objectives, or even one's own attitude. Adjustments may need to be made after one class or session before the next is taught or even in the middle of a single learning experience. Consider, for example, evaluation of the process of teaching a newly diagnosed juvenile insulin-dependent diabetic and her parents how to administer insulin. Would you facilitate learning better by first injecting yourself with normal saline so they can see you maintain a calm expression? If you had planned to have the parent give the first injection, but the child seems less fearful, might you consider revising your teaching plan to let the child first perform self-injection?

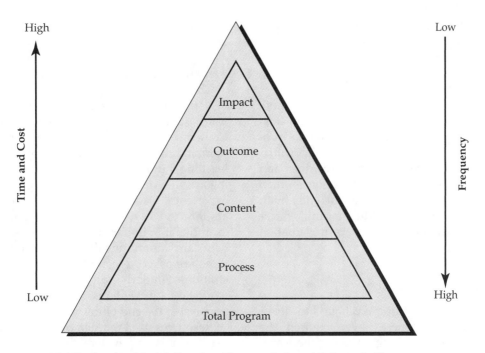

**FIGURE 15–1    RSA Evaluation Model** Reprinted by permission of Roberta S. Abruzzese.

Process evaluation is integral to the education process itself. It "forms" an educational activity because evaluation is an ongoing component of assessment, planning, and implementation. As part of the education process, this ongoing evaluation helps the nurse anticipate and prevent problems before they occur or identify problems as they arise.

Consistent with the purpose of process evaluation, the primary question is, "How can teaching be improved to facilitate learning?" The nurse's teaching effectiveness, the teaching process, and the learner's responses are monitored on an ongoing basis. Abruzzese (1978) describes process evaluation as a "happiness index." While teaching and learning are ongoing, learners are asked their opinions about faculty, learning/course objectives, content, teaching and learning methods, physical facilities, and administration of the learning experience. Specific questions could include:

• Am I giving the patient time to ask questions?

• Is the information I am giving in class consistent with information included in the handouts?

• Does the patient look bored? Is the room too warm?

• Should I include more opportunities for return demonstration?

The scope of process evaluation generally is limited in breadth and time period to a specific learning experience such as a class or workshop, yet is sufficiently detailed to include as many aspects of the specific learning experience as possible while they occur. Learner behavior, teacher behavior, learner–teacher interaction, learner response to teaching materials and methods, and characteristics of the environment are all aspects of the learning experience within the scope of process evaluation. All learners and all teachers participating in a learning experience should be included in process evaluation. If resources are limited and participants include a number of different groups, a representative sample of individuals from each group rather than everyone from each group may be included in the evaluation.

Resources usually are less costly and more readily available for process evaluation than for other types such as impact or total program evaluation. Although process evaluation occurs more frequently—during and throughout every learning experience—than any other type, it occurs concurrently with teaching. The need for additional time, facilities, and dollars to conduct process evaluation is consequently decreased.

## Content Evaluation

The purpose of *content evaluation* is to determine whether learners have acquired the knowledge or skills taught during the learning experience. Abruzzese (1978) describes content evaluation as taking place immediately after the learning experience to answer the guiding question, "To what degree did the learners learn what was imparted?" or "To what degree did learners achieve specified objectives?" Asking a patient to give a return demonstration or asking participants to complete a cognitive test at the completion of a one-day seminar are common examples of content evaluation.

Content evaluation is depicted in the RSA Model as the level "in between" process and outcome evaluation levels. In other words, content evaluation can be considered as focusing on how the teaching–learning process affected immediate, short-term outcomes. To answer the question, "Were specified objectives met as a result of teaching?", requires that the evaluation be designed differently from an evaluation to answer the question, "Did learners achieve specified objectives?" Evaluation designs will be discussed in some detail later in this chapter. An important point

to be made here, however, is that evaluation questions must be carefully considered and clearly stated because they dictate the basic framework for design and conduct.

The scope of content evaluation is limited to a specific learning experience and to specifically stated objectives for that experience. Content evaluation occurs at a circumscribed point in time, immediately after completion of teaching, but encompasses all teaching–learning activities included in that specific learning experience. Data are obtained from all learners targeted in a specific class or group. For example, if both parents and the juvenile diabetic are taught insulin administration, all three are asked to complete a return demonstration. Similarly, all nurses attending a workshop are asked to complete the cognitive post-test at the end of the workshop.

Resources used to teach content can also be used to carry out evaluation of how well that content was learned. For example, equipment included in teaching a patient how to change a dressing can be used by the patient to perform a return demonstration. In the same manner, a pretest used at the beginning of a continuing education seminar can be readministered as a post-test at seminar completion to measure change.

## Outcome (Summative) Evaluation

The purpose of *outcome evaluation* is to determine the effects or outcomes of teaching efforts. Outcome evaluation is also referred to as *summative evaluation* because its intent is to "sum" what happened as a result of education. Guiding questions in outcome evaluation include the following:

- Was teaching appropriate?
- Did the individual(s) learn?
- Were behavioral objectives met?
- Did the patient who learned a skill before discharge use that skill correctly once home?

Just as process evaluation occurs concurrently with the teaching–learning experience, outcome evaluation occurs after teaching has been completed or after a program has been carried out.

Outcome evaluation measures changes occurring as a result of teaching and learning. Abruzzese (1978) differentiates outcome evaluation from content evaluation by focusing outcome evaluation on measuring more long-term change that "persists after the learning experience" (p. 243). Changes can include institution of a new process, habitual use of a new technique or behavior, or integration of a new value or attitude. Which changes you will measure usually will be dictated by the objectives established as a result of the initial needs assessment.

The scope of outcome evaluation depends in part on the changes being measured, which, in turn, depend on the objectives established for the educational activity. As mentioned earlier, outcome evaluation focuses on a longer time period than does content evaluation. Whereas evaluating accuracy of a patient's return demonstration of a skill prior to discharge may be appropriate for content evaluation, outcome evaluation should include measuring a patient's competency with a skill in the home setting after discharge. Similarly, nurses' responses on a workshop post-test may be sufficient for content evaluation, but if the workshop objective states that nurses will be able to incorporate their knowledge into practice on the unit, outcome evaluation should include measuring nurses' knowledge or behavior some time after they have returned to the unit. Abruzzese (1978) suggests that outcome data be collected six months after baseline data to determine whether a change has really taken place.

Resources required for outcome evaluation are more costly and sophisticated than those for process or content evaluation. Compared to the resources required for the first two types of evaluation in the RSA Model, outcome evaluation requires greater expertise to develop measurement and data collection strategies, more time to conduct the evaluation, knowledge of baseline data establishment, and ability to conduct reliable and valid comparative data after the learning experience. Postage to mail surveys and time and personnel to carry out observation of nurses on the clinical unit or to complete patient/family telephone interviews are specific examples of resources that may be necessary to conduct an outcome evaluation.

## Impact Evaluation

The purpose of *impact evaluation* is to determine the relative effects of education on the institution or the community. Put another way, the purpose of impact evaluation is to obtain information that will help decide whether continuing an educational activity is worth its cost. Examples of questions appropriate for impact evaluation include "What is the effect of the education program on subsequent nursing staff turnover?" and "What is the effect of the cardiac discharge teaching program on long-term frequency of rehospitalization among patients who have completed the program?"

The scope of impact evaluation is broader, more complex, and usually more long-term than that of process, content, or outcome evaluation. Whereas outcome evaluation would focus on whether specific teaching resulted in achievement of specified outcomes, for example, impact evaluation would go beyond that to measure the effect or worth of those outcomes. In other words, outcome evaluation would focus on a course objective, whereas impact evaluation would focus on a course goal. Consider, for example, a class on the use of body mechanics. The outcome objective is that staff members will demonstrate proper use of body mechanics in providing patient care. The goal is to decrease back injuries among the hospital's direct-care providers. This distinction between outcome and impact evaluation may seem subtle, but it is important to the appropriate design and conduct of an impact evaluation.

Resource requirements for conducting an impact evaluation are extensive and may be beyond the scope of an individual nurse educator. Literature on evaluation describes impact evaluation as being most like evaluation research (Abruzzese, 1978; Hamilton, 1993; Waddell, 1992). (The distinction between evaluation and evaluation research will be addressed later in this chapter.) "Good" science is rarely inexpensive and never quick; good impact evaluation shares the same characteristics. The resources needed to design and conduct an impact evaluation generally include reliable and valid instruments, trained data collectors, personnel with research and statistical expertise, equipment and materials necessary for data collection and analysis, and access to populations who may be culturally or geographically diverse. Because impact evaluation is so expensive and time-intensive, this type of evaluation should be targeted toward courses and programs where learning is critical to patient well-being or to safe, high-quality, cost-effective healthcare delivery (Puetz, 1992).

Conducting an impact evaluation may seem a monumental task, but do not let that stop you from undertaking the effort. Rather, plan ahead, proceed carefully, and obtain the support and assistance of colleagues. Keeping in mind the purpose for conducting an impact evaluation should be helpful in maintaining the level of commitment needed throughout the process. The current managed care environment requires justification for every health dollar spent. The value of patient and staff education may be intuitively evident, but the positive impact of education must be demonstrated if it is to be funded.

## Program Evaluation

The purpose of *program evaluation* can be generically described as "designed and conducted to assist an audience to judge and improve the worth of some object" (Johnson & Olesinski, 1995, p. 53). The "object" in this case is an educational program. Using the framework of the RSA Model (Abruzzese, 1978), the purpose of total program evaluation is to determine the extent to which all activities for an entire department or program over a specified period of time meet or exceed goals originally established. Guiding questions appropriate for a total program evaluation from this perspective might be "To what extent did programs undertaken by members of the nursing staff development department during the year accomplish annual goals established by the department?" or "How well did patient education activities implemented throughout the year meet annual goals established for the institution's patient education program?"

The scope of program evaluation is broad, generally focusing on overall goals rather than on specific objectives. While the term *program* could be defined as an individual educational offering (Albanese and Gjerde, 1987), the resource requirements for conducting a program evaluation generally are too extensive to justify the effort on less than a broad scale. Abruzzese (1978) describes the scope of program evaluation as encompassing all aspects of educational activity (e.g., process, content, outcome, impact) with input from all the participants (e.g., learners, teachers, institutional representatives, community representatives). The time period over which data are collected may extend from several months to one or more years, depending on the time frame established for meeting the goals to be evaluated.

Resources required for program evaluation may include the sum of resources necessary to conduct process, content, outcome, and impact evaluations. A program evaluation may require significant expenditures for personnel if the evaluation is conducted by an individual or team external to the organization. Additional resources required may include time, materials, equipment, and personnel necessary for data entry, analysis, and report generation.

As stated earlier, the RSA Model remains useful as a general framework for categorizing basic types of evaluation: process, content, outcome, impact, and program. As depicted in the model, differences between these types are, in large part, a matter of degree. For example, process evaluation occurs most frequently; impact evaluation occurs least frequently. Content evaluation focuses on immediate effects of teaching; outcome evaluation concentrates on more long-term effects of teaching. Conduct of process evaluation requires fewer resources compared with impact evaluation, which requires extensive resources for implementation. The RSA Model further illustrates one way that process, content, outcome, and impact evaluations can be considered together as components of total program evaluation.

Clinical examples of how different types of evaluation relate to one another can be found in Haggard's (1989) description of three dimensions in evaluating teaching effectiveness for the patient and in Rankin and Stallings's (2001) four levels of evaluation of patient learning. The three dimensions described by Haggard and the four levels identified by Rankin and Stallings are consistent with the basic types of evaluation included in Abruzzese's RSA Model, as shown in Table 15–1. As can be seen from Table 15–1, models developed from an education theory base, such as the RSA Model, have much in common with models developed from a patient care theory base, exemplified by the other two models.

At least one important point about the difference between the RSA and other models needs to be mentioned, however. That difference is depicted in the learner evaluation model shown in Figure 15–2. This learner-focused model emphasizes the continuum of patient health/learner performance from needs assessment to patient health/learner performance once an adequate level of health status/performance has been regained or achieved. Both models have value in focusing and planning any type of evaluation but are especially important for impact and program evaluations.

**TABLE 15–1   Comparison of levels/types of evaluation across staff/patient education evaluation models**

| Abruzzese (1978) | Haggard (1989) | Rankin & Stallings (2001) |
|---|---|---|
| Process | Patient assimilation of information during teaching | Patient-education intervention |
| Content | Patient information retention after teaching | Patient/family performance following learning |
| Outcome | Patient use of information in day-to-day life | Patient/family performance at home |
| Impact | N/A | Overall self-care and health maintenance |
| Program | N/A | N/A |

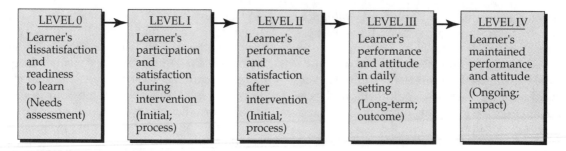

FIGURE 15–2    **Five Levels of Learner Evaluation**  SOURCE: Based on S. H. Rankin & K. D. Stallings (2001). *Patient Education: Principles and Practices*, 4th ed. Philadelphia: Lippincott.

## ◼ DESIGNING THE EVALUATION

The design of an evaluation is created within the framework, or boundaries, already established by focusing the evaluation. In other words, the design must be consistent with the purpose, questions, and scope and must be realistic given available resources. Evaluation design includes at least three interrelated components: structure, methods, and instruments.

### Designing Structure

An important question to be answered in designing an evaluation is "How rigorous should the evaluation be?" The obvious answer is that all evaluations should have some level of rigor. In other words, all evaluations should be systematic and carefully and thoroughly planned or structured before they are conducted. How rigor is translated into design structure depends on the questions to be answered by the evaluation, the complexity of the scope of the evaluation, and the expected use of evaluation results. The more the questions address cause and effect, the more complex the scope. Likewise, the more critical and broad-reaching the expected use of results, the more the evaluation design should be structured from a research perspective.

**Evaluation Versus Research**   Evaluation and research are neither synonymous nor mutu-

ally exclusive activities. The extent to which they are either very different or indistinguishable from each other depends on the type of evaluation and type of research considered. Ruzicki (1987) makes the following distinction between the two:

> While both research and evaluation involve objective, systematic collection of data, evaluation is conducted to make decisions in a given setting. Research is designed so that it can be generalized to other settings and replicated in other settings. Furthermore, research seeks new knowledge, examines cause and effect relationships, tests hypotheses, whereas evaluation determines mission achievement, examines means-end processes, and assesses attainment of objectives (p. 234).

This argument holds true when comparing "basic" research to process evaluation, for example. Basic research is defined as tightly controlled experimental studies of cause and effect conducted for the purpose of generating new knowledge. This new knowledge may or may not eventually influence practice. Process evaluation occurs concurrently with an educational intervention and is conducted in an uncontrolled or real-world setting for the purpose of making change as soon as the need for change is identified.

Differences between research and evaluation have become less distinct over the past several years with the advent of "applied" research, with the acceptance of qualitative measures and methods as legitimate research, and with the increasing importance given to results of outcome, impact, and program evaluations. The purpose for conducting applied research is to positively affect change in practice. There is little difference between this purpose and the purpose for conducting evaluation. *Evaluation research,* which is one type of applied research, can be defined as "a process of applying scientific procedures to accumulate reliable and valid data on the manner and extent to which specified activities produce outcomes or effects" (Hamilton, 1993, p. 148). Using this definition, Hamilton identifies program accreditation, program cost analysis, and outcome of treatment as appropriate for use of evaluation research designs and methods. Hamilton further describes impact evaluation as appropriate for use of quasi-experimental and experimental research design structures. A number of other authors support some use of research designs and data collection methods for outcome, impact, and program evaluations (Albanese & Gjerde, 1987; Berk & Rossi, 1990; Holzemer, 1992; Puetz, 1992; Waddell, 1992).

Of course, not all outcome, impact, and program evaluations should be conducted as research studies. Some important differences do exist between evaluation and evaluation research. One of the most significant relates to the influence of a primary audience. As discussed earlier in this chapter, the primary audience, or the individual or group requesting the evaluation, is a major component in focusing an evaluation. The evaluator must design and conduct the evaluation consistent with the purpose and related questions identified by the primary audience. Evaluation research, by contrast, does not have an identified primary audience. The researcher has autonomy to develop a protocol to answer a question posed by the researcher.

A second difference between evaluation and evaluation research is one of timing. The necessary timeline for usability of evaluation results may not be sufficient to prospectively develop a research proposal and obtain institutional review board approval prior to beginning data collection.

Given the discussion of evaluation versus evaluation research, how are decisions about level of rigor of an evaluation actually translated into an evaluation structure? The structure of an evaluation design depicts the number of groups to be included in the evaluation, the number of evaluations or periods of evaluation, and the time sequence between an educational intervention and evaluation of that intervention. A "group" can comprise one individual, as in the case of one-to-one nurse–patient teaching, or several individuals, as in the case of a nursing in-service program or workshop.

A process evaluation might be conducted during a single patient education activity where the educator observes patient behavior during instruction/demonstration and engages the patient in questions and answers upon completion of each new instruction. Because the purpose of process evaluation is to facilitate better learning while that learning is going on, education and evaluation occur concurrently in this case.

Evaluation also may be conducted after an educational intervention. This structure is probably the most commonly employed in conducting educational evaluations, although it is not necessarily the most appropriate. On completion of an educational activity, participants may be asked to fill out a satisfaction survey to provide data for a process evaluation, or they may be given a cognitive test to provide data for a content evaluation. If the purpose of conducting a content evaluation is to determine whether learners know the content just taught, a cognitive post-test or immediate return demonstration is adequate. If the purpose of conducting the evaluation is to determine whether after a class learners know specific content that they did not know before attending that class, then a structure that begins with collection of baseline data is more appropriate. Collection of baseline data, which can be compared with data collected at one or more points in time after learners have completed the educational activity, provides an opportunity to measure whether change has occurred. The ability to measure change in a particular skill or level of knowledge, for example, also requires that the same instruments be used for data collection at both points in time. Data collection will be discussed in more detail later in this chapter.

If the purpose of conducting an evaluation is to determine whether learners know content or can perform a skill as a result of an educational intervention, the most appropriate structure will include at least two groups: one receiving education and one not receiving education. Both groups are evaluated at the same time, even though only one group receives education. The group receiving the new education program is called the treatment or experimental group, and the group receiving standard care or the traditional education program is called the comparison or control group. The two groups may or may not be "equivalent." Equivalent groups are those with no known differences between them prior to some intervention, whereas nonequivalent groups may be different from one another in several ways. For example, patients on Nursing Unit A may receive an educational pamphlet to read prior to attending a class, while patients on Nursing Unit B attend the class without first reading the pamphlet. Because patients on the two units probably are different in many ways—age and diagnosis, for example—besides which educational intervention they received, they would be considered nonequivalent groups.

Use of the term *nonequivalent* is common to discussions of traditional research designs.

Quasi-experimental designs, such as "nonequivalent control group" designs, should be among those considered in planning an outcome, impact, or program evaluation. Especially if the purpose of an evaluation is to demonstrate that an education program "caused" fewer patient returns to the clinic or fewer nurses to leave the institution, for example, the evaluation structure must have the rigor of evaluation research.

Another type of quasi-experimental design, called a time-series design, might include only one group of learners from which evaluative data are collected at several points in time both before and after receiving an educational intervention. If data collected before the education consistently demonstrate lack of learner ability to comply with a treatment regimen, whereas data collected after the education consistently demonstrate a significant improvement in patient compliance with that regimen, the evaluator could argue that the education was the reason for the improvement in this case.

In more recent years, pluralistic designs have appeared in the literature as approaches especially suited for evaluation of projects that have a community base, that include participants from diverse settings or perspectives, or that require both program processes and outcomes to be included in the evaluation (Billings, 2000; Gerrish, 2001; Hart, 1999). As the term implies, a *pluralistic design* uses a variety of sources and methods for obtaining evaluative data, often including both qualitative and quantitative evidence. Because these designs are comprehensive, resource-intensive, and long-term in nature, they are most appropriate for program evaluation.

This chapter does not provide an exhaustive description of evaluation designs. Rather, it is intended to increase awareness of the value and usefulness of these designs, especially when the results of an evaluation will be used to make major financial or programmatic decisions. The literature on evaluation of nursing staff education and patient education has become an increasingly rich source of examples of how to conduct rigorous evaluation. A literature search that includes many or all of the following journals is a must for planning evaluation of healthcare education in a cost-conscious and outcome-focused healthcare environment: *Evaluation and the Health Professions, Journal of Continuing Education in Nursing, Adult Education Quarterly, Health Education Quarterly, Nurse Educator, Journal of Nursing Staff Development, Health Education Research, Nursing Management, Nursing Research, Research in Nursing and Health*, and *Journal of Advanced Nursing*.

## Evaluation Methods

Evaluation focus provides the basis for determining the evaluation design structure. The design structure, in turn, provides the basis for determining evaluation methods. Evaluation methods include those actions that are undertaken to carry out the evaluation according to the design structure. All evaluation methods deal in some way with data and data collection. Answers to the following questions will assist in selection of the most appropriate, feasible methods for conducting a particular evaluation in a particular setting and for a specified purpose:

- What types of data will be collected?
- From whom or what will data be collected?
- How, when, and where will data be collected?
- By whom will data be collected?

**Types of Data to Collect** Evaluation of healthcare education includes collection of data about people, about the educational program or activity, and about the environment in which the educational activity takes place. Process, outcome, impact, and program evaluations require data about all three: the people, the program, and the environment. Content

evaluations may be limited to data about the people and the program, although this limitation is not necessary. Types of data that are collected about people can be classified as physical, cognitive, affective, or psychomotor. Data that are collected about educational activities or programs generally include such program characteristics as cost, length, number of educators required, amount and type of materials required, teaching–learning methods used, and so on. Data that are collected about the environment in which a program or activity is conducted generally include such environmental characteristics as temperature, lighting, location, layout, space, and noise level.

Given the possibility that an unlimited and overwhelming amount of data could be collected, how do you decide what data should be collected? The most straightforward answer to this question is that data should be collected that will answer evaluation questions posed in focusing the evaluation. The likelihood that you will collect the right amount of the right type of data to answer evaluation questions can be significantly improved by (1) remembering that any data you collect, you are obligated to use and (2) using operational definitions. An operational definition of a word or phrase is a definition that is written in measurement terms.

Functional health status, for example, can be theoretically defined as an individual's ability to independently carry out activities of daily living without self-perceived undue difficulty or discomfort. Functional health status can be operationally defined as an individual's composite score on the SF-36 survey instrument (Ware et al., 1978; Stewart et al., 1988). The SF-36, which has undergone years of extensive reliability and validity testing with a wide variety of patient populations and in several languages, is generally considered the "gold standard" for measuring functional health status from the individual's perspective.

Similarly, patient compliance can be theoretically defined as the patient's regular and consistent adherence to a prescribed treatment regimen. For use in an outcome evaluation of a particular educational activity, patient compliance might be operationally defined as the patient's demonstration of unassisted and error-free completion of all steps in the sterile dressing change as observed in the patient's home on three separate occasions at two-week time intervals.

As you can see from these examples, an operational definition states exactly what data will be collected. In the first example, measurement of functional health status will require collection of patient survey data using a specific self-administered questionnaire. The second example provides even more information about data collection than does the first, by including where and how many times the patient's performance of the dressing change is to be observed, as well as stating that criteria for compliance include both unassisted and error-free performance on each occasion.

In addition to being categorized as describing people, programs, or the environment, data can be categorized as quantitative or qualitative. Quantitative data are numeric and generally are expressed in statistics such as mean, median, ratio, $F$ statistic, $t$ statistic, or chi-square. Numbers can be used to answer questions of how much, how many, how often, and so on in terms that are commonly understood by the audience for the evaluation. Mathematical analysis can demonstrate with some level of precision and reliability whether a learner's knowledge or skill has changed since completing an educational program, for example, or how much improvement in a learner's knowledge or skill is the result of an educational program. Qualitative data include feelings, behaviors, words, and phrases and generally are expressed in themes or categories. Qualitative data can be described in quantitative terms, such as percentages or counts, but this transformation eliminates the richness and insight that the use of qualitative data can offer. Qualitative data can be used as background to better interpret quantitative data, especially if the evaluation is intended to measure such value-laden or conceptual terms as *satisfaction* or *quality.*

Any evaluation may be strengthened by collecting both quantitative and qualitative data. For example, an evaluation to determine whether a stress reduction class resulted in decreased work stress for participants could include participants' qualitative expressions of how stressed they feel plus quantitative pulse and blood pressure readings. Because collection of both quantitative and qualitative data, while intuitively appealing, is resource-intensive, be certain that the focus of the evaluation justifies such an undertaking.

**From Whom or What to Collect Data**   Data can be collected directly from the individuals whose behavior or knowledge is being evaluated, from surrogates or representatives of these individuals, or from documentation or databases already created. Whenever possible, plan to collect at least some data directly from individuals being evaluated. In the case of process evaluation, data should be collected from all learners and all educators participating in the educational activity. Content and outcome evaluations should include data from all learners.

Because impact and program evaluations have a broader scope than do the first three types of evaluation, collecting data from all individuals who participated in an educational program over an extended period of time may be impossible due to the inability to locate participants or a lack of sufficient resources to gather data from such a large number of people. When all participants cannot be counted or located, data may be collected from a subset, or sample, of participants who are considered to represent the entire group. If an evaluation is planned to collect data from a sample of participants, be careful to include participants who are representative of the entire group. A random selection of participants from whom data will be collected will minimize bias in the sample but cannot guarantee representativeness.

Consider the example of an impact evaluation conducted to determine whether a five-year program supporting home-based health education actually improved the general health status of individuals in the community served by the program. Suppose all members of the community could be counted. A random sample of community members could be generated by first listing and numbering all members' names, then drawing numbers using a random numbers table until a 10% sample is obtained. Such a method for selecting the sample of community members would eliminate intentional selection of those individuals who were the most active program participants and who might therefore have a better health status than does the community as a whole. At the same time, the 10% random sample could unintentionally include only those individuals who did not participate in the health education program. Data collected from this sample of nonparticipants would be equally as misleading as data collected from the first sample. A more representative sample for this evaluation should include both participants and nonparticipants, ideally in the same proportions in the sample as in the community.

Preexisting databases should never be used as the only source of evaluative data unless they were created for the purpose of that evaluation. Even though these data were collected for a different purpose, they may be helpful for providing additional information to the primary audience for the evaluation. Data already in existence generally are less expensive to obtain than are original data. The decision whether to use preexisting data depends on whether they were collected from people of interest in the current evaluation and whether they are consistent with operational definitions used in the current evaluation.

## How, When, and Where to Collect Data

Methods for how data can be collected include the following:

- Observation
- Interview
- Questionnaire or written examination
- Record review
- Secondary analysis of existing databases

Which method is selected depends, first, on the type of data being collected and, second, on available resources. Whenever possible, data should be collected using more than one method. Using multiple methods will provide the evaluator, and consequently the primary audience, with more complete information about the program or performance being evaluated than could be accomplished using a single method.

Observations can be conducted by the evaluator in person or can be videotaped for viewing at some later time. In the combined role of educator-evaluator, the nurse educator who is conducting a process evaluation can directly observe a learner's physical, verbal, psychomotor, and affective behaviors so that they can be responded to in a timely manner. Use of videotape or a nonparticipant observer also can be beneficial for picking up the educator's own behaviors of which the educator is unaware, but which might be influencing the learner.

The timing of data collection, or when data collection takes place, has already been addressed both in discussion of different types of evaluation and in descriptions of evaluation design structures. Process evaluation, for example, generally occurs during and immediately after an educational activity. Content evaluation takes place immediately after completion of education. Outcome evaluation occurs some time after completion of education, after learners have returned to the setting where they are expected to use new knowledge or perform a new skill. Impact evaluation generally is conducted from weeks to years after the educational program being evaluated because the purpose of impact evaluation is to determine what change has occurred within the community or institution as a whole as a result of an educational program.

Timing of data collection for program evaluation is less obvious than for other types of evaluation, in part because a number of different descriptions of what constitutes a program evaluation can be found both in the literature and in practice. As discussed earlier, Abruzzese (1978) describes data collection for program evaluation as occurring over a prolonged period because program evaluation is itself a culmination of process, content, outcome, and impact evaluations already conducted.

Where an evaluation is conducted can have a major effect on evaluation results. Be careful not to make the decision about where to collect data on the basis of convenience for the data collector. An appropriate setting for conducting a content evaluation may be in the classroom or skills laboratory where learners have just completed class instruction or training. An outcome evaluation to determine whether training has improved the nurse's ability to perform a skill with patients on the nursing unit, however, requires that data collection—in this case, observation of the nurse's performance—be conducted on the nursing unit. Similarly, an outcome evaluation to determine whether discharge teaching in the hospital enabled the patient to provide self-care at home requires that data collection, or observation of the patient's performance, be conducted in the home. What if available resources are insufficient to allow for home visits by the evaluator? To answer this question, keep in mind that the focus of the evaluation is on performance by the patient, not performance by the evaluator. Training a family member, a visiting nurse, or even the patient to observe and record patient performance at home is preferable to bringing the patient to a place of convenience for the evaluator.

**Who Collects Data**   Evaluative data are most commonly collected by the educator who is conducting the class or activity being evaluated because that educator is already present and interacting with learners. Combining the role of evaluator with that of educator is one appropriate method for conducting a process evaluation because evaluative data are integral to the teaching–learning process. Inviting another educator or a patient representative to observe a class can provide additional data from the perspective of someone who does not have to divide his or her attention between teaching and evaluating. This second, and perhaps less biased, input can strengthen legitimacy and usefulness of evaluation results.

Data can also be collected by the learners themselves, by other colleagues within the department or institution, or by someone from outside the institution. Puetz's (1992) description of data collection using a participant evaluation team is an example of data collection that includes learners. The evaluation team is composed of a small number of randomly selected individuals who are scheduled to attend an educational program. Team members are introduced to other program participants at the beginning of the class, join other participants during the program, and collect data through self-report as well as through observation and interaction with others during breaks.

When selecting who will collect data, keep in mind that the individuals chosen to carry out this task become an extension of the evaluation instrument. If the data that are collected are to be reliable, unbiased, and accurate, the data collectors must be unbiased and sufficiently expert at the task. Use of unbiased expert data collectors is especially important for collecting observation and interview data, because these data in part depend on the subjective interpretation of the data collector. Other data can also be affected by who collects those data. For example, if staff nurses are asked to complete a job satisfaction survey and their head nurse is asked to collect the surveys for return to the evaluator, what problems do you think might occur? Might some staff nurses be hesitant to provide negative scores on certain items, even though they hold a negative opinion? Likewise, physiological data can be altered, however unintentionally, by the data collector. Consider, for example, an outcome evaluation to determine whether a series of biofeedback classes given to young executives can reduce stress as measured by pulse and blood pressure. How might some executives' pulse and blood pressure results be affected by a data collector who is extremely physically attractive or outwardly angry?

Use of trained data collectors from an external agency is, in most cases, not a financially viable option. The potential for a data collector to bias data can be minimized using a number of less expensive alternatives, however. First, limit the number of data collectors as much as possible, as this step will automatically decrease person-based variation. Ask individuals assisting you with data collection to wear similar neutral colors, to avoid cologne, and to speak in a moderate tone. Because "moderate tone," for example, may not be interpreted the same way by everyone, hold at least one practice session or "dry run" with all data collectors prior to actually conducting the evaluation. Whenever possible, ask for help with data collection from someone who has no vested interest in results and who will be perceived as unbiased and nonthreatening by those providing the data. Interview scripts to be read verbatim by the interviewer can ensure that all patients or staff being interviewed will be asked the same questions.

With the advent of continuous quality improvement as an expectation of daily activity in healthcare organizations, healthcare professionals are obligated to become more knowledgeable about principles of measurement and ways to implement measurement techniques in their work setting (Joint Commission on Accreditation of Healthcare Organizations, 1995). One benefit that this change in practice has for the nurse educator is that more people within the organization have some expertise in data collection and are motivated to help with data collection activities. Another potential benefit is that data collection activities are likely to already be a part of practice. Not only might the nurse educator have readily available individuals to assist with data collection, but the educator might also have readily available and usable instruments and data.

Use of a portfolio as a method for evaluation of an individual's learning over time has been documented in the literature for more than 25 years, primarily from an academic perspective (Appling et al., 2001; Ball et al., 2000; Cayne, 1995; Roberts et al., 2001). Although formal education of nursing students is not the focus of this text, other uses of portfolios are relevant to the role of the practice-based nurse as educator. Individual completion of a professional portfolio is a current requirement for recertification in some nursing specialties in the United States and for periodic registration in the United Kingdom (Ball, 2000; Serembus, 2000). In light of the increasing demands on today's professionals to maintain currency in their competence to practice, Serembus (2000) suggests that a practice portfolio may soon be a requirement for relicensure in the United States.

Given the importance of a nurse's portfolio to his or her career status, the nurse educator may find several colleagues asking for assistance in creating and maintaining a portfolio that will provide a strong base of evaluative evidence demonstrating that nurse's continuing professional development and consequent impact on practice. Perhaps the best suggestion the nurse educator might offer—and heed—is to clarify the focus of the portfolio as determined by the requiring organization (in this case, the "primary audience") and as stated in that organization's criteria for portfolio completion. Is the focus more on process evaluation, outcome evaluation, or both? Specifically, is the nurse expected to demonstrate "reflective practice"? If so, what does the organization accept as evidence of "reflective practice"?

One reason why focus clarification is so challenging is because there is no consistent description of how portfolios are to be used or what they are to contain. In its simplest form, a practice portfolio comprises a collection of information and materials about one's practice that have been gathered over time. The issue of whether this collection is intended to demonstrate previous learning or whether the process of collecting is itself a learning experience continues to foster debate (Cayne, 1995; Roberts, 2001). Central to this issue is the notion of reflective practice. First coined by Schön (1987), the term *reflective practice* still does not have a commonly agreed-upon definition (Cotton, 2001; Hannigan, 2001; Teekman, 2000). Schön describes two key components of reflective practice as *reflection-in-action* and *reflection-on-action*. Reflection-in-action occurs when the nurse introspectively considers a practice activity while performing it so change for improvement can be made at that moment. Reflection-on-action occurs when the nurse introspectively analyzes a practice activity after its completion so as to gain insights for the future (Cotton, 2001). From an evaluation perspective, these components are similar to formative and summative evaluation, indicating that reflective practice has more than one focus.

Given the complexity of attempting to address multiple foci with the use of a single evaluation method—the practice portfolio—it is not surprising that use of portfolios has inspired such controversy. To the extent that a portfolio is required to include physical documentation as evidence of reflective practice, an introspective activity, the argument by some that portfolios are not adequately reliable or valid for use in evaluation of learning (Ball et al., 2000; Cayne, 1995) is also not surprising.

## Evaluation Instruments

This chapter is intended to present key points to consider in selection, modification, or construction of evaluation instruments. Whenever possible, an evaluation should be conducted using existing instruments, because instrument development requires considerable expertise, time, and expenditure of resources. Construction of an original evaluation instrument, whether it is in the form of a questionnaire or a type of equipment, also requires rigorous testing for reliability and validity. Timely provision of evaluative information for making decisions rarely allows the luxury of the several months to several years needed to develop a reliable, valid instrument.

The initial step in instrument selection is to conduct a literature search for evaluations similar to the evaluation being planned. A helpful place to begin is with the same journals listed earlier in this chapter. Instruments that have been used in more than one study should be given preference over an instrument developed for a single use, because instruments used multiple times generally have been more thoroughly tested for reliability and validity. Once a number of potential instruments have been identified, each instrument must be carefully critiqued to determine whether it is, in fact, appropriate for the evaluation planned.

First, the instrument must measure the performance being evaluated exactly as that performance has been operationally defined for the evaluation. For example, if satisfaction with a continuing education program is operationally defined to include a score of 80% or higher on five specific program components (such as faculty responsiveness to questions, relevance of content, and so on), then the instrument selected to measure participant satisfaction with the program must include exactly those five components and must be able to be scored in percentages.

Second, an appropriate instrument should have documented evidence of its reliability and validity with individuals who are as closely matched as possible with the people from whom you will be collecting data. If you will be evaluating the ability of older adult patients to complete activities of daily living, for example, you would not want to use an instrument developed for evaluating the ability of young orthopedic patients to complete routine activities. Similarities in reading level and visual acuity also should exist if the instrument being evaluated is a questionnaire or scale that participants will complete themselves.

Existing instruments being considered for selection also must be affordable, must be feasible for use in the location planned for conducting data collection, and should require minimal training on the part of data collectors.

The evaluation instrument most likely to require modification from an existing tool or development of an entirely new instrument is a cognitive test. The primary reason for constructing such a test is that it must be consistent with content actually covered during the educational program or activity. The intent of a cognitive test is to be comprehensive and relevant and to fairly test the learner's knowledge of content covered. Use of a test blueprint is one of the most useful methods for ensuring comprehensiveness and relevance of test questions because the blueprint enables the evaluator to be certain that each area of course content is included in the test and that content areas emphasized during instruction are similarly emphasized during testing.

## Barriers to Evaluation

If evaluation is so crucial to healthcare education, why is evaluation often an afterthought or even overlooked entirely? The reasons given for not conducting evaluations are many and varied but rarely, if ever, insurmountable. To overcome barriers to evaluation, they first must be identified and understood; then the evaluation must be designed and conducted in a way that will minimize or eliminate as many identified barriers as possible.

Barriers to conducting an evaluation can be classified into three broad categories:

- Lack of clarity
- Lack of ability
- Fear of punishment or loss of self-esteem

**Lack of Clarity**  Lack of clarity most often results from an unclear, unstated, or ill-defined evaluation focus. Undertaking any action is difficult if the performer does not know the purpose for taking that action. Undertaking an evaluation certainly is no different. Often evaluations are attempted to determine the quality of an educational program or activity, yet quality is not defined beyond some vague sense of "goodness." What is *goodness* and from whose perspective will it be determined? Who or what has to demonstrate evidence of goodness? What will happen if goodness is or is not evident? Inability to answer these or similar questions creates a significant barrier to conducting an evaluation. Not knowing the purpose of an evaluation or what will be done with evaluation results, for example, can become a barrier for even the most seasoned evaluator.

Barriers in this category have the greatest potential for successful resolution because the best solution for lack of clarity is to provide clarity. Recall that evaluation focus includes five components: audience, purpose, questions, scope, and resources. To overcome a potential lack of clarity, all five components must be identified and made available to those conducting the evaluation. A clearly stated purpose must explain why the evaluation is being conducted. Part of the answer to this question consists of a statement detailing what decisions will be made on the basis of evaluation results. Clear identification of who constitutes the primary audience is as important as a clear statement of purpose. It is from the perspective of the primary audience that terms such as *quality* should be defined and operationalized. While the results of the evaluation will provide the information on which decisions will be made, the primary audience will actually make those decisions.

**Lack of Ability**   Lack of ability to conduct an evaluation most often results from insufficient knowledge of how to conduct the evaluation or insufficient or inaccessible resources needed to conduct the evaluation. Clarification of evaluation purpose, questions, and scope is often the responsibility of the primary audience. Clarification of resources, however, is the responsibility of both the primary audience and the individuals conducting the evaluation. The primary audience members are accountable for providing the necessary resources—personnel, equipment, time, facilities, and so on—to conduct the evaluation they are requesting. Unless these individuals have some expertise in evaluation, they may not know what resources are necessary. The persons conducting the evaluation, therefore, must accept responsibility for knowing what resources are necessary and for providing that information to the primary audience. The person asked or expected to conduct the evaluation may be as uncertain about necessary resources as is the primary audience, however.

Lack of knowledge of what resources are necessary or lack of actual resources may form a barrier to conducting an evaluation that can be difficult, although not impossible, to overcome. Lack of knowledge can be resolved or minimized by enlisting the assistance of individuals with needed expertise through consultation or contract (if funds are available), through collaboration, or indirectly through literature review. Lack of other resources—time, money, equipment, facilities, and so

on—should be documented, justified, and presented to those requesting the evaluation. Alternative methods for conducting the evaluation, including the option of making decisions in the absence of any evaluation, also should be documented and presented.

**Fear of Punishment or Loss of Self-Esteem**
Evaluation may be perceived as a judgment of personal worth. Individuals being evaluated may fear that anything less than a perfect performance will result in punishment or that their mistakes will be seen as evidence that they are somehow unworthy or incompetent as human beings. These fears form one of the greatest barriers to conducting an evaluation. Unfortunately, the fear of punishment or of being seen as unworthy may not easily be overcome, especially if the individual has had past negative experiences. Consider, for example, traditional quality assurance monitoring, where results were used to correct deficiencies through punitive measures. To give another example, how many times has an educator interpreted learner dissatisfaction with a teaching style as learner dislike for the educator as a person? How many times have pediatric patients' parents said, "If you don't do it right, the doctor won't let you go home . . . and we will be very disappointed in you"? Every one of us probably has experienced "test anxiety" at some point in our own education.

The first step in overcoming this barrier is to realize that the potential for its existence may be close to 100%. Individuals whose performance or knowledge is being evaluated are not likely to say overtly that evaluation represents a threat to them. Rather, they are far more likely to demonstrate self-protective behaviors or attitudes that can range from failure to attend a class that has a post-test, to providing socially desirable answers on a questionnaire, to responding with hostility to evaluation questions. An individual may intentionally choose to "fail" an evaluation as a method for controlling the uncertainty of success.

The second step in overcoming the barrier of fear or threat is to remember that "the person is more important than the performance or the product" (Narrow, 1979, p. 185). If the purpose of an evaluation is to facilitate better learning, as in process evaluation, focus on the process. Consider the example of teaching a newly diagnosed diabetic how to administer insulin. The educator has carefully and thoroughly explained each step in the process of insulin administration, observing the patient's intent expression and frequent head nods during the explanation. When the patient tries to demonstrate the steps, however, he is unable to begin. Why? One answer may be that the use of an auditory teaching style does not match the patient's visual learning style. Another possibility might be that too many distractions are present in the immediate environment, making concentration on learning all but impossible.

A third step in overcoming the fear of punishment or threatened loss of self-esteem is to point out achievements, if they exist, or to continue to encourage effort if learning has not been achieved. Give praise honestly, focusing on the task at hand.

Finally, and perhaps most importantly, use communication of information to prevent or minimize fear. Lack of clarity exists as a barrier for those who are the subjects of an evaluation as much as for those who will conduct the evaluation. If learners or educators know and understand the focus of an evaluation, they may be less fearful than if such information is left to their imaginations. Remember that failure to provide certain information may be unethical or even illegal. For example, any evaluative data about an individual that can be identified with that specific person should be collected only with the individual's informed consent. The ethical and legal importance of informed consent as a protection of human rights is a central concern of institutional review boards. Indeed, institutional review board approval is a prerequisite to initiation of virtually every experimental medical intervention conducted on patients or families.

## CONDUCTING THE EVALUATION

To conduct an evaluation means to implement the evaluation design by using the instruments chosen or developed according to the methods selected. How smoothly an evaluation is implemented depends primarily on how carefully and thoroughly the evaluation was planned. Planning is not a complete guarantee of success, however. Three methods to minimize the effects of unexpected events that occur when carrying out an evaluation are to (1) conduct a pilot test first, (2) include "extra" time, and (3) keep a sense of humor.

Conducting a pilot test of the evaluation entails trying out the data collection methods, instruments, and plan for data analysis with a few individuals who are the same as or very similar to those who will be included in the full evaluation. A pilot test must be conducted if any newly developed instruments are planned for the evaluation, so as to assess reliability, validity, interpretability, and feasibility of those new instruments. Also, a pilot test should be carried out prior to implementing a full evaluation that will be expensive or time-consuming to conduct or on which major decisions will be based. Process evaluation generally is not amenable to pilot testing unless a new instrument will be used for data collection. Pilot testing should be considered prior to conducting outcome, impact, or program evaluations, however.

Including "extra" time during the conduct of an evaluation means leaving room for the unexpected delays that almost invariably occur during evaluation planning, data collection, and translation of evaluation results into reports that will be meaningful and usable by the primary audience. Because those delays not only will occur but also are likely to occur at inconvenient times during the evaluation, keeping a sense of humor is vitally important.

An evaluator with a sense of humor is more likely to maintain a realistic perspective in reporting results that include negative findings, too. An audience with a vested interest in positive evaluation results may blame the evaluator if results are lower than expected.

## ANALYZING AND INTERPRETING DATA COLLECTED

The purposes for conducting data analysis are (1) to organize data so that they can provide meaningful information and (2) to provide answers to evaluation questions. *Data* and *information* are not synonymous terms. That is, a mass of numbers or a mass of comments does not become information until it has been organized into coherent tables, graphs, or categories that are relevant to the purpose for conducting the evaluation.

Basic decisions about how data will be analyzed are dictated by the nature of the data and by the questions used to focus the evaluation. As described earlier, data can be quantitative or qualitative. Data also can be described as continuous or discrete. Age and level of anxiety are examples of continuous data; gender and diagnosis are examples of discrete data. Finally, data can be differentiated by level of measurement. All qualitative data are at the nominal level of measurement, meaning they are described in terms of categories such as "health focused" versus "illness focused." Quantitative data can be at the nominal, ordinal, interval, or ratio level of measurement. The level of measurement of the data determines what statistics can be used to analyze those data. A useful suggestion for deciding how data will be analyzed is to enlist the assistance of someone with experience in data analysis.

Analysis of data should be consistent with the type of data collected. In other words, all data analysis must be rigorous, but not all

data analysis need include use of inferential statistics. For example, qualitative data, such as verbal comments obtained during interviews and written comments obtained from open-ended questionnaires, are summarized or "themed" into categories of similar comments. Each category or theme is qualitatively described by directly quoting one or more comments that are typical of that category. These categories then may be quantitatively described using descriptive statistics such as total counts and percentages.

Different qualitative methods for analyzing data are emerging as they gain legitimacy in a scientific environment once ruled by traditional experimental quantitative methods. One use of qualitative methods in evaluation is called fourth-generation evaluation (Hamilton, 1993), or naturalistic or constructivist evaluation. Perhaps most beneficial in conducting a process evaluation, fourth-generation evaluation focuses on teacher–learner interaction and observation of that interaction by the teachers and learners present. As the term *constructivist* might imply, evaluation is an integral component of the education process; that is, evaluation helps construct the education. Data collection, analysis, and use of results occur concurrently. Teacher and learner questions and responses are observed and recorded during an education program. These observations are summarized at the time of occurrence and throughout the program, and then are used to provide immediate feedback to participants in the educational activity.

The first step in analysis of quantitative data consists of organization and summarization using statistics such as frequencies and percentages that describe the sample or population from which the data were collected. A description of a population of learners, for example, might include such information as response rate and frequency of learner demo-

| TABLE 15–2   Demographic comparison of survey respondents to total course participants using group averages | | |
|---|---|---|
| Learner Demographics | Survey Respondents ($n = 50$) | All Course Participants ($N = 55$) |
| Age | 27.5 years | 25.5 years |
| Length of time employed | 3.5 years | 7.5 years |
| Years of post-high school education | 2.0 years | 2.0 years |

graphic characteristics. Table 15–2 presents an example of how such information might be displayed.

The next step in analysis of quantitative data is to select the statistical procedures appropriate for the type of data collected that will answer questions posed in planning the evaluation. Again, a good suggestion is to enlist the assistance of an expert.

## REPORTING EVALUATION RESULTS

Results of an evaluation must be reported if the evaluation is to be of any use. Such a statement seems obvious, but how many times have you heard that an evaluation was being conducted but never heard anything more about it? How many times have you participated in an evaluation but never seen the final report? How many times have you conducted an evaluation yourself but not provided anyone with a report on findings? Almost all of us, if we are honest, would have to answer even the last question with a number greater than zero.

Reasons for not reporting evaluation results are diverse and numerous. Ignorance of who should receive the results, belief that the results are not important or will not be used, inability to translate results into language useful for producing the report, and fear that results will be misused are four major reasons

for why evaluative data may often never get from the spreadsheet to the customer.

Following a few guidelines when planning an evaluation will significantly increase the likelihood that results of the evaluation will be reported to the appropriate individuals or groups, in a timely manner, and in usable form:

1. Be audience focused.
2. Stick to the evaluation purpose.
3. Stick to the data.

### Be Audience Focused

The purpose for conducting an evaluation is to provide information for decision making by the primary audience. The report of evaluation results must, therefore, be consistent with that purpose. One rule of thumb to use: Always begin an evaluation report with an executive summary that is no longer than one page. No matter who the audience members are, their time is important to them. A second important guideline is to present evaluation results in a format and language that the audience can use and understand without additional interpretation. This statement does not mean that technical information should be excluded from a report to a lay audience; rather, it means that such information should be written using nontechnical terms. Graphs and charts generally are easier to understand than are tables of numbers, for example. If a secondary audience of technical experts also will receive a report of evaluation results, include an appendix containing the more detailed or technically specific information in which they might be interested. Third, make every effort to present results in person as well as in writing. A direct presentation provides an opportunity for the evaluator to answer questions and to assess whether the report meets the needs of the audience. Finally, include specific recommendations or suggestions for how evaluation results might be used.

## Stick to the Evaluation Purpose

Keep the main body of an evaluation report focused on information that fulfills the purpose for conducting the evaluation. Provide answers to the questions asked. Include the main aspects of how the evaluation was conducted, but avoid a diary-like chronology of the activities of the evaluators.

## Stick to the Data

Maintain consistency with actual data when reporting and interpreting findings. Keep in mind that a question not asked cannot be answered and that data not collected cannot be interpreted. If you did not measure or observe a teacher's performance, for example, do not draw conclusions about the adequacy of that performance. Similarly, if the only measures of patient performance were those conducted in the hospital, do not interpret successful inpatient performance as successful performance by the patient at home or at work. These examples may seem obvious, but "conceptual leaps" from the data collected to the conclusions drawn from those data are an all-too-common occurrence. One suggestion that decreases the opportunity to overinterpret data is to include evaluation results and interpretation of those results in separate sections of the report.

A discussion of any limitations of the evaluation is an important part of the evaluation report. For example, if several patients were unable to complete a questionnaire because they could not understand it or because they were too fatigued, say so. Knowing that evaluation results do not include data from patients below a certain educational level or physical status will help the audience realize that they cannot make decisions about those patients based on the evaluation. Discussion of limitations also will provide useful information for what not to do the next time a similar evaluation is conducted.

## SUMMARY

The process of evaluation in healthcare education involves gathering, summarizing, interpreting, and using data to determine the extent to which an educational activity is efficient, effective, and useful for those who participate in that activity as learners, teachers, or sponsors. Five types of evaluation were discussed in this chapter: process, content, outcome, impact, and program evaluations. Each of these types focuses on a specific purpose, scope, and questions to be asked of an educational activity or program to meet the needs of those who ask for the evaluation or who can benefit from its results. Each type of evaluation also requires some level of available resources for the evaluation to be conducted.

The number and variety of evaluation models, designs, methods, and instruments are experiencing an exponential growth as the importance of evaluation becomes more evident in today's healthcare environment. A number of guidelines, rules of thumb, and suggestions have been included in this chapter's discussion of how a nurse educator might go about selecting the most appropriate model, design, methods, and instruments for a particular type of evaluation. Perhaps the most important point to remember was made at the beginning of this chapter: Each aspect of the evaluation process is important, but all of them are meaningless if the results of evaluation are not used to guide future action in planning and carrying out educational interventions.

## REVIEW QUESTIONS

1. How is the term *evaluation* defined?
2. How does the process of evaluation differ from the process of assessment?
3. What is the first and most crucial step in planning any evaluation?
4. What are the five (5) basic components included in determining the focus of an evaluation?
5. What are the five (5) basic types (levels) of evaluation in order from simple to complex identified in Abruzzese's RSA Evaluation Model?
6. How does *formative evaluation* differ from *summative evaluation* and what is another name for each of these two types of evaluation?
7. What is the purpose of each type (level) of evaluation as described by Abruzzese in her RSA Evaluation Model?
8. What data collection methods can be used in conducting an evaluation of educational interventions?
9. What are the three (3) major barriers to conducting an evaluation?
10. When and why should a pilot test be conducted prior to implementing a full evaluation?
11. What are the three (3) guidelines to follow in reporting the results of an evaluation?

## REFERENCES

Abruzzese, R.S. (1978). Evaluation in nursing staff development. In *Nursing Staff Development: Strategies for Success*. St. Louis: Mosby–Year Book.

Albanese, M. A. & Gjerde, C. L. (1987). Evaluation. In H. VanHoozer et al. (eds.), *The Teaching Process: Theory and Practice in Nursing*. Norwalk, CT: Appleton-Century-Crofts.

Appling, S. E., Naumann, P. L., & Berk, R. A. (2001). Using a faculty evaluation triad to achieve evidence-based teaching. *Nursing and Health Care Perspectives, 22*(5), 247–251.

Ball, E., Daly, W. M., & Carnwell, R. (2000). The use of portfolios in the assessment of learning and competence. *Nursing Standard, 14*(43), 35–37.

Berk, R. A. & Rossi, P. H. (1990). *Thinking About Program Evaluation*. Newbury Park, CA: Sage.

Billings, J. R. (2000). Community development: A critical review of approaches to evaluation. *Journal of Advanced Nursing, 31*(2), 472–480.

Cayne, J. (1995). Portfolios: A developmental influence? *Journal of Advanced Nursing, 21*(2), 395–405.

Cotton, A. H. (2001). Private thoughts in public spheres: Issues in reflection and reflective practices in nursing. *Journal of Advanced Nursing, 36*(4), 512–559.

Dilorio, C., Price, M. E., & Becker, J. K. (2001). Evaluation of the neuroscience nurse internship program: The first decade. *Journal of Neuroscience Nursing, 33*(1), 42–49.

Gerrish, K. (2001). A pluralistic evaluation to explore people's experiences of stroke services in the community. *Health & Social Care in the Community, 7*(4), 248–256.

Haggard, A. (1989). Evaluating patient education. In *Handbook of Patient Education*. Rockville, MD: Aspen.

Hamilton, G. A. (1993). An overview of evaluation research methods with implications for nursing staff development. *Journal of Nursing Staff Development, 9*(3), 148–154.

Hannigan, B. (2001) A discussion of the strengths and weaknesses of "reflection" in nursing practice and education. *Journal of Clinical Nursing, 10*(2), 278–283.

Hart, E. (1999). The use of pluralistic evaluation to explore people's experiences of stroke services in the community. *Health & Social Care in the Community, 7*(4), 248–256.

Holzemer, W. (1992). Evaluation methods in continuing education. *Journal of Continuing Education in Nursing, 23*(4), 174–181.

Johnson, J. H. & Olesinski, N. (1995). Program evaluation: Key to success. *Journal of Nursing Administration, 25*(1), 53–60.

Joint Commission on Accreditation of Healthcare Organizations. (1995). *Accreditation Manual for Hospitals.* Oakbrook Terrace, IL: Joint Commission on Accreditation of Healthcare Organizations.

Koch, T. (2000). "Having a say": Negotiation in fourth-generation evaluation. *Journal of Advanced Nursing, 31*(1), 117–125.

Narrow, B. (1979). *Patient Teaching in Nursing Practice: A Patient and Family-centered Approach.* New York: Wiley.

Puetz, B. E. (1992). Evaluation: Essential skill for the staff development specialist. In K. J. Kelly (ed.), *Nursing Staff Development: Current Competence, Future Focus.* Philadelphia: Lippincott.

Rankin, S. H. & Stallings, K. D. (2001). *Patient Education: Principles and Practices,* 4th ed. Philadelphia: Lippincott.

Roberts, P., Priest, H., & Bromage, C. (2001). Selecting and utilizing data sources to evaluate health care education. *Nurse Researcher, 8*(3), 15–29.

Ruzicki, D. A. (1987). Evaluating patient education—a vital part of the process. In C. E. Smith (ed.), *Patient Education: Nurses in Partnership with Other Health Professionals.* Orlando, FL: Grune & Stratton.

Schön, D. A. (1987). *Educating the Reflective Practitioner. Towards a New Design for Teaching and Learning in the Professions.* London: Jossey-Bass.

Serembus, J. F. (2000). Teaching the process of developing a professional portfolio. *Nurse Educator, 25*(6), 282–287.

Stewart, A. L., Hays, R. D., & Ware, J. E. (1988). The MOS Short-Form General Health Survey: Reliability and validity in a patient population. *Medical Care, 26*(7), 724.

Teekman, B. (2000). Exploring reflective thinking in nursing practice. *Journal of Advanced Nursing, 31*(5), 1125–1135.

Tolson, D. (1999). Practice innovation: A methodological maze. *Journal of Advanced Nursing, 30*(2), 381–390.

Waddell, D. (1992). The effects of continuing education on nursing practice: A meta-analysis. *Journal of Continuing Education in Nursing, 23*(4), 164–168.

Walker, E. & Dewar, B. J. (2000). Moving on from interpretivism: An argument for constructivist evaluation. *Journal of Advanced Nursing, 32*(3), 713–720.

Ware, J. E., Jr., Davies-Avery, A., & Donald, C. A. (1978). *Conceptualization and Measurement of Health for Adults in the Health Insurance Study: Vol. V, General Health Perceptions.* Santa Monica, CA: RAND.

# Readability and Comprehension Tests

## HOW TO USE THE SPACHE GRADE-LEVEL SCORE FORMULA

1. For short passages, test the entire piece. For longer passages, test a minimum of three randomly selected samples of 100 words each. (If the 100-word mark in the sample falls after the midpoint of the sentence, count the sentence as a part of the sample.)

2. Average sentence length (a) can be determined by counting the number of words in the sample and dividing by the number of sentences. If a sentence is punctuated by a period, question mark, exclamation point, semicolon, or colon, count it as an independent sentence.

3. Count the number of words not on the Dale List (b) according to the following guidelines:

   - Count a word only once, even if it appears again or with variable endings later in the sample.
   - Do not count first names.
   - Do not count plurals or possessive endings of nouns.
   - Do not count regular verb forms (*-ing*, *-ed*, *-es*), but do count irregular verb forms.
   - Count adjective or adverb endings (*-ly*, *-er*, *-est*).
   - Count a group of words that consists of repetition of a single word (e.g., "oh, oh, oh"; "look, look, look") as a single sentence regardless of punctuation.
   - Do not count familiar letters like A, B, C.

4. Apply the formula:

$$GL = 0.141(a) + 0.086(b) + 0.839$$

   where GL is grade level, (a) is average sentence length, and (b) is the number of words not listed on the Dale List.

   In other words, multiply the average sentence length in a sample of 100 words by 0.141. Then multiply the percent of words outside the Dale "Easy Word List" by 0.086. To these figures, add a constant, 0.839. The sum represents the estimated reading difficulty of the book. This will be a figure such as 2.267, which, when rounded off as 2.3, designates a book equal in difficulty to readers of school text-books commonly used in the third month of second grade. When using this formula, it is suggested that at least three samples from the reading material be scored and the results averaged for a more reliable estimate of reading difficulty (Spache, 1953; Spadero, 1983).

## HOW TO USE THE FLESCH FORMULA

1. To test a whole piece of writing, take three to five 100-word samples of an article or twenty-five to thirty 100-word samples of a book. For short pieces, test the entire selection. Do not pick "good" or "typical" samples, but choose every third paragraph or every other page. In a 100-word sample, find the sentence that ends nearest to the 100-word mark; that may be, for example, at the 94th or the 109th word. Start each sample at the beginning of a paragraph, but do not use an introductory paragraph as part of the sample. Count contractions and hyphenated words as one word; count numbers and letters separated by space as words.

2. Figure the average sentence length (SL) by counting the number of words and dividing by the number of sentences. In counting sentences, follow units of thought marked off by periods, colons, semicolons, question marks, or exclamation points.

3. Determine word length (WL) by counting the number of syllables in each word in the sample as they are normally read aloud (i.e., two syllables for $ ["dollars"] and four syllables for *1918* ["nineteen-eighteen"]. It helps to read silently aloud while counting. Divide the syllables by the number of words in the sample and multiply by 100.

4. Apply the formula:

$$RE = 206.835 - 0.846 \, WL - 1.015 \, SL$$

where RE is the reading ease score, WL is the average word length measured as syllables per 100 words, and SL is the average sentence length in words (Flesch, 1948; Spadero, 1983; and Spadero et al., 1980).

The reading ease score ranges from zero (practically unreadable) to 100 (very easy for any literate person) with interpretations in between (Table A–1).

## HOW TO USE THE FOG FORMULA

1. Count 100 words in succession (W). If the selection is long, choose several samples of 100 words from the text, and average the results.

2. Count the number of complete sentences (S). If the 100th word falls past the midpoint of a sentence, include this sentence in the count.

3. Divide the words (W) by the number of sentences (S).

4. Count the number of words having three or more syllables (A), but do not count verbs ending in *-ed* or *-es* that make a word have a third syllable, do not

| TABLE A–1 | Reading ease scores | | | |
|---|---|---|---|---|
| READING EASE SCORE | SYLLABLES PER 100 WORDS | AVERAGE SENTENCE LENGTH | DIFFICULTY LEVEL | GRADE LEVEL |
| 0–30 | 192 or more | 29 or more | Very difficult | College grad |
| 30–50 | 167 | 25 | Difficult | College |
| 50–60 | 155 | 21 | Fairly difficult | 10–12 |
| 60–70 | 147 | 17 | Standard | 8–9 |
| 70–80 | 139 | 14 | Fairly easy | 7 |
| 80–90 | 131 | 11 | Easy | 6 |
| 90–100 | 123 or less | 8 or less | Very easy | 5 |

SOURCE: Adapted from Flesch, R. (1948). A new readability yardstick. *Journal of Applied Psychology, 32*(3), 230; and Spadero, D.C. (1983). Assessing readability of patient information materials. *Pediatric Nursing, 9*(4), 275.

count capitalized words, and do not count combinations of simple words, such as *butterfly*.

5. Apply the formula:

$$GL = (W/S + A) \times 0.4$$

In other words, to find the GL (grade level), divide the number of words (W) by the number of complete sentences (S) in the sample 100-word passage, add the number of words having three or more syllables (A), and multiply the result by a constant of 0.4 (Gunning, 1968; Spadero, 1983; Spadero et al., 1980).

## HOW TO USE THE FRY READABILITY GRAPH

1. Select three 100-word sample passages from near the beginning, middle, and end of a book, article, pamphlet, or brochure. Skip all proper nouns as part of the 100-word count. Fewer than three samples and passages of less than 30 sentences can be used, but the user should be aware that there is necessarily a sacrifice in both reliability and validity.

2. Count the total number of sentences in each 100-word sample (estimating to the nearest tenth of a sentence for partial sentences).

3. Average the sentence counts of the three sample passages.

4. Count the total number of syllables in each 100-word sample. Count one syllable per vowel sound; for example, *cat* has one syllable, *blackbird* has two, and *continental* has four. Caution: Do not be fooled by word size (e.g., *polio* [three syllables], *through* [one syllable]). Endings such as -*y*, -*ed*, -*el*, or -*le* usually make a syllable (e.g., *ready* [two syllables], *bottle* [two syllables]). Graph users sometimes have trouble determining syllables. The clue is to believe what you hear (speech sounds), not what you see (e.g., *wanted* is a two-syllable word, but *stopped* is a one-syllable word). Count proper nouns, numerals, and initials or acronyms as words. A word is a symbol or group of symbols bounded by a blank space on either side. Thus, *1945*, *&*, and *IRS* are all words. Each symbol

should receive a syllable count of one (i.e., the date *1945* is one word with four syllables, and the initials *IRS* is one word with three syllables).

5. Average the total number of syllables for the three samples.

6. Plot on the graph the average sentence count and the average word count to determine the appropriate grade level of the material. For example,

|  | NUMBER OF SYLLABLES | NUMBER OF SENTENCES |
|---|---|---|
| 1st hundred words | 153 | 6.3 |
| 2nd hundred words | 161 | 5.9 |
| 3rd hundred words | <u>139</u> | <u>5.2</u> |
| Average count = | 453 ÷ 3 = 151 | 17.4 ÷ 3 = 5.8 |

In the example, the average number of syllables is 151, and the average number of sentences is 5.8. When plotted on the graph (Figure A–1), the point falls within

FIGURE A–1   **Fry Readability Graph—Extended**   SOURCE: Edward Fry, Rutgers University Reading Center, New Brunswick, NJ.

the approximate grade level of 9, which shows the materials to be at the ninth-grade readability level. If the point when plotted falls in the gray area, grade-level scores are invalid (Fry, 1968; Fry, 1977; Spadero et al., 1980).

## HOW TO USE THE SMOG FORMULA

### Passages Longer Than 30 Sentences

1. Count 10 consecutive sentences near the beginning, 10 consecutive sentences from the middle, and 10 consecutive sentences from the end of the selection to be assessed. A sentence is any independent unit of thought punctuated by a period, question mark, or exclamation point. If a sentence has a colon or semi-colon, consider each part as a separate sentence.

2. From the 30 randomly selected sentences, count the words containing three or more syllables (polysyllabic), including repetitions. Abbreviated words should be read aloud to determine their syllable count (e.g., *Sept.* = *September* = three syllables). Letters or numerals in a string beginning or ending with a space or punctuation mark should be counted if, when read aloud in context, at least three syllables can be distinguished. Do not count words ending in -ed or -es if the ending makes the word have a third syllable. Hyphenated words are counted as one word. Proper nouns should be counted.

3. Approximate the reading grade level from the SMOG Conversion Table (Table A–2), or calculate the reading grade level by estimating the nearest perfect square root of the number of words with three or more syllables and then adding a constant of 3 to the square root. For example, if the total number of polysyllabic words was 53, the nearest perfect square would be 49. The square

| Table A–2    SMOG Conversion Table | |
|---|---|
| **WORD COUNT** | **GRADE LEVEL** |
| 0–2 | 4 |
| 3–6 | 5 |
| 7–12 | 6 |
| 13–20 | 7 |
| 21–30 | 8 |
| 31–42 | 9 |
| 43–56 | 10 |
| 57–72 | 11 |
| 73–90 | 12 |
| 91–110 | 13 |
| 111–132 | 14 |
| 133–156 | 15 |
| 157–182 | 16 |
| 183–210 | 17 |
| 211–240 | 18 |

SOURCE: Developed by: Harold C. McGraw, Office of Educational Research, Baltimore County Public Schools, Towson, MD.

---

### [1](Mastectomy:) A Treatment for Breast Cancer

[2]You've been (diagnosed) as having breast cancer and your doctor has (recommended) a (mastectomy.)
[3]If you're like most women, you (probably) have many concerns about this treatment for breast cancer.
[4](Surgery) of any kind is a (frightening) (experience,) but (surgery) for breast cancer raises special concerns.
[5]You may be (wondering) if the (surgery) will cure your cancer, how you'll feel after (surgery) —and how you're going to look.

[6]It's not (unusual) to think about these things. [7]More than (100,000) women in the United States will have (mastectomies) this year. [8]Each of them will have (personal) concerns about the impact of the (surgery) on her life.

[9]This booklet is designed to ease some of your fears by letting you know what to expect—from the time you enter the (hospital) to your (recovery) at home. [10]It may also help the special people in your life who are concerned about your (well-being.)

---

FIGURE A–2    **Example of Counting Words with Three or More Syllables**

root of 49 would be 7. By adding a constant of 3, the reading level would be tenth grade.

Figure A–2 is an example of how to count all the words containing three or more syllables in a set of 10 sentences taken from one of the many pamphlets designed and distributed by the National Cancer Institute of the National Institutes of Health, Public Health Service, U.S. Department of Health and Human Services, entitled *Mastectomy: A Treatment for Breast Cancer* (1987, p. 1).

In Figure A–2, there are 20 words with three or more syllables. Note, the word *United* is not counted as a three-syllable word because only the *-ed* ending makes it polysyllabic (see rule 2). For this passage of 10 sentences, the grade level is eleventh grade.

## Passages Shorter Than 30 Sentences

1. Count the number of sentences in the material and the number of words containing three or more syllables.
2. In the left-hand column of Table A–3, locate the number of sentences. Then in the column opposite, locate the conversion number.
3. Multiply the word count found in Step 1 by the conversion number. Locate this number in Table A–2 to obtain the corresponding grade level.

*Example:* If the material is 25 sentences long and 15 words of three or more syllables were counted in this material, the conversion number in Table A–3 for 25 sentences is 1.2. Multiply the word count of 15 by 1.2 to get 18. For the word count of 18, the grade level in Table A–2 is 7. Therefore, the material is at a seventh-grade reading level.

| Table A–3   SMOG conversion for samples with fewer than 30 sentences | |
| --- | --- |
| NUMBER OF SENTENCES IN SAMPLE MATERIAL | CONVERSION NUMBER |
| 29 | 1.03 |
| 28 | 1.07 |
| 27 | 1.1 |
| 26 | 1.15 |
| 25 | 1.2 |
| 24 | 1.25 |
| 23 | 1.3 |
| 22 | 1.36 |
| 21 | 1.43 |
| 20 | 1.5 |
| 19 | 1.58 |
| 18 | 1.67 |
| 17 | 1.76 |
| 16 | 1.87 |
| 15 | 2.0 |
| 14 | 2.14 |
| 13 | 2.3 |
| 12 | 2.5 |
| 11 | 2.7 |
| 10 | 3 |

## HOW TO USE THE CLOZE TEST

### How to Construct a Cloze Test

1. Select a prose passage (one without reference to figures, tables, charts, or pictures) from printed educational materials currently in use such as pamphlets, brochures, manuals, or instruction sheets. Be sure the material is typical of what is normally given to patients but has not been previously read by them. The chosen passage should include whole paragraphs so that readers benefit from complete units of thought.

2. Leave the first and last sentences intact, and delete every fifth word from the other sentences for a total of about 50 word deletions. Do not delete proper nouns, but delete the word following the proper noun. Replace all deleted words with a line or blank space, all of equal length.

### How to Score a Cloze Test

1. Count as correct only those words that *exactly* replace the deleted words (synonyms are not to be counted as a correct answer).

2. Inappropriate word endings such as *-s*, *-ed*, *-er*, and *-ing* should be counted as incorrect.

3. The raw score is the number of exact word replacements.

### High Blood Pressure

High blood pressure, also called hypertension, affects 37 million Americans—many of them older than 55. A dangerous, silent killer, __1__ can lead to stroke, __2__ attack and heart or __3__ failure. Yet, in most __4__, no one knows what __5__ high blood pressure. Body __6__, emotions, heredity, overweight, and __7__ high-sodium (salt) diet may __8__ something to do with __9__ blood pressure, but scientists __10__ uncertain. It has long __11__ recognized as a major __12__ factor in stroke and __13__ attack—cardiovascular diseases which __14__ nearly 1 million deaths __15__ year.

To understand high __16__ pressure, it is necessary __17__ know something about how __18__ heart and blood vessels __19__. Your heart is a __20__ that acts like a __21__. The left side of __22__ heart receives oxygen-rich blood __23__ the lungs and pumps __24__ through the arteries to __25__ parts of your body, __26__ it with nutrients and __27__. Blood that has distributed __28__ nutrients and oxygen returns __29__ the right side of __30__ heart which pumps it __31__ the pulmonary artery to __32__ lungs where it absorbs __33__, and then the process __34__ again.

The force exerted __35__ your blood flowing against __36__ walls of the blood __37__ is blood pressure. The __38__ action of your heart __39__ the force. Your blood __40__ varies from moment to __41__ depending upon the situations __42__ activities in which you __43__ involved. For example, when __44__ become excited, the small __45__ that nourish your tissues __46__. The heart must pump __47__ harder to force the __48__ through the arteries, causing __49__ blood pressure to rise. __50__ the blood pressure will __51__ to normal when you __52__. Because of these changes in blood pressure, the doctor will usually take several blood pressure readings over a period of time before making a diagnosis of high blood pressure.

**FIGURE A–3  Sample Cloze Test**  SOURCE: Adapted from American Heart Association (1983) *An older person's guide to cardiovascular health*, National Center, 7320 Greenville Avenue, Dallas, TX 75231. The information from this booklet is not current and is used for illustrative purposes only.

4. Divide the raw score by the total number of blank spaces to determine the percentage of correct responses. For example, if the passage has 50 blanks and the patient correctly filled in 25 blanks (10 were incorrect responses and 15 spaces were left blank), divide 25 by 50, and the percentage score would be 50%.

5. A score of 60% or above indicates the patient is fully capable of understanding the material. A score of 40% to 60% indicates the patient needs supplemental instruction. A score below 40% indicates that the material as written is too difficult for the patient to understand.

The following are the words that were deleted from the sample Cloze test in Figure A-3.

| | | | |
|---|---|---|---|
| 1. it | 13. heart | 25. all | 37. vessels |
| 2. heart | 14. cause | 26. supplying | 38. pumping |
| 3. kidney | 15. a | 27. oxygen | 39. creates |
| 4. cases | 16. blood | 28. its | 40. pressure |
| 5. causes | 17. to | 29. to | 41. moment |
| 6. chemistry | 18. the | 30. your | 42. or |
| 7. a | 19. work | 31. through | 43. are |
| 8. have | 20. muscle | 32. the | 44. you |
| 9. high | 21. pump | 33. oxygen | 45. arteries |
| 10. remain | 22. your | 34. begins | 46. constrict |
| 11. been | 23. from | 35. by | 47. even |
| 12. risk | 24. it | 36. the | 48. blood |

*Note:* Words are listed in missing order. Hyphenated words are counted as one word; words in parentheses are counted as a word.

# Resources and Organizations for Special Populations

## Blindness

**National Diabetes Information Clearinghouse**
Box NDIC
9000 Rockville Pike
Bethesda, MD 20892
(301) 468-2162

**Resource Persons for Diabetes and Vision Impairment**
VIP Special Interest Group
AADE
444 North Michigan Avenue
Suite 1240
Chicago, IL 60611-3901

*List of members of American Association of Diabetes Educators (AADE) who possess specialized skills for working with visually impaired persons. List was compiled by the Visually Impaired Persons (VIP) Special Interest Group for the AADE and is available from that special interest group.*

**Resources for Visually Impaired Diabetics**
Vision Foundation Inc.
818 Mt. Auburn Street
Watertown, MA 02172

*The Vision Foundation publication is revised annually and is available for $4 prepaid for either large-print or cassette edition.*

## Deafness

**The National Academy of Gallaudet College**
Florida Avenue at 7th Street N.E.
Washington, DC 20002

*Training programs; assistance in developing training programs; publications on working with deaf patients.*

**The National Center for Law and the Deaf**
Gallaudet College
Florida Avenue at 7th Street N.E.
Washington, DC 20002

*Guidelines for services for deaf patients; assistance in developing such guidelines.*

**The Registry of Interpreters for the Deaf**
814 Thayer Avenue
Silver Spring, MD 20910

*Information on interpreting and interpreters; referral to local agencies and state chapters of the Registry of Interpreters for the Deaf for assistance in locating interpreters.*

## Disability Services

**Clearinghouse on Disability Information**
U.S. Department of Education
Switzer Building Room 3132
Washington, DC 20202
(202) 731-1241

**Information Center for Individuals with Disabilities**
Fort Point Place First Floor
27–43 Wormwood Street
Boston, MA 02210-1606
(617) 727-5540

**Library of Congress National Library Service for the Blind and Physically Handicapped**
1291 Taylor Street NW
Washington, DC 20542
(202) 707-5100
(800) 424-9100
(TDD 202) 707-0744

## Head Injury

**National Head Injury Foundation**
1776 Massachusetts Avenue NW
Suite 100
Washington, DC 20036
(202) 296-6443

## Healthcare-Related Federal Agencies

**National Institute on Disability and Rehabilitation Research**
U.S. Department of Education
400 Maryland Avenue SW
Room 3060
Washington, DC 20202
(202) 732-1134

**Rehabilitation Services Administration**
Department of Human Services
605 G Street NW
Room 101M
Washington, DC 20001
(202) 727-3211

## Learning Disabilities

**A.D.D. Warehouse**
300 Northwest 70th Avenue
Suite 102
Plantation, FL 33317
(305) 792-8944

**Association for Children and Adults with Learning Disabilities**
4156 Library Road
Pittsburgh, PA 15234
(412) 341-8077

**Attention Disorders Association of Parents and Professionals Together (ADAPPT)**
P.O. Box 293
Oak Forest, IL 60452
(312) 361-4330

## Mental Health

**Mental Health Law Project**
1101 15th St. NW
Suite 1212
Washington, DC 20005

**National Mental Health Association**
1012 Prince Street
Alexandria, VA 22314-2971

## Mental Retardation

**Mental Retardation Association of America**
211 East 300 South
Suite 212
Salt Lake City, UT 84111

**National Association of Developmental Disabilities Councils**
1234 Massachusetts Avenue NW
Suite 103
Washington, DC 20005

## Neuromuscular Disorders

**Amyotrophic Lateral Sclerosis Association**
21021 Ventura Boulevard
Suite 321
Woodland Hills, CA 91364
(818) 990-2151

**Epilepsy Foundation of America**
4351 Garden City Drive
Landover, MD 20785
(301) 459-3700

**Guillain-Barré Syndrome Foundation International**
P.O. Box 262
Wynnewood, PA 19096
(215) 667-0131

**Muscular Dystrophy Association**
810 7th Avenue
New York, NY 10019
(212) 586-0808

**Myasthenia Gravis Foundation, Inc.**
53 W. Jackson Boulevard
Suite 660
Chicago, IL 60604
(312) 427-6252

**National Ataxia Foundation**
15500 Wayzata Boulevard
Suite 750
Wayzata, MN 55391
(612) 473-7666

**National Multiple Sclerosis Society**
205 E. 42nd Street
New York, NY 10017
(800) 624-8236

**Parkinson's Disease Foundation**
William Black Medical Research Building
Columbia Presbyterian Medical Center
650 W. 168th Street
New York, NY 10032
(800) 457-6676
(212) 923-4700

**United Cerebral Palsy Foundation Associations**
7 Penn Plaza, Suite 804
New York, NY 10001
(212) 268-6655

Spinal Cord

**National Spinal Cord Injury Association**
600 W. Cummings Park
Suite 2000
Woburn, MA 01801
(617) 935-2722

**New England Paralyzed Veterans of America**
1600 Providence Highway
Suite 101R
Walpole, MA 02081
(508) 660-1181

**Paralyzed Veterans of America**
801 18th Street NW
Washington, DC 20006
(202) 872-1300

Stroke

**National Institute of Neurological and Communicative Disorders and Stroke**
Building 31
Room 8A52
9000 Rockville Pike
Bethesda, MD 20892

**National Stroke Association**
300 E. Hampden Avenue
Suite 240
Englewood, CO 80110-2654
(303) 762-9922

**Stroke Clubs International**
805 12th Street
Galveston, TX 77550
(409) 762-1022

ADAPTIVE COMPUTERS

The following is a partial list of computer software and other adaptive equipment available to people with disabilities.

*The Alliance for Technology Access (ATA), formerly called the National Special Education Alliance, is a growing network of nonprofit resource centers located around the country that specializes in using computers to help individuals with disabilities. For more information on the ATA contact:*

**Foundation for Technology Access**
1307 Solano Avenue
Albany, CA 94706
(415) 528-0747

**TSI/VTEK**
455 N. Bernardo Avenue
Mountain View, CA 94039-7455
(800) 227-8418

*Large Print Display Processor, Braille Display Processor, Optacon II*

## Blindness

*Some Braille printers are able to print both Braille and standard text on the same page. This feature enables individuals who are blind to share their printed work with people who are sighted.*

**American Thermoform Corp.**
2311 Travers Avenue
City of Commerce, CA 90040
(213) 723-9021
Ohtsuki Printer (Braille)

**Enabling Technologies**
3102 S.E. Jay Street
Stuart, FL 33497
(407) 283-4817
Romeo Brailler

**Duxbury Systems, Inc.**
435 King Street
P.O. Box 1504
Littleton, MA 01460
(508) 486-9766

*Duxbury Braille Translator (software)*

## Head-Controlled Mouse

**Prentke Romich Company**
1022 Heyl Road
Wooster, OH 44691
(800) 642-8255

*Headmaster Workstation*

**Pointer Systems, Inc.**
One Mill Street
Burlington, VT 05401
(800) 537-1562

*Freewheel*

## Outliners (Thought Processors)

*In many instances, outlining software can be used in place of a word processor, and for people with learning disabilities, outlining software may be the best place to start almost any kind of writing.*

**Symmetry Corporation**
761 E. University Drive, #C
Mesa, AZ 85203
(800) 624-2485
Acta Advantage

**MECC**
3490 Lexington Avenue North
St. Paul, MN 55126
(612) 481-3500
MECC Outliner

## Computerized Speech Tools

**American Speech-Language and Hearing Association**
10801 Rockville Pike
Rockville, MD 20852
(301) 897-5700

**United States Society for Augmentative and Alternative Communication**
c/o Barkley Memorial Center
University of Nebraska
Lincoln, NE 68588
(402) 472-5463

## Voice Recognition Systems

*Voice recognition systems hold enormous potential for individuals with movement limitations; they effectively control the computer without any physical interaction taking place between the person and computer.*

**Articulate Systems, Inc.**
2380 Ellsworth Street
Berkeley, CA 94720
(415) 549-1013
Voice Navigator

**Voice Connection**
17835 Skypark Circle
Suite C
Irvine, CA 92714
(714) 261-2366
IntroVoice

Newsletters and Magazines

**Assistive Device News**
Central Pennsylvania Special
Education Regional Resource Center
150 South Progress Avenue
Harrisburg, PA 17109
(717) 367-1161

*The Assistive Device News is published by the Pennsylvania Assistive Device Center located at the Elizabethtown Hospital and Rehabilitation Center. The newsletter contains information about technology solutions for individuals with physical impairments.*

**Augmentative Communication News**
One Surf Way
Suite 215
Monterey, CA 93940
(408) 649-3050

*The Augmentative Communication News is a professional journal that focuses on augmentative communication, integration theory, technology, assessment, treatment, and the education of users who rely on augmentative communication systems.*

# Glossary

**4MAT system**  A learning style model based on Kolb's model combined with right/left brain research.

**abstract conceptualization**  A term used by Kolb as one of two ways of processing information; known as the "thinking" mode.

**accommodator**  One of the four learning style types according to Kolb's theory, combining the learning modes of concrete experience and active experimentation.

**acculturation**  Describes an individual's adaptation to the customs, values, beliefs, and behaviors of a new country or culture.

**active experimentation**  A term used by Kolb as one of two ways of processing information; known as the "doing" mode.

**acuity**  The degree of complexity of a patients' illness state, indicating a high level of required care.

**adaptive computing**  The professional services and the technology (both hardware and software) that make computing technology accessible for persons with disabilities.

**adherence**  Commitment or attachment to a prescribed, predetermined regimen.

**affective domain**  One of three domains in the taxonomy of behavioral objectives; deals with attitudes, values, and beliefs.

**ageism**  Prejudice against the older adult that perpetuates the negative stereotyping of aging as a period of decline.

**aids**  See *instructional materials/tools*.

**analogue**  A type of model that uses analogy to explain something by comparing it to something else. The model performs like the real object, although its actual appearance may differ. A dialysis machine and the use of a description of a pump to explain how the kidneys and heart work respectively are examples of analogues.

**andragogy**  The art and science of helping adults learn; a term coined by Malcolm Knowles to describe his theory of adult learning.

**animistic thinking**  The tendency of preschoolers to endow inanimate objects with life and consciousness; the belief that objects possess human characteristics.

**appearance**  As an important feature of instructional tools, it is the way printed and display materials look to the reader. Appearance is a vital element in determining the effectiveness of media in capturing and holding the learner's attention through adequate use of white space, minimal use of words to convey the message, use of illustrations to break up blocks of print, and use of contrasts in color or shading.

**assess**  To gather, summarize, and interpret pertinent data about the learner to make a decision or plan.

**assessment phase**  The first phase of the educational cycle, which provides the foundation for the rest of the educational process.

**assessment**  The process of systematically collecting data to determine the relative magnitude, importance, or value of needs, problems, and strengths of the learner to decide a direction for action.

**assimilation**  The willingness of a person emigrating to a new culture to gradually adopt and incorporate the characteristics of the prevailing culture.

**assimilator**  One of the four learning style types, according to Kolb's theory, combining the learning modes of abstract conceptualization and reflective observation.

**attention deficit disorder (ADD)**   A disorder of children with prominent attentional difficulties as demonstrated by inattention and impulsivity that are signs of developmentally inappropriate behavior.

**audio learning resources**   Instructional tools whose chief characteristic is exploitation of the learners' sense of hearing as a mechanism for teaching. Audiotapes and recorders are examples.

**audiovisual materials (tools)**   Nonprint instructional media that can influence all three domains of learning and stimulate the senses of hearing and/or sight to help convey the message to the learner. This category includes five major types: projected, audio, video, telecommunications, and computer formats.

**augmented feedback**   An opinion or conveyance of a message through oral or body language by the teacher to the learner about how well he or she performed a psychomotor skill.

**autonomy**   The right to self-determination.

**avoidance conditioning**   A type of negative reinforcement whereby an unpleasant stimulus is anticipated rather than directly applied and the person avoids doing something they do not want to do when faced with a fearful event.

**barriers to education**   Those factors that impede the nurse's ability to deliver educational services.

**behavioral (learning) objectives**   Intended outcomes of the education process that are action oriented rather than content oriented and learner centered rather than teacher centered.

**behaviorist learning**   One of the five major learning theories. According to behaviorists, the focus for learning is mainly on what is directly observable, and learning is viewed as the product of the stimulus conditions (S) and the responses (R) that follow. It is sometimes termed the S-R model of learning.

**beneficence**   The principle of doing good.

**bodily-kinesthetic intelligence**   A term used by Gardner to describe children who learn by processing knowledge through bodily sensations.

**brain injury**   Irreversible cerebral cell damage to neurons and axons resulting in degrees of difficulty with learning.

**brain preference indicator (BPI)**   A learning style instrument used to determine hemispheric dominance.

**breach of contract**   Failure, without legal excuse, to perform a promise. Violation of a binding agreement or obligation in the performance of professional duties.

**causal thinking**   The ability of school-aged children to understand cause and effect through logic, concrete thinking, and inductive and deductive reasoning.

**chronic illness**   A disease or disability that is permanent and can never be completely cured. It constitutes the number one medical malady of people in this country and affects the physical, psychosocial, economic, and spiritual aspects of an individual's life.

**clientele factors**   As one of three main categories of elements in any instructional setting, client variables may positively or negatively influence the success of teaching strategies and learning outcomes in the delivery of healthcare education.

**Cloze procedure**   A standardized test to measure comprehension of written materials (particularly recommended for health education literature) based on systematically deleting every fifth word from a portion of a text and having the reader fill in the blanks.

**cognitive ability**   The extent to which information can be processed, indicative of the level at which the learner is capable of learning; of major importance when designing instruction.

**cognitive development perspective**   Focuses on the qualitative changes in perceiving, thinking, and reasoning as individuals grow and mature based on how external events are conceptualized, organized, and represented within each person's mental framework or schema.

**cognitive development**   The process of acquiring more complex and adaptive ways of thinking as an individual grows from infancy to adulthood according to Piaget's four stages of cognitive maturation: sensorimotor, preoperational, concrete operations, and formal operations.

**cognitive domain**   One of three domains in the taxonomy of behavioral objectives; deals with aspects of behavior focusing on the way in which someone thinks in acquiring facts, concepts, principles, etc.

**cognitive learning**  One of the five major learning theories, according to a cognitive theorist's perspective, in order to learn, individuals change as a result of the way they perceive, process, interpret, and organize information based on what is already known; the reorganization of information leads to new insights and understanding.

**commercially prepared materials**  Predesigned, cost-effective printed educational materials that are widely available on a wide range of topics for purchase by educators as supplements to teaching-learning, such as brochures, pamphlets, books, posters, etc.

**compliance**  Submission or yielding to predetermined goals through regimens prescribed or established by others.

**comprehension**  The degree to which individuals understand what they have read or heard; the ability to grasp the meaning of a verbal or nonverbal message.

**computer literacy**  The ability to use the necessary computer hardware and software to meet the needs for information.

**computer-assisted instruction (CAI)**  A nontraditional, individualized instructional method of self-study using the high technology of the computer to deliver an educational activity. The interactive capability of CAI holds enormous potential for reinforcing learning, primarily in the cognitive domain, and its efficacy is dependent on programmatic software, hardware, and the learner's familiarity with and motivation to use this technology.

**concrete experience**  A term used by Kolb to describe a dimension of perceiving; known as the "feeling" mode.

**concrete operations period**  As defined by Piaget, this is the third stage in the cognitive development of children when the school-aged child (ages 6 to 12 years) is capable of logical thought processes and the ability to reason but the child is still incapable of abstract thinking.

**concrete sequential**  A term used by Gregoric to describe learners who tend to operate in a highly structured, conservative manner. Details and time schedules are critical to these learners.

**confidentiality**  A binding social contract or covenant; a professional obligation to respect privileged information between the health professional and the client.

**Constructivism**  See *Social Constructivist Perspective*

**consumer informatics**  A discipline that analyzes consumers' needs for information, studies and implements methods of making information accessible to consumers, and models and integrates consumer preferences into medical information systems. Also referred to as *consumer health informatics.*

**content evaluation**  A systematic assessment taking place immediately after the learning experience to determine the degree to which learners have acquired the knowledge or skills taught during a teaching/learning session.

**content**  The actual information that is communicated to the learner through various teaching methods and tools.

**contracting**  A popular, relatively recent means of facilitating learning through informal or formal agreements that delineate and promote learning objectives.

**converger**  One of the four learning style types according to Kolb's theory, combining the learning modes of abstract conceptualization and active experimentation.

**corpus callosum**  The connector between the two hemispheres of the brain.

**cosmopolitan orientation**  Persons with a worldly perspective on life who are receptive to new ideas and opportunities to learn new ways of doing things; a component of experiential readiness.

**cost benefit**  "Money well spent." Cost of services (e.g., education) ensures return of satisfied clients and stability of the economic base of a healthcare facility.

**cost recovery**  Occurs when revenues generated are equal to or greater than expenditures.

**cost savings**  Monies realized through decreased use of expensive services, shortened length of stay, or fewer complications resulting from preventive services or patient education.

**cost-benefit analysis**  The relationship between cost and outcomes that can be expressed in monetary terms; also called a *cost-benefit ratio.*

**cost-benefit ratio**  Relationship (expressed as a ratio) of program costs to economic benefits gained by the healthcare institution.

**cost-effectiveness analysis**  The efficiency of an educational offering when an actual monetary value cannot be assigned to a program.

**crystallized intelligence**  The intellectual ability developed over a lifetime, which includes such elements as vocabulary, general information, understanding of social interactions, arithmetic reasoning, and capacity to evaluate experiences, which tends to increase over time as a person ages.

**cuing**  Using prompts and reminders to get a learner to perform routine tasks by focusing on an appropriate combination of time and situation.

**cultural assessment**  An organized, systematic appraisal of beliefs, values, and practices of an individual or group to determine client needs as a basis for planning nursing care interventions.

**cultural awareness**  The process of becoming sensitive to the interactions with other cultural groups by examining one's biases and prejudices toward others of another culture or ethnic background.

**cultural brokerage**  Also known as *cultural negotiation*, this process involves translating messages, instructions, and belief systems between the nurse and client to determine the health problem(s) and preferred treatment(s).

**cultural competence**  The ability to demonstrate knowledge and understanding of another person's culture and accept and respect cultural differences by adapting interventions to be congruent with that specific culture when delivering care.

**cultural diversity**  Interacting with others who represent different cultures from one's own culture.

**cultural encounter**  The process of exposing oneself in nursing practice to cross-cultural interactions with clients of diverse cultural backgrounds.

**cultural knowledge**  The process of acquiring an educational foundation about various cultural world views.

**cultural literacy**  The ability of knowing how to communicate with someone from another culture without having to explain undertones,

voice intonations, and message contexts during a conversation.

**cultural relativism**  The values and behaviors every human group assigns to its conventions, which arise out of its own historical background and can only be accurately interpreted and understood in the light of that group's cultural world view.

**cultural skill**  The process of learning how to conduct an accurate cultural assessment.

**culturally Competent Model of Care**  A model for conducting a thorough and sensitive cultural assessment that includes the four components of cultural awareness, cultural knowledge, cultural skill, and cultural encounter.

**culture**  A complex concept that is an integral part of each person's life and includes knowledge, beliefs, values, morals, customs, traditions, and habits acquired by the members of a society.

**culturological assessment**  A systematic appraisal or examination of the cultural beliefs, values, and practices of individuals, groups, and communities to determine explicit needs and intervention practices within the cultural context of the people being evaluated.

**delivery system**  The physical form of instructional materials, including durable equipment used to present these materials, such as film and projectors, audiotapes and tape players, and computer programs and computers.

**demonstration materials**  Tools that stimulate the senses by combining sight with touch, smell, and sometimes even taste with the advantage of helping to teach cognitive and psychomotor skill development. Major forms of media in this category include many types of nonprint media, such as models, real equipment, diagrams, charts, posters, displays, photographs, and drawings.

**demonstration**  A traditional instructional method by which the learner is shown by the teacher how to perform a particular psychomotor skill.

**deontological**  The ethical notion of the "Golden Rule" promulgated by the sixteenth-century philosopher Immanuel Kant.

**desirable needs**  Learning needs of the client that are not life dependent but related to well-being and can be met by the overall ability of nursing staff to provide quality care.

**determinants of learning**  Consist of learning needs, readiness to learn, and learning styles.

**developmental disability**  A disorder that manifests itself during the developmental period when a child demonstrates subaverage general intellectual functioning with concurrent deficits in adaptive behaviors. Sometimes referred to as mental retardation or developmental delay.

**developmental stages**  Milestones marking changes in the physical, cognitive, and psychosocial growth of an individual over time from infancy to old age.

**digital divide**  The gap between those individuals who have access to information technology resources and those who do not.

**direct costs**  Tangible, predictable costs associated with expenditures for personnel, equipment, etc.

**disability**  Inability to perform some key life functions; often used interchangeably with the term *functional limitation.*

**discharge planning**  An interdisciplinary process, highly dependent on patient educational interventions for effectiveness, by which members of the healthcare team (often led by nurses) plan and coordinate services for the purpose of providing continuity of care to patients and their families between various care settings.

**discrimination learning**  The ability to differentiate, with more and varied practice, among similar stimuli.

**displays**  Type of demonstration materials, frequently regarded as static, which may be permanently installed or portable. Included in this category are chalkboards, flip charts, and posters.

**distance learning**  A flexible telecommunications method of instruction using video or computer technology to transmit live, on-line, or taped messages directly between the instructor and the learner who are separated from one another by time and/or location.

**diverger**  One of the four learning style types according to Kolb's theory, combining the learning modes of concrete experience and reflective observation.

**domains of learning**  Cognitive, psychomotor, and affective are the three domains in which learning occurs.

**Dunn and Dunn Learning Style Inventory**  A self-reporting instrument that is used in the identification of how individuals prefer to function, learn, concentrate, and perform in learning activities.

**duty**  Responsibility; professional expectation.

**dysarthria**  Difficulty with voluntary muscle control of speech due to damage to the central or peripheral nervous system that controls muscles essential to speaking and swallowing. Types of dysarthria include flaccid, spastic, ataxic, hypokinetic, or mixed. Persons with degenerative neurologic diseases often suffer with this disorder.

**education process**  A systematic, sequential, planned course of action that parallels the nursing process and consists of two interdependent operations, teaching and learning, which form a continuous cycle to include assessment of the learner, establishment of a teaching plan, implementation of teaching methods and tools, and evaluation of the learner, teacher, and education program.

**education**  An overall umbrella term used to describe the process, including the components of teaching and instruction, of producing observable or measurable behavioral changes (in knowledge, attitudes, and/or skills) in the learner through planned educational activities.

**educational contracting**  See *learning contract.*

**educational objectives**  See *instructional objectives*

**educator role**  The teaching role a nurse assumes in supporting, encouraging, and assisting the learner to put learning of behaviors (knowledge, skills, and attitudes) into meaningful parts and wholes to reach an optimum potential of functioning.

**edutainment**  Computer games as educational software that are disguised in a game format.

**e-learning**  An abbreviation for electronic learning, which professional development and training organizations have capitalized on by using the power of computer technology to provide learning solutions for workforce training; it involves the use of technology-based tools and processes to provide for customized learning anytime or anywhere.

**e-mail**   An Internet-based activity that is a quick, inexpensive, and increasingly popular way to communicate asynchronously via the computer.

**embedded figures test (EFT)**   A test designed to measure how a person's perception of the environment (field independence/dependence) is influenced by the context in which it appears.

**emoticons**   Symbols commonly used to represent emotions, such as a ☺ (smiley face) or ;) (winking), by people who are sending e-mail messages.

**emotional readiness**   A state of psychological willingness to learn, which is dependent on such factors as anxiety level, support system, motivation, risk-taking behavior, frame of mind, and psychosocial developmental stage.

**environmental factors**   As one of three main categories of elements in any instructional setting, variables in the environment may positively or negatively influence the success of teaching strategies and learning outcomes in the delivery of health education.

**escape conditioning**   An individual's response that causes an unpleasant or uncomfortable stimulation to cease.

**ethical rights and duties**   A term that refers to the norms or standards of behavior of healthcare professionals.

**ethics**   Guiding principles of human behavior.

**ethnicity**   A dynamic and complex concept referring to how members of a group perceive themselves and how, in turn, they are perceived by others in relation to the population subgroup's common heritage of customs, characteristics, language, and history.

**ethnocentrism**   A concept in which the belief is held that one's own culture is superior and all other cultures are less sophisticated.

**ethnomedical**   A cultural orientation delineating the nature and consequences of illness problems and disease interventions rather than adhering to the biomedical orientation of defining diseases and illness interventions. In this context, the concept of illness incorporates the relationship of humans with their universe, bridging culture with a sensitivity toward the daily practices inherent within specific ethnic groups.

**evaluation research**   Scientific inquiry applied to a specific program or activity to determine processes, outcomes, and/or their relationship.

**evaluation**   A systematic and continuous process by which the significance of something is judged; the process of collecting and using information to determine what has been accomplished and how well it has been accomplished to guide decision making.

**experiential readiness**   A state of willingness to learn based on such factors as an individual's past experiences with learning, cultural background, previous coping mechanisms, and locus of control.

**expressive aphasia**   An absence or impairment of the ability to communicate through speech or writing due to a dysfunction in the Broca's area of the brain, which is the center of the cortex that controls motor abilities.

**external locus of control**   An individual's motivation to learn comes from outside oneself, attributing success or failure of an action to luck, the nature of the task, or to the efforts of someone else.

**extraversion-introversion (EI)**   Terms used to describe behavior that reflects an orientation to either the outside world of people or to the inner world of concepts and ideas; one of four dichotomous preference dimensions in the Myers-Briggs Type Indicator.

**extrinsic feedback**   A response provided by the teacher through the sharing of opinion or the conveying of a message through body language about how well a learner has performed; often used in relation to psychomotor skill performance.

**field dependence**   One of two styles of learning in the cognitive domain identified by Witkin in which a person's perception of the environment is immersed in and influenced by the surrounding field.

**field independence**   One of two styles of learning in the cognitive domain identified by Witkin in which a person's perception of the environment is separate from the surrounding field.

**fixed costs**   Predictable and controllable expenses that remain stable over time.

**Flesch formula**   An objective, statistical measurement tool for readability of written materials between fifth grade and college level, based on a count of the two basic language elements of average sentence length in words of selected samples and of average word length measured as syllables per 100 words of sample.

**fluid intelligence** The intellectual capacity to perceive relationships, to reason, and to perform abstract thinking, which declines over time as degenerative changes occur with aging.

**focus groups** Optimally 4 to 12 potential learners grouped together for the purpose of identifying points of view or knowledge about a certain topic. A facilitator leads the discussion by asking questions.

**Fog formula** An index appropriate for use in determining readability of materials from fourth grade to college level based on average sentence length and the percentage of multisyllabic words in a 100-word passage.

**formal operations period** As defined by Piaget, this is the fourth and final stage of cognitive development in which the adolescent (ages 12 to 18 years) is capable of abstract thought, internalization of ideas, complex logical reasoning, and understanding causality.

**formal settings** Scheduled sessions in which teaching-learning takes place.

**format** The general physical appearance of a book, pamphlet, or other printed materials, which includes such characteristics as the type face, the margins, the organization of information, the quality of the paper, etc.

**formative evaluation** Also referred to as *process evaluation*. It is a systematic and continuous assessment of success of the teaching process made during the implementation of materials, methods, and activities to control, ensure, or improve the quality of performance in delivery of an educational program.

**Four-Step Appraisal of Needs** A systematic approach for assessing learning needs of caregivers and the healthcare organizations in which they practice.

**Fry formula** A measurement tool for testing the readability of materials (especially books, pamphlets, and brochures) at the level of first grade through college by using a graph to plot the number of syllables of words and the number of sentences in three 100-word samples.

**functional illiteracy** The lack of fundamental education skills needed by adults to read, write,

or comprehend information below the fifth-grade level of difficulty to function effectively in today's society; the inability to read well enough to understand and interpret written information for use as intended.

**functional magnetic resonance imaging (FMRI)** A type of advanced technology that has revolutionized the field of neuroscience by making colorful images on computer monitors of the brain to determine the possible areas of nerve activity involved in the processes of thinking, emotions, and recall.

**gaming** A nontraditional instructional method requiring the learner to participate in a competitive activity (which may or may not reflect reality) with preset rules.

**Gardner's seven types of intelligence** A theory that describes the styles of learning in children.

**gender-related cognitive abilities** A comparison between the sexes as to how males and females act, react, and perform in situations affecting every sphere of life as a result of genetic and environmental influences on behavior.

**gerogogy** The art and science of teaching the elderly.

**Gestalt perspective** Emphasizes the importance of perception in learning, with a focus on the configuration or organization of a pattern of stimuli.

**goal** A desirable outcome to be achieved by the learner at the end of the teaching–learning process; goals are global and more future oriented and long-term in nature than the specific, short-term objectives that lead step by step to the final achievement of a goal.

**Gregorc Style Delineator** A self-analysis instrument designed to assess a person's learning style with respect to perceiving, ordering, processing, and relating information.

**group discussion** A commonly employed, traditional method of instruction whereby a group of learners (ideally 3 to 20 people) gather together to exchange information, feelings, and opinions with each other and the teacher; the activity is learner centered and subject centered.

**habilitation** Includes all the activities and interactions that enable individuals with a disability to develop new abilities to achieve their maximum potential.

**hardware**   Part of the delivery system for many types of media (e.g., computers, projectors, tape players).

**Health Belief Model**   A framework or paradigm used to explain or predict health behavior composed of the interaction between individual perceptions, modifying factors, and likelihood of action.

**health education**   A participatory educational approach, often used interchangeably with the term *patient education* or *client education*, aimed at preventing disease, promoting positive health, and incorporating the physical, mental, and social aspects of learning needs.

**health literacy**   Refers to how well an individual can read, interpret, and comprehend health information for maintaining an optimal level of wellness.

**Health Promotion Model**   A framework that describes the interaction of health-promoting factors including cognitive perceptual factors, modifying factors, and likelihood of participation in health promoting behaviors.

**healthcare setting**   One of three classifications of instructional settings, in which the delivery of health care is the primary or sole function of an institution, organization, or agency. Examples: hospitals, visiting nurse associations, public health departments, outpatient clinics, physician offices, health maintenance organizations, extended-care facilities, and nurse-managed centers.

**healthcare team**   An interdisciplinary group of healthcare professionals and nonprofessionals who provide services to the patient and family members in an attempt to maximize optimal health and well-being of the client to whom their activities are directed.

**healthcare-related setting**   One of three classifications of instructional settings, in which healthcare-related services are offered as a complementary function of a quasihealth agency. Examples: American Heart Association, American Cancer Society, Muscular Dystrophy Association, and Leukemia Society of America.

**hearing impairment**   A complete loss or a reduction in sensitivity to sounds by persons who are deaf or hard of hearing.

**hidden costs**   Costs that cannot be predicted or accounted for until after the fact.

**hierarchy of needs**   Theory of human motivation based on integrated wholeness of the individual and levels of satisfaction of basic human needs organized by potency.

**historically underrepresented groups**   A more politically sensitive and correct term to substitute for the term *minority.*

**humanistic learning**   One of the five major learning theories, which views learning as being facilitated by curiosity, needs, a positive self-concept, and open situations where freedom of choice and individuality are promoted and respected.

**ideology**   Thoughts, attitudes and beliefs that reflect the social needs and desires of an individual or ethnocultural group.

**illiteracy**   The total inability of adults to read, write, or comprehend information.

**illusionary representations**   A category of instructional materials that depict realism, such as dimensionality. Examples are photographs, drawings, and audiotapes, which depend on imagination to fill in the gaps and offer the learner experiences that simulate reality.

**iloralacy**   The inability to understand simple oral language.

**imaginary audience**   A belief or obsession by adolescents that everyone is focusing on them and their activities, which has considerable influence over teenagers' behavior.

**impact evaluation**   The process of assessing outcomes or effects of an educational activity that extend beyond the activity itself to address organizational and/or societal effects.

**indirect costs**   Costs that may be fixed but are not necessarily directly related to an educational activity (e.g., heating, electricity, housekeeping).

**informal settings**   Unplanned or spontaneous sessions in which teaching-learning takes place.

**informatics**   See *consumer informatics.*

**Information Age**   The present period of time, in which sweeping advances in computer and information technology have transformed the economic, social, and cultural life of society.

**information literacy**   The ability to access, evaluate, organize, and use information from a variety of sources.

**information processing perspective** Emphasizes the process of memory functioning in the way information is encountered, organized, stored, and retrieved.

**input disability** A general category of learning disability that refers to the process of receiving and recording information in the brain, which includes visual, auditory, perceptual and integrative processing, such as dyslexia and short- and long-term memory disorders.

**instruction** Often used interchangeably with teaching, it is in fact one aspect of teaching that involves the communicating of information about a specific skill in the cognitive, affective, or psychomotor domain with the objective of producing learning.

**instructional materials/tools** The resources or vehicles used to help communicate information, which include both print and nonprint media, to aid teaching-learning by stimulating the various senses such as vision and hearing. These are intended to supplement, not replace, actual teaching. Synonymous terms are *educational aids* or *audiovisual materials*.

**instructional method** A traditional or nontraditional technique or approach used by the teacher to bring the learner into contact with the content to be learned; a way or a process to communicate and share information with the learner.

**instructional objectives** Intended outcomes of the education process that are in reference to an aspect of a program or a total program of study that are content-oriented and teacher-centered; also referred to as educational objectives.

**instructional setting** A situation or area in which health teaching takes place as classified on the basis of what relationship health education has to the primary function of an organization, agency, or institution in which the teaching occurs.

**instructional strategy** See *teaching strategy*.

**internal locus of control** Individuals are motivated from within to learn, attributing success or failure to their own ability or effort.

**Internet** A huge global computer network, of which the World Wide Web is a component, established to allow transfer (exchange) of information from one computer to another; it provides a diverse range of services used to deliver information to large numbers of people and to enable people to communicate with one another, such as via e-mail, real-time chat, electronic discussion groups, or Usenet newsgroups.

**interpersonal intelligence** A term used by Gardner to describe children who learn best in groups.

**intrapersonal intelligence** A term used by Gardner to describe children who learn well with independent self-paced instruction.

**intrinsic feedback** A response that is generated within the self, giving learners a sense of or a feel for how they have performed; often used in relation to a psychomotor skill performance.

**judgment-perception (JP)** Terms used to describe behavior that reflects the way a person comes to a conclusion about something or becomes aware of something; one of four dichotomous preference dimensions in the Myers-Briggs Type Indicator.

**justice** The equal distribution of benefits and burdens.

**knowledge deficit** A gap in what a learner needs or wants to know; this category of nursing diagnosis can include learning needs in the cognitive, affective, and psychomotor domains.

**knowledge readiness** A state of willingness to learn dependent on such factors as the learner's present knowledge base, the level of learning capability, and the preferred style of learning.

**Kolb's Learning Style Inventory** An experiential learning model that includes four modes of learning reflecting the dimensions of perception and processing.

**law** A clearly stated pronouncement of a binding custom, enforceable by a controlling body.

**layout** The arrangement of printed and/or graphic information on a flat surface. Effective use of white space, graphics, and wording will depend heavily on this arrangement.

**learner characteristics** One of the three major variables that refers to the learner's perceptual abilities, reading ability, self-direction, and learning style, which must be considered when making appropriate choices of instructional materials.

**learning contract** A mutually-agreed-on specific plan of action between the learner and educator clearly defining the specific behavioral objectives and predetermined goal to be achieved as a result of instruction. Also referred to as an educational contract.

**learning curve** Also sometimes referred to as the *experience curve*, it is a record of an individual's improvement in psychomotor skill development made by measuring his or her ability at different stages during a specified time period, which includes six stages: negligible progress, increasing gains, decreasing gains, plateau, renewed gains, and approach to limit.

**learning disability (LD)** A generic term that refers to a heterogeneous group of disorders manifested by significant difficulties with learning. Inattention and impulsivity are signs indicating developmentally inappropriate behavior.

**learning needs** Gaps in knowledge that exist between a desired level of performance and the actual level of performance; what the learner needs to know.

**learning styles** The manner by which (how) individuals perceive and then process information. Certain characteristics of style are biological in origin, whereas others are sociologically developed as a result of environmental influences.

**learning theory** A coherent framework and set of integrated constructs and principles that describe, explain, or predict how people learn.

**learning** A conscious or unconscious permanent change in behavior as a result of a lifelong, dynamic process by which individuals acquire new knowledge, skills, and/or attitudes that can be measured and can occur at anytime or in any place due to exposure to environmental stimuli.

**lecture** The oldest, most commonly used, and most traditional instructional method by which the teacher verbally transmits information in a highly structured format directly to a group of learners.

**legal rights and duties** A term that refers to rules governing behavior or conduct of healthcare professionals that are enforceable under threat of punishment or penalty, such as a fine, imprisonment, or both.

**legally blind** A person's vision is 20/200 or less in the better eye with correction, or if visual field limits in both eyes are within 20 degrees diameter.

**linguistic intelligence** A term used by Gardner to describe children who have highly developed auditory skills and think in words.

**listening test** A standardized test to measure comprehension using a selected passage from an instructional material written at approximately the fifth-grade level that is read aloud at a normal rate to determine what a person understands and remembers when listening.

**listserv** An automated mailing list software program that copies messages and distributes them to all subscribers.

**literacy** The ability of adults to read, understand, and interpret information written at the eighth-grade level or above. An umbrella term used to describe socially required and expected reading and writing abilities; the relative ability of persons to use printed and written material commonly encountered in daily life.

**locus of control (LOC)** The location of control of behaviors as either self-directed or directed by others. Persons with internal or external locus of control differ particularly in the degree of responsibility taken for their own actions (see also *Internal Locus of Control* and *External Locus of Control*).

**logical-mathematical intelligence** A term used by Gardner to describe children who are strong in exploring patterns, categories, and relationships of objects.

**low literacy** The ability of adults to read, write, and comprehend information between the fifth and the eighth-grade level of difficulty (also referred to as marginally literate or marginally illiterate).

**malpractice** Failure to exercise an accepted degree of professional skill or learning by one rendering professional services that results in injury, loss, or damage to the recipient of those services.

**mandatory needs** Requisites to be learned for survival or situations where the learner's life or safety is threatened.

**marginally literate** A term to describe a person with low literacy skills; also known as *marginally illiterate.*

**media characteristics** One of the three major variables that refers to the form through which information will be communicated, which must be considered when making appropriate choices of instructional materials.

**media/medium** The form in which information or ideas are conveyed to learners.

**mental illness** A mental disability that may be acute or chronic, which affects a member or members of one in five families in the United States.

**message** See *content.*

**minority groups** The four major groups in this country include Blacks, Hispanics, Asian/Pacific Islanders, and American Indians as defined by the U.S. Census Bureau; a more politically sensitive term is *historically underrepresented groups.*

**models** Three-dimensional instructional tools that allow the learner to immediately apply knowledge and psychomotor skills by observing, examining, manipulating, handling, assembling, and disassembling objects while the teacher provides feedback. Replicas, analogues, and symbols are all types of models that enhance instruction by means that range from concrete to abstract.

**moral rights and duties** A term that refers to an internal value system, a certain "moral fabric," that is expressed externally in ethical behaviors of healthcare professionals; often used interchangeably with the terms *morality* and *morals.*

**morals** Synonymous with *ethics;* a value system.

**motivation** A psychological force that moves a person to take action in the direction of meeting a need or goal, evidenced by willingness or readiness to act.

**motivational axioms** Premises on which an understanding of motivation is based, such as a state of optimum anxiety, learner readiness, realistic goal setting, learner satisfaction/success, and uncertainty-reducing or uncertainty-maintaining dialogue.

**motivational incentives** Factors that influence motivation in the direction of the desired goal.

**musical intelligence** A term used by Gardner to describe children who are talented in playing musical instruments, singing, dancing, and keeping rhythm and who often learn best with music playing in the background.

**Myers-Briggs Type Indicator (MBTI)** A self-report inventory that uses forced-choice questions and word pairs to measure four dichotomous dimensions of behavior.

**needs assessment** The process of determining through data collection what a person, group, organization, or community must learn or wants to learn to provide appropriate education programs to meet the required or desired needs of the learners.

**negligence** Doing or nondoing of an act, pursuant to a duty, that a reasonable person in the same circumstances would or would not do; the acting or the nonacting is the proximate cause of injury to another person or property.

**noncompliance** Nonsubmission or resistance of the individual to follow a prescribed, predetermined regimen.

**non-healthcare setting** One of three classifications of instructional settings in which health care is an incidental or supportive function of an organization, such as a business, industry, and school system.

**nonmalfeasance** The notion of doing no harm.

**nonprint instructional materials** Include the full range of audio and visual instructional materials, including demonstrations and displays.

**numeracy** The ability to read and interpret numbers.

**nurse practice acts** Legal provisions of each state defining nursing and the standards of nursing practice, usually including patient teaching as a professional responsibility to protect the public from incompetent practitioners.

**Nurse-Client Negotiations Model** A model developed for the purpose of cultural assessment and planning for care of culturally diverse people that recognizes the popular, professional, and folk arenas (sectors) as concepts to bridge the gap between the scientific perspectives of the nurse and the cultural perspectives of the client.

**nursing process** A model for nursing practice using the problem-solving approach, which includes the phases of assessment, nursing diagnosis, planning, implementation, and evaluation of patient care that parallels the *educational process.*

**objectives (behavioral)** Statements defining specific health activities, quantitatively measurable and descriptive of the intended results (rather than the process) of instruction, to be competently achieved by the learner in a finite period of time. Well-stated objectives reflect the characteristic components of performance, condition, and criteria.

**obstacles to learning**   Those factors that negatively affect the ability of the learner to attend to and process information.

**one-to-one instruction**   A common, traditional instructional method for exchange of information whereby the teacher delivers individual verbal instruction of learning activities in a format designed specifically to meet the needs of a particular learner.

**operant conditioning**   Focuses on the behavior of an organism as a result of a positive or negative reinforcer (stimulus or event) applied after a response that strengthens the probability that the response will be performed again; nonreinforcement and punishment decrease the likelihood that a response will continue to be performed.

**oral literacy**   The ability to comprehend the spoken word.

**organizational factors**   As one of three main categories of elements in any instructional setting, variables in the organization may positively or negatively influence the success of teaching strategies and learning outcomes in the delivery of health education.

**outcome evaluation**   See *summative evaluation.*

**outcome**   The result of actions that may be intended or unintended; synonymous with stated goals.

**output disability**   A general category of learning disability that refers to orally responding and performing physical tasks, which include language and motor disorders.

**pacing**   The speed at which information is presented to a learner.

**parochial orientation**   Persons who demonstrate close-mindedness in thinking, conservativeness, and less willingness to learn new material and who place trust in traditional authority figures; a component of experiential readiness.

**patient education**   A process of assisting consumers of health care to learn how to incorporate health-related behaviors (knowledge, skills, and/or attitudes) into everyday life with the purpose of achieving the goal of optimal health.

**pedagogy**   The art and science of helping children to learn.

**PEMs**   See *printed education materials.*

**personal fable**   A belief by adolescents that they are invincible and invulnerable to outside forces.

**physical maturation**   Change in an individual's physical characteristics as a result of normal body growth and development during the aging process.

**physical readiness**   A state of willingness to learn that is dependent on such factors as measures of physical ability, complexity of task, health status, and gender.

**pooled ignorance**   Lack of knowledge or information about issues or problems prior to a group discussion session, whereby clients cannot adequately learn from one another if they do not possess a basic, accurate understanding of a subject to draw on for purposes of discourse.

**portfolio**   A method for evaluation of an individual's learning over time.

**Positron emission tomography (PET)**   A type of technology that has revolutionized the field of neuroscience by making images of the brain to detect which possible areas of the brain are used for cognating, feeling, and remembering.

**possible needs**   "Nice to know" information that is not essential at a given point in time or in situations in which learning is not directly related to daily activities.

**posters**   A type of display that combines print and nonprint media to help convey a message.

**poverty circle (cycle of poverty)**   A process whereby parents who are of low income and educational level produce children of low income and educational attainment, who grow up and repeat the process with their own children; a situation in which generation after generation are born into poverty by many factors, such as poor health care, limited resources, family stress, and low-paying jobs.

**precausal thinking**   Unawareness by preschoolers of causation by invisible and mechanical forces.

**PRECEDE-PROCEED Model**   A comprehensive epidemiological health promotion, planning, and evaluation model used in educational and environmental development.

**preoperational period**  As defined by Piaget, this is the second key milestone in the cognitive development of children when the child of the preschool age group (3 to 6 years) is acquiring language skills and gaining experience but thinking is precausal, animistic, egocentric, and intuitive, with only a vague understanding of relationships and multiple classifications of objects.

**presentation**  The form in which the message (content) is put forth, occurring along a continuum from real objects to symbols.

**printed education materials (PEMs)**  As the most common type of teaching tools, these include handouts, leaflets, books, pamphlets, brochures, and instruction sheets, which may be purchased or instructor developed.

**process evaluation**  See *formative evaluation*.

**Prochaska's Change Model**  See *Stages of Change Model*.

**Productivity Environmental Preference Survey (PEPS)**  The assessment tool used in the adult version of the Dunn and Dunn Learning Style Inventory.

**program evaluation**  A systematic assessment to determine the extent to which all activities for an entire department or program over a specified time period have accomplished the goals originally established.

**programmed instruction**  A type of self-study tool, usually printed or computerized, that takes the learner through the learning task step by step.

**projected learning resources**  Audiovisual instructional formats that depend primarily on the learners' sense of sight as the means through which messages are received. These resources require equipment to project images, usually in a darkened room, and include movies, slides, overhead transparencies, and others.

**Propositional reasoning**  The ability to think abstractly and use complex logical reasoning, which begins in the adolescent stage of development.

**psychodynamic learning**  One of the five major learning theories. Largely a theory of motivation stressing emotions rather than cognition and responses; this perspective emphasizes the importance of conscious and unconscious forces derived from earlier childhood experiences and conflicts that guide and change behavior.

**psychomotor domain**  One of three domains in the taxonomy of behavioral objectives, which is concerned with the physical activities of the body, such as coordination, reaction time, and muscular control, related to the acquisition of a skill or task.

**psychosocial development**  The process of psychological and social adjustment as an individual grows from infancy to adulthood according to Erickson's eight stages of the psychological and social maturation of humans: trust versus mistrust; autonomy versus shame and doubt; initiative versus guilt; industry versus inferiority; identity versus role confusion; intimacy versus isolation; generativity versus self-absorption and stagnation; and ego integrity versus despair.

**readability**  The level of reading difficulty at which printed teaching tools are written. A measure of those elements in a given text of printed material that influence with what degree of success a group of readers will be able to read and understand the information; the ease, or, conversely, the difficulty, with which a person can understand or comprehend the style of writing of a selected printed passage.

**readiness to learn**  The time when the learner is receptive to learning and is willing and able to participate in the learning process; preparedness or willingness to learn.

**reading**  Also known as *word recognition*, it is the process of transforming letters into words and being able to pronounce them correctly.

**realia**  The most concrete form of stimuli that can be used to deliver information. Example: a real person or a model being used to demonstrate a procedure such as breast self-examination.

**REALM (Rapid Estimate of Adult Literacy in Medicine)**  A reading skills test to measure a patient's ability to read medical and health-related vocabulary.

**receptive aphasia**  An absence or impairment of the ability to comprehend what is read or heard due to a dysfunction in the Wernicke's area of the brain, which controls sensory abilities. Although hearing is unimpaired, the person is unable to understand the significance of the spoken word and is unable to communicate verbally.

**reflective observation** A term used by Kolb to describe a dimension of perceiving; known as the "watching" mode.

**reflective practice** A notion of evaluation that includes the two components of *reflection-in-action*, when the nurse introspectively considers a practice activity while performing it so change for improvement can be made at that moment (formative evaluation), and *reflection-on-action*, when the nurse introspectively analyzes a practice activity after completion so as to gain insights for the future (summative evaluation).

**rehabilitation** The relearning of previous skills, which often requires an adjustment to altered functional abilities and altered lifestyle.

**repetition** A technique that strengthens learning by aiding in retention of information of new or difficult material through reinforcement of important points.

**replica** A facsimile constructed to scale that resembles the features or substance of the original object. It may be examined or manipulated by the learner to get an idea of how something works. Example: resuscitation dolls.

**respondeat superior** Master-servant rule; "let the master respond and answer."

**respondent conditioning** Emphasizes the importance of stimulus conditions and the associations formed in the learning process whereby, without thought or awareness, learning takes place when a newly conditioned stimulus (CS) becomes associated with a conditioned response (CR); also termed classical or Pavlovian conditioning.

**return demonstration** A traditional instructional method by which the learner attempts to perform a psychomotor skill, with cues or prompting as needed from the teacher.

**revenue generation** Income realized over and above costs; also called profit.

**role-modeling** The use of self as a role model, often overlooked as an instructional method, whereby the learner acquires new behaviors and social roles by identification with the role model.

**role-playing** A nontraditional method of instruction by which learners participate in an unrehearsed dramatization, acting out an assigned part of a character as they think the character would act in reality.

**SAM (Suitability Assessment of Materials)** An evaluation instrument designed to measure the appropriateness of print materials, illustrations, and video- and audiotaped instructions for a given patient population.

**selective attention** The process of recognizing and selecting appropriate and inappropriate stimuli.

**self-composed instructional materials** Printed instructional materials composed by individual instructors for the purposes of supplementing teaching.

**Self-Efficacy Theory** A framework that describes the belief that one is capable of accomplishing a specific behavior.

**self-instruction** A nontraditional method of instruction used by a teacher to provide or design teaching materials and activities that guide the learner in independently achieving the objectives of learning.

**self-study materials** Written materials that are designed to allow the learner to independently master understanding of concepts or tasks.

**sensing-intuition (SN)** Describes how individuals perceive the world, either directly through the five senses or indirectly by way of the unconscious; one of four dichotomous preference dimensions in the Myers-Briggs Type Indicator.

**sensorimotor period** As defined by Piaget, this is the first key milestone in the cognitive development of children in the age group of infancy to toddlerhood when learning is enhanced through movement and manipulation of objects in the environment via visual, auditory, tactile, olfactory, taste, and motor stimulation.

**sensory deficits** A category of common physical disabilities that includes, in particular, hearing and visual impairments.

**silent epidemic** A term used to describe the literacy problem in the United States; also known as the *silent barrier* or *silent disability*.

**simulation laboratories** A type of learning laboratory that contains real equipment in a lifelike setting, but that allows the learner to practice manipulating and using this equipment as a prelude to performing a task in a real-life situation. Frequently used to supplement the learning of psychomotor skills.

**simulation** A nontraditional method of instruction whereby an artificial or hypothetical experience is created that engages the learner in an activity reflecting real-life conditions but without the risk-taking consequences of an actual situation.

**skill inoculation** The opportunity for repeated practice of a behavioral task.

**SMOG formula** A relatively easy to use, popular, valid test of readability based on 100% comprehension of printed material from grade 4 to college level.

**social cognition perspective** An aspect of cognitive theory that highlights the influence of social factors on perception, thought, motivation, and behaviors.

**Social constructivist perspective** One of the more recent orientations of the cognitive learning theory that emphasizes the increasingly popular belief that learning and human development are significantly influenced by the constantly changing social and cultural context in which people live.

**social learning** One of five major learning theories, this theory is seen as a mixture of behaviorist, cognitive, and psychodynamic influences; much of learning is a social process that occurs by observation and watching other people's behavior to see what happens to them. Role-modeling is a central concept of this theory, with cognitive or psychodynamic aspects of internal processing and motivation sometimes considered in the learning process.

**socioeconomic status (SES)** Variation in health status, health behavior, or learning abilities among individuals of different social and economic levels.

**software** Computer programs and other instructional materials such as videotapes and overhead transparencies.

**Spache Grade-Level Score** A readability formula specifically designed to judge materials written for children at grade levels below the fourth grade (elementary grades first through third).

**spatial intelligence** A term used by Gardner to describe children who learn by images and pictures.

**spinal cord injury** Traumatic insult to the spinal cord resulting in alterations or complete disruption of normal motor, sensory, and autonomic functions.

**spontaneous recovery** A response, which appears to be extinguished, reappears at any time (even years later), especially when stimulus conditions are similar to those in the initial learning experience.

**staff education** A process of assisting nursing staff personnel to acquire knowledge, skills, or attitudes in nursing practice for the purpose of maintaining or improving their ability to deliver quality care to the consumer.

**Stages of Change Model** A model developed by Prochaska that informs the phenomenon of health behaviors of the learner, particularly applied to addictive and problem behaviors, and includes the six distinct stages of change: precontemplation, contemplation, preparation, action, maintenance, and termination.

**stereotyping** An oversimplified conception, opinion, or belief about some aspect of an individual or group.

**stimulus generalization** The tendency of initial learning experiences to be easily applied to other similar stimuli.

**story typing** A strategy used for low-level readers whereby, while audiotaping, patients listen to oral instruction, then repeat it in their own words, and the message is transcribed into a typed version using the patient's own phrases.

**subcultures** Ethnocultural groups of people who have experiences different from those of the dominant culture.

**Suitability Assessment of Materials** See SAM.

**summative evaluation** Systematic assessment of the degree to which individuals have learned or objectives have been met as a result of education intervention; also referred to as outcome evaluation.

**support system** Resources and significant others, such as family and friends, on whom the patient relies or is dependent for information or assistance in managing activities of daily living and who may serve as a positive or negative influence on teaching efforts.

**syllogistic reasoning** The ability of school-aged children to consider two premises and draw a logical conclusion from them.

**symbol** A type of model that conveys a message to the learner through the use of abstract constructs, like words, that stand for the real thing. Cartoons and printed materials are examples of symbolic forms of a message.

**symbolic representations** Numbers and words, symbols written and spoken to convey ideas or represent objects, which are the most common form of communication and yet are the most abstract types of messages.

**tailoring** Coordinating a patient's treatment regimens into their daily schedules by allowing new tasks to be associated with old behaviors.

**task characteristics** One of the three major variables defined by the behavioral objectives in the cognitive, affective, and psychomotor domains of learning, which must be considered when making appropriate choices of instructional materials.

**taxonomic hierarchy** See *taxonomy*.

**taxonomy** A form of hierarchical classification of cognitive, affective, and psychomotor domains of behaviors according to their degree or level of complexity.

**teachable moment** As defined by Havighurst, that point in time when the learner is most receptive to a teaching situation; it can occur at any hour that a patient, family member, staff member, or nursing student has a question or needs information.

**teaching plan** Overall blueprint or outline for instruction clearly defining the relationship between the essential components of behavioral objectives, instructional content, teaching methods and tools, time frame for teaching, and methods of evaluation that fit together in a logical pattern of flow to achieve a predetermined goal.

**teaching strategy** An overall plan of action for instruction that anticipates barriers and resources of the learning experience to achieve specific behavioral objectives.

**teaching** As one component of the educational process, it is a deliberate, intentional act of communicating information to the learner in response to identified learning needs with the objective of producing learning to achieve desired behavioral outcomes.

**telecommunications learning resources** Instructional tools used to help convey information via electrical energy from one place to another such as telephones, televisions, and computers.

**telecommunications** Technological devices for the deaf (TDD).

**teleological** The ethical notion purported by John Stuart Mill that, given the alternatives, choices should be made that result in the greatest good for the greatest number of people.

**telepractice** The provision of nursing, medical, and other types of technology-facilitated healthcare services to clients at a distance.

**Theory of Reasoned Action** A framework that is concerned with prediction and understanding of human behavior within a social context.

**Therapeutic Alliance Model** An interpersonal provider-patient model that addresses the continuum of compliance, adherence, and collaboration in therapeutic relationships.

**thinking-feeling (TF)** An approach used by individuals to arrive at judgments through impersonal, logical, subjective, or empathetic processes; one of four dichotomous preference dimensions in the Myers-Briggs Type Inventory.

**TOFHLA** A relatively new instrument for measuring patients' literacy level by using actual hospital materials, such as prescription labels, appointment slips, and informed consent documents, to determine their reading and numeracy skills.

**tools** See *instructional materials/tools*.

**transcultural nursing** A formal area of study and practice comparing and analyzing different cultures and subcultures with respect to cultural care, health practices, and illness beliefs with the goal of using these insights to provide culture-specific and culture-universal care to diverse groups of people.

**transductive reasoning** Thinking by preschoolers that is from the particular to the particular, rather than inductive or deductive.

**transfer of learning** The effects of learning one skill on the subsequent performance of another related skill; includes *self-transfer, near transfer,* and *far transfer.*

**triad communication**   A technique of involving a third person, such as a family member, significant other, or caregiver, in the communication pattern of the nurse and the client to serve as a listener and learner in the teaching situation for the purpose of assisting the client in understanding content, encouraging family or caregiver involvement and support, and enhancing client compliance with treatment regimens.

**usenet**   A global discussion system made up of a cooperative network of computers that distribute and archive messages posted to topic-specific electronic discussion groups called newgroups.

**variable costs**   Not predictable, volume-related expenses.

**veracity**   Truth telling; honesty.

**visual impairment**   A reduction or complete loss of vision due to infection, accident, poisoning, or congenital degeneration of the eye(s). See *legally blind.*

**World Wide Web**   A computer network of information servers around the world that are connected to the Internet; it is a technology-based educational resource that was created as a virtual space for the display of information.

**WRAT (Wide Range Achievement Test) technique**   A word recognition screening test used to assess a person's ability to recognize and pronounce a list of words out of context as a criterion for measuring comprehension of written materials. Level I test is designed for children ages 5 to 12 years; level II is intended to test persons over 12 years of age.

# Author Index

# Subject Index